The Integrative Neurobiology of Affiliation

The Integrative Neurobiology of Affiliation

Edited by C. Sue Carter, I. Izja Lederhendler, and Brian Kirkpatrick

A Bradford book

The MIT Press
Cambridge, Massachusetts
London, England

All the materials in this book originally appeared in *The Integrative Neurobiology of Affiliation,* Volume 807, December 1996 (ISBN: 1573310581), published by the New York Academy of Sciences. The MIT Press edition is an abridged version of the original NYAS volume. The MIT Press has exclusive license to sell this English-language edition throughout the world.

This book was printed and bound in the United States of America.

Library of Congress Cataloging-in-Publication Data

The integrative neurobiology of affiliation / edited by C. Sue Carter, I. Izja Lederhendler, and Brian Kirkpatrick.
p. cm.
"A Bradford book."
Represents the partial proceedings of a conference by the same title published in 1997.
Includes bibliographical references.
ISBN 0-262-53158-5 (pbk.: alk. paper)
1. Neuropsychology—Congresses. 2. Affiliation (Psychology)—Physiological aspects—Congresses. I. Carter, Carol Sue, 1944– . II. Lederhendler, I. Izja. III. Kirkpatrick, Brian.
QP360.I565 1999
571.7′19—dc21 98-36500
CIP

Contents

IV Neuroendocrine Perspectives on Social Behavior

V Clinical Perspectives on Social Behavior

Introduction

This volume of the *Annals of the New York Academy of Sciences* represents the proceedings of a conference sponsored by The National Institute of Mental Health with additional support from The National Institute for Child Health and Human Development and the National Science Foundation. The conference was held in Washington, DC, in March 1996. The central purpose and theme of this meeting was to examine the biological and especially the neural substrates of affiliation and related social behaviors. It was particularly appropriate that one way The National Institute of Mental Health chose to celebrate its fiftieth anniversary was through this optimistic theme–striving to improve our understanding of human interactions.

Affiliation refers to social behaviors that bring individuals closer together. This includes such forms of positive association as attachment, parent-offspring interactions, pair-bonding, and coalitions. Affiliations provide a social matrix within which other behaviors, including reproduction and aggression, may occur. Reproductive and aggressive behaviors also reduce the distance between individuals, but their expression is regulated, in part, by a positive social fabric based on affiliations.

Affiliation, treated as an independent topic, received little attention prior to 1990. However, a review of recent Medline citations revealed a 10-fold increase in research on "affiliation" between 1971 and 1994, while studies of "aggression" declined slightly during that period (Levine *et al.*). Since a variety of terms may be used to describe social behavior, it is likely that this analysis underestimates contemporary interest in this topic.

Social behavior and, to a lesser extent, affiliation previously have been described in the context of psychology, sociology, anthropology, psychiatry, and evolutionary biology. However, little attention has been directed at the regulatory physiology and neural processes that subserve affiliative behaviors. In fact, scientists have only recently recognized a set of biological substrates frequently associated with the expression of such behaviors.

Because research on social behavior does not fall within well-defined scientific boundaries, one goal of this conference was to bring together scientists with interdisciplinary and integrative perspectives on the neurobiology of affiliation. The integrative framework facilitates interactions between researchers who study behavior in the context of natural history with those who study the nervous system. We sought to provide an open forum which could strengthen integrative research by discussing both analytic and synthetic findings and by discussing not only what is known, but also what may be absent in our understanding of affiliative behaviors.

It has been argued that affiliative behaviors evolved from reproductive behaviors (Crews) and indeed, affiliative behaviors must serve the purposes of reproduction. The interdependence of these classes of behavior was further emphasized in cases in which behaviors aimed at providing for self-defense and immediate survival must be inhibited to permit sexual and parental behaviors. From the individual's point of view, the need for increased proximity associated with mating may be regarded as potentially dangerous. Monogamy, or other forms of social bonds or coalitions, may be significant in providing comparatively secure social environments for reproduction and other positive social behaviors such as parental behavior.

Complex behavior systems capable of reducing conflict and maximizing cooperation have been observed in animals as diverse as spotted hyenas (Glickman *et al.*) and chimpanzees (De Waal and Aureli). The evolutionary importance of such systems is powerfully illustrated by the fact that physiological processes, such as the production of gonadal sex steroids (Wingfield *et al.*) or sperm (Dixson), are correlated with social organization in diverse species of birds and mammals.

Social experiences can affect the subsequent expression of affiliative behaviors and can alter various physiological processes. Documentation of the effects of early social experiences is abundant in the nonhuman primate and human literature (Levine *et al.*; Kraemer; Keverne *et al.*; Carlson and Earls; Grossman *et al.*; Kupfer and Frank). For example, in primates, early attachment experiences with a mother or other caregiver may have long-lasting consequences for the development of both cognitive and emotional systems (Kraemer). Research with squirrel monkeys reveals striking increases in activity within the adrenal axis following separation from either a parent or peer and conversely has demonstrated the capacity of social companionship to buffer these physiological effects (Levine *et al.*; Mendoza and Mason).

Dramatic examples of the physiological consequences of the social environment in adult animals come from studies in nonhuman primates. In rhesus monkeys, sexual experience with females in the group may allow males to develop affiliative relationships (Wallen and Tannenbaum). The importance of social behavior for reproductive success also is illustrated in the common marmoset. This species usually exhibits a social system built around a monogamous breeding pair where ovulation is inhibited in socially subordinate females. The mechanisms for this social inhibition of reproduction remain unknown, but increased stress or suppression of gonadotropin-releasing hormone have been excluded (Abbott *et al.*).

Physiological studies of social, sexual, parental, and aggressive behavior typically have emphasized the role of the central nervous system (CNS) in these behaviors. An emergent theme in these studies is the role of specific neural tissues in approach and avoidance behaviors in the presence of social stimuli. Neuroanatomical systems for maternal behavior in domestic rats are particularly well characterized. Based on research in rats, it has been proposed that parental behavior requires the suppression of fearful or aversive responses in the presence of infants and a concurrent approach towards stimuli that previously elicited these responses. Areas including the hypothalamus and limbic system may regulate social approach and avoidance. Systems based in the medial amygdala (MA) have been implicated in avoidance, whereas those integrated by the medial preoptic area (MPOA) and ventral portion of the bed nucleus of the stria terminalis (VBST) may regulate social approach (Numan and Sheehan). The MA and its neurochemical connections to the lateral septum (De Vries and Villalba) also have been implicated in male parental behavior in another rodent, the prairie vole. In studies of golden hamsters, these same brain regions also have been implicated in male sexual behavior (Newman *et al.*). Although parallels between parental behavior and sexual behavior have been noted, the system of overlapping neural circuits and mechanisms for these behaviors remain incompletely described. A variety of behaviors, such as parenting and sexual behavior, may involve common neural systems and regulatory processes.

Monogamy is a common social system in birds (Wingfield *et al.*) but rare in mammals. However, adult social attachments and pair bonds have been documented in monogamous mammalian species, including New World primates (Mendoza and Mason) and rodents, such as prairie voles. Monogamous social systems offer a unique opportunity to study well-defined social attachments and to model underlying neuroendocrine (Carter *et al.*) and molecular and cellular (Insel *et al.*; Witt) processes for affiliative behaviors.

Analyses of the mechanisms responsible for social bond formation have focused recently on several neuropeptides including the endogenous opiates, oxytocin and vasopressin. Endogenous opiates, and in particular the endorphins, can alleviate separation distress and other emotional processes (Panksepp *et al.*), and endogenous opiates have been implicated in the induction and maintenance of maternal behavior in several species including rodents and sheep (Keverne *et al.*). Oxytocin also has been implicated in these behaviors as well as in maternal behavior in rats (Pedersen), selective filial bonding in sheep (Keverne *et al.*), selective affiliations in rats (Panksepp *et al.*), pair-bond formation in prairie voles (Carter *et al.*; Insel *et al.*), and nonspecific social contact in several species (Witt). Oxytocin also plays a major role in the regulation of pain responses and autonomic nervous system functions including blood pressure and digestion (in part through effects on the vagus nerve). Oxytocin may be an important component of the antistress effects that are associated with both positive social interactions and lactation (Uvnäs-Moberg; Carter and Altemus).

Vasopressin, which is structurally similar to oxytocin, has been implicated in male parental behavior. Vasopressin synthesis is facilitated by androgens, whereas at least some oxytocin receptors are estrogen dependent. Dynamic interactions between oxytocin and vasopressin could contribute to gender differences such as those that are common in parental responses (DeVries and Villalba). The effects of stress on pair-bond formation in prairie voles also are sexually dimorphic, possibly due to gender differences in neuropeptides including oxytocin and vasopressin (Carter *et al.*).

Mammalian social behaviors rely on both the CNS and the autonomic nervous system (ANS). The role of the ANS, including the vagus nerve, and its representations within the brain are particularly interesting. The well-known functions of the vagus to coordinate visceral demands, including oxygenation, metabolism, and digestion, and reproductive activities, are all the more significant given our recent understanding that the vagus nerve and associated neuropeptides may coordinate these functions with social interactions and emotional expressions. The vagus is composed of two subsystems, an evolutionarily earlier portion associated with vegetative functions and a more recently evolved component that may play a role in complex social behaviors (Porges). The complex functions of the vagus facilitate social interactions, communication, and emotional regulation while inhibiting self-defense functions associated with the "vegetative" vagus and the sympathetic components of the ANS. Both oxytocin and vasopressin are implicated in autonomic functions, providing important neurochemical substrates that could influence emotions (Uvnäs-Moberg).

Studies of cognitive contributions to the expression of social behavior face special challenges. The subject matter of particular interest is critical, yet because it exists exclusively as neural representations of past experience and anticipatory behaviors, it is relatively difficult to study. The mechanisms through which cognition regulates and integrates the emotions and behavioral expression in different social contexts are largely unknown.

Cognition, by its nature, comprises processes that determine important differences among individuals. It is therefore compelling to ask about the role of cognition in determining why some individuals adapt successfully to social stressors while others do not. What role does communication play? The neurobiology of communication, therefore, not only offers a unique perspective on brain development and organization, but also is a model system for the study of socially regulated internal states such as stress.

In mammals, and particularly in primates, social behavior is less dependent on hormonal and emotional control, with a corresponding increase in cognitive regulation. In primates, for example, the emphasis in mother-infant bonding turns from complex perinatal regulators to maternal decision-making, accompanied by increased neocortical size. Among primate species, the relative amount of brain tissue devoted to neocortex and hippocampus is positively correlated with the social complexity typical for a species. New findings using transgenic mice suggest that sex differences exist in the degree of parental contribution to various brain regions. Maternal genomic imprinting (selective activation of some genes and inactivation of others) differentially directs cortical development, while paternally imprinted cells primarily appear in hypothalamic-limbic structures (Keverne *et al.*). These startling results have implications for our understanding of the cognitive regulation of social processes, such as the integration of executive and emotional functions, which are just beginning to be understood.

Comparative work on primate communication in New World monkeys reveals patterns of selective learning which in turn determine subsequent plasticity in adult vocal skills (Snowdon). These skills are maintained by mechanisms of attention and reinforcement, based on social interactions. Vocal communication is common in birds, and remarkable comparability exists in the developmental sequencing of human language and birdsong (Hall *et al.*). Although vocal learning evolved independently in birds and humans, in both cases there is a gradual emancipation from deterministic control systems and increasing dependence on environmental/sensory factors. Whether the similar patterns of developmental stages and transitions in primate and avian systems result from convergent patterns of neural development remains to be determined. Parakeets, for example, use multiple systems to sequentially coordinate auditory feedback and song expression in specialized forebrain nuclei (Brauth *et al.*).

It has been proposed that comparable neural systems in humans control the sequential motor patterning underlying vocalization.

More mechanistic approaches to understanding the acquisition of vocal communication systems are illustrated by studies of the cellular and receptor-based systems that constrain learning and memory for birdsong (Nordeen). These studies also illustrate the unique advantages of studies of avian vocalization for understanding general processes through which early experience may influence neural and behavioral development. For example, an important hypothesis to emerge from neurobiological studies of birdsong proposes that adult patterns of social behavior may be shaped through the selective elimination of synapses, allowing adult neuronal circuitry to be specified by sensory experience.

The expression of complex behaviors such as aggression or conflict avoidance allows us to focus our attention on the important intersection between cognitive and emotional systems. Conflict or its resolution emerges from a balance between internal states (emotional systems) and social decision-making processes (anticipatory affiliative behaviors, empathic fear/anxiety reduction, and social risk assessment) (De Waal and Aureli). In the context of a group, aggression is more readily understood as a negotiating tool rather than a deterministic activity isolated from other social behaviors.

Genes, and the mechanisms by which they are regulated, probably predispose some individuals to depression, schizophrenia, and other nervous system disorders; however, social experiences throughout the life span may alter the expression of these diseases and their clinical course (Kupfer and Frank). Autism (Grossman *et al.*) and certain forms of schizophrenia (the deficit syndrome) (Kirkpatrick) are defined by dysfunctional social behaviors and in some cases a failure to develop affiliations. Findings of increased stress hormone levels in children in Romanian orphanages (Carlson and Earls) emphasize the vulnerability of human infants to social deprivation. Animal studies of the neurobiology of stress provide the framework for understanding what happened to these children and more importantly provide a rational basis for treatment. Careful examination of the behavioral, cognitive, and emotional details of the social expression of psychopathology in people, such as vocalizations, gaze aversion, or perserverative movements, may inspire appropriate studies in nonhuman primates or other animals. Thus, exploration of the neuropharmacological and neuroanatomical substrates of comparable behavior patterns from a cross-species, interdisciplinary perspective may, in turn, lead to new therapeutic approaches.

SUMMARY

The research presented at this conference, including a series of excellent posters from junior investigators, documents the pervasive importance of affiliation and other social behaviors. Affiliative behaviors interact with, but are distinct from reproductive and aggressive behaviors. Patterns of social behaviors tend to be more species-typical than the behaviors associated with reproduction or aggression. However, neural circuits necessary for approach or avoidance also are necessary for the expression of various types of affiliative behavior such as maternal behavior or pair-bond formation. Furthermore, candidate neurochemical systems have been identified that contribute to various types of affiliative behavior. For example, studies revealing new behavioral functions for steroid hormones of the adrenal axis, such as corticosterone, and neuropeptides, including the endorphins, oxytocin and vasopressin, extend our general knowledge of neurobiology; they may also lead to studies that expand our understanding of social behavior and the connections to systems that regulate emotions.

The work represented in this volume also has important implications for the study of serious neuropsychiatric disorders. For example, episodes of certain of these disorders can be induced by social stressors; in other disorders, a marked decrease in affiliative behaviors is a prominent feature of the patients' difficulties. Futhermore, abnormalities in animal systems implicated in the neurobiology of affiliation (oxytocin, vasopressin, and the hypothalamic-pituitary-adrenal system) have also been documented for major depression in humans.

Animal models, such as those described at this conference, offer evolutionary perspectives, from which it is possible to extract general principles. At the same time, our understanding of the mechanistic and neurobiological substrates of both constructive and destructive social behaviors is increasing. At the conference, the evolutionary and mechanistic perspectives converged on the theme that studies of affiliative behaviors cannot be fully interpreted in isolation from other social behaviors; neither can they effectively be isolated from the biological and social contexts that shape their expression. Advances in this research area seem dependent on integrating experimental research across levels of analysis. Although this task is challenging, we are confident that an awareness of integrative principles can lead to new and important research opportunities.

C. Sue Carter, I. Izja Lederhendler, and Brian Kirkpatrick

I

The Evolutionary Point of View

1

Species Diversity and the Evolution of Behavioral Controlling Mechanisms

D. Crews

> *"We have evolved a nervous system that acts in the interest of our gonads, and one attuned to the demands of reproductive competition."*[1]

Modern molecular genetic methods have undoubtedly opened many doors to the study of the neurobiological bases of behavior. A wholly molecular approach, however, yields little information about the ontogeny or adaptation of behavior. For this, we must turn to organismal studies and ecological and evolutionary analyses. At the most fundamental level, the study of diverse species provides us with a perspective different from that which has emerged from studies of man and other domesticated animals. This appreciation of variety keeps us from becoming wedded prematurely to a particular paradigm. Because genes always function within cells, cells within organs, organs within animals and, ultimately, animals within environments that are ever-changing, the need exists for studies that integrate the different levels of biological organization, from genes to Gaia. These two elements, diversity and integration, greatly aid efforts to better understand past, present, and perhaps even future behavior. This approach also leads to new discoveries in the relationships among molecular biology, physiology, and behavior as well as evolutionary biology and behavioral ecology.

Before discussing the neurobiology of social and sexual behaviors and how they may have evolved, it is first useful to review some of the evolutionary forces that lead to species diversity.

EVOLUTIONARY FORCES LEADING TO DIVERSITY

A successful strategy for investigating and making sense of diversity is to look for generalities. By comparing various organisms, we find themes that recur throughout all

The research discussed here was supported by a National Institute of Mental Health MERIT Award and a National Institute of Mental Health Research Scientist Award.

Address for correspondence: David Crews, Department of Zoology, University of Texas at Austin, Austin, Texas 78712 (tel: 512/471–1113; fax: 512/471–6078: e-mail address: crews@bull.zo.utexas.edu).

animals. When closely related species are compared, it becomes possible to trace the progressive specialization of traits and thus illuminate the course of evolution.[2] Three concepts should guide the reader. The first considers the primary function of sexual behavior and the importance of mate compatibility. The second concerns the distinction between natural selection and sexual selection. The third regards the nature of the constraints that shape the evolution of reproductive processes.

Reproductive Synergism

In terms of evolution, reproduction is the single most important element in an individual's life, more important even than the length of an individual's survival. Simply put, if an individual does not reproduce, its genes will not be represented in future generations.

Reproduction has been the impetus for the evolution of many specialized behaviors, serving to coordinate hormonal, gonadal, and behavioral events. Detailed analyses indicate that these behaviors tend to be ritualized, stereotyped, and characteristic of the species. Reproduction occurs only when the participants both send and receive appropriate signals, so that each phase of reproduction depends on preceding events and, at the same time, sets the stage for what follows (FIG. 1). The act of choosing the best mate is of utmost importance, for it is the interaction between the paired individuals that stimulates the physiological changes necessary for reproduction (e.g., maturation and release of each individual's gametes).

The importance of mate choice is seen particularly well in long-lived species in which an individual's lifetime reproductive success can be monitored. For example, most kittiwake gulls pair for life.[3] Some individuals, however, have a different mate the next breeding season. In about half of these instances, mates are changed because the original partner has died. In the other half, the pair will have "divorced" and will select a new mate. The cause of divorce can be traced to the failure of the pair to hatch at least one egg the preceding year. Not only do successful pairs fledge more young, but they also produce eggs faster, indicating that females in these pairs reach breeding condition earlier. In canvasback ducks, only females allowed to stay with their self-chosen partner lay eggs; females paired with males chosen by humans lack the characteristic pituitary and gonadal hormone changes associated with ovulation.[4]

Natural Selection versus Sexual Selection

Darwin considered natural selection and sexual selection to be different processes. Both are primary forces driving the evolution of traits. Natural selection generally results in heritable traits that are adaptational responses to changes in the environment, and the resulting variation both between and within species is shaped by differential survivorship. Sexual selection, on the other hand, arises from interactions among individuals as they compete for mating opportunities. Females often choose males on the basis of the morphological and/or behavioral characteristics they display. Natural and sexual selections often act in opposite directions on male traits, favoring,

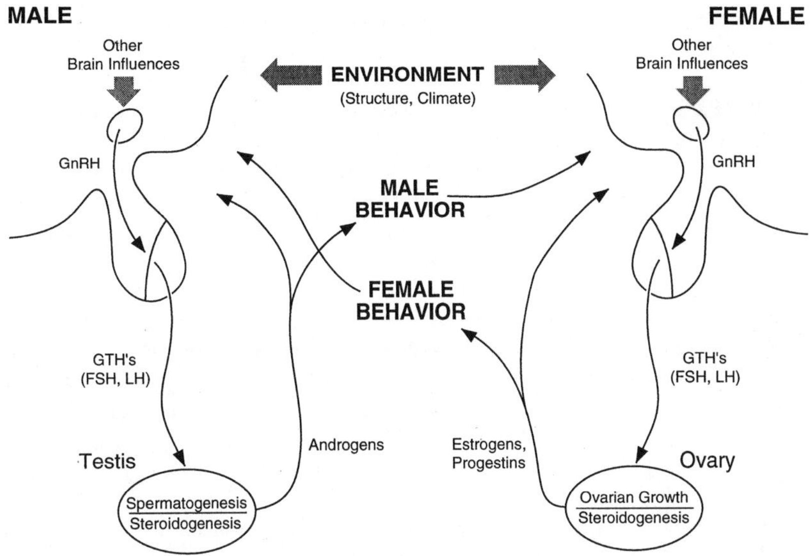

FIGURE 1. Dynamic relationship between internal and external environments in the control of mating behavior in vertebrates. The behavior of the male and the female helps to synchronize the maturation and release of the sperm and eggs so that fertilization occurs. Changes in the climate, ecology, or behavior of conspecifics initiate and modulate gonadal and hormonal changes during reproduction. Thus, hormones regulate behavior in the individual animal and are themselves affected by other stimuli, including the behavior and, indirectly, the physiology of its mate. In such a dynamic system each successive phase of reproduction depends on preceding events and at the same time sets the stage for the following phase. (Reproduced with permission from ref. 2.)

for instance, drab plumage (natural selection) on the one hand, and colorful plumage (sexual selection) on the other.

Constraints on Reproduction

It is often said that sexual behavior in vertebrates is dependent upon the nature and pattern of gonadal steroid hormone secretion. This conclusion stems primarily from the species most studied rather than reflecting a universal principle. Indeed, species differ in their hormone-behavior relations in ways that often can be traced to adaptational responses to physical and social environments. Reproduction is constrained by (1) the immediate environment, (2) limitations inherent in developmental and physiological processes, and (3) evolutionary history.[2,5–7]

Environmental Constraints. The evolution of reproductive seasons is determined by environmental factors selecting for those individuals that reproduce during optimum conditions and selecting against those individuals that bear young during times of food scarcity or other adverse conditions. This has been termed the *ultimate* causation of breeding seasons and includes factors such as adequate food, availability of nesting materials, and predation pressure. *Proximate* causation refers to those stimuli used by the organism that actually initiate, maintain, and terminate breeding and include seasonal fluctuations in day length, temperature, moisture, and the like.[8] The responsiveness of the neuroendocrine system to proximate cues may vary seasonally, reflecting endogenous circadian and circannual rhythms. Environmental constraints are especially severe in harsh environments. Here species typically exhibit an explosive or opportunistic pattern of reproduction in which all breeding activity is compressed into a few days or weeks.

Developmental and Physiological Constraints. Developmental and physiological processes may also constrain when animals breed and shape the mechanisms controlling reproduction. For example, in most species sperm cannot be produced in less than 6 weeks. Although some mice and ground squirrels can produce sperm in as little as 31 days, they appear to be the only exceptions to this rule. A similar time constraint applies to the production of eggs, although some small rodents can generate eggs in less than 1 week. In ectotherms (cold-blooded vertebrates), eggs commonly require many months or even years to mature.

A related constraint is the temperature dependence of gonadal activity. In ectotherms, gamete production and hormone secretion will not occur at cold temperatures, presenting a problem for species living at high altitudes or latitudes. For these animals, mating must occur as early in the spring as possible so that young can be born and grow sufficiently to survive the next winter. In some species males produce sperm during the summer and then store them through the winter, enabling them to inseminate females immediately on emergence from hibernation. In hibernating mammals spermatogenesis occurs during periodic arousals from dormancy. In harsh environments where proximate factors are rare and aperiodic, a third strategy is evident whereby gametes are maintained in an almost completely developed state. Thus, in the zebra finch breeding occurs immediately when it rains.[6,7]

Physiological constraints can also arise out of developmental constraints. In addition to hormones produced by the individual's own gonads during embryogenesis and throughout life, significant amounts of hormones are contained in the mother's milk.[9,10] Another source of hormones is found in the fetal environment. For example, in mammalian species (including humans), the fetus's position relative to other fetuses within the uterus affects its level of exposure to androgen. Androgens excreted by male fetuses expose fetuses located between two males to higher levels of exogenous androgen compared to fetuses located between two females.[11–13] These hormone differences resulting from intrauterine position can account for many of the differences among individuals of the same sex. For example, female mice which develop *in utero* between two males (2M females) have a masculinized phenotype, are less attractive to males, and are more aggressive to female stimulus animals than are females which develop between two females (2F females).[12,13] In addition to being less attractive and more aggressive, 2M female gerbils mature later and have lower estrogen levels and higher androgen levels than 2F females.[11] Finally, brain metabolic activity in the sexually dimorphic area of the preoptic area (POA), a region involved in the regulation of sex-typical behaviors in this species,[14] is greater in 2M female than in 2F female gerbils.[15]

Self-contained, the shelled egg traditionally was thought to be immune from maternal or uterine influences known to affect the mammalian embryo. However, the yolk in egg-laying species is a significant repository of circulating hormones, reflecting the hormonal profile of the mother. This is a form of "hormonal inheritance"[16] in that the endocrine state of the mother influences the hormonal content of the egg and thus the development of the young. In female striped bass, the circulating concentrations of various steroid and protein hormones are greatest at the time the eggs are yolking and have an important impact on the growth and development of the fry.[17,18] In the Japanese quail, circulating steroid levels in the female are correlated with steroid levels in the yolk and, in turn, the degree of sexual differentiation of the embryo.[19] In the zebra finch and the canary, testosterone content in yolk varies predictably across eggs within a clutch, and these differences correlate with subsequent behavioral differences in the adult.[20]

An important and as yet unresolved question is whether these effects may be transgenerational. In mammals, 2M female gerbils produce litters with male-biased sex ratios,[21] indicating that hormones experienced *in utero* affect the reproduction of the next generation. It is important to note that these examples of hormonal inheritance represent nongenomic heritable effects distinct from genomic inheritable effects.[22]

In many reptiles an individual's gonadal sex is determined not by chromosomes at fertilization, but by the temperature experienced during the middle of embryogenesis, a process known as temperature-dependent sex determination (TSD). In TSD, incubation temperature modulates expression of genes encoding steroidogenic enzymes and sex steroid hormone receptors, so that the resulting sex steroid hormone milieu determines gonadal sex.[23]

In the leopard gecko, the relation between incubation temperature and the secondary sex ratio is shaped like a bell curve with 26°C producing only female hatchlings, 30°C producing a female-biased sex ratio, 32.5°C producing a male-biased sex ratio, and 35°C producing all females. The temperature experienced as an egg affects the rate of growth[24] as well as the morphology,[25] physiology,[24,26] brain metabolic activity,[27] the size of brain nuclei,[27] and the aggressive and sexual behaviors[28,29] of the adult. For example, females from a male-biased incubation temperature are masculinized in their growth rate, adult body size and morphology, physiology, brain metabolism, and sociosexual behavior compared to females from lower incubation temperatures (FIG. 2). Taken together, these data suggest that incubation temperature, not gonadal steroids, is the primary organizer of brain and behavior in TSD species.

Evolutionary History. The evolutionary history, or phylogeny, of the species is another source of constraints, predisposing the emergence of certain mechanisms and not others. Applying this principle to reproductive physiology, we might predict that closely related species sharing a similar reproductive pattern but living in different environments will exhibit similarities in the neuroendocrine mechanisms underlying reproduction. For example, garter snakes are a large genus that radiated throughout the New World after crossing the Bering Strait. All garter snakes exhibit a dissociated reproductive pattern (to be discussed) and appear to possess the same neuroendocrine mechanisms controlling mating behavior.[30] On the other hand, distantly related species sharing similar challenges do not necessarily have similar neuroendocrine mechanisms. For example, garter snakes have a different neuroendocrine mechanism controlling mating behavior compared to most mammals.

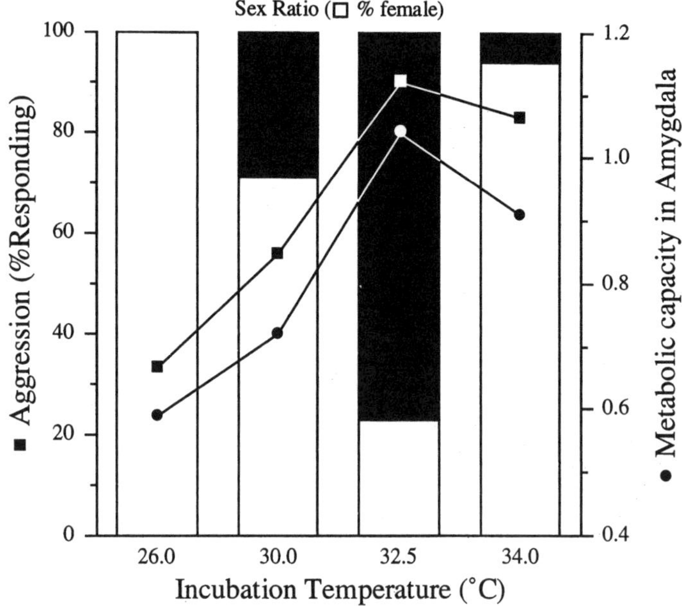

FIGURE 2. Relationship between sex ratio, aggressive behavior, and cytochrome oxidase activity in the amygdala in female leopard geckos. Sex in the leopard gecko is determined by the incubation temperature of the egg; the sex ratio produced at the temperatures indicated is reflected in the bar graph. The proportion of females responding aggressively towards a courting male is indicated by *squares*. Cytochrome oxidase activity in the amygdala of females from these same incubation temperatures is shown in *circles*. Thus, embryonic experience with temperature affects the level of aggressive behavior and brain metabolism in the amygdala of adult females.

DIVERSITY IN THE PROXIMATE MECHANISMS CONTROLLING SEXUAL BEHAVIOR: A BRIEF SURVEY

At some level, all behaviors are mediated by hormones. That is to say, steroid hormones, neurotransmitters, neuropeptides, and brain protein hormones modulate the activity of the neuronal circuits that subserve specific behaviors. What actually initiates these behaviors and the neurochemistry that underlies them, however, can vary from organism to organism.

Proximate Stimuli Activating Sexual Behavior

In many vertebrates, elevated plasma levels of gonadal steroid hormones are necessary if proximate stimuli are to activate sexual activity. In these animals, the sex hormones alter the perceptions of the individual, and stimuli take on new meanings.[31] Other organisms, however, circumvent this reliance on gonadal steroid hormones, relying instead on various proximate cues from the environment or from other animals to activate sexual behavior.

Mixed Reproductive Strategies

If environmental, physiological, and phylogenetic constraints can influence reproductive processes, such as when gametes are produced, gonadal steroid hormones are secreted, and mating behavior is performed, the neuroendocrine mechanisms controlling each of these processes are likely to have undergone corresponding adaptations.

There appear to be four basic reproductive strategies in vertebrates. In most domesticated species, both the male and the female have an associated reproductive pattern. That is, a temporal association exists between the growth of the gonad and gamete maturation, hormone secretion, and the display of mating behavior. Also in some species both sexes exhibit a dissociated reproductive pattern; that is, peak gonadal activity and sex steroid secretion do not coincide with the display of mating behavior. Most exciting from a biological standpoint are the species in which the sexes differ in their reproductive strategies. In these species, one of two things can happen. The male can produce sperm before breeding and store them until mating occurs. Alternatively, the male mates when the sperm mature, and the female stores the sperm in her reproductive tract until a later date. In this latter instance, the act of mating initiates gonadal growth in the female. Species with mixed reproductive strategies hold promise for untangling the ecological and evolutionary forces on reproductive behavior because the sexes differ fundamentally in the organization and activation of neuroendocrine mechanisms controlling behavior.

Mixed reproductive strategies can also be found within the same sex. For example, in rodents, individuals within a population may utilize different proximate cues for regulating gonadal activity: photoperiod may be important in some individuals; in others, it may be temperature or food.[32] Such individual differences in the required proximate cue can be adaptive, resulting in a fine-tuning of reproduction in the population to its environment.

Another fascinating discovery is that of alternative mating tactics.[33] This refers to the fact that in some species individuals of the same sex, usually males, may display distinctly different phenotypes. For example, in the sound-producing teleost fish, the plains midshipman, there are two types of males, the typical territory-holding phenotype and a smaller, noncalling male; these two phenotypes also differ in their neurobiology.[34]

Many of these alternative mating tactics appear to arise from environmental and/ or developmental alterations and are not heritable. For example, in the red-sided garter snake, male courtship is elicited by an estrogen-dependent pheromone released from the skin of the female, often causing many males to congregate about the female, forming a ''mating ball.'' Some males (called she-males) mimic females and release the same attractiveness pheromone.[35,36] These female mimics have a decided mating advantage in that they confuse the other males in the mating ball by providing a second source of the attractiveness pheromone, whereas to the she-male, there is only a single source.[35] Behavioral and morphological studies reveal that she-males court and mate with females, have the male homogametic chromosomal constitution, and have fully functional testes and accessory sex structures. Interestingly, circulating concentrations of testosterone (T) are much higher in she-males than in normal males.[35] This seeming paradox is explained by the high concentration of aromatase, an enzyme that converts T to estradiol (E2), in the liver and skin of she-males.[37] This latter point is important when the effects of estrogen administration are considered. Injecting exogenous E2 causes adult males to secrete the attractiveness pheromone into their circulation, but not to release it through the skin.[38] Hence, they are not courted. However, E2 administration to neonatal males causes them to both secrete and release the pheromone, thereby eliciting courtship from other males.[39] Garter snakes are viviparous, and the percentage of she-males in the population is similar to the percentage of males found between two females *in utero*. Thus, she-males appear to result from a developmental process similar to that of the intrauterine position effect in rodents.[11–13] In other species having alternative mating tactics, the different morphs have a genetic basis. Only in a few instances have these alternative mating tactics been found to have a genetic basis. For example, in ruffed grouse satellite males, which display plumage and mating behavior different from those of territory-holding males, the different tactics arise from a polymorphism in a single gene locus.[40]

Finally, some of the most fascinating examples of behavioral and physiological diversity are found in coral reef fish. Some species have ovotestes and trade behavioral roles for each spawning act (simultaneous hermaphrodites). Others undergo a sex change in adulthood (sequential hermaphrodites), with some functioning first as males and then as females later in life (protandry), whereas other species first function as female, then as male (protogyny). Recently a small goby was found to exhibit repeated sex change throughout the course of its life.

Perhaps the best studied sex-changing fish is the bluehead wrasse. In this small protogynous fish most males in a group are small and drab (initial color phase males), with a single large, brightly colored male (terminal phase males) who is dominant and does most of the breeding. Within minutes of removing the dominant male, the largest fish will begin to display male-typical behaviors. Within days a change in physiology occurs, and within weeks the gonads change from ovaries to testes. This suggests that it is the individual's perception of its social environment that initiates the sex change. Recent studies indicate that ovariectomized females will exhibit the same behavioral changes, even inducing gravid females to spawn in response to their courtship, indicating that the behavior, not the gonads, is essential for sex change.[41]

EVOLUTION OF SEXUAL BEHAVIOR

Up to this point we have concentrated on the diversity of species and some of the factors that led to this diversity. What about the mechanisms underlying species differences in behavior? Social behavior emerged from sexual (reproductive) behaviors. It follows that sexual behaviors will involve more ancient regions of the brain (e.g., the limbic system), whereas the regulation of more complex social behaviors will incorporate these regions in addition to more recently evolved portions of the brain.

Origin of Sexual Behavior

If asked, most people would say that sexual reproduction evolved from asexual reproduction. A common argument is that as male and female reproductive physiologies became more distinct and complex, it was necessary to better synchronize the male and the female, hence leading to the appearance of sex-typical behavior patterns capable of acting as neuroendocrine primers. This line of reasoning assumes further that the presence of two gonadal sexes predates the evolution of sexual behavior.

Is this paradigm correct? As pointed out by Beach,[42] the concept of sexual behavior is defined by the concept of male and female. Because of the tautology inherent in present definitions of sexual behavior, it is useful to use another term. I suggest the term "facilitatory behavior," defined as any social signal that leads to increased reproductive output of all interacting individuals. Universal characters are evolutionarily more ancient than less widespread characters. It is also likely that such pervasive characters are ancestral and hence more basic to life.

As already stated, predation, competition, food supply, and the availability of suitable nesting sites are ultimate factors in determining when and where animals reproduce. Most synchronously reproducing species are social, and social cues, along with other environmental stimuli, serve as proximate factors affecting cycles of reproduction. This sociality or group facilitation of reproduction is widespread, occurring in all life forms, because it confers certain advantages, such as increasing an individual's protection against environmental toxins, heightening detection of predators, and stimulating population growth.[43] The advantages of synchronous breeding and sociality apply equally to sexual and asexual organisms. It is well known that in vertebrates the courtship behavior of the male stimulates the reproductive physiology of the female (Fig. 1). This facilitatory process is even seen in parthenogenetic or all-female vertebrates; indeed, if such stimulation does not occur, egg production is reduced to below normal levels.[44] In microorganisms such as bacteria, population growth is characterized by a lag phase of gradual population growth which ends after a certain threshold density is achieved. This is followed by a log phase in which population growth is exponential before stabilizing, the stationary phase. The duration of the lag phase can be shortened if new microorganisms are cultured in conditioned medium that previously contained a colony in the log phase. Similarly, if two asexual protozoans are incubated together, the rate of division is considerably more than double that in a culture started with a single individual.

In cellular slime molds, plurality is a prerequisite for reproduction. Individual amebae are dispersed in the soil until the food supply (bacteria) is depleted. At that time, the amebae begin to aggregate, attracted by the pulsatile secretion of cyclic AMP from a few "founder" cells. The free-living cells become concentrated into central cell masses and, when sufficiently large, form a sausage-shaped slug. The slug is both light and heat sensitive and moves towards the surface. Eventually, the slug rights itself, and the leading (now upper) third of the cells begin to differentiate into a rigid stalk. The remaining cells flow upwards to the top of the stalk where they form a small sphere known as the fruiting body. It is these cells that are dispersed by wind or by contact with a passing organism, starting a new generation.

However, almost all asexual life forms existing today evolved from sexual forms.[45] The only organisms believed to have always been asexual are the stromatolites, the blue-green algae. It is therefore significant that stromatolites are found in very large,

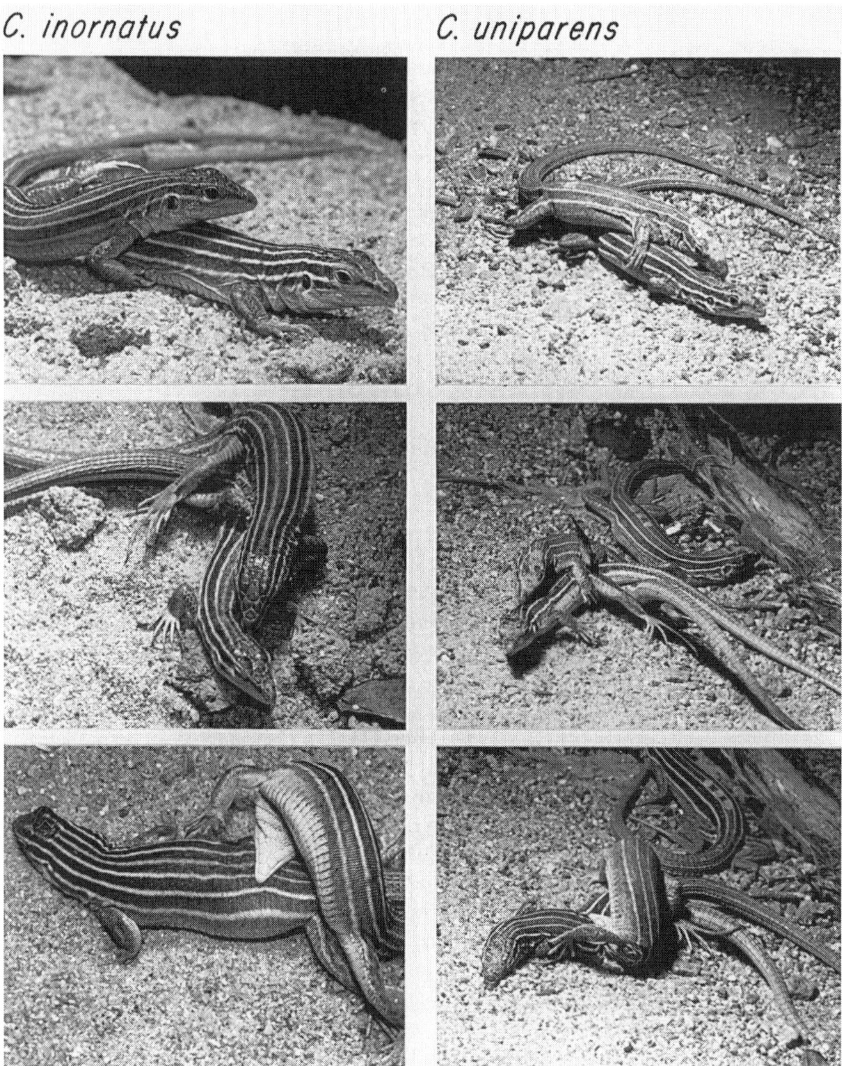

FIGURE 3. *Legend is on facing page.*

dense clusters and rely on aggregative behavior to reproduce. The fact that facilitation of reproduction is found in both sexual and asexual life forms indicates that it is an ancestral trait. Indeed, the diversity of organisms exhibiting behavioral facilitation is greater than the diversity of organisms exhibiting meiosis. Thus, behavioral facilitation is likely more fundamental (ancient) than sexual reproduction. On the basis of this evidence, I propose that facilitatory behavior arose first or, to revert to common terminology, that sexual behavior evolved before sex.[46]

FIGURE 3. Sexual and pseudosexual behavior in whiptail lizards. (**Left**) The mating sequence in the sexual whiptail lizard (*C. inornatus*), the maternal ancestor of the all-female parthenogenetic whiptail. The male approaches and investigates the female with his bifid (split) tongue, an action that presumably indicates involvement of chemical senses. If the female is sexually receptive, she stands still for the male, allowing him to mount her back. Usually just before the male mounts the female, he grips with his jaws either a portion of the skin on the female's neck or her foreleg. As the male rides the female, he scratches her sides and presses her body against the substrate. The male then begins to maneuver his tail beneath the female's tail, attempting to appose their cloacal regions. During mating, one of two hemipenes is intromitted into the female's cloaca. With intromission, the male shifts his jaw-grip from the female's neck to her pelvic region, thereby assuming a contorted copulatory posture termed the *doughnut.* This posture is maintained for 5-10 minutes, after which the male rapidly dismounts and leaves the female. (**Right**) A similar sequence in the descendant parthenogenetic whiptail lizard (*C. uniparens*). During pseudosexual behavior, one individual will approach and mount another individual, and after riding for a few minutes, the mounting (male-like) individual will swing its tail beneath that of the mounted (female-like) individual, apposing the cloacal regions. At the same time the mounting individual will shift its jaw-grip from the neck to the pelvic region of the mounted individual, forming the doughnut posture. Because parthenogens are morphologically female, there are no hemipenes and intromission does not occur. (Reproduced with permission from ref. 64.)

An Animal Model System to Study the Evolution of the Neuroendocrine Control of Sex-Typical Behaviors

How do the neural mechanisms that subserve behavior evolve, and how can we incorporate the great diversity in species-typical behaviors into our experimental approach? If the neuroendocrine mechanisms controlling sociosexual behaviors of living species could be compared with those of their ancestors, this question could be answered. However, because the ancestors of most animals are extinct, other approaches to this question must be used which yield approximations at best. The whiptail lizard offers a rare opportunity in that representatives of both the ancestral and the descendant species still exist. This "snapshot" of evolution in essence enables study of the evolutionary process directly.[47]

About one third of the species of whiptail lizards are parthenogenetic with all individuals having ovaries; the species of the genus are gonochoristic (separate sexes in separate individuals). Despite this loss of males, both male-like and female-like sexual behaviors are observed in the parthenogens (FIG. 3).

Because gonadal sex has been dissociated from sexuality in the parthenogen, the fundamental nature of sexuality can be probed without the complication of gender.[25] Furthermore, the whiptail lizard enables examination of two issues in behavioral neuroscience from a new perspective: first, how the cellular mechanisms that control sexual behaviors might have evolved and second, how the neuroendocrine mechanisms that subserve sex-typical behaviors differ.

Although parthenogenetic whiptail species descended directly from gonochoristic whiptail species, they differ in an important aspect of their reproductive biology, namely, the circulating concentrations of E2 in reproductively active parthenogenetic whiptails are approximately fivefold lower than those in reproductively active females

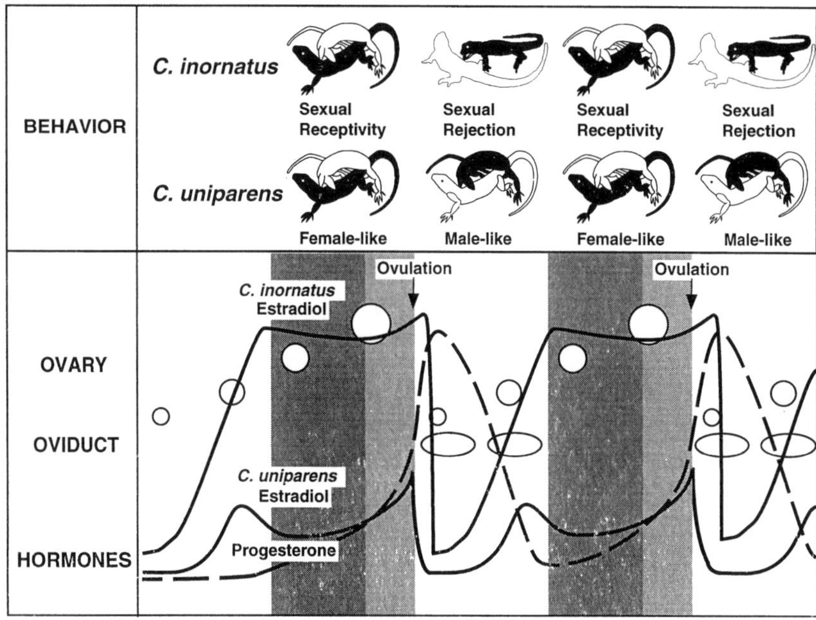

FIGURE 4. Schematic illustration of the relationship between ovarian development, circulating concentrations of sex steroid hormones, and reproductive behavior in the ancestral sexual and the descendant parthenogenetic whiptail species. Note (1) that species differences exist in circulating concentrations of estradiol, and (2) that unlike female whiptails which typically exhibit sexual receptivity only during vitellogenesis and aggressively reject male courtship advances during the postovulatory period, the parthenogenetic whiptail alternates between expressing female-like receptive behavior and male-like mounting and copulatory behavior, depending on the gonadal and hormonal condition. (Reproduced with permission from ref. 50.)

of the sexual species (FIG. 4). Because changes in the circulating concentrations of sex steroid hormones can have dramatic effects on endocrine physiology and behavior, the difference in plasma E2 levels between the descendant parthenogenetic and the ancestral sexual whiptail lizard might be expected to be accompanied by differences in estrogen-dependent phenomena. Indeed, an inverse relation exists between the behavioral sensitivity to sex hormones, sex steroid receptor gene expression, and circulating sex steroid hormone concentration. As in other vertebrates, the ventromedial hypothalamus is involved in the hormonal induction of receptive behavior in whiptail lizards.[48,49] Lower dosages of exogenous estrogen are required to induce receptive behavior in parthenogens than in females of the sexual ancestral species[50] because of a greater sensitivity to estrogen at the molecular level. Not only are the circulating concentrations of E2 correlated with estrogen-receptor mRNA (ER-mRNA) in the POA, but the species differ in the ability of estrogen to upregulate progesterone receptor-mRNA in the ventromedial hypothalamus (FIG. 5). Thus, species differences in neuroendocrine mechanisms can be attributed to: (1) sensitivity to sex hormones and (2) hormone-dependent regulation of sex steroid hormone receptor

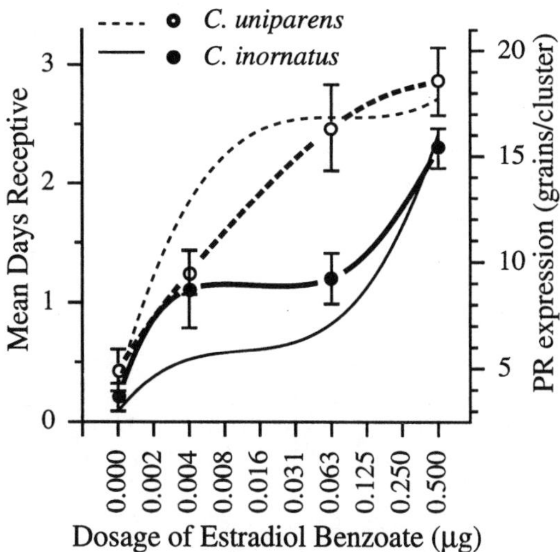

FIGURE 5. Species differences in the induction of sexual receptivity (*thin lines*) and progesterone receptor-mRNA expression (*thick lines*) by estradiol benzoate (EB) in ovariectomized individuals of the ancestral sexual and descendant parthenogenetic species. Ovariectomized animals were given a single injection of EB and either they were tested daily for receptivity for 4 days following the injection or brains were removed 24 hours after treatment and analyzed using *in situ* hybridization. *Vertical error bars* represent standard errors of the mean. (Reproduced with permission from ref. 50.)

gene expression. With this in mind, predictions can be made about the molecular neuroendocrinology of species with different patterns of reproductive physiology (FIG. 6).

Why is ER-mRNA expression in the POA higher in the descendant parthenogenetic whiptail than in its ancestral sexual species? One possibility is the increased gene dosage resulting from the triploid nature of the genome. Polyploid species differ physiologically and ecologically from their diploid relatives because of increased gene dosage and hence higher enzyme levels. Allozyme analysis of sexual (diploid) and parthenogenetic (triploid) whiptails demonstrates that each of the three sets of chromosomes actively transcribes genes at rates proportional to the gene dosage, rather than one chromosome set becoming inactivated as might be expected. Triploidy, therefore, could result in increased sensitivity to E2 not only by increasing the basal rate of ER production, but also by increasing estrogen-dependent gene transcription as the target gene number is increased.

Individual parthenogenetic whiptails show primarily female-like pseudosexual behavior during the preovulatory stage when plasma E2 concentrations are relatively high and progesterone levels relatively low. On the other hand, male-like pseudocopulatory behavior occurs in the postovulatory phase when plasma levels of E2 are low and levels of progesterone are high (FIG. 7). Interestingly, neither testosterone nor dihydrotestosterone is detectable in the circulation of the parthenogen, although they

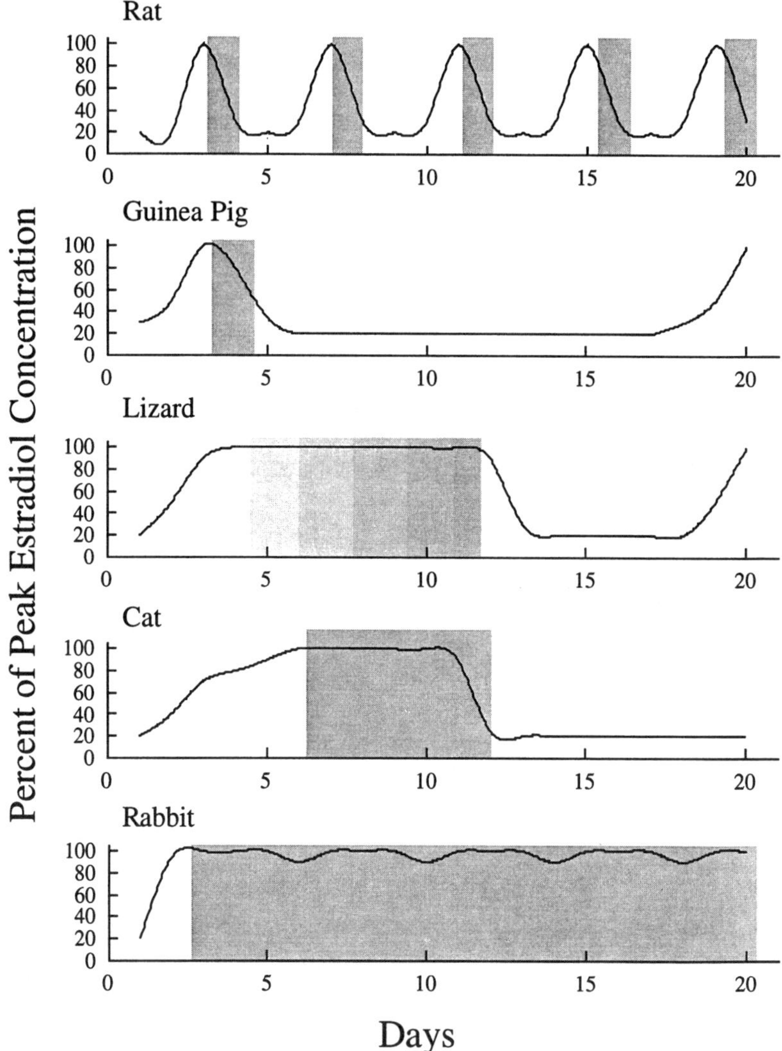

FIGURE 6. Relationship between circulating levels of ovarian hormones and sexual receptivity in several representative vertebrates. The species shown differ in the duration and frequency of their follicular phase as reflected in the circulating estradiol concentrations. *Shaded areas* represent the period of behavioral estrus. It is predicted that the estrogenic regulation of estrogen receptor-mRNA expression in the ventromedial nucleus of the hypothalamus would differ in species with brief follicular phases as in the rat and mouse compared to species with extended or overlapping follicular phases and/or behavioral estrus as in the lizard, cat, and rabbit. (Reproduced with permission from ref. 50.)

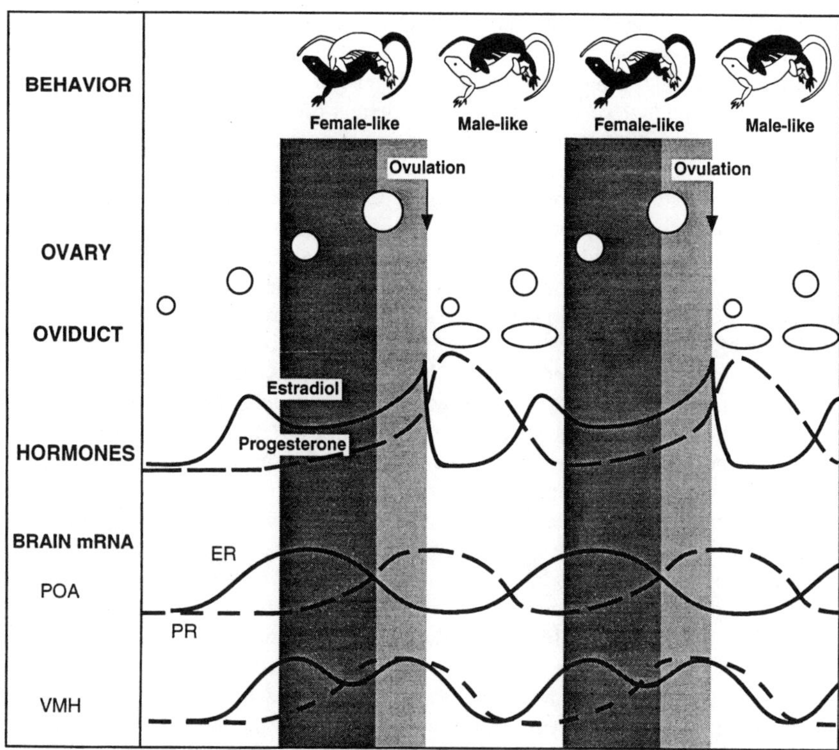

FIGURE 7. Relation among male-like and female-like pseudosexual behavior, ovarian state, and circulating levels of estradiol and progesterone during different stages of the reproductive cycle of the parthenogenetic whiptail lizard. The transition from receptive to mounting behavior occurs at ovulation (*arrow*). Also shown are the changes in estrogen receptor (ER)- and progesterone receptor (PR)-mRNA concentration in the preoptic area (POA) and the ventromedial hypothalamus (VMH).

retain a sensitivity to androgens and a distribution of androgen receptor similar to that seen in the sexual ancestral species.[51]

An important concept in behavioral neuroendocrinology is that changes in behavior commonly occur at transitions in the ratio in circulating levels of hormones. The close parallel between the severalfold rise in progesterone levels at ovulation suggests that it may be the hormone responsible for the expression of pseudocopulatory behavior. Supporting evidence is that (1) exogenous progesterone elicits pseudocopulatory behavior in ovariectomized parthenogens, and (2) intrahypothalamic progesterone implants into the preoptic area/anterior hypothalamus (POAH) elicit mating behavior in both castrated males of the sexual species and ovariectomized parthenogens as well as upregulating androgen receptor gene expression in the preoptic area/anterior hypothalamus.

As in other species with an associated reproductive pattern, courtship behavior in males of the sexual ancestral species depends on testicular androgens. How could an androgen-dependent mechanism subserving male-typical mating behavior in the sexual ancestral species evolve to become a progesterone-dependent mechanism underlying male-like behavior in the parthenogenetic descendant species? Evolution depends on *individual variation;* without it there would be no basis from which to evolve. It turns out that some males of the sexual ancestral species are sensitive to progesterone.[47] That is, in about one third of castrated males, administration of exogenous progesterone *restores* the complete repertoire of male-typical sexual behavior. It is clear that progesterone does not act as a precursor and that a metabolite of progesterone is responsible for activating male sexual behavior. Administration of the synthetic agonist R5020 (which induces progesterone receptor function) stimulates sexual behavior in castrated males, whereas administration of the synthetic antagonist RU486 (which blocks progesterone receptor function) abolishes sexual behavior in castrated, progesterone-treated males. Other work reveals that (1) progesterone plus androgen (testosterone or dihydrotestosterone) synergize to stimulate sexual behavior in males much like E2 plus progesterone synergize to elicit sexual receptivity in females,[52] and (2) the androgen receptor of the sexual species is similar to that of mammals in its specificity and kinetics.[53] Furthermore, it appears that progesterone acts via the progesterone receptor and not the androgen receptor. Intrahypothalamic implantation of progesterone into the POAH upregulates androgen receptor in the preoptic area, amygdala, and lateral septum of progesterone-sensitive males, but not of progesterone-insensitive males. In contrast, progesterone receptor-mRNA abundance is lower in the POAH of progesterone-sensitive males than of progesterone-insensitive males (FIG. 8). Because intact, unimplanted males representing these two populations do not have differential baseline abundance of androgen receptor- or progesterone receptor-mRNA in these nuclei,[54] it appears that progesterone differentially regulates its own receptor and androgen receptor in areas of the brain involved in the control of male-typical sexual behavior and that the nature of this regulation shows interindividual variability.

Thus, in the sexual ancestral species individual variation in the sensitivity to progesterone seems to have served as the substrate for the evolution of the novel hormone-brain-behavior relationship observed in the parthenogen. That is, because reproduction requires reciprocal behavioral stimulation, the elevation of progesterone following ovulation presented a reliable and appropriately timed stimulus that, given the lack of androgens, could be coopted to trigger mounting behavior in the parthenogen. Evidence that this has indeed occurred is indicated by the finding that exogenous E2 upregulates progesterone receptor-mRNA in the preoptic area of the parthenogen, but not in females of the ancestral sexual species (FIG. 9).

But is this behavioral responsiveness to progestin in males specific only to reptiles? Dogma is that progesterone inhibits sexual behavior in male vertebrates. However, recent studies indicate that progesterone has a functional role in males. For example, 17α, 20β-dihydroxyprogesterone stimulates spawning behavior in castrated rainbow trout.[55] In male rats, the diurnal rhythm in progesterone secretion is pronounced, with peak progesterone levels coinciding with the period of greatest copulatory activity.[56] When progesterone is administered in physiological dosages rather than the pharmacological dosages usually used, some castrated male rats will mate with receptive females; when progesterone is combined with subthreshold dosages of testosterone, all castrated males mount, a response that is blocked by the progesterone antagonist

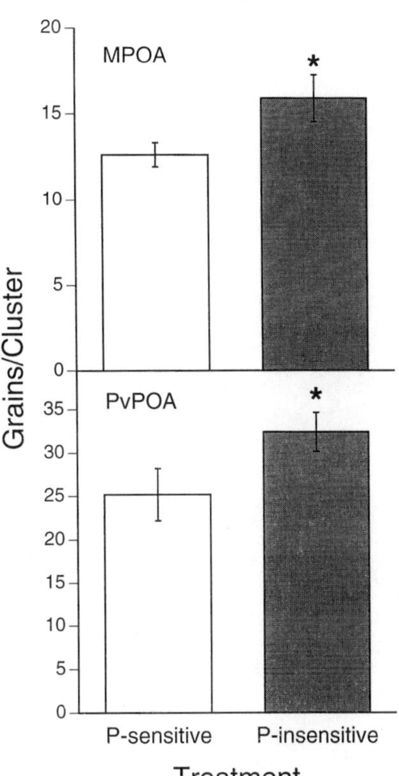

FIGURE 8. Abundance of progesterone receptor-mRNA measured as average number of silver grains per cluster in the medial preoptic area (MPOA) and the periventricular preoptic area (PvPOA) of castrated progesterone-sensitive and progesterone-insensitive males of the ancestral sexual species following intra-hypothalamic implants of progesterone. *Vertical error bars* represent standard errors of the mean.

RU486.[57,58] Thus, although progesterone has long been known to be involved in the control of female-typical sexual behavior, comparative studies have revealed a previously unsuspected role of progesterone in the control of male sexual behavior.

The parthenogenetic lizard also allows the neural bases of sex differences to be examined in a new way. As mentioned, the neural circuits underlying sex-typical mating behaviors of the sexual ancestral species have been retained in the parthenogenetic descendants. In sexually reproducing vertebrates the male and female brains differ in some ways, including the size of nuclei involved in the control of sexual behavior. Thus, in sexual whiptail lizards, the POAH, which is involved in the control of male-typical mounting behavior, is larger in males than in females (FIG. 10).[59] The ventromedial hypothalamus, which is involved in the control of female-typical receptivity, is larger in females. During hibernation or following castration, the POAH shrinks and the ventromedial hypothalamus enlarges (that is, these brain areas become female-like); a similar relationship exists at the neuronal level.[60] This indicates clearly that in the ancestral sexual species structural dimorphisms develop in the adult and, furthermore, that testicular androgens control the seasonal growth of these areas. Finally, the patterns of brain metabolism during courtship in the ancestral sexual species and pseudocopulation in the parthenogenetic descendant are similar.[61]

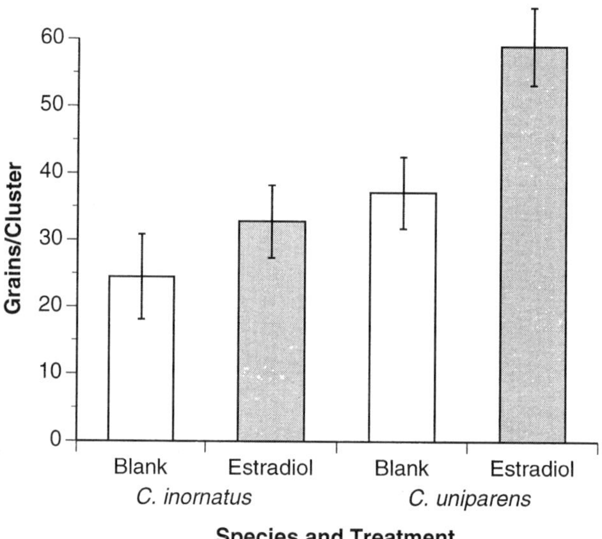

2-Way ANOVA comparison

Source	F-ratio	P value
species	8.352	0.008
treatment	4.569	0.043
speciesXtreatment interaction	1.093	0.307

FIGURE 9. Evolution of a novel neuroendocrine mechanism controlling male-typical mounting and copulatory behavior. Depicted is the abundance of progesterone receptor-mRNA measured as the average number of silver grains per cluster in the preoptic area (POA) of the ancestral sexual (*Cnemidophorus inornatus*) and descendant parthenogenetic (*C. uniparens*) whiptail lizard. *Box* (*below*) contains statistical comparisons.

These data might lead one to conclude that the brain of the parthenogen is bisexual, resembling both the male and the female of the ancestral sexual species. This is a reasonable hypothesis, given that the parthenogen exhibits both male-like and female-like "sexual" behaviors. Surprisingly, this is not the case. The POAH and ventromedial hypothalamus of the parthenogenetic whiptail is similar in size to those of females of the sexual ancestral species, even in those individuals that are exhibiting male-like pseudocopulatory behavior naturally or under hormone treatment.[59,60] Furthermore, no difference in neuron somata size exists in those individuals exhibiting male-like pseudosexual behavior than in those exhibiting female-like pseudosexual behavior. Even if parthenogens are treated with androgen so that they exhibit only male-like pseudosexual behavior and assume coloration patterns and glandular

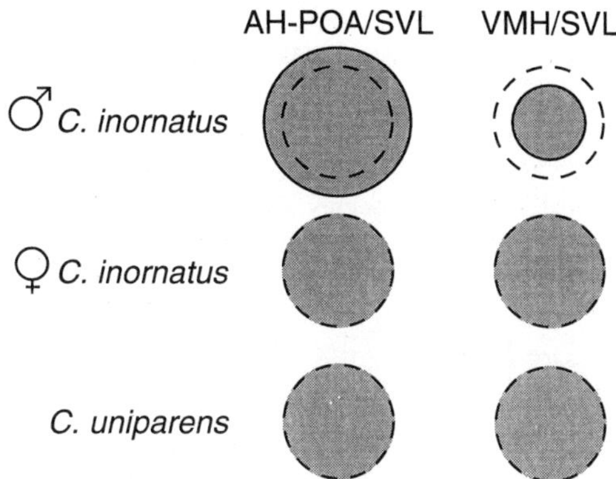

FIGURE 10. Schematic representations of the volumes of the sexually dimorphic areas in the brain relative to body size in the ancestral sexual and descendant parthenogenetic whiptail lizard. To aid in comparison, the volume of the anterior hypothalamus-preoptic area (AH-POA) and the ventromedial hypothalamus (VMH) of female *C. inornatus* is represented as a *bold outline* in other drawings to indicate significant differences. (Reproduced with permission from ref. 2.)

excretions similar to those of males of the sexual ancestral species, the brain remains unchanged.

Such findings raise questions as to the meaning of sexual dimorphisms in the vertebrate brain. For example, we hear today that homosexuals and transsexuals behave as they do because their brain is different from that of heterosexuals. However, the parthenogen clearly retains the ability to express male-like pseudosexual behaviors, but it does so *not* because it has a masculinized POAH, but because it has coopted the progesterone surge to trigger the masculine behavioral potential that remains in a feminized brain. In other words, behavioral differences need not be paralleled by structural differences in the brain and it is not the size, but the activity, of brain areas that matters.

SUMMARY AND CONCLUSIONS

One of the first things that we are impressed by is the great variety of animals, particularly their behaviors and their physiologies. With so many differences, are there any generalities? With the establishment of evolutionary theory, evidence of "unity in diversity" comes with discoveries of common anatomical features, the cell cycle, conservation of intermediary metabolism, and the genetic code, to name but a few. In vertebrates there appears to be a conservation of the neural circuits underlying sexual behavior, but it is still too early to state the extent to which this concept can be extended to the hormonal mechanisms underlying behavior.

Much of our conceptual understanding of behavioral neuroendocrinology stems from extensive studies on relatively few species. When an evolutionary perspective is applied to behavioral neuroscience, the breadth and validity of our assumptions about the mechanisms that control species-typical behaviors are challenged. This is not the same thing as saying that there are few unitary explanations that apply to all mammals, amniotes, or even vertebrates. Considerable information has been gathered about the neuroendocrine bases of behavior in a few species, but to uncover truly broad generalizations, we must look with equal intensity and rigor at other organisms.

The pattern of evolution is best illustrated in the diversity of organisms, and the ecological and evolutionary perspective illuminates the utility of various "experiments of nature." By studying (1) closely related species that live in different habitats, we can see if the adaptational responses are similar, and (2) distantly related species that live in the same habitat, we can see if the solutions are analogous. The unique qualities of each species also give us a deeper understanding of the constraints in fundamental processes. When basic conflicts exist, control mechanisms adapt or the species goes extinct. Interestingly, although the neural circuits themselves do not degenerate, they are either no longer used or coopted for other functions.[62,63]

ACKNOWLEDGMENT

I thank John Branch for reading this manuscript.

REFERENCES

1. GHISELIN, M. T. 1974. The Economy of Nature and the Evolution of Sex. University of California Press. Berkeley, CA.
2. CREWS, D. 1992. *In* Introduction to Behavioral Endocrinology. J. Becker, S. M. Breedlove & D. Crews, Eds.: 143-186. MIT Press/Bradford Books, Cambridge, MA.
3. THOMAS, C. S. & J. C. COULSON. 1988. *In* Reproductive Success. T. H. Clutton-Brock, Ed.: 251-262. University of Chicago Press. Chicago, IL.
4. BLUHM, C. K. 1985. *In* The Endocrine System and the Environment. B. K. Follett, S. Ishii & A. Chandola, Eds. Japanese Scientific Society Press, Tokyo.: 247-264. Springer-Verlag. Berlin.
5. CREWS, D. 1984. Horm. Behav. **18:** 22-28.
6. CREWS, D. & M. C. MOORE. 1986. Science **231:** 121-125.
7. WHITTIER, J. M. & D. CREWS. 1987. *In* Hormones and Reproduction in Fishes, Amphibians, and Reptiles. D. O. Norris & R. E. Jones, Eds.: 385-409. Plenum Press. New York.
8. WINGFIELD, J. C., R. E. HEGNER, A. M. DUFTY & G. F. BALL. 1990. Am. Nat. **136:** 829-846.
9. KACSOH, B., L. C. TERRY, J. S. MEYERS, W. R. CROWLEY & C. E. GROSVENOR. 1989. Endocrinology **125:** 1326-1336.
10. KOLDOVSKY, O. 1995. Am. Zool. **35:** 446-454.
11. CLARK, M. M., D. CREWS & B. G. GALEF. 1991. Physiol. Behav. **49:** 239-243.
12. VOM SAAL, F. S. 1981. J. Reprod. Fertil. **62:** 633-650.
13. VOM SAAL, F. S. 1991. *In* Heterotypical Behavior in Man and Animals. M. Haug, P. F. Brain & C. Aron, Eds.: 42-70. Chapman and Hall. London, England.
14. YAHR, P. 1995. *In* Neurobiological Effects of Sex Steroid Hormones. P. E. Micevych & R. P. Hammer, Eds.: 40-56. Cambridge University Press. Cambridge, England.
15. JONES, D., F. GONZALEZ-LIMA, D. CREWS, B. G. GALEF & M. M. CLARK. 1996. Physiol. Behav. In press.
16. CREWS, D., T. W. WIBBELS & W. H. N. GUTZKE. 1989. Gen. Comp. Endocrinol. **75:** 159-166.
17. BERN, H. A. 1990. Am. Zool. **30:** 877-885.
18. SCHRECK, C. B., M. S. FITZPATRICK, G. W. FEIST & C.-G. YEOH. 1991. *In* Proceedings of the Fourth International Symposium of Reproductive Physiology of Fish. A. P. Scott, J. P. Sumpter, D. E. Kime & M. S. Rolfe, Eds. Fish Symp **91:** 256-258. Sheffield.
19. ADKINS-REGAN, E., M. A. OTTINGER & J. PARK. 1995. J. Exp. Zool. **271:** 466-470.
20. SCHWABL, H. 1993. Proc. Natl. Acad. Sci. USA **90:** 11446-11450.
21. CLARK, M. M., P. KARPIUK & B. G. GALEF. 1993. Nature **364:** 712.
22. KIRKPATRICK, M. & R. LANDE. 1989. Evolution **43:** 485-503.

23. Crews, D., J. M. Bergeron, D. Flores, J. J. Bull, J. K. Skipper, A. Tousignant & T. Wibbels. 1994. Dev. Genet. **15:** 297-312.
24. Tousignant, A. & D. Crews. 1995. J. Morphol. **224:** 1-12.
25. Crews, D. 1988. Psychobiology **16:** 321-334.
26. Gutzke, W. H. N. & D. Crews. 1988. Nature **332:** 832-834.
27. Coomber, P., F. Gonzalez-Lima & D. Crews. 1996. J. Comp. Neurol. Submitted.
28. Flores, D. L. & D. Crews. 1995. Horm. Behav. **29:** 458-473.
29. Flores, D. L., A. Tousignant & D. Crews. 1994. Physiol. Behav. **55:** 1067-1072.
30. Crews, D. 1990. *In* Hormones, Brain and Behaviour in Vertebrates. J. Balthazart, Ed.: 1-14. S. Karger AG. Basel.
31. Beach, F. A. 1983. Can. J. Psychol. **37:** 193-210.
32. Bronson, F. H. 1989. Mammalian Reproductive Biology. University of Chicago Press. Chicago.
33. Moore, M. C. 1991. Horm. Behav. **25:** 154-179.
34. Bass, A. 1992. Trends Neurosci. **15:** 139-145.
35. Mason, R. T. & D. Crews. 1985. Nature **316:** 59-60.
36. Mason, R. T., H. M. Fales, T. H. Jones, L. K. Pannell, J. W. Chinn & D. Crews. 1989. Science **245:** 290-293.
37. Mason, R. T. & R. W. Krohmer. 1995.
38. Garstka, W. R. & D. Crews. 1981. Science **214:** 681-683.
39. Crews, D. 1985. Physiol. Behav. **35:** 569-575.
40. Lank, D. B., C. M. Smith, O. Hanotte, T. Burke & F. Cooke. 1995. Nature **378:** 59-62.
41. Godwin, J., R. Warner & D. Crews. 1996. Science. Submitted.
42. Beach, F. A. 1979. *In* Sex, Hormones and Behaviour. R. Potter & J. Whelan, Eds. Ciba Foundation Symposium **62:** 113-143. Excerpta Medica. Amsterdam.
43. Allee, W. C. 1938. Cooperation Among Animals. Henry Schuman. New York, NY.
44. Skipper, J. S., L. J. Young, J. M. Bergeron, M. T. Tetzlaff, C. T. Osborn & D. Crews. 1993. Proc. Natl. Acad. Sci. USA **90:** 7172-7175.
45. Charlesworth, B. 1991. Science **251:** 1030-1033.
46. Crews, D. 1982. Psychoneuroendocrinology **7:** 259-270.
47. Crews, D. 1989. *In* Evolution and Ecology of Unisexual Vertebrates. R. Dawley & J. Bogart, Eds.: 132-143. New York State Museum. Albany, NY.
48. Wade, J. & D. Crews. 1991. Horm. Behav. **25:** 342-353.
49. Kendrick, A., M. Rand & D. Crews. 1995. Brain Res. **680:** 226-228.
50. Young, L. J. & D. Crews. 1995. Trends Endocrinol. Metab. **6:** 317-323.
51. Young, L. J., G. F. Lopreato, K. Horan & D. Crews. 1994. J. Comp. Neurol. **347:** 288-300.
52. Lindzey, J. & D. Crews. 1992. Gen. Comp. Endocrinol. **86:** 52-58.
53. Lindzey, J. & D. Crews. 1993. Horm. Behav. **27:** 269-281.
54. Crews, D., J. Godwin, E. A. Prediger, M. Grammer & R. Sheppard. J. Neurosci. In press.
55. Mayer, I., N. R. Liley & B. Borg. 1994. Horm. Behav. **28:** 181-190.
56. Kalra, P. S. & S. P. Kalra. 1977. Endocrinology **101:** 1821-1827.
57. Witt, D. M., L. J. Young & D. Crews. 1994. Psychoneuroendocrinology **19:** 553-562.
58. Witt, D. M., L. J. Young & D. Crews. 1995. Physiol. Behav. **57:** 307-313.
59. Crews, D., J. Wade & W. Wilczynski. 1990. Brain Behav. Evol. **36:** 262-270.
60. Wade, J., J.-M. Huang & D. Crews. 1993. J. Neuroendocrinol. **5:** 81-93.
61. Rand, M. S. & D. Crews. 1994. Brain Res. **655:** 163-167.
62. Kavanau, L. J. 1990. Anim. Behav. **39:** 758-767.
63. Wilczynski, W. 1984. Am. Zool. **24:** 755-763.
64. Crews, D. 1987. *In* Psychobiology of Reproductive Behavior. D. Crews, Ed.: 88-119. Prentice-Hall Inc. Englewood Cliffs, NJ.

2

Ecological Constraints and the Evolution of Hormone-Behavior Interrelationships

John C. Wingfield, Jerry Jacobs, and Nigella Hillgarth

Behavioral endocrinologists traditionally have focused on the hormones that influence behavior and their underlying mechanisms. Less well studied are potential ecological constraints on interactions of hormones and behavior and their possible implications for evolution of diverse patterns of behavior throughout the life cycle. For example, Crews[1–3] and Crews and Moore[4] point out that in many vertebrate species, maturation of gonads and sexual behavior are uncoupled. In some cases, sexual behavior is expressed when the gonads are inactive. In males, stored spermatozoa are used during copulation, and females also can store sperm until their ovaries develop and ovulation occurs. Thus, sex steroid hormones secreted into the blood would be appropriate signals by which sexual behavior is activated in the associated case (where gonad maturation and sexual behavior coincide), but not necessarily in the dissociated case (where sexual behavior occurs when the gonads, and presumably sex steroid hormone secretion, are inactive). Crews and his associates[1–4] suggest that hormonal control of different patterns of sexual behavior may be diverse as a result of ecological factors that provide selection for specific mechanisms in *one* population at *one* time in its life history. It is therefore possible, perhaps probable, that different mechanisms have evolved to regulate similar behavior at different stages in the life cycle of the same population or even at the same stage in other populations. The purpose of this communication is to point out that although there may be many ecological constraints, they fall under two main groups: (1) Patterns of behavior vary in relation to life cycle. Sexual behavior may be expressed at different times in the life cycle (as just cited). Some species show territorial behavior for restricted periods during the reproductive season, whereas others may be territorial year round. The context of territorial aggression changes as stages in the life cycle progress, but qualitatively and even quantitatively the behavior remains the same (to be discussed). Thus, a hormone signal to activate a behavioral trait may be appropriate at one stage in the life cycle but not at another. (2) Potential ecological ''costs'' that a hormonal signal may have in terms of overall fitness,[5–7] especially if that hormone has effects on physiology and morphology *in addition* to behavior.

Preparation of this manuscript and much of the authors' research was funded by the National Science Foundation, particularly grants OPP-9300771 and DCB-9005081 to J.C.W.

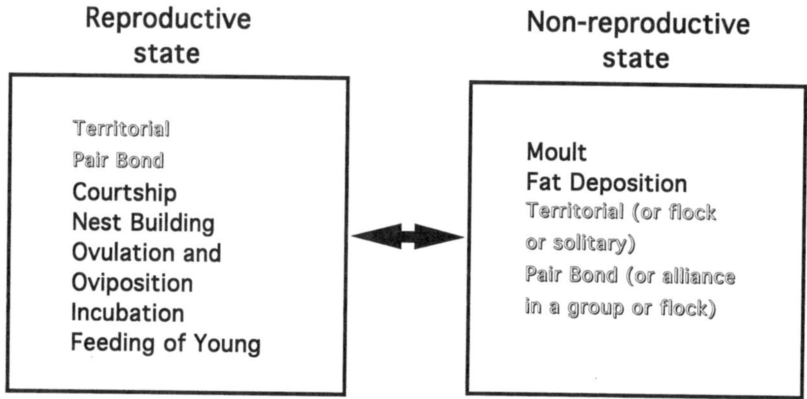

FIGURE 1. A simple example of two interchangeable life history states in a seasonally breeding population. Each has a unique set of substates defined by characteristic morphological, physiological, and behavioral traits. Note, however, that territorial and pair bond behaviors may be shared in both states (*open type*), whereas others appear specific (*bold type*). Finite state machine theory predicts that although some behaviors appear to be shared, the hormone control mechanisms that activate those behaviors in each state may be different.[11]

To illustrate these points we focus on the interrelationship of testosterone and aggression over territories and access to mates. In these cases an individual may exclude conspecifics from its territory with the exception of the mate. Members of a pair often will defend a territory together, whereas some species breed in cooperative groups that share and defend a joint territory.[8,9] Such affiliative behavior gives rise to potential conflicts, aggression towards other conspecifics but tolerance of one, the mate, or a few in the case of territorial groups. Examples of territorial aggression, interrelationships with testosterone, and pair bonds come from birds, our primary research animals. Additionally, avian behavioral ecology is particularly well known, and their endocrinology has been studied extensively under field conditions.[10]

LIFE HISTORY STATES AND TEMPORAL PATTERNS OF BEHAVIOR

Before we launch into ecological constraints on the interrelationships of testosterone, aggression, and pair bonds, it is first necessary to introduce the concept of "life history states" as a way of analyzing the progression of stages in the life cycles of individuals within populations. Transitions between these states are what determine patterns of behavior and potentially provide us with a theoretical framework from which to determine mechanisms of hormone control. A very simple example is given in FIGURE 1 of two life history states, reproductive and nonreproductive. The theory of finite state machines[11] assumes that these states have a unique set of substates that have characteristic combinations of morphological, physiological, and behavioral traits. These are only expressed in that specific state and probably have a unique set of neural and endocrine mechanisms that control their activation.[11] Within the reproductive state (FIG. 1) are many substates such as nest building behavior, ovulation, and parental care. Obviously these would not be expressed in the nonreproductive state (i.e., winter). Nonetheless, some behavioral patterns appear to be shared. Many avian species are territorial in both reproductive and nonreproductive states. Others may be paired or be members of a stable group in both states (FIG. 1). Observations indicate that these behaviors are similar in both states, leading to the assumption that hormonal control mechanisms may also be similar.[12] By contrast, the theory of finite state machines[11] predicts that they are different. We review evidence for the ecological bases of territorial and pairing behavior in reproductive and nonreproductive states as a test of the finite state machine model in general and discuss how this approach may shed light on the evolution of hormone-behavior interactions.

ECOLOGICAL CONSTRAINTS IN RELATION TO PATTERNS OF TERRITORIALITY AND MAINTENANCE OF PAIR BONDS

Any behavioral traits that are expressed in predictable patterns require regulatory mechanisms. Typically, hormone secretions activate behavioral traits in three major ways.[13,14] (1) Hormones that are secreted in a paracrine fashion and act entirely centrally as neurotransmitters or neuromodulators; (2) hormones that are secreted into the blood (i.e., true endocrine), enter the CNS, and start organizational effects or activate behavior; (3) A combination of both 1 and 2 where a blood-borne hormone may act on neurotransmitters/neuromodulators that in turn regulate behavior. Here we focus on the activational effects (2 above) of the sex steroid hormone testosterone on territorial aggression in birds as well as in relation to pair bonds.

It has been known for many decades that aggression associated with a breeding territory or access to mates is regulated by circulating levels of testosterone.[15,16] Once testosterone enters the brain, it may be aromatized to estradiol or reduced to 5-alpha-dihydrotestosterone within neurons. These metabolites of testosterone then bind to intracellular receptors[17] and influence behavior. However, it is important to note that unlike hormones that are secreted and act entirely centrally, blood-borne hormones virtually always have additional physiological and morphological actions. This is particularly true for testosterone (FIG. 2) which has marked effects on behavior (sexual and aggressive in reproductive contexts),[15,16] but it is also essential for completion of spermatogenesis.[18] Additionally, testosterone has morphological effects on the development of accessory glands (vas deferens etc.) and some secondary sex characters.[9,19] On the basis of these well documented actions of testosterone, activation of territorial behavior by elevated circulating testosterone levels in a reproductive state would obviously be appropriate. On the other hand, activation of territorial behavior by testosterone would be highly inappropriate in the nonbreeding season because of additional effects on reproductive physiology and morphology.

It is also now clear that high plasma levels of testosterone are immunosuppressive[20–22] (FIG. 2). This may have first arisen as a mechanism to suppress actions of the immune system within the testes, because as developing spermatozoa become haploid, they develop surface proteins that are recognized as foreign by cells of the immune system. Thus, suppression of immune responses within the testes enhances

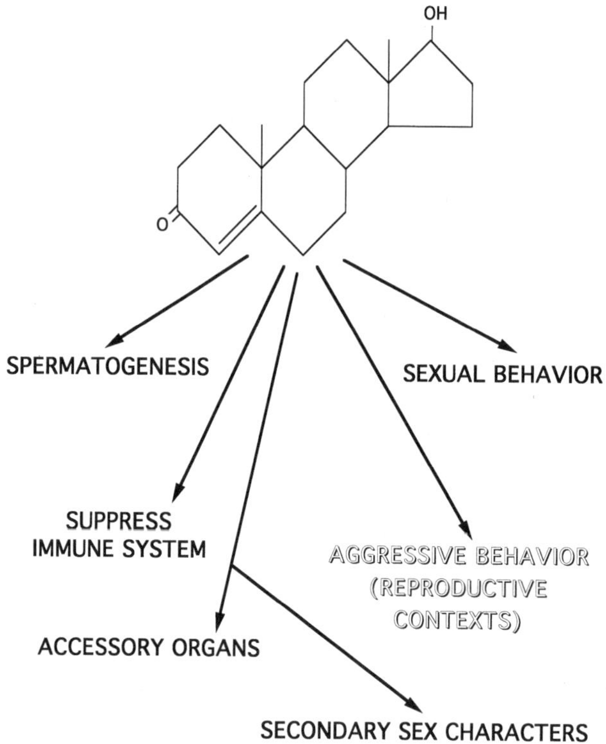

FIGURE 2. Known biological actions of the steroid hormone testosterone. These effects can be behavioral, morphological, and physiological. Many actions may include enzymatic conversion to active metabolites such as estradiol or dihydrotestosterone (DHT). Compiled from refs. 15, 16, 19, 20, 21, and 23.

fertility. Problems arise when testosterone is secreted into the blood and then has the potential to inhibit the immune system throughout the organism.[23]

Such diverse effects of a single hormone such as testosterone pose problems for the regulation of territorial aggression and pair bonds that are expressed in diverse patterns in different taxa. As just suggested,[5–7,24] these problems include: (1) Inappropriate expression of physiological and morphological effects when the hormone is secreted in different life history states (even though the behavior regulated by that hormone may be appropriate); (2) ''Costs,'' in terms of reduced overall fitness such as increased mortality, reproductive failure, and other potentially deleterious effects. Next we discuss patterns of territorial aggression and pair bond behavior in relation to testosterone secretion in male birds and address the ''costs'' later.

Patterns of Territorial Behavior

Although it has long been known that testosterone can activate aggressive behavior associated with territory establishment and maintenance,[15,16] correlations of circulating

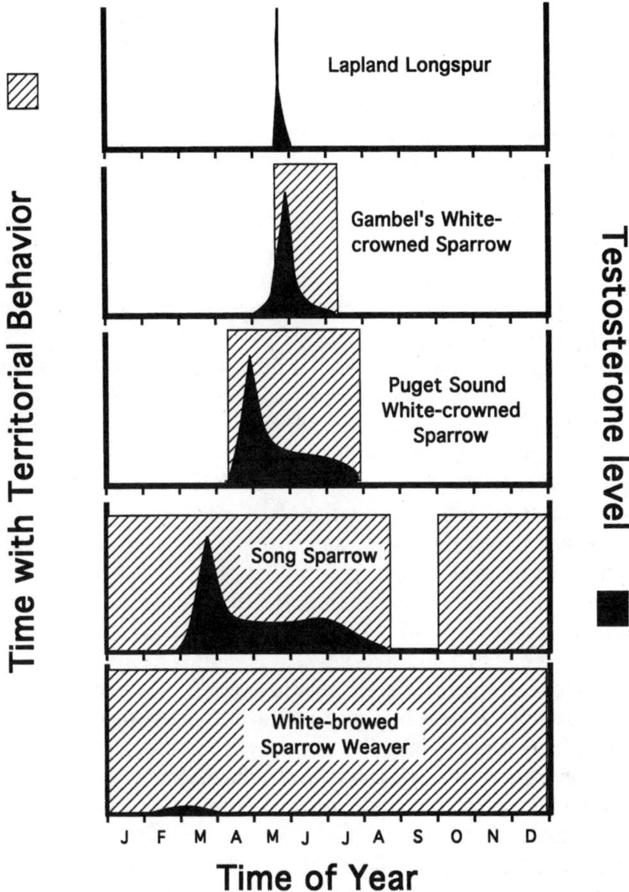

FIGURE 3. Patterns of territorial behavior (*shaded blocks*) and of circulating testosterone (*black curves*) in various avian taxa: Lapland longspur (*Calcarius laponnicus*)[25]; Gambel's white-crowned sparrow (*Zonotrichia leucophrys gambelii*)[26]; Puget Sound white-crowned sparrow (*Z. l. pugetensis*),[27] song sparrow (*Melospiza melodia*),[28] and white-browed sparrow-weaver (*Plocepasser mahali*).[29] In highly seasonal species, elevated circulating levels of testosterone correlate well with expression of territorial behavior. In those species in which territorial aggression is expressed less seasonally (lower two panels), circulating testosterone levels are less well coordinated with the behavior, especially outside the breeding season.

levels of testosterone with periods of territorial behavior have been less consistent.[8,9] Why should testosterone apparently activate territorial aggression in some taxa but not others? Possible clues come from a summary of field studies presented in FIGURE 3. Data from three species in the top panels of FIGURE 3 (arctic to temperate climates) are territorial during the breeding season only. During the rest of the year they form flocks. Breeding seasons in the arctic are so short that many populations have only 5-

6 weeks to initiate and complete breeding. In the arctic passerine *Calcarius lapponicus*, territorial behavior is extremely brief (a few days) and high circulating levels of testosterone are similarly short lived[25] (top panel, FIG. 3). Throughout the rest of the breeding season, males of this species are not territorial. Gambel's white-crowned sparrow, *Zonotrichia leucophrys gambelii*, breeds further south in the subarctic zone of Alaska. Here the period of territorial behavior is longer and paralleled by high circulating levels of testosterone[26] (second panel, FIG. 2). Further south still, the Puget Sound white-crowned sparrow, *Z. l. pugetensis*, breeds at mid-latitudes and is multiple brooded. The breeding season spans April to July, during which males are territorial and plasma levels of testosterone are similarly high[27,28] (third panel, FIG. 3). Data from these three taxa indicate that high circulating levels of testosterone match periods of territorial aggression precisely.

The lower two panels of FIGURE 3 tell a different story. Rufous song sparrows, *Melospiza melodia morphna*, also breed at mid-latitude and have a slightly longer breeding season than do *Z. l. pugetensis*. Circulating levels of testosterone are high throughout this period (fourth panel, FIG. 3). During the pre-basic molt (August to September), males remain in their territories but show no aggression if challenged by a simulated territorial intrusion consisting of a decoy male and a broadcast of tape-recorded songs.[28] Accordingly, plasma levels of testosterone are undetectable.[28] Note that in September and October, male rufous song sparrows once again express territorial aggression, but without any increase in testosterone levels in the blood. They continue to express territorial aggression (as assessed by simulated territorial intrusion) through the winter and into the next breeding season[28] (FIG. 3). Castration of free-living male song sparrows in October has no effect on their ability to maintain territories even during the next breeding season.[12] Clearly, neither testosterone nor other gonadal hormones are required to express territorial aggression in this species. Further investigations show that although this taxon is nonmigratory, the reproductive and nonreproductive territories of individual males may not always be the same. At a study site in western Washington State, breeding and nonbreeding territories are up to 100 m apart, and some overlap partially.[30] These data suggest that territorial aggression in the reproductive and nonreproductive state (e.g., FIG. 1) may be similar in postures and vocalizations, but in context may be different. Perhaps it is not surprising that control mechanisms may also be different in the two states.

These data raise the question of whether testosterone has any effect on the expression of territorial aggression in rufous song sparrows. High levels of testosterone during the breeding season may increase persistence of territorial aggression, especially after a territorial intrusion. Territorial males in spring continue to patrol their territories and sing at a high frequency even after a simulated intrusion has been terminated and the decoy removed. In contrast, removal of a simulated territorial intrusion in the autumn is accompanied by immediate cessation of territorial behavior. Implants of testosterone into free-living, territorial males in autumn reinstate the "persistence" of territorial aggression compared with that of controls.[12] Although territorial aggression can be activated in the absence of testosterone in this species, persistence of aggression in the presence of a simulated territorial intrusion or after the "intruder" has been removed is indeed testosterone dependent.

Many species of birds are territorial throughout their lives, including the period of molt. An example is given in panel 5 (bottom panel) of FIG. 3 using data obtained from free-living white-browed sparrow weavers, *Plocepasser mahali,* sampled in a tropical dry forest in Zambia, Africa. This species lives in cooperative groups with a dominant male and female that are mated and up to 9 additional members that do not breed, but do help defend the group territory. Plasma levels of testosterone are virtually undetectable in all males throughout the year[29] (FIG. 3). Dominant breeding males show a slight elevation of circulating testosterone in mid-breeding season (FIG. 3), but this is not correlated with any obvious change in behavior. Experimental manipulations using simulated group territorial intrusions or removal of breeding males with respective controls result in violent changes in territorial aggression and dominance-subordinance relationships but no change in testosterone levels.[31,32] Curiously, testosterone levels in the testes are identical to those of north temperate species.[29] Furthermore, injection of chicken gonadotropin releasing hormone-1 results in massive increases in plasma levels of luteinizing hormone but only a slight elevation of testosterone.[29] These data suggest that the hypothalamo-pituitary-gonad axis of the white-browed sparrow weaver is functional, but that very little testosterone is actually released into the blood. Territorial aggression in this species is constant year round and apparently independent of testosterone regulation.

The comparisons made in FIGURE 3 clearly suggest that only when territorial aggression and reproduction coincide exactly do patterns of testosterone levels in blood match expression of the behavior directly. When territorial aggression is expressed at other times, additional control mechanisms must be in operation.

Patterns of Pair Bond Formation and Maintenance

In many avian species it is generally thought that testosterone regulates male courtship behavior and formation of sexual pair bonds,[15] although other central mechanisms are also important (Carter, this volume). In those species in which pair bonds are maintained only for the breeding season, then the duration of pair bond maintenance is correlated with high circulating levels of testosterone. This relationship is obvious for the three taxa of seasonally breeding and migratory species in FIGURE 4 (top 3 panels). Variation in time here is due to different lengths of the breeding season, as described above. For the other two species, pair bonds and other affiliative behavior appear to be far more complex. In rufous song sparrows, high plasma levels of testosterone are found throughout the breeding season when sexual pair bonds are maintained[28] (panel 4, FIG. 4). During the molt, males show no obvious associations with other individuals, and circulating levels of testosterone are undetectable. However, males become territorial again in the autumn and frequently appear paired. Testosterone levels remain low[28] (FIG. 4). Closer examination of these "pairs" reveals that less than 30% are male-female pairs, the rest being male-male associations or groups of up to seven birds of mixed sexes on a territory. Many of these may have been "floaters" (a term used to describe nonterritorial members of a population) that are tolerated on several adjacent territories.[30] Of the male-female pairs that are territorial during the autumn, only one pair subsequently bred together. All others eventually mate and breed with different partners. Furthermore, if female rufous song sparrows are given implants of estradiol to make them sexually receptive in the autumn, territorial males fail to form pair bonds with them.[33] Although rufous song

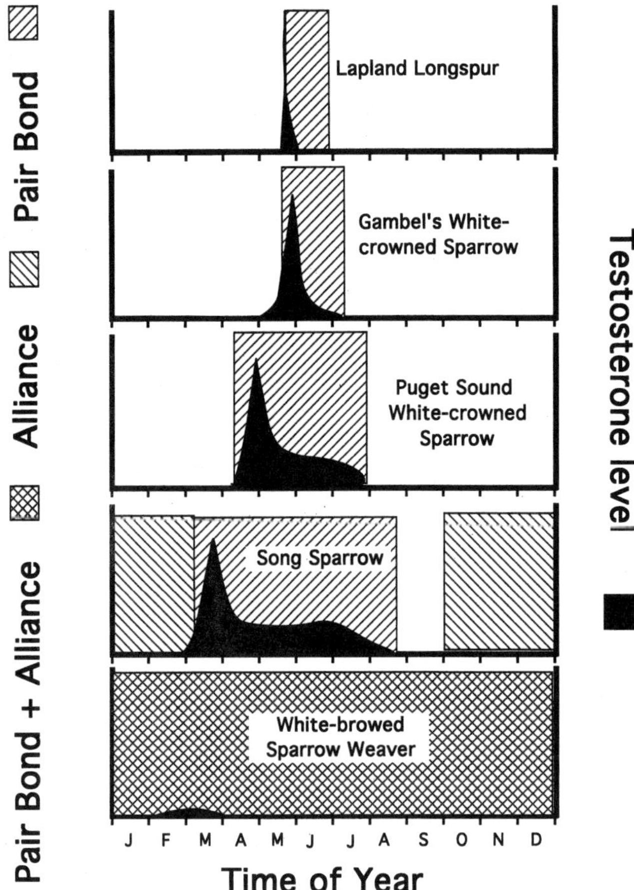

FIGURE 4. Patterns of affiliative behavior (*shaded blocks*) and of circulating testosterone (*black curves*) in various avian taxa. Affiliation can be a true pair bond between a breeding male and female, an alliance (apparent pair bond but not reproductive in context), or both can occur simultaneously in cooperative groups: Lapland longspur (*Calcarius laponnicus*)[25]; Gambel's white-crowned sparrow (*Zonotrichia leucophrys gambelii*)[26]; Puget Sound white-crowned sparrow (*Z. l. pugetensis*),[27] song sparrow (*Melospiza melodia*),[28] and white-browed sparrow-weaver (*Plocepasser mahali*).[29] High circulating levels of testosterone occur simultaneously with pair bonds in reproductive contexts and not with nonreproductive alliances.

sparrows are territorial throughout much of the year, the context of those territories changes from reproductive in spring and early summer to a territorial ''alliance'' in the nonreproductive season. Here again we see an example of similar behavior (apparent pair bonds) but with different contexts in each life history state.

The white-browed sparrow weaver shows an even more complex pattern of affiliative behavior while being territorial year round (Fig. 4, bottom panel). These birds are cooperative breeders and form groups that can be stable for many months or even years. Typically they consist of a breeding male and female (sexual pair bond) as well as a group of nonbreeding birds of both sexes that form a territorial group. These auxiliary members help defend the group territory, and some may feed young (i.e., helpers-at-the-nest). Thus, we have an example here of simultaneous sexual pair bonds and territorial alliances (FIG. 4, bottom panel). Note, however, that testosterone levels in blood remain virtually undetectable throughout the year[29] (FIG. 4). In this species, neither sexual pair bonds or alliances with other individuals appear to be dependent on testosterone.

It would be intriguing to explore potential central mechanisms (e.g., effects of arginine vasotocin; see Carter, this volume) underlying these two types of affiliative behavior (sexual pair bonds versus territorial alliances). Here we see examples of both types of affiliation within a population, thus avoiding potential phylogenetic differences inherent when comparing two unrelated taxa. Similar powerful comparisons are being made with different populations of *Microtus* that show monogamous versus no, or polygamous, pair bonds (Carter, this volume).

Autumn "Sexuality"

Data from the species in FIGURES 3 and 4 are representative of over 50 avian species now studied in the field or in seminatural conditions. They allow us to begin asking questions about *why* different hormone mechanisms appear to be regulating superficially similar behavioral traits. They also allow us to formulate more penetrating hypotheses to explore mechanisms further as well as to gain insight into how these diverse patterns evolved. From FIGURES 3 and 4 it is clear that both territorial aggression and pair bond maintenance may occur in different life history states, and endocrine profiles that support experimental evidence in one state may fail to do so in another. Finite state machine theory may indeed be useful in analyzing life history states and point out where mechanisms underlying the regulation of behavior in various taxa, or within a taxon at different states in the life cycle, may be expected to be similar or different. To test this possibility we suggest that in those avian species in which autumnal territorial aggression and pair formation are sexual in context, then plasma levels of testosterone should also be high in this apparently nonreproductive state. Four avian species that show autumn territorial aggression and/or pair bonding in sexual contexts in autumn (these territories are actual breeding territories and the mates subsequently breed together) also have autumnal peaks of circulating testosterone (FIG. 5). Five avian species in which autumnal territoriality and pair bonding are not sexual in context show no such peak in testosterone. Note that all species show the normal spring peak of circulating testosterone at the beginning of the breeding season (FIG. 5).

This simple test is a useful indicator that a theoretical approach using finite state machine theory and natural history data may actually be predictive of potential hormone mechanisms, but further testing in the laboratory is now needed. Mechanisms at the receptor and metabolite level are also critical (see below). These data in the context of finite-state machine theory now suggest the hypothesis (FIG. 6) that in species with autumnal peaks of testosterone secretion, the nonreproductive state may be very short in duration and restricted to the period of prebasic molt. The reproductive

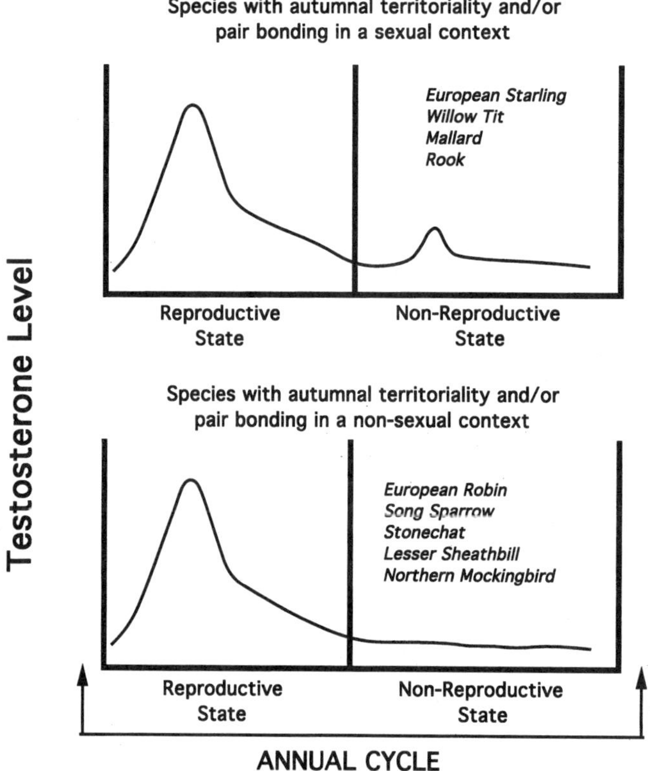

FIGURE 5. Patterns of circulating testosterone levels in avian species showing autumnal territoriality and/or pair bonding in a sexual context (**top panel**) and nonsexual context (**lower panel**). Autumn in these cases falls within the apparent nonreproductive state (i.e., these birds had regressed gonads). Scientific names for species listed are: European starling (*Sturnus vulgaris*); willow tit (*Parus montanus*); mallard (*Anas platyrhynchos*); rook (*Corvus frugilegus*); European robin (*Erithacus rubecula*); song sparrow (*Melospiza melodia morphna*); stonechat (*Saxicola torquata*); lesser sheathbill (*Chionis minor*); and northern mockingbird (*Mimus polyglottos*). Data compiled from refs. 28, 35–41.

state is now very long with its inception in autumn. Those species that show territorial behavior and alliances in nonreproductive contexts may have a much longer nonreproductive state. Preparations for breeding, the onset of the reproductive state, do not begin until spring (Fig. 6). This suggests different control mechanisms for temporal patterns of reproductive function compared to those in species with no autumnal peaks of testosterone. These ideas are testable and may lead to new understanding not only of controlling patterns of behavior, but also of how the life cycle is organized.

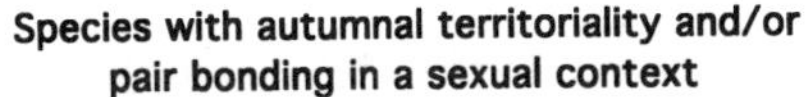

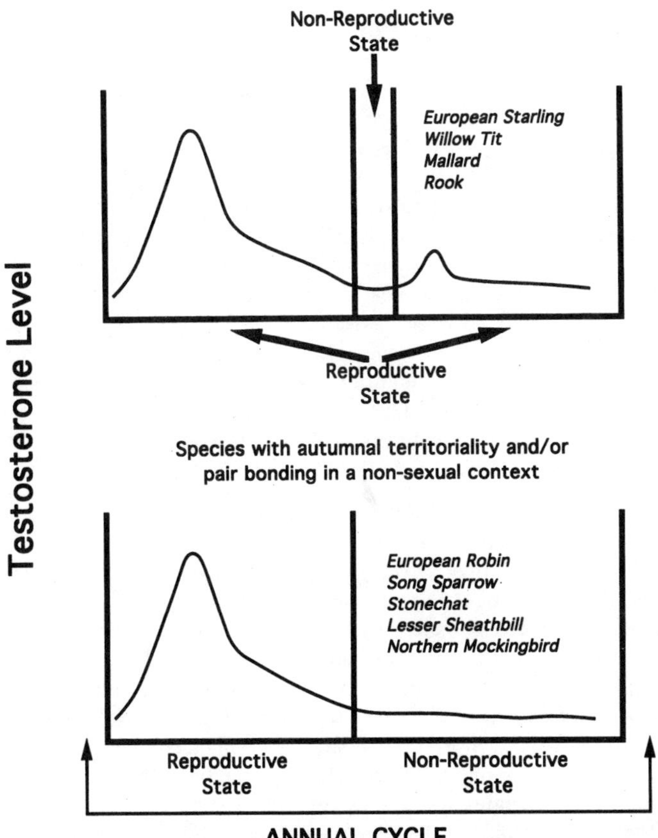

FIGURE 6. A new interpretation of the patterns of life history states based on finite state machine theory and the data presented in FIGURES 3-5. In those species showing autumnal territoriality and/or pair bonding in a sexual context (**top panel**), the reproductive state may be very long, taking up most of the year. Preparations for breeding may begin in autumn. The nonreproductive state becomes very short in duration, perhaps spanning only the period of prebasic molt. In those species in which autumnal territoriality and pairing (alliances) are not sexual in context, the nonreproductive state is much longer. Preparations for breeding may not occur until the next spring. Clearly the central and endocrine mechanisms underlying these strikingly different temporal patterns of life history states may not be the same. See text for details.

ECOLOGICAL CONSTRAINTS IN RELATION TO "COSTS" OF HIGH CIRCULATING LEVELS OF TESTOSTERONE

As a blood-borne hormone, testosterone has a spectrum of effects on reproductive morphology, physiology, and behavior (FIG. 2). Recently, however, it has become clear that high circulating levels of testosterone can have deleterious effects, direct and indirect, that in turn can reduce overall fitness[5–7,24,46] (see also ref. 47). Potential "costs" of high plasma levels of testosterone outside the normal breeding season are the many behavioral, physiological, and morphological actions that are important for reproductive function, but are inappropriate in the nonbreeding season (see above). Even within the breeding season there also may be "costs" associated with high testosterone levels that potentially may reduce fitness. It is presumably beneficial to have high circulating levels of testosterone during at least parts of the breeding season, but considerable evidence suggests that males of most avian species maintain plasma levels of testosterone at concentrations well below what they can actually secrete.[48,49] Similarly, among females, androgen levels tend to be low because of potential "costs" associated with masculinization; however, female spotted hyenas (*Crocuta crocuta*) have taken advantage of this by mimicking male genitalia presumably to obtain dominance status and thus gain the benefits of male help in raising young.[50,51] These exceptions notwithstanding, prolonged high levels of testosterone clearly are deleterious, and mechanisms have evolved to avoid these costs. Wingfield[24] tentatively identified six types, and we add a seventh here:

1. *Direct energetic costs:* Testosterone may have direct effects on metabolic rate (e.g., oxygen consumption), although this point needs further clarification in wild species. In Japanese quail (*Coturnix japonica*), castrated males have reduced oxygen consumption, but implants of testosterone fail to reverse this.[52] On the other hand, in free-living birds there is increasing evidence that experimentally induced high levels of testosterone result in loss of body mass and fat depots.[5,53] Reduced energy reserves can be deleterious, especially in the nonbreeding season.
2. *Indirect energetic costs:* Effects of testosterone on behavior, especially elevated activity associated with territorial aggression, male-male competition, courtship, etc. can increase oxygen consumption and glucose and fat utilization, simultaneously reducing time spent foraging to replenish energy stores.[24,49,54,55]
3. *Predation:* Conspicuous behavior associated with courtship and territorial aggression (e.g., singing, chases, prominent perches) can increase mortality due to predation as well as attract predators to the nest. In brown-headed cowbirds (*Molothrus ater*), implants of testosterone increase over-winter mortality versus controls.[55] However, these effects may not be universal, because implants of testosterone into dark-eyed juncos (*Junco hyemalis*) do not reduce fitness or survival in males if the implants are removed after the end of the breeding season. Note that if testosterone treatment is extended into the nonreproductive state, survival is impaired compared to that of controls.[47]
4. *Wounding:* Combat resulting from male-male aggression always has the potential for injury. Male brown-headed cowbirds treated with testosterone develop severe injuries presumably from escalated fighting. Similarly, in red-winged blackbirds (*Agelaius phoeniceus*), testosterone treatment of males results in larger and greater numbers of wounds than those in controls.[49]

5. *Conflict with parental care:* In many avian species, males provide significant parental care, resulting in marked increases in reproductive success. Evidence is mounting that high plasma levels of testosterone interfere with expression of parental care in males, resulting in reduced reproductive success. Experimental elevation of testosterone in males while they are feeding young has been shown to decrease the provisioning rate in pied flycatchers (*Ficedula hypoleuca*), house sparrows (*Passer domesticus*), yellow-headed blackbirds (*Xanthocephalus xanthocephalus*), and dark-eyed juncos.[6,49,56,57] These effects are often, but not always, accompanied by reduced reproductive success. They may depend to some extent on whether the female can compensate for reduced feeding by the male.[49]

6. *Conflict with pair formation and courtship:* Testosterone-induced aggression in males may lead to attacks against females which are counterproductive for pair formation. This is a viable possibility as a ''cost,'' but more experimentation is required. In white-crowned and song sparrows, testosterone treatment actually results in an increase in the number of mates versus control males.[53] Nonetheless, further analysis reveals that this finding is perhaps due to an increase in territory size so that more than one female can settle. In male red-winged blackbirds, testosterone implants have no effect on the rate at which males are able to attract females.[49]

7. *Immunosuppression:* High physiological levels of testosterone suppress the development of immune responses. For example, a group of male chickens (*Gallus gallus*) with levels of testosterone approximately 6 ng/ml of plasma have reduced development of autoimmune responses versus those in another group with testosterone titers at 2-3 ng/ml.[58-60] A recent investigation in white-crowned sparrows shows that to maintain normal peak breeding concentrations in blood, males implanted with testosterone have significantly lower secondary immune responses to sheep red blood cell antibodies than do controls given empty implants (Hillgarth and Wingfield, in preparation).

Elevated plasma levels of testosterone may have indirect effects on morphology owing to immunosuppression.[20] Although there are many examples of vertebrates with high testosterone levels that have significantly elevated rates of infection than congeners with lower circulating concentrations, several studies have also shown that parasites and disease also affect the development of secondary sex characteristics such as wattles and combs in jungle fowl (*Gallus gallus*)[61] as well as display aggressive behavior. Therefore, high blood levels of testosterone can be costly in terms of morphological expression as well as physiology and behavior.

Taken together, the problems associated with expression of superficially similar behavior (territoriality and pair bonding) in different life history states and the secretion of hormones in more than one state can present considerable problems in organization of the life cycle. The ''costs'' associated with these may reduce overall fitness significantly, thus suggesting strong selection for mechanisms that allow flexibility in the temporal patterns of life history states but also maximize fitness. Even within closely related taxa, diverse patterns of behavior whose expressions are dictated by environmental constraints may have resulted in evolution of different mechanisms. Finally, this brings us to the possible implications of this comparative approach to behavioral endocrinology and how ecological constraints may have influenced the evolution of hormone-behavior interactions.

IMPLICATIONS FOR MECHANISMS UNDERLYING HORMONE-BEHAVIOR INTERACTIONS

Knowledge of how and why animals interact in their natural habitat and application of field endocrinology techniques that allow us to follow hormone changes accompanying patterns of behavior is a powerful combination that allows us to correlate endocrine events with behavior of individuals in their natural habitat. These data provide us with realistic trends that in turn shed new light on apparent paradoxes of multiple expression of similar behavioral traits (i.e., in different life history states) without common hormone mechanisms. Experimental manipulations of the hormonal state in the field have been even more powerful in establishing potential common themes or where traditional thinking needs to be revised.[9,12] It may also be possible to assess phylogenetic effects in diverse hormone-behavior mechanisms. Comparing closely related taxa that live and breed in different habitats (e.g., populations of the same species that live in high elevations or latitudes versus more temperate climes) and express the same behavioral traits in different patterns and contexts would indicate whether hormone mechanisms have diversified so as to "streamline" the life history cycle and maximize fitness. Conversely, species that are not closely related but live in similar habitats could be compared to determine if hormone control mechanisms are similar (convergent evolution) or if each species has solved similar problems by different mechanisms.[62] It should also be noted that these approaches are entirely testable. Controlling for simple phylogenetic differences is particularly important and will identify where ecological constraints are critical. This may in turn allow us to predict where and when specific mechanisms underlying hormone-behavior interactions occur as well as how they evolved. But what implications do these data have for mechanisms at the cell and molecular level?

Receptors and Hormone Metabolism within Target Cells

Considerable evidence indicates that some steroid hormones can be metabolized to alternate, biologically active forms within target cells that then bind to different receptors. For example, testosterone has four potential fates within cells.[15] (1) Direct actions of testosterone after binding to a receptor specific for that steroid hormone; (2) Aromatization to estradiol-17β which then acts through estrogen receptors; (3) 5α reduction to 5α-dihydrotestosterone which may have its own receptor; and (4) 5β reduction to 5β-dihydrotestosterone which apparently has no biological action. (This step may be a deactivation shunt.)

Clearly any of these pathways can be used to modify a cell's response to testosterone. Aromatization has received considerable attention both in development and during seasonal reproduction in relation to sexual behavior and song in birds. Furthermore, the brain apparently may be a major site for aromatase activity, resulting in significant production of estradiol in some species. The substrate for aromatization can be testosterone itself or any other aromatizable androgen.[63] This raises the possibility that temporal or population changes in the cellular distribution of aromatase could significantly alter the responsiveness of a tissue to testosterone. Alternatively, secretion of an aromatizable androgen other than testosterone could reduce other morphological, physiological, and behavioral effects of testosterone but still activate estrogen-dependent processes within cells that express aromatase.[64] In white-crowned sparrows, it was suggested that expression of reproductive behaviors (especially song) in the nonbreeding season may be regulated by estrogens, because aromatase activity in the telencephalon is high in autumn and winter.[17] Such studies coupled with distribution of testosterone receptors will be critical in the future. The avian models just cited may be ideal for these studies by focusing on diverse patterns of behavior related to ecological constraints rather than variation due to phylogeny.

Deactivation of Behavior

In many vertebrates, particularly in the tropics, territorial aggression may be expressed throughout much of the life cycle or breeding seasons may span much of the year (Figs. 3 and 4). In these populations it was suggested that many behavioral patterns associated with reproduction and territorial aggression may be independent of hormonal activation.[12] In other words, they may be "hard wired" and the frequency of expression regulated by paracrine secretions and neurotransmitters within the brain. At least preliminary evidence now exists that other hormones may "deactivate" the expression of specific behavior for restricted periods such as stress-induced abandonment of reproduction. In song sparrows, Wingfield and Silverin[65] showed that implants of corticosterone that deliver a pulse of corticosterone for approximately 2 days result in marked suppression of territorial aggression, even though plasma levels of testosterone remained within the normal range for that time of year. Furthermore, in the side-blotched lizard (*Uta stansburiana*), implants of testosterone increase the size of the home range, but simultaneous implants of corticosterone block this effect.[66] These data suggest that corticosterone may truly deactivate behavior associated with maintaining a home range rather than have an indirect effect to decrease plasma levels of testosterone. Corticosterone has since been shown to also decrease sexual behavior and parental behavior; however, whether this occurs through a direct mechanism or indirectly through suppression of other hormones that have appropriate activational effects remains to be determined.[65,67] The possibility that other hormones (e.g., endorphins) may deactivate reproductive and associated behaviors for short periods during molt, for example, also remains to be determined outside of the laboratory and in the natural habitat. This area of research may prove to be a highly productive especially given the diverse patterns of behavior within the closely related species described above.

SUMMARY

Vertebrates show a diverse array of social behaviors. Equally complex are the mechanisms by which these behavioral patterns are regulated by hormones and the effects of behavioral interactions on hormone secretion. Nonetheless, comparative field and laboratory experiments indicate that general underlying themes, including mechanisms, may exist. For example, comparative studies in birds reveal that testosterone activates a type of aggression, territorial behavior, in those species that are territorial only during the breeding season. Territoriality at other times appears to be independent of sex steroid control, although qualitatively and quantitatively the behavior appears identical. Similarly, formation of pair bonds appears to be complex. In some populations such bonds are sexual, whereas in others they appear to be alliances possibly for joint defense of a territory. In cooperative groups of birds, pair bonds and alliances may exist simultaneously. Testosterone appears to be important for activation of the courtship behavior that leads to formations of sexual pair bonds. However, many investigations indicate that pair bonds in nonsexual contexts are not regulated by testosterone. Hormonal mechanisms underlying the establishment of alliances (if any) remain unknown. Clearly, these complex behavioral patterns due to seasonal changes and variation in context pose important questions for control mechanisms.

One obvious question is, why this diversity in control mechanisms? It appears that there are evolutionary "costs" to high circulating levels of testosterone. They can be energetic costs or may involve increased predation risk or reduced survival after wounding. In males that express parental behavior, high circulating testosterone levels interfere with parental care, resulting in reduced reproductive success. Thus, regulation of testosterone secretion must balance the need to compete with other males as well as provide parental care. High circulating levels of testosterone for prolonged periods are also known to suppress the immune system. This latter effect may have profound implications for the development of androgen-dependent secondary sex characteristics that have evolved through sexual selection.

There are several ways to avoid potential "costs" of hormone secretion at inappropriate times. A hormone may be metabolized at its target cell to another form that then binds to a different receptor (e.g., aromatization of testosterone to estradiol). Also receptors may be downregulated in tissues that would otherwise respond inappropriately in a specific life history state. On the other hand, multiple hormone mechanisms may have evolved to activate behavioral traits at the right time and in the correct context. When a behavioral trait is expressed throughout the life cycle, hormones may potentially deactivate behavior for short periods.

With detailed investigations of organisms in their natural environment we can determine the potential ecological costs underlying hormone-behavior interactions that, in turn, shed light on their evolution. These data also indicate a number of problems for hormonal control mechanisms, but also indicate trends, alternatives, and hopefully in the future a more complete understanding of common mechanisms underlying behavioral endocrinology at the cell and molecular level. Only then will we be able to predict when and where specific mechanisms of hormone-behavior interactions operate and how they evolved.

REFERENCES

1. Crews, D. 1984. Gamete production, sex hormone secretion, and mating behavior uncoupled. Horm. Behav. **18:** 22–28.
2. Crews, D. 1987. Diversity and the evolution of behavioral controlling mechanisms. *In* Psychobiology of Reproductive Behavior: An Evolutionary Perspective. D. Crews, Ed.: 88–119.
3. Crews, D. 1992. Diversity of hormone-behavior relations in reproductive behavior. *In* Behavioral Endocrinology. J. B. Becker, S. M. Breedlove & D. Crews, Eds.: 143–186.

4. Crews, D. & M. C. Moore. 1986. Evolution of mechanisms controlling mating behavior. Science **231:** 121-125.
5. Ketterson, E. D., V. Nolan, Jr., L. Wolf, C. Ziegenfus, A. M. Dufty Jr., G. F. Ball & T. S. Johnsen. 1991. Testosterone and avian life histories: The effect of experimentally elevated testosterone on corticosterone and body mass in dark-eyed juncos. Horm. Behav. **25:** 489-503.
6. Ketterson, E. D., V. Nolan, Jr., L. Wolf & C. Ziegenfus. 1992. Testosterone and avian life histories: Effects of experimentally elevated testosterone on behavior and correlates of fitness in the dark-eyed junco (*Junco hyemalis*). Am. Nat. **140:** 980-999.
7. Nolan, V. Jr., E. D. Ketterson, C. Ziegenfus, D. P. Cullen & C. R. Chandler. 1992. Testosterone and avian life histories: Effects of experimentally elevated testosterone on prebasic molt and survival in male dark-eyed juncos. Condor **94:** 364-370.
8. Wingfield, J. C. & M. Ramenofsky. 1985. Hormonal and environmental control of aggression in birds. *In* Neurobiology. R. Gilles & J. Balthazart, Eds.: 92-104. Springer-Verlag. Berlin.
9. Wingfield, J. C., G. F. Ball, A. M. Dufty, Jr., R. E. Hegner & M. Ramenofsky. 1987. Testosterone and aggression in birds: Tests of the "challenge hypothesis." Am. Sci. **75:** 602-608.
10. Wingfield, J. C. & D. S. Farner. 1993. The endocrinology of wild species. *In* Avian Biology. D. S. Farner, J. R. King & K. S. Parkes, Eds. Vol. 9: 163-237. Academic Press. New York.
11. Jacobs, J. 1996. Using a Finite State Machine Model to Understand Organismal Responses to Changes in the Environment. Ph.D. Thesis, University of Washington, Seattle, Washington.
12. Wingfield, J. C. 1994. Control of territorial aggression in a changing environment. Psychoneuroendocrinology **19:** 709-721.
13. Becker, J. B., S. M. Breedlove & D. Crews, Eds. 1992. Behavioral Endocrinology. Massachusetts Institute of Technology Press. Cambridge, MA.
14. Nelson, R. J. 1995. An Introduction to Behavioral Endocrinology. Sinauer Assoc. Inc. Sunderland, MA.
15. Balthazart, J. 1983. Hormonal correlates of behavior. *In* Avian Biology. D. S. Farner, J. R. King & K. C. Parkes, Eds. Vol. 7: 221-365. Academic Press. New York, NY.
16. Harding, C. F. 1983. Hormonal influences on avian aggressive behavior. *In* Hormones and Aggressive Behavior. B. Svare, Ed.: 435-467. Plenum Press. New York, NY.
17. Schlinger, B. A., R. H. Slotow & A. P. Arnold. 1992. Plasma estrogens and brain aromatase in winter white-crowned sparrows. Ornis Scand. **23:** 292-297.
18. Gorbman, A., W. W. Dickhoff, S. R. Vigna, N. B. Clark & C. L. Ralph. 1983. Comparative Endocrinology. Wiley. New York, NY.
19. Witschi, E. 1961. Sex and secondary sexual characters. *In* Biology and Comparative Physiology of Birds. A. J. Marshall, Ed. Vol. 2: 115-168. Academic Press. New York.
20. Folstad, I. & A. J. Karter. 1992. Parasites, bright males and the immunocompetence handicap. Am. Nat. **139:** 603-622.
21. Wedekind, C. & I. Folstad. 1994. Adaptive or non-adaptive immunosuppression by sex hormones? Am. Nat. **143:** 936-938.
22. Hillgarth, N. & J. C. Wingfield. 1996. Parasites and sexual selection—endocrinological aspects. *In* Host-Parasite Evolution—Avian Models. D. Clayton & J. Moore, Eds. Oxford University Press. Oxford. In press.
23. Hillgarth, N., M. Ramenofsky & J. C. Wingfield. 1996. Testosterone and sexual selection. Behav. Ecol. Sociobiol. In press.
24. Wingfield, J. C. 1990. Interrelationship of androgens, aggression and mating systems. *In* Endocrinology of Birds: Molecular to Behavioral. M. Wada, S. Ishii & C. G. Scanes, Eds.: 187-205. Jap. Sci. Soc. Press. Springer-Verlag, Tokyo and Berlin.

25. HUNT, K., J. C. WINGFIELD, L. B. ASTHEIMER, W. A. BUTTEMER & T. P. HAHN. 1995. Temporal patterns of territorial behavior and circulating testosterone in the Lapland longspur and other Arctic passerines. Am. Zool. **35:** 274-284.
26. WINGFIELD, J. C. & D. S. FARNER. 1978. The annual cycle in plasma irLH and steroid hormones in feral populations of the white-crowned sparrow, *Zonotrichia leucophrys gambelii.* Biol. Reprod. **19:** 1046-1056.
27. WINGFIELD, J. C. & D. S. FARNER. 1978. The endocrinology of a naturally breeding population of the white-crowned sparrow (*Zonotrichia leucophrys pugetensis*). Physiol. Zool. **51:** 188-205.
28. WINGFIELD, J. C. & T. P. HAHN. 1994. Testosterone and territorial behavior in sedentary and migratory sparrows. Anim. Behav. **47:** 77-89.
29. WINGFIELD, J. C., R. E. HEGNER & D. LEWIS. 1991. Circulating levels of luteinizing hormone and steroid hormones in relation to social status in the cooperatively breeding white-browed sparrow weaver, *Plocepasser mahali,* J. Zool. Lond. **225:** 43-58.
30. WINGFIELD, J. C. & D. MONK. 1992. Control and context of year-round territorial aggression in the non-migratory song sparrow, *Melospiza melodia morphna.* Ornis Scand. **23:** 298-303.
31. WINGFIELD, J. C., R. E. HEGNER & D. LEWIS. 1992. Hormonal responses to removal of a breeding male in the cooperatively breeding white-browed sparrow weaver, *Plocepasser mahali.* Horm. Behav. **26:** 145-155.
32. WINGFIELD, J. C. & D. LEWIS. 1993. Hormonal and behavioral responses to simulated territorial intrusion in the cooperatively breeding white-browed sparrow weaver, *Plocepasser mahali.* Anim. Behav. **45:** 1-11.
33. WINGFIELD, J. C. & D. MONK. 1994. Behavioral and hormonal responses of male song sparrows to estrogenized females during the non-breeding season. Horm. Behav. **28:** 146-154.
34. BURGER, A. E. & R. P. MILLAR. 1980. Seasonal changes of sexual and territorial behavior and plasma testosterone levels in male lesser sheathbills (*Chionis minor*). Z. Tierpsychol. **52:** 397-406.
35. DAWSON, A. 1983. Plasma gonadal steroid levels in wild starlings (*Sturnus vulgaris*) during the annual cycle and in relation to the stages of breeding. Gen. Comp. Endocrinol. **49:** 286-294.
36. DONHAM, R. S. 1979. Annual cycle of plasma luteinizing hormone and sex hormones in male and female mallards (*Anas platyrhynchos*). Biol. Reprod. **21:** 1273-1285.
37. GWINNER, E., T. RÖDL & H. SCHWABL. 1994. Pair territoriality of wintering stonechats: Behavior, function and hormones. Behav. Ecol. Sociobiol. **34:** 321-327.
38. LINCOLN, G. A., P. A. RACEY, P. J. SHARP & H. KLANDORF. 1980. Endocrine changes associated with spring and autumn sexuality of the rook, *Corvus frugilegus.* J. Zool. Lond. **190:** 137-153.
39. LOGAN, C. A. & J. C. WINGFIELD. 1990. Autumnal territorial aggression is independent of plasma testosterone in mockingbirds. Horm. Behav. **24:** 568-581.
40. LOGAN, C. A. & J. C. WINGFIELD. 1995. Hormonal correlates of breeding status, nest construction and parental care in multiple-brooded Northern Mockingbirds, *Mimus polyglottos.* Horm. Behav. **29:** 12-30.
41. PAULKE, E. & E. HAASE. 1978. A comparison of seasonal changes in the concentrations of androgens in the peripheral blood of wild and domestic ducks. Gen. Comp. Endocrinol. **34:** 381-390.
42. SCHWABL, H. & E. KRINER. 1991. Territorial aggression and song of male European robins (*Erithacus rubecula*) in autumn and spring: Effects of antiandrogen treatment. Horm. Behav. **25:** 180-194.
43. SILVERIN, B., P. A. VIEBKE & J. WESTIN. 1989. Hormonal correlates of migration and territorial behavior in juvenile willow tits during autumn. Gen. Comp. Endocrinol. **75:** 148-156.

44. SILVERIN, B., P. A. VIEBKE & J. WESTIN. 1986. Seasonal changes in plasma levels of LH and gonadal steroids in free-living willow tits, *Parus montanus.* Ornis Scand. **17:** 230-236.
45. SILVERIN, B., P. A. VIEBKE & J. WESTIN. 1984. Plasma levels of luteinizing hormone and steroid hormones in free-living winter groups of willow tits (*Parus montanus*). Horm. Behav. **18:** 367-379.
46. MARLER, C. A. & M. C. MOORE. 1988. Evolutionary costs of aggression revealed by testosterone manipulations in free-living male lizards. Behav. Ecol. Sociobiol. **23:** 21-26.
47. KETTERSON, E. D., V. NOLAN, JR., M. J. CAWTHORN, P. G. PARKER & C. ZIEGENFUS. 1996. Phenotypic engineering: Using hormones to explore the mechanistic and functional bases of phenotypic variation in nature. Ibis **138:** 70-86.
48. WINGFIELD, J. C., R. E. HEGNER, A. M. DUFTY, JR. & G. F. BALL. 1990. The "challenge hypothesis": Theoretical implications for patterns of testosterone secretion, mating systems and breeding strategies. Am. Nat. **136:** 829-846.
49. BELETSKY, L. D., D. F. GORI, S. FREEMAN & J. C. WINGFIELD. 1995. Testosterone and polygyny in birds. *In* Current Ornithology. D. M. Power, Ed. Vol. **12:** 1-42. Plenum Press. New York, NY.
50. GLICKMAN, S. E., L. G. FRANK, K. E. HOLECAMP, L. SMALE & P. LICHT. 1993. Costs and benefits of "androgenization" in the female spotted hyena: The natural selection of physiological mechanisms. *In* Perspectives in Ethology, Volume 10: Behavior and Evolution. P. P. G. Bateson *et al.,* Eds.: 87-117. Plenum Press. New York.
51. FRANK, L. G., M. L. WELDELE & S. E. GLICKMAN. 1995. Masculinization costs in hyenas. Nature **377:** 584-585.
52. HÄNSSLER, I. & R. PRINZINGER. 1979. The influence of the sex hormone testosterone on body temperature and metabolism of the male Japanese quail (*Coturnix coturnix japonica*). Experentia **35:** 509-510.
53. WINGFIELD, J. C. 1984. Androgens and mating systems: Testosterone-induced polygyny in normally monogamous birds. Auk **101:** 665-671.
54. HÖGSTAD, O. 1987. It is expensive to be dominant. Auk **104:** 333-336.
55. DUFTY, A. M., JR. 1989. Testosterone and survival: A cost of aggressiveness? Horm. Behav. **23:** 185-193.
56. SILVERIN, B. 1980. Effects of long-acting testosterone treatment on free-living pied flycatchers, *Ficedula hypoleuca,* during the breeding period. Anim. Behav. **28:** 906-912.
57. HEGNER, R. E. & J. C. WINGFIELD. 1987. Effects of experimental manipulation of testosterone levels on parental investment and breeding success in male house sparrows. Auk **104:** 462-469.
58. GAUSE, W. C. & J. A. MARCH. 1986. Effect of testosterone treatments for varying periods on autoimmune development and on specific infiltrating leukocyte populations in the thyroid gland of obese strain chickens. Clin. Immunol. Immunopathol. **39:** 664-678.
59. MARCH, J. A. & C. G. SCANES. 1994. Neuroendocrine-immune interactions. Poultry Sci. **73:** 1049-1061.
60. HILLGARTH, N. & J. C. WINGFIELD. 1996. Testosterone and immunosuppression in vertebrates: Implications for parasite-mediated sexual selection. *In* Parasites and Pathogens: Effects on Host Hormones and Behavior. N. E. Beckage, Ed. Chapman and Hall. In press.
61. ZUK, M., R. THORNHILL, J. D. LIGON & K. JOHNSON. 1990. Parasites and mate choice in red jungle fowl. Am. Zool. **30:** 235-244.
62. CREWS, D. 1996. Species diversity and the evolution of behavior controlling mechanisms. Ann. N.Y. Acad. Sci., this volume.
63. SCHLINGER, B. A. & A. P. ARNOLD. 1991. Brain is a major site of estrogen synthesis in a male songbird. Proc. Natl. Acad. Sci. USA **88:** 4191-4194.
64. SCHLINGER, B. A. 1994. Estrogens to song: Picograms to sonograms. Horm. Behav. **28:** 191-198.

65. Wingfield, J. C. & B. Silverin. 1986. Effects of corticosterone on territorial behavior of free-living song sparrows, *Melospiza melodia.* Horm. Behav. **20:** 405-417.
66. DeNardo, D. F. & B. Sinervo. 1994. Effects of steroid hormone interaction on activity and home range size of male lizards. Horm. Behav. **28:** 273-287.
67. Moore, F. L. & R. T. Zoeller. 1985. Stress-induced inhibition of reproduction: Evidence of suppressed secretion of LHRH in an amphibian. Gen. Comp. Endocrinol. **60:** 252-258.

3

Evolutionary Perspectives on Primate Mating Systems and Behavior

Alan F. Dixson

Animal mating systems are diverse and complex; a number of authors have attempted to classify these systems and to explain their evolutionary bases, for example, in birds,[1] insects,[2] mammals,[3] and vertebrates in general.[4,5] Rather than attempt to review all possible animal mating systems and then to place the primates within some universally acceptable scheme, I have chosen to define only those mating systems that occur in prosimians, monkeys, and apes. Human mating systems may also be set in context within this framework. Two important considerations are, first, does a female usually mate with one male or with multiple partners during her ovarian cycle and, second, are sexual relationships long-term and relatively exclusive or short-term and nonexclusive. This line of reasoning results in the recognition of five mating systems (TABLE 1): (1) monogamy, (2) polygyny, (3) polyandry, (4) multimale-multifemale, and (5) dispersed or nongregarious. In monogamous, polygynous, and polyandrous primate groups, females have longer-term sexual relationships either with a single male or in the case of polyandry with two or more partners. By contrast, in multimale-multifemale and dispersed mating systems, females mate with a number of partners in a more labile, nonexclusive manner.

Rees and Harvey[6] cautioned that "any species-specific mating system classification is likely to be an unfair representation of the true gametic pattern." Therefore, it would be incorrect to "straightjacket" each primate species into one of the five mating systems. First, we must acknowledge that more than one mating system can occur within a single species, that is, monogamy and polyandry in certain marmosets or tamarins (family *Callitrichidae*) or polygyny, monogamy, and polyandry in *Homo sapiens.* To address this problem I shall adopt the approach that a given species has a "primary mating system" and one or more "secondary systems." Second, it must be kept in mind that any particular mating system is not impermeable to external pressures that affect sexual interactions. "Extrapair" copulations occur outside monogamous pairings, for instance, as was been amply documented in many avian species.[7] Extrapair copulation was described for the monogamous titi monkey (*Callicebus moloch*), but we have no notion of its frequency in other monogamous primate species or its consequences in terms of reproductive success. The occurrence of such additional matings does not alter the fact that the primary system is one of pair formation and monogamy. Likewise in the case of female defense polygyny, resident males may be ousted during "takeovers" by nongroup males (as in the Hanuman

TABLE 1. Classification Scheme for Primate Mating Systems

Number of Males Mating per Female Cycle	Type of Sexual Relationship	Mating System	Examples
One	Long-term, exclusive	Monogamy	*Indri, Aotus, Callicebus, Symphalangus Hylobates*
One	Long-term, exclusive[a] but other females also mate with the resident male	Polygyny	*Theropithecus, Papio hamadryas, Nasalis, Gorilla*
Two or more	Long-term, exclusive	Polyandry	*Saguinus fuscicollis*[b]: *Callithrix humeralifer*[b]
Two or more	Short-term, not exclusive, gregarious	Multimale-multifemale	*Propithecus, Macaca,* most *Papio* spp, *Cercocebus, Saimiri, Lagothrix, Pan*
Two or more	Short-term, not exclusive, non-gregarious	Dispersed	*Microcebus, Daubentonia,* most *Galago,* spp, *Perodicticus*

[a] The single male mates with other females in the ''harem'' unit.
[b] Monogamy also occurs in these callitrichid species and is probably the primary mating system in many cases.

langur[8] or gelada[9]). Lone males living outside multimale-multifemale groups may enter groups and mate with resident females (Japanese macaque[10]). Young males in such multimale-multifemale groups often emigrate and attempt to gain acceptance in neighboring groups; females may exhibit some degree of preference for mating with these new males (baboons[11]). Within any given mating system, sexual selection favors those individuals that maximize their lifetime reproductive success. In this regard a bewildering array of mating "tactics" may be observed in various primates. Males and females may pursue different tactical paths, and given the dichotomy in "parental investment" between the two sexes,[12] we should expect differences and conflicts to occur. As an example, the multipartner matings that occur in multimale-multifemale primate groups are far from being totally indiscriminate or "promiscuous." Thus, a temporary "consortship[5]" may occur between particular partners during the fertile phase of the female's cycle (e.g., baboons[13] and chimpanzees[14]), and females may exhibit sexual preferences for certain males (pigtailed macaque[15]) and vice-versa (rhesus macaque[16]). Long-term alliances between particular males and females have been described in yellow baboons,[17] and these influence mate choice by females when they enter breeding condition.

Intrasexual competition and social rank can also have powerful effects on mating frequency and reproductive success. In this brief review I deal with three aspects of intermale competition as they relate to mating frequencies and reproductive success. First, relationships between dominance rank and reproductive success are considered, with special reference to the use of DNA fingerprinting techniques to reveal paternity of offspring in primate groups. Second, the reproductive strategies of subordinate males will be considered, and particularly the suppression of secondary sexual development which occurs in males of certain species when intermale competition is pronounced. Finally, given that females also exert "choice" in mating contexts and that females may mate with multiple partners in many primates, it is necessary also to consider the subject of "sperm competition[18]" and its effect on male reproductive success in various mating systems.

GENETIC ASSESSMENT OF MALE REPRODUCTIVE SUCCESS

Behavioral measurements of mating success provide only an imperfect guide to male reproductive success. Under natural conditions, only a fraction of the total sexual activity in primate social groups is ever observed or recorded. When a female mates with multiple partners, paternity cannot be gauged using behavioral data alone, because the female's reproductive tract provides the final arena for sperm competition. Some mating tactics, such as "sneaky" copulations by lower-ranking males, are by their very nature difficult to observe or quantify. Genetic assignment of paternity is required to measure male reproductive success and to understand the relative success rates of the various tactics employed by males throughout the life span. The discovery of DNA fingerprinting by Jeffreys *et al.*[19,20] has revolutionized this field. This technique, originally developed for work on human beings, has been used to study the mating systems of numerous animals, including birds,[21] carnivores,[22,23] and nonhuman primates.[24,25] Although primate studies are still at a relatively early stage, important information has been obtained on relationships between male dominance rank, mating success, and reproductive success in several monkey species. Some of this information is reviewed below.

To commence with an extreme example, I shall describe some observations on male dominance and reproductive success in the mandrill (*Mandrillus sphinx*). This is the largest and most brightly colored of all monkeys; adult male mandrills may weigh over 30 kg (2-3 times as much as adult females) and they are magnificently adorned with red and blue "sexual skin" on the rump, genitalia, and face. In their natural habitat, the lowland rainforests of Gabon and Congo, mandrills occur in large multimale-multifemale groups which sometimes fragment into smaller units. Solitary males have also been recorded.[26-28] The mating system of the mandrill has frequently, and incorrectly, been classified as polygynous, the smaller units being assumed to represent harems such as those that occur in hamadryas baboons and geladas.[29,30] However, no published account on wild mandrills contains robust data on either their sexual behavior or their mating system. Studies of a large, semifree-ranging mandrill group in Gabon have shown that adult males do not establish one-male units. Instead, a number of resident males associate with females year round and compete for copulations during the annual mating season. "Solitary" males haunt the fringes of the group and engage in "sneaky" or opportunistic matings.[31] Male rank and mating success are positively correlated in this mandrill group as reflected in the reproductive success of high-ranking, group-associated individuals (FIG. 1). Over a 5-year period, two of the three resident adult males sired all offspring for which it was possible to assign paternity by means of DNA fingerprinting. None of the three solitary males or three subadults in the social group is known to have sired offspring during this period; however, a number of them copulated with the 12 resident females. FIGURE 1 also shows that the original alpha male in the group sired 80-100% of offspring born between 1987 and 1989. He was then deposed and occupied the second-ranking position in the group. Loss of alpha status resulted in a reduction in reproductive success, but this effect was gradual; the deposed male continued to sire 67% and 25% of infants born during the next 2 years. It was observed that certain females continued to associate with and to invite copulations from the previously dominant male. In this regard it is relevant to consider that such a previously high-ranking individual still possesses the same genotype as that during the period of his alpha status; indeed, he has a proven "track record" and should, in theory, still be attractive to females.

To place these observations in context, one must keep in mind that this group occupied a 6-hectare rainforested enclosure and numbered 57 individuals by the end of the study. In the wild, where a multimale-multifemale mandrill group numbers 300-400 and has a home range of about 30 km^2, there may be considerably greater latitude for alternative mating tactics and greater reproductive success in subordinate or solitary males. Dominant males do not "herd" or "guard" a harem of females; instead, each individual female is followed and mate-guarded throughout the late follicular phase of the menstrual cycle when her sexual skin swelling is maximal. An analysis of such mate-guarding behavior and reproductive success during a single annual mating season is shown in FIGURE 2. The data refer to the last 6 days of maximum swelling, plus the day of sexual skin deflation ("breakdown") during conception cycles in 12 females. It is likely that ovulation occurs during this period, as this is known to be the case in baboons.[32] FIGURE 2 shows that the most dominant,

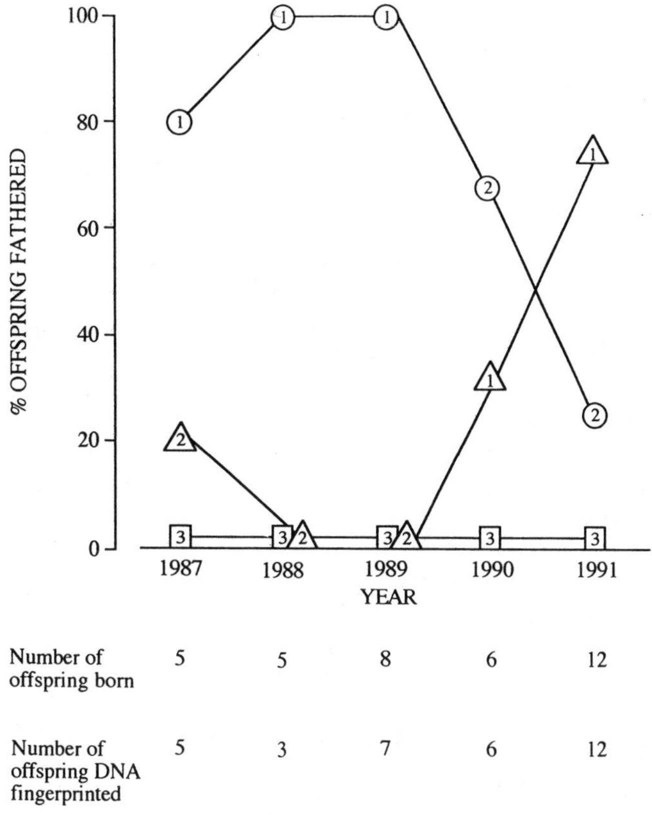

FIGURE 1. Association between rank and paternity for three group-associated adult male mandrills (nos. 7, 14, and 15), showing effects of rank changes on percentages of infants sired each year between 1987 and 1991. Each male is represented by a separate symbol (male 7: O; male 14: Δ; male 15: □), and his rank (1, 2, or 3) is written inside the symbol. Numbers of offspring born and DNA fingerprinted are given for each year of the study. Further explanation is provided in the text. Data are from ref. 31.

group-associated male (no. 14) mate-guarded and copulated with 11 of the 12 females during the periovulatory phase. He accounted for 24 (i.e., 77%) of ejaculations observed. The second ranking male (no. 7) mate-guarded three females, for shorter periods, and accounted for 13% of ejaculatory mounts. Only two other males were observed to copulate during the presumptive periovulatory period, a solitary male (no 13, on two occasions) and a resident subadult (no. 5B, once). DNA fingerprinting of offspring resulting from these conception cycles showed that male 14 had sired nine infants, whilst male 7 accounted for the remaining three. Thus, even in this situation in which a rigid male dominance hierarchy existed and females were guarded intensively, there were instances in which behavioral observations failed to predict paternity accurately. As an example, only male 14 was seen to guard or mate with

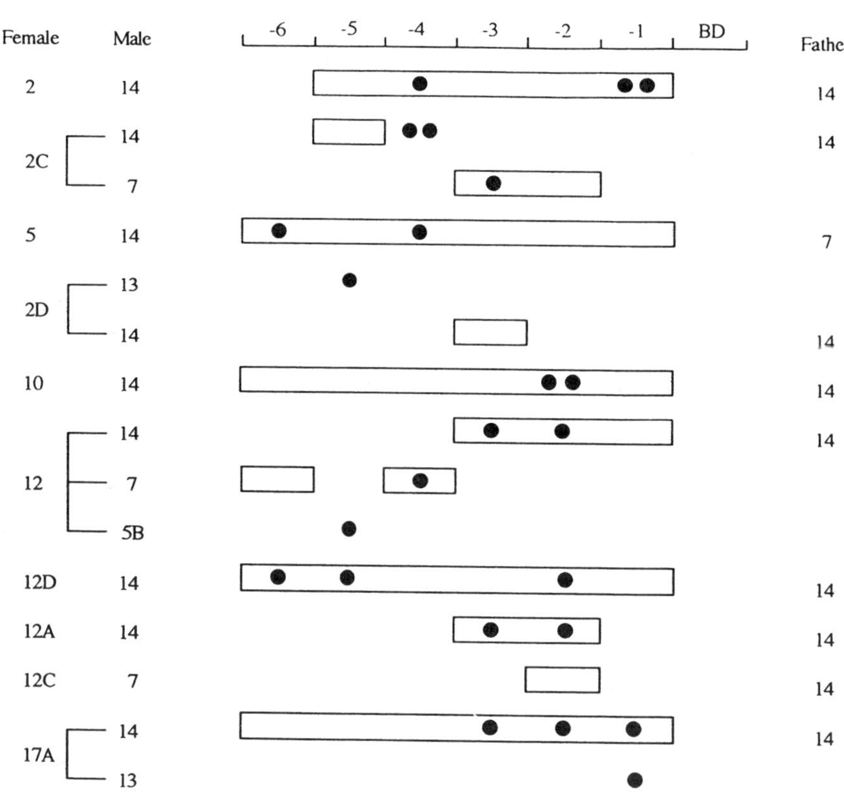

FIGURE 2. Mating behavior and reproductive success in a group of mandrills during a single annual reproductive cycle. Individual females are identified in the extreme *left hand column* and those males that engaged in sexual activity are shown in the *adjacent column*. Sexual behavior was scored during the 7 days leading up to and including the day of sexual skin breakdown (BD), which includes the periovulatory period. Mate guarding activity (during which the male follows and closely associates with a specific female) is indicated by the *open boxes*, and the occurrence of ejaculatory mounts by *closed circles*. The male identified from DNA fingerprints as being the father of the resulting infant (only conception cycles are shown) is given in the *right hand column*. Data are from ref. 31.

females 5 and 6, yet male 7 sired the resulting offspring. It appears likely that some degree of "female choice" operates in these situations. Females sometimes terminated guarding episodes by persistently avoiding and running from males. Likewise, females were observed to solicit copulations from certain males, whilst refusing mount attempts by others. Given the variety of alternative mating tactics employed by male primates and the additional variable of female choice or preferences for particular partners, it should not surprise us to discover that male rank does not correlate perfectly with mating success or reproductive success. Some brief descriptions of DNA fingerprinting studies in macaques will be useful in order to emphasize these points.

Several studies have examined relationships between male rank and reproductive success in rhesus monkey groups.[33-35] The results generally indicate that a positive relationship exists between the two variables, but the effect is not as pronounced as is that described for the mandrill. Berard *et al.*[33] determined paternity for 11 of 15 infants born during a single year into a semifree-ranging rhesus monkey group on the island of Cayo Santiago. The two highest ranking of 11 resident males sired four (i.e., 36%) of these offspring, whilst males ranked at positions six, eight, and nine in the hierarchy accounted for one offspring each. Extragroup males also copulated with females during the annual mating season, and three of these succeeded in siring four infants. Because extragroup males (including individuals of low rank in their home groups) enjoyed significant reproductive success, this study provides genetic evidence for the value of mating season mobility in macaque males.[36] Using captive groups of rhesus monkeys and much larger samples, both Smith[34] and Bercovitch and Nurnberg[35] demonstrated more clear-cut effects of male rank. In Bercovitch and Nurnberg's study, just 8 of 21 males sired offspring in a large captive group (n = 150) occupying a 1-acre corral. Dominant males were reproductively most successful, and an "ensemble of traits" including large body size, good condition (high fat reserves), and voluminous testes characterized these successful individuals.

Paul *et al.*'s[37] study of rank, mating effort, and reproductive success in male Barbary macaques also indicates a complex relationship between male rank and reproductive success. Data were collected on a large group of monkeys during 4 consecutive years. Several groups shared a 14.5-hectare enclosure, and it was possible to determine parentage for 75 of 83 offspring born into the focal group. In all years, a positive correlation occurred between male rank and mating success, and for 3 of these years, rank and reproductive success were also positively correlated. However, this latter relationship disappeared if subadult males were excluded from the analysis; with some exceptions, males aged 4-7 years also had poor mating success. Longer-term studies of paternity over a 14-year period in this captive population confirm that subadult Barbary macaques have much poorer reproductive success than do adults, and many in this age-band fail to sire any offspring despite being fertile in the physiological sense.[38] Even older males (aged 8-10 years) that succeeded in mating with females sometimes sired no offspring. Among younger males, however, there were a few 6- or 7-year-olds that achieved significant reproductive success. Paul *et al.*[37] noted that whilst dominant males forced such younger males to the periphery of the group during the day, some of them succeeded in acquiring access to females at dawn, dusk, or nighttime "when low visibility and the difficulty of manoeuvering in the sleeping trees reduced the effectiveness of the older males' coalitions.''

In the Barbary macaque, rank changes among males are fairly frequent, and females copulate with many partners during the periovulatory period. Hence, ''sperm competition'' rather than dominance rank alone may have very important effects on the outcome for paternity, and the distinct possibility exists that frequent copulations and depletion of sperm reserves might affect the fertility of males.

A final example of research that has combined DNA fingerprinting to determine paternity with measurements of male dominance rank and sexual activity concerns longtailed macaques (*Macaca fascicularis*) at Ketambe in Sumatra.[39,40] This remarkable study involved observing and trapping three groups of longtailed macaques under natural conditions in the rainforest. Previous work on this population by van Noordwijk and van Schaik[41] had established how a male longtailed macaque's mating success alters across his life span. De Ruiter *et al.*'s results[39,40] confirm a striking effect of alpha rank on male reproductive success in longtailed macaque groups. Second ranking or ''beta'' males also sired more offspring than did others, and these authors noted that beta males were often individuals that had previously occupied alpha rank in their groups. In longtailed macaques, some males emigrate from their groups at 8-10 years of age and undergo a period of solitary life and rapid growth before challenging for alpha status. This strategy is believed to be crucial for attainment of full reproductive potential.[41]

Interesting as these studies on macaques and mandrills are, they refer to just a handful of Old World monkey species that have multimale-multifemale mating systems. Genetic analysis of polygynous, monogamous, or dispersed primate mating systems are virtually nonexistent. It is assumed in monogamous species, such as the lesser apes, callitrichids, owl monkeys, titi monkeys, and indris, that the resident male in a family group sires all offspring; the impact of extrapair copulations has yet to be assessed in such cases. In nocturnal prosimians such as the mouselemurs, galagos, and lorises, the dynamics of the mating system are unknown. In my view, females mate with multiple partners in many of these species, and sperm competition is important, as in diurnal anthropoids which live in multimale-multifemale social groups (to be described). Among the polygynous primates, DNA fingerprinting information was obtained on free-ranging patas monkeys (*Erythrocebus patas*) by Oshawa *et al.*[42] Multimale influxes into single male units of patas monkeys sometimes occur during the annual mating season.[43] In Oshawa *et al.*'s study the resident male in a single group had to contend with ''sneak'' copulations by outsiders as well as an influx of five intruders during one mating season. The resident sired six of nine offspring (i.e., 66%) born under these conditions. These limited data support the view that female defense polygyny offers a reproductive advantage to resident males in one-male units. It would be most surprising if this was not the case. However, a vast amount of work remains to be done, combining field observations of behavior with genetic assessments of reproductive success. This combination of techniques should allow functional dissection of primate mating systems and measurements of how various reproductive strategies translate into reproductive success across the life span.

INTERMALE COMPETITION AND DELAYED SECONDARY SEXUAL DEVELOPMENT

In the previous section it was noted that when intermale competition for mating opportunities is pronounced, high-ranking adult males may achieve greater mating success than subordinates, especially subadult individuals that have yet to attain full size and reproductive condition. This is the case in multimale-multifemale and polygynous mating systems. In some cases, and they may be more widespread among primates than currently realized, the result is suppression of development of secondary sexual characters in adolescent and young adult males. This "strategy" may have disadvantages in that less brightly colored or adorned males might be less sexually attractive to females; however, little is known about this aspect of "female choice" in primates. An advantage may accrue to a suppressed individual in lessening the risk of aggressive conflict with dominant males, delaying investment in "costly" secondary sexual adornments and yet allowing some opportunity for occasional matings. In some of these cases it seems clear that the hypothalamic-pituitary-testicular axis is active and that spermatogenesis occurs despite reduction in growth of certain secondary sexual traits. Examples are shown in TABLE 2. In the mandrill, for instance, group-associated adult males in a semifree-ranging colony had brighter red and blue sexual skin on the face and rump, larger testes, and higher circulating testosterone levels than did peripheral or solitary individuals (FIG. 3). Group-associated males also had a more stocky appearance and possessed large deposits of fat around the rump and flanks; hence, the term "fatted" males was applied to them, by contrast with the leaner, "nonfatted" solitary males.[44] The greater reproductive success of high-ranking fatted males in this semifree-ranging mandrill group has already been described. Another well-documented example concerns the orangutan (*Pongo pygmaeus*) in which suppression of growth of the cheek "flanges," throat sac, and long hair can occur in maturing captive males, when a fully developed adult male is present.[45] This delay in full secondary sexual growth does not mean that such males are infertile or sexually inactive, however. Spermatogenesis and increased testosterone secretion occur at between 6 and 7 years of age in captivity,[46] and in the wild such "nonflanged" males pursue females and attempt forced copulations.[47] Other less well documented examples of secondary sexual suppression are listed in TABLE 2. In the bald uakari (*Cacajao calvus*), some males develop rapidly at puberty, exhibiting testicular enlargement, loss of hair on the head, reddening of the skin on the face and scalp, as well as growth of distinctive bulging temporal muscles. Other males in the same social group may take several years to undergo these changes in genital and secondary sexual development.[48] In the black howler (*Alouatta caraya*), some maturing males retain for a time the brown pelage color found in juveniles and in adult females of this species. Such males are sometimes sexually active despite their immature appearance, although their reproductive success is not known.[49]

TABLE 2 also includes examples of possible reproductive suppression in nocturnal prosimians which have dispersed, nongregarious, mating systems. In these cases, exemplified by *Galago demidoff* and *G. moholi,* it is not brightly colored secondary sexual structures that are retarded, because nocturnal primates do not possess such visual adornments. Rather it is body weight that is affected, and there may also be effects on development of scent-marking glands. Dominant or "A males" are heavier

TABLE 2. Examples of Suppression of Secondary Sexual Development in Male Primates: Possible Effects of Intermale Competition

Species	Traits Affected	Mating System[a]	Sources
Prosimians			
Galago demidoff	Body weight of subordinate male is 75% of that found in dominants	D	50
G. moholi	Body weight of "B" males is 93% of that in dominant, territorial "A" males	D	51
New World Monkeys			
Cacajao calvus	Muscular temporal "bulges" on head of adult male develop more slowly and testicular growth is retarded	MM	48
Alouatta caraya	Retention of (brown) juvenile coat color, rather than transition to adult (black) pelage	MM/PG?	49
Old World Monkeys			
Nasalis nasalis	Delayed growth of adult male's large nose in all-male groups or in maturing offspring in captive group	PG	71 72
Cercopithecus neglectus	Retention of juvenile (russet/grey) pelage in presence of dominant male	MG/PG	73
Macaca fascicularis	Attainment of full body weight is delayed until males emigrate	MM	41
Mandrillus sphinx	Muted secondary sexual color, smaller testes, and lower plasma testosterone in subordinate, peripheral and solitary males	MM	44
Apes and Man			
Pongo pygmaeus	Delayed cheek flange, vocal sac, and hair growth in maturing males, when fully developed male is present	D?	45
Homo sapiens	Pubertal development: growth of external genitalia, pubic hair, larynx, and masculinity show great individual variation. Are social factors involved?	PG/MG	74

[a] Mating systems: MG = monogamous; PG = polygynous; MM = multimale/multifemale; D = dispersed.

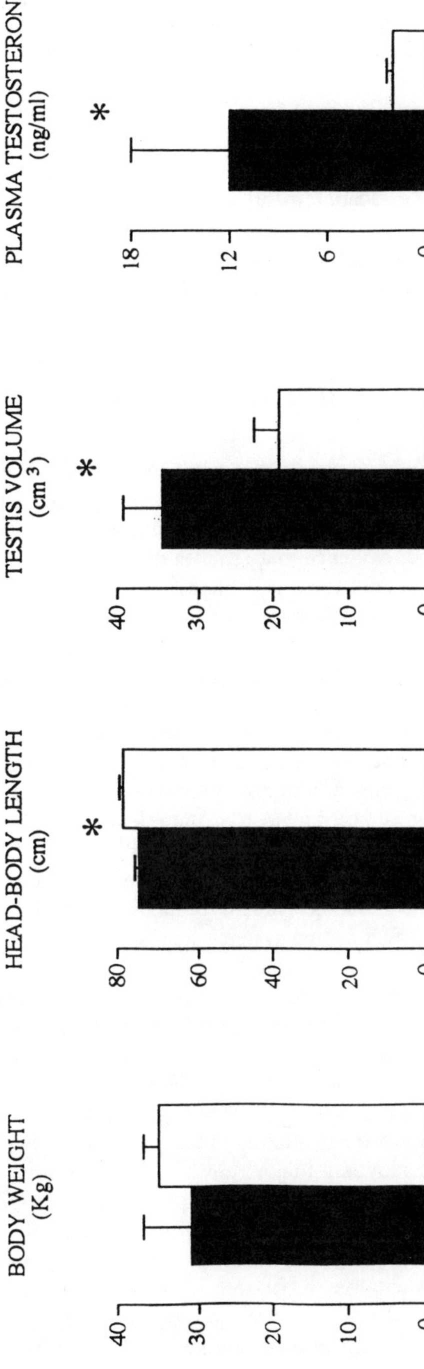

FIGURE 3. Comparisons of body weight, head body length, volume of left testis, and plasma testosterone levels in three "fatted" adult male mandrills (*closed bars*) and three nonfatted individuals (*open bars*). $^*p < 0.05$ (Mann-Whitney U test). Data are means + SEM and are taken from refs. 31 and 44.

and succeed in occupying larger home ranges with more ready access to the ranging areas of neighboring females.[50,51] In the mouselemur (*Microcebus murinus*), dominant males produce a urinary pheromone which causes reproductive suppression in subordinates.[52]

In the examples just described for diurnal anthropoids and nocturnal prosimians, it may be presumed that suppression of secondary sexual development is likely to represent a transient phase in the lifetime reproductive strategy of the male. If an opportunity to occupy a vacant territory arises, full development of secondary sexual characters may then proceed. This is the case, for instance, in the mandrill in which removal of dominant males results in the development of sexual skin and attainment of the "fatted" condition in a previously subordinate individual (author's unpublished observations).

SPERM COMPETITION AND ASSOCIATED PHENOMENA

In 1970, Parker[18] wrote a classic paper in which he proposed that when a female mates with multiple partners, then sexual selection might operate at the genitalic level because of competition between spermatozoa of rival males. As far as the primates are concerned, evidence that females mate with a number of males during the fertile phase of the ovarian cycle is strongest for those species that have multimale-multifemale mating systems (Table 3). In association with this, relative testes size is greater in anthropoids which live in multimale-multifemale groups than in those that are monogamous or polygynous.[53,54] Increased testes size relative to body weight is due primarily to the greater volume of seminiferous tubules required to produce larger numbers of spermatozoa, because sperm competition has favored males that can produce maximum numbers of gametes per ejaculate.[55] Both seasonally breeding and nonseasonally breeding multimale-multifemale species exhibit larger relative testes sizes; the effect is not due to a requirement to produce large numbers of gametes during a restricted annual mating season.[56]

The occurrence of multiple matings in females of those primate species that have dispersed, nongregarious mating systems remains a matter for speculation. Most primates that have dispersed mating systems are nocturnal prosimians; males typically occupy larger homeranges that overlap relatively little, but exhibit extensive overlap with a number of female range areas.[51] Prosimians are distinguished by the occurrence of relatively brief periods of female sexual receptivity, and a number of males may congregate around an individual female when she is in estrus (e.g., *Galago crassicaudatus;*[57] *G. senegalensis;*[51] *Daubentonia madagascariensis*[58]). It is also the case that many nocturnal prosimians, including pottos, lorises, mouselemurs, and galagos, have very large testes in relation to body weight.[54,59] For these reasons sperm competition has likely played a major role in the evolution of the mating systems of these primates; behavioral and DNA fingerprinting studies will be required to test this hypothesis.

The importance of sperm competition in primates with multimale-multifemale mating systems and its putative importance in certain nocturnal prosimians does not mean that such selection pressure is totally absent in monogamous or polygynous forms. However, sperm competition is unlikely to be significant in a monogamous

TABLE 3. Evidence for Multiple-Partner Matings by Females in Multimale-Multifemale Primate Groups[a]

Species	Type of Study	Numbers of Males Mated per Female	Source
Prosimians			
Lemur catta	Field study	3-5	75
Propithecus verreauxi	Field study	1-2	76
New World Monkeys			
Alouatta palliata	Field study	>1	77
Ateles paniscus	Field study	>1	78
Brachyteles arachnoides	Field study	4	79
Cebus apella	Field study	1-7	80
Old World Monkeys			
Cercopithecus aethiops	Field study	>1	81
Miopithecius talapoin	Field study	>1	82
Papio ursinus	Field study	1-3	83
Papio cynocephalus	Field study	>1	84
Papio anubis	Field study	>1	85
		1-3	17
Cercocebus albigena	Field study	>1	86
Mandrillus sphinx	Semi-free ranging	1-3	31
Macaca mulatta	Field study	1-11 ($\bar{x}$ 3.2)	87
	Field study	x 3.8	88
	Field study	>1	89
	Field study	1-9 ($\bar{x}$ 3 or 4)	90
Macaca fuscata	Semi-free ranging	>1	91
	Captive group	3-19 ($\bar{x}$ 10.7)[b]	92
Macaca fascicularis	Field study	>1	93
Macaca radiata	Captive group	>1	94
Macaca sylvanus	Field study	3-11 ($\bar{x}$-6.0)	95
	Field study	5-11 ($\bar{x}$-7.12)	96
Macaca nemestrina	Captive group	1-5 ($\bar{x}$-2.5)	97
Apes			
Pan troglodytes	Field study	8+	98
	Field study	>1	99
Pan paniscus	Field study	>1	100
	Field study	>1	101

[a] Cases in which multipartner matings occur but the number of males involved is unknown are indicated by >1. Data in this table refer to matings during a single ovarian cycle, including the presumptive period of ovulation. Copulations occurring during pregnancy are not considered.

[b] These data refer to numbers of male partners during a single mating season and not necessarily during a single ovarian cycle.

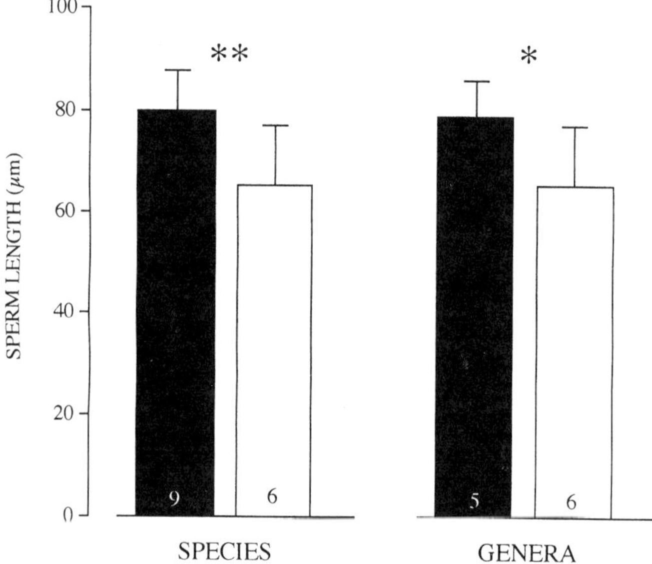

FIGURE 4. Comparison of sperm length in primates having large testes in relation to body weight (*closed bars*) and those having small testes in relation to body weight (*open bars*). Species with large relative testes size are: *Macaca nemestrina, M. fascicularis, M. arctoides, M. mulatta, Papio anubis, P. cynocephalus, Saimiri sciureus, Cercopithecus aethiops,* and *Pan troglodytes.* Species with small relative testes size are: *Callithrix jacchus, Theropithecus gelada, Hylobates lar, Pongo pygmaeus, Gorilla gorilla,* and *Homo sapiens.* Comparisons at the specific and generic level are statistically significant; $*p < 0.05$; $**p = 0.02$ (Mann-Whitney U test). Data are from ref. 63.

species, such as the gibbon, or a polygynous form, such as the gorilla, by comparison with multimale-multifemale species such as macaques, baboons, or chimpanzees. Man is primarily a monogamous/polygynous primate, and in association with this, human testes are relatively small in relation to body weight.[53] Human sperm reserves are more readily depleted by multiple ejaculations[60] than in the chimpanzee.[61] Attempts to account the evolution of human sexuality in relation to sperm competition are unconvincing.[62]

A variety of features of male reproductive anatomy, physiology, and behavior have been molded by sexual selection in relation to sperm competition, and a few examples may be quoted here. Not only relative testes size, but also sperm length is greater in primates that are "polyandrous" (used here to mean that females mate with multiple partners) than in monandrous forms.[63] Thus, anthropoids with multimale-multifemale mating systems and larger relative testes size also have significantly longer gametes than do monogamous or polygynous species with relatively small testes (Fig. 4). Few primate species have been examined, however, and the need exists to collect further data and to test this hypothesis more rigorously. The implication is that longer gametes confer some advantage due to their ability to swim more rapidly

TABLE 4. Hourly Frequencies of Ejaculation in Primates with Multimale-Multifemale (MM), Polygynous (PG), or Monogamous (MN) Mating Systems[a]

Species	Study Type	Males (n)	Ejaculation Range	Ejaculation Mean	Mating System
Lemur catta[b]	F	5	1-1.75	1.35	MM
Callithrix jacchus	CG	6	0.095-0.202	0.155	MN
Aotus lemurinus	CG	5	–	0.07	MN
Papio ursinus	F	–	–	0.75	MM
Papio cynocephalus	F	9	0.41-1.46	0.83	MM
Mandrillus sphinx[b]	SF	6	0-3	0.85	MM
Macaca mulatta[b]	CG	–	0-0.69	0.38	MM
Macaca fascicularis	CG	–	0-1.33	0.69	MM
Macaca radiata[b]	CG	–	0.44-2.44	0.97	MM
Macaca arctoides	CG	18	0-11	1.91	MM
Macaca sylvanus[b]	F	21	0-4.14	2.28	MM
Macaca nigra	CG	1	–	0.63	MM
Macaca thibetana[b]	F	7	0-0.9	0.45	MM
Erythrocebus patas[b]	F	5	0.19-0.74	0.43	MM[c]
Theropithecus gelada	F	–	–	0.18	PG
Symphalangus syndactylus	F	–	–	0.005	MN
Pan paniscus	F	5	0.19-0.42	0.27	MM
Pan troglodytes	F	–	0.03-1.14	0.52	MM
Gorilla gorilla	F	3	0.32-0.38	0.35	PG
Homo sapiens	NA	3,342	0-0.119	0.025	PG/MN

Abbreviations: F = field study; CG = captive group(s); SF = semifree-ranging group; NA = North American population. Data on *M. sphinx* include the author's unpublished obervations, and mean frequency relates to the highest-ranking male in the group.

[a] Data from ref. 102.

[b] A species with pronounced mating seasonality.

[c] *E. patas* is classified as an MM species, because in this study influxes of additional males during the mating season created a multimale-multifemale group.

in the oviduct and thus to attain fertilization under competitive conditions. The notion that different physiological types of sperm might occur, such as "egg-getter" sperm or "kamikaze" sperm, in human ejaculates remains highly speculative,[64] particularly because there is no evidence for such specializations in nonhuman primates (such as macaques and chimpanzees) where intense sperm competition is known to occur.

It is logical to suggest that sperm competition might favor males that sustain higher ejaculatory frequencies with females during the periovulatory period in order to increase the total numbers of gametes introduced into the female tract. This appears to be the case in primates (TABLE 4). Species with multimale-multifemale mating systems copulate at much higher frequencies (mean ± SEM: 0.879 ± 0.157 ejaculations per hour) than do the polygynous or monogamous species (0.131 ± 0.052 ejaculations) listed in this table. Differences between the two groups are statistically significant at both the species and the genus level, as shown in FIGURE 5.

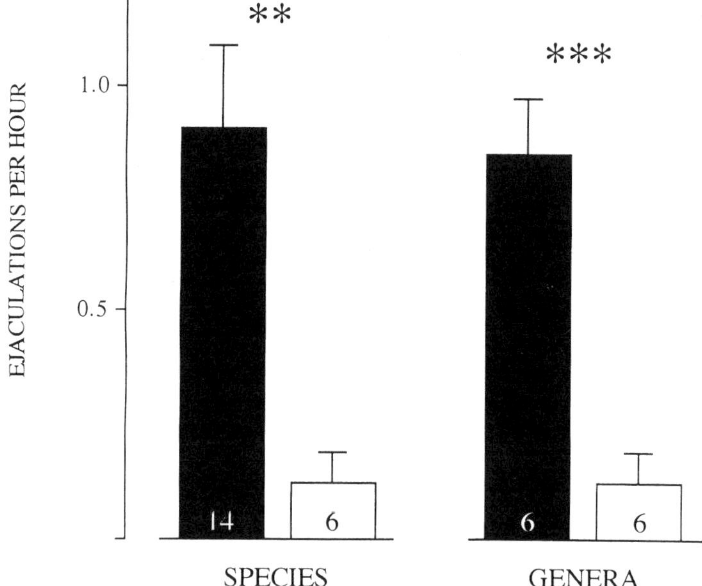

FIGURE 5. Mean hourly frequencies of ejaculation in ''monandrous'' primate species and genera (polygynous and monogamous mating systems as indicated by *open bars*) compared to ''polyandrous'' species and genera (multimale-multifemale mating system as indicated by *closed bars*). $^{**}p < 0.002$; $^{***}p < 0.001$ (Mann-Whitney U test). Numbers of species and genera are indicated at the foot of each histogram. Data are from TABLE 4.

Comparative studies of many primate species have also shown that complex penile morphologies and copulatory patterns are more prevalent in those species in which sperm competition is likely (i.e., multimale-multifemale and dispersed mating systems[54,59,65]). Sexual selection has favored the evolution of multiple intromission or prolonged single intromission patterns of copulation under these circumstances. Specializations such as elongation of the penis, the presence of a longer baculum, and more complex distal penile morphologies are more prevalent in those primates in which females mate with multiple partners during the fertile period. Indeed, female influences on the evolution of these masculine genital specializations have probably been of paramount importance.

Eberhard[66] suggested that in those animal species in which females mate with multiple partners, the penis may function as an ''internal courtship device,'' encouraging sperm transport or storage and thus increasing the likelihood of successful fertilization. Small adaptive features of penile morphology or behavior that are advantageous during copulation thus become subject to rapid sexual selection by ''female choice'' in the same manner as do some masculine secondary sexual characteristics (e.g., plumage of peacocks or argus pheasants[67]). Eberhard's theory has been applied successfully to studies of mating systems and genital evolution in primates.[54] In Old World anthropoids, for example, females of some species develop prominent sexual

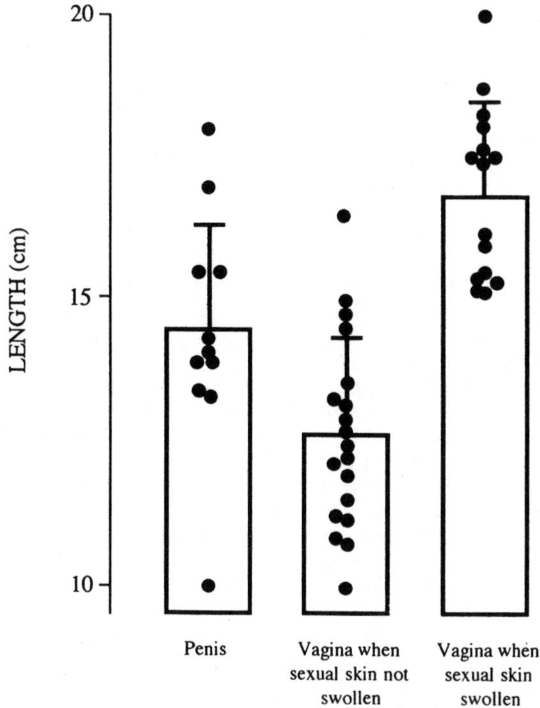

FIGURE 6. Measurements of penile erection and vaginal length in adult chimpanzees. Sexual swelling results in elongation of the vaginal canal with consequent inability of many males to contact the female's cervix during intromission. Data are individual values, with the overall mean and standard deviation indicated by the histogram and bar. Data are from ref. 70.

skin swellings during the periovulatory phase of the menstrual cycle. This is the case in mandrills (as already described above) and also in baboons, mangabeys, talapoins, some macaques, some African colobines (e.g., *Colobus badius*), and chimpanzees.[68] Sexual skin swellings are visually attractive to males and stimulate their sexual arousal.[69] However, the swelling also causes marked lengthening of the female's vaginal canal (by up to 50% in the chimpanzee; FIG. 6), and this in turn has resulted in sexual selection for penile elongation in adult males.[70] Female choice doubtless operates at many levels during and after copulation, and a major challenge for future studies of sperm competition will be to understand precisely how the ejaculates of rival males interact within the female's reproductive system and how "female choice" operates at the level of the vagina, uterus, uterotubal junction, and oviduct.

ACKNOWLEDGMENTS

My thanks to the Medical Research Council (UK) and to CIRMF in Gabon for support of various studies cited in this review.

REFERENCES

1. EMLEN, S. T. & L. W. ORING. 1977. Science **197:** 215-223.
2. THORNHILL, R. & J. ALCOCK. 1983. The Evolution of Insect Mating Systems. Harvard University Press. Cambridge, MA.
3. CLUTTON-BROCK, T. H. 1989. Proc. Roy. Soc. Lond. B **236:** 339-372.
4. ALCOCK, J. 1984. Animal Behavior. An Evolutionary Approach. Sinauer. Sunderland, MA.
5. DAVIES, N. B. 1991. Mating systems. *In* Behavioral Ecology, An Evolutionary Approach. J. R. Krebs & N. B. Davies, Eds. Blackwell. London.
6. REES, J. A. & P. H. HARVEY. 1991. The evolution of animal mating systems. *In* Mating and Marriage. V. Reynolds & J. Kellett, Eds.: 1-45. Oxford University Press. Oxford.
7. BIRKHEAD, T. R. & A. P. MOLLER. 1992. Sperm Competition in Birds. Academic Press. London.
8. SUGIYAMA, Y. 1967. Social organization of Hanuman langurs. *In* Social Communication among Primates. S. A. Altmann, Ed. University of Chicago Press. Chicago.
9. DUNBAR, R. I. M. 1984. Reproductive Decisions. Princeton University Press. Princeton.
10. TOKUDA, K. 1961. Primates **3:** 1-40.
11. PUSEY, A. E. & C. PACKER. 1987. Dispersal and philopatry. *In* Primate Societies. B. B. Smuts *et al.*, Eds.: 250-266. University of Chicago Press. Chicago.
12. TRIVERS, R. 1972. Parental investment and sexual selection. *In* Sexual Selection and the Descent of Man. B. Campbell, Ed.: 136-179. Heinemann. London.
13. SEYFARTH, R. M. 1978. Behaviour **64:** 204-226.
14. TUTIN, C. E. G. 1979. Behav. Ecol. Sociobiol. **6:** 29-38.
15. EATON, G. G. 1973. Social and endocrine determinants of sexual behaviour in simian and prosimian females. *In* Proc. 4th Congress of the International Primatological Society. Vol. 2. Primate Reproductive Behaviour. C. H. Phoenix, Ed. Karger. Basel.
16. HERBERT, J. 1968. Anim. Behav. **16:** 351-353.
17. SMUTS, B. B. 1985. Sex and Friendship in Baboons. Aldine. New York.
18. PARKER, G. A. 1970. Biol. Rev. **45:** 525-567.
19. JEFFREYS, A. J., W. WILSON & S. L. THEIN. 1985. Nature Lond. **314:** 67-73.
20. JEFFREYS, A. J., W. WILSON & S. L. THEIN. 1985. Nature Lond. **316:** 76-79.
21. BURKE, T. & M. BRUFORD. 1987. Nature Lond. **327:** 149-152.
22. PACKER, C., D. A. GILBERT, A. E. PUSEY & S. J. O'BRIEN. 1991. Nature Lond. **351:** 562-565.
23. AMOS, W., S. TWISS, P. P. POMEROY & S. S. ANDERSON. 1993. Proc. Roy. Soc. Lond. B **252:** 199-207.
24. MARTIN, R. D., A. F. DIXSON & E. J. WICKINGS. 1992. Paternity in Primates, Genetic Tests and Theories. Karger. Basel.
25. DE RUITER, J. R. & M. INOUE. 1993. Primates **34:** 553-555.
26. HOSHINO, J., A. MORI, H. KUDO & M. KAWAI. 1984. Primates **25:** 295-307.
27. JOUVENTIN, P. 1975. Terre et Vie **29:** 493-532.
28. KUDO, H. 1987. Primates **28:** 289-308.
29. STAMMBACK, E. 1987. Desert, forest and montane baboons: Multilevel societies. *In* Primate Societies. B. Smuts *et al.*, Eds.: 112-120. Chicago University Press. Chicago.
30. ROLDAN, E. R. S. & M. GOMENDIO. 1995. Folia Primatol. **64:** 225-230.
31. DIXSON, A. F., T. BOSSI & E. J. WICKINGS. 1993. Primates **34:** 525-532.
32. WILDT, D. E., U. DOYLE, S. C. STONE & R. M. HARRISON. 1977. Primates **18:** 261-270.
33. BERARD, J. D., P. NURNBERG, J. T. EPPLEN & J. SCHMIDTKE. 1993. Primates **34:** 481-489.
34. SMITH, D. G. 1993. Primates **34:** 471-480.
35. BERCOVITCH, F. & P. NURNBERG. 1996. J. Reprod. Fertil. In press.
36. LINBURG, D. G. 1969. Science **166:** 1176-1178.
37. PAUL, A., J. KUESTER, A. TIMME & J. ARNEMANN. 1993. Primates **34:** 481-502.
38. KUESTER, J., A. PAUL & J. ARNEMANN. 1995. Primates **36:** 461-476.

39. De Ruiter, J. R., W. Scheffrahn, G. Trommelen, A. G. Uitterlinden, R. D. Martin & J. A. R. A. M. van Hooff. 1992. *In* Paternity in Primates, Genetic Tests and Theories. R. D. Martin, A. F. Dixson & E. J. Wickings, Eds.: 171-190. Basel. Karger.
40. De Ruiter J. R., J. van Hooff & W. Scheffrahn. 1994. Behaviour **129:** 204-224.
41. van Noordwijk, M. A. & C. P. van Schaik. 1985. Anim. Behav. **33:** 849-861.
42. Ohsawa, H., M. Inoue & O. Takenaka. 1993. Primates **34:** 533-544.
43. Chism, J. B. & T. E. Rowell. 1986. Ethology **72:** 31-39.
44. Wickings, E. J. & A. F. Dixson. 1992. Physiol. Behav. **52:** 909-916.
45. Kingsley, S. 1982. Causes of non-breeding and the development of the secondary sexual characters in the male orang-utan: A hormonal study. *In* The Orang-utan: Its Biology and Conservation. L. De Boer, Ed. W. Junk. The Hague.
46. Dixson, A. F., J. Knight, H. D. M. Moore & M. Carman. 1982. Int. Zoo Yearb. **22:** 222-227.
47. Galdikas, B. M. 1985. Am. J. Primatol. **8:** 87-99.
48. Fontaine, R. 1981. The uakaris, genus Cacajao. *In* Ecology and Behavior of Neotropical Primates. A. F. Coimbra-Filho & R. A. Mittermeier, Eds. Academia Brasiliera de Ciencias. Rio de Janeiro.
49. Neville, M. K., K. E. Glander, F. Braza & A. B. Rylands. 1988. The howling monkeys, genus *Alouatta. In* Ecology and Behavior of Neotropical Primates. R. A. Mittermeier, A. B. Rylands, A. Coimbra-Filho & G. A. B. Fonseca, Eds. Vol. **2:** 349-453. W. W. F. Washington, DC.
50. Charles-Dominique, P. 1977. Ecology and Behaviour of Nocturnal Prosimians. Duckworth. London.
51. Bearder, S. K. 1987. Lorises, bushbabies and tarsiers: Diverse societies in solitary foragers. *In* Primate Societies. B. Smuts *et al.,* Eds.: 11-24. Chicago University Press. Chicago.
52. Perret, M. 1992. Folia Primatol. **59:** 1-25.
53. Harcourt, A. H., P. H. Harvey, S. G. Larson & R. V. Short. 1981. Nature **293:** 55-57.
54. Dixson, A. F. 1987. J. Zool. Lond. **213:** 423-443.
55. Moller, A. P. 1988. J. Hum. Evol. **17:** 479-488.
56. Harcourt, A. H., A. Purvis & L. Liles. 1995. Funct. Ecol. **9:** 468-476.
57. Clark, A. B. 1985. Int. J. Primatol. **6:** 581-600.
58. Sterling, E. J. 1993. Patterns of range use and social organization in aye-ayes (*Daubentonia madagascariensis*) on Nosy Mangabe. *In* Lemur Social Systems and Their Ecological Basis. P. M. Kappeler & P. M. Ganshorn, Eds.: 1-10. Plenum. New York.
59. Dixson, A. F. 1995. Sexual selection and the evolution of copulatory behaviour in nocturnal prosimians. *In* Creatures of the Dark: The Nocturnal Prosimians. L. Alterman, G. A. Doyle & M. K. Izard, Eds. Plenum. New York.
60. Freund, M. 1963. J. Reprod. Fertil. **6:** 269-286.
61. Marson, J. D. Gervais, S. Meuris, R. W. Cooper & P. Jouannet. 1989. J. Reprod. Fertil. **85:** 43-50.
62. Baker, R. R. & M. A. Bellis. 1993. Anim. Behav. **46:** 887-909.
63. Dixson, A. F. 1995. Folia Primatol. **61:** 221-227.
64. Baker, R. R. & M. A. Bellis. 1988. Anim. Behav. **36:** 936-939.
65. Dixson, A. F. 1991. Sexual selection, natural selection and copulatory patterns in male primates. Folia Primatol. **57:** 96-101.
66. Eberhard, W. G. 1985. Sexual Selection and Animal Genitalia. Harvard University Press. Cambridge, MA.
67. Darwin, C. 1871. The Descent of Man and Selection in Relation to Sex. John Murray. London.
68. Dixson, A. F. 1983. Adv. Stud. Behav. **13:** 63-106.
69. Girolami, L. & C. Bielert. 1987. Int. J. Primatol. **8:** 651-661.
70. Dixson, A. F. & N. I. Mundy. 1994. Arch. Sex Behav. **23:** 267-280.
71. Hollihn, U. 1973. Int. Zoo Yearb. **13:** 185-188.

72. BENNETT, E. L. & A. C. SEBASTIAN. 1988. Int. J. Primatol. **9:** 233-255.
73. KINGDON, J. S. 1980. Trans. Zoo. Soc. Lond. **35:** 425-475.
74. TANNER, J. M. 1992. Human growth and development. *In* The Cambridge Encyclopedia of Human Evolution. S. Jones, R. Martin & D. Pilbeam, Eds.: 98-105. Cambridge University Press. Cambridge.
75. KOYAMA, N. 1988. Primates **29:** 163-175.
76. RICHARD, A. 1976. Patterns of Mating Behaviour in Propithecus Verteauxi. *In* Prosimian Behaviour. R. D. Martin, G. A. Doyle & A. C. Walker, Eds. Duckworth. London.
77. JONES, C. B. 1985. Primates **26:** 130-142.
78. ROOSMALEN, M. G. M. & L. KLIEN. 1988. The spider monkeys, genus *Ateles. In* Ecology and Behaviour of Neotropical Primates, Vol 2. R. A. Mittermeir, A. B. Rylands, A. Coimbra-Filho & G. A. B. Fonseca, Eds.: 455-537. W. W. F. Washington, DC.
79. MILTON, K. M. 1985. Behav. Ecol. Sociobiol. **17:** 53-59.
80. JANSON, C. H. 1984. Z. Tierpsychol. **65:** 177-200.
81. ANDELMAN, S. J. 1987. Am. Nat. **129:** 785-799.
82. ROWELL, T. E. & A. F. DIXSON. 1975. J. Reprod. Fertil. **43:** 419-434.
83. HALL, K. R. L. 1962. Proc. Zool. Soc. Lond. **139:** 283-327.
84. HAUSFATER, G. 1975. Contrib. Primatol. **7:** 1-50.
85. SCOTT, N. J. 1984. Reproductive behavior of adolescent female baboons. *In* Female Primates: Studies by Women Primatologists. M. F. Small, Ed.: 77-102. Alan Liss. New York.
86. WALLIS, S. J. 1983. Int. J. Primatol. **4:** 153-166.
87. CONOWAY, C. H. & C. B. KOFORD. 1965. J. Mammal. **45:** 577-588.
88. LOY, J. 1971. Oestrous behavior of free-ranging rhesus monkeys. Primates **12:** 1-31.
89. LINBURG, D. G. 1983. Mating behavior and estrus in the Indian rhesus monkey. *In* Perspectives in Primate Biology. K. P. Seth, Ed.: 45-61. Today & Tomorrow. New Delhi.
90. MANSON, J. H. 1992. Anim. Behav. **44:** 405-416.
91. WOLFE, L. D. 1984. Japanese macaque female sexual behavior. *In* Female Primates: Studies by Women Primatologists. M. Small, Ed.: 141-157. Liss. New York.
92. HANBY, J., L. ROBERTSON & C. H. PHOENIX. 1971. Folia Primatol. **16:** 123-143.
93. VAN NOORDWIJK, M. A. 1985. Z. Tierpsychol. **70:** 279-296.
94. GLICK, B. B. 1980. Ontogenetic and psychobiological aspects of the mating activities of male *Macaca radiata. In* The Macaques: Studies in Ecology, Behavior and Evolution. D. Linburg, Ed.: 345-360. Van Nostrand Reinhold. New York.
95. TAUB, D. M. 1980. Female choice and mating strategies among wild Barbary macaques (*Macaca sylvanus*). *In* The Macaques: Studies in Ecology, Behavior and Evolution. D. Linburg, Ed.: 287-344. Van Nostrand Reinhold. New York.
96. MÉNARD, N., W. SCHEFFRAHN, D. VALET, C. ZIDANE & C. REBER. 1992. Application of blood protein electrophresis and DNA fingerprinting to the analysis of paternity and social characteristics of wild Barbary macaques. *In* Paternity in Primates: Genetic Tests and Theories. R. D. Martin, A. F. Dixson & E. J. Wickings, Eds. Karger. Basel.
97. TOKUDA, K., R. C. SIMMS & J. D. JENSEN. 1968. Primates **9:** 283-294.
98. GOODALL, J. 1986. The Chimpanzees of Gombe: Patterns of Behavior. Belknap. Cambridge, MA.
99. HASEGAWA, T. & M. HAIRAIWA-HASEGAWA. 1990. Sperm competition and mating behavior. *In* The Chimpanzees of the Mahale Mountains, Sexual and Life History Strategies. T. Nishida, Ed.: 115-132. Tokyo University Press. Tokyo.
100. FURUICHI, T. 1987. Primates **28:** 309-318.
101. KANO, T. 1992. The Last Ape: Pygmy Chimpanzee Behavior and Ecology. Tokyo University Press. Tokyo.
102. DIXSON, A. F. 1995. Folia Primatol. **64:** 146-152.

4

Emotion: An Evolutionary By-Product of the Neural Regulation of the Autonomic Nervous System

Stephen W. Porges

A new theory, the polyvagal theory of emotion, is presented which links the evolution of the autonomic nervous system to affective experience, emotional expression, vocal communication, and contingent social behavior. The polyvagal theory is derived from the well-documented phylogenetic shift in the neural regulation of the autonomic nervous system that expands the capacity of the organism to control metabolic output. The theory emphasizes the phylogenetic dependence of the structure and function of the vagus, the primary nerve of the parasympathetic nervous system. Three phylogenetic stages of neural development are described. The first stage is characterized by a primitive unmyelinated vegetative vagal system that fosters digestion and responds to novelty or threat by reducing cardiac output to protect metabolic resources. Behaviorally, this first stage is associated with immobilization behaviors. The second stage is characterized by a spinal sympathetic nervous system that can increase metabolic output and inhibit the primitive vagal system's influence on the gut to foster mobilization behaviors necessary for "fight or flight." The third stage, which is unique to mammals, is characterized by a myelinated vagal system that can rapidly regulate cardiac output to foster engagement and disengagement with the environment. The myelinated vagus originates in a brainstem area that evolved from the primitive gill arches and in mammals controls facial expression, sucking, swallowing, breathing, and vocalization. It is hypothesized that the mammalian vagal system fosters early mother-infant interactions and serves as the substrate for the development of complex social behaviors. In addition, the mammalian vagal system has an inhibitory effect on sympathetic pathways to the heart and thus promotes calm behavior and prosocial behavior.

The polyvagal theory of emotion proposes that the evolution of the autonomic nervous system provides the organizing principle to interpret the adaptive significance of affective processes. The theory proposes that the evolution of the mammalian autonomic nervous system, and specifically the brainstem regulatory centers of the vagus and other related cranial nerves, provides substrates for emotional experiences and affective processes that are necessary for social behavior in mammals. In this context, the evolution of the nervous system limits or expands the ability to express

The preparation of this manuscript was supported in part by grant HD 22628 from the National Institute of Child Health and Human Development and grant MCJ 240622 from the Maternal and Child Health Bureau.

emotions, which in turn may determine proximity, social contact, and the quality of communication. The polyvagal construct has been previously introduced[1] to document the neurophysiological and neuroanatomical distinction between the two vagal branches and to propose their unique relation with behavioral strategies. This report elaborates on the polyvagal construct and proposes that affective strategies are derivative of the evolutionary process that produced the polyvagal regulation.

There is a consensus that affect is expressed in facial muscles and in organs regulated by the autonomic nervous system. However, with the exception of work by Cannon,[2,3] which focused on the sympathetic-adrenal system as the physiological substrate of emotion, the presumed neural regulation of affective state has not been investigated. Even contemporary researchers investigating affective signatures in the autonomic nervous system[4–7] have tacitly accepted Cannon's assumption that emotions reflect responses of the sympathetic nervous system.

Unlike the architectural dictum that form (i.e., structure) follows function, *the function of the nervous system is derivative of structure.* The flexibility or variability of autonomic nervous system function is totally dependent on the structure. By mapping the phylogenetic development of the structures regulating autonomic function, it is possible to observe the dependence of autonomic reactivity on the evolution of the underlying structure of the nervous system. The phylogenetic approach highlights a shift in brainstem and cranial nerve morphology and function from an oxygen-sensitive system (i.e., the primitive gill arches) to a system that regulates facial muscles, cardiac output, and the vocal apparatus for affective communication.

CANNON'S BLUNDER

Cannon emphasized the idea that emotions were expressions of sympathetic-adrenal excitation. In limiting emotional experiences solely to the mobilization responses associated with sympathetic-adrenal activity, Cannon denied the importance of visceral feelings and neglected the contribution of the parasympathetic nervous system. Cannon's views were not compatible with earlier statements on the importance of visceral feedback and the parasympathetic nervous system. For example, in *The Expression of Emotions in Man and Animals,* Darwin[8] acknowledged the importance of the bidirectional neural communication between the heart and the brain via the "pneumogastric" nerve. This, the 10th cranial nerve, is now called the vagus nerve and is the major component of the parasympathetic nervous system.

> ... when the mind is strongly excited, we might expect that it would instantly affect in a direct manner the heart; and this is universally acknowledged and felt to be the case. Claude Bernard also repeatedly insists, and this deserves especial notice, that when the heart is affected it reacts on the brain; and the state of the brain again reacts through the pneumogastric [vagus] nerve on the heart; so that under any excitement there will be much mutual action and reaction between these, the two most important organs of the body (p.69).

For Darwin, emotional state represented a covariation between facial expression and autonomic tone. However, he did not elucidate the specific neurophysiological mechanisms. Our current knowledge of the neuroanatomy, embryology, and phylogeny of the nervous system was not available to Darwin. At that time it was not known that vagal fibers originated in several medullary nuclei, that branches of the vagus exerted control over the periphery through different feedback systems, and that the function of the branches of the vagus followed a phylogenetic principle. However, Darwin's statement is important, because it emphasizes afferent feedback from the heart to the brain, independent of the spinal cord and the sympathetic nervous system, as well as the regulatory role of the vagus in the expression of emotions.

The autonomic nervous system is related to visceral state regulation and the regulation of behaviors associated with mobilization or immobilization. For example, sympathetic excitation is clearly linked to mobilization. In vertebrates, the sympathetic nervous system is characterized by a trunk or column of ganglia paralleling the segmentation of the spinal cord. Skeletal motor pathways to the limbs are paralleled by sympathetic fibers to facilitate the metabolically demanding behaviors related to fight and flight. In fact, from Cannon's perspective and to many who followed, the sympathetic nervous system due to its mobilizing capacity was the component of the autonomic nervous system associated with emotion. This, however, neglected the autonomic components of affective experiences that were metabolically conservative, including processes such as signaling via facial expressions and vocalizations or specific immobilization responses.

AUTONOMIC DETERMINANTS OF EMOTION

Over the last 100 years we have learned much about the autonomic nervous system, its evolutionary origins, and how it relates to emotion. Initially, we can distinguish among three components of the autonomic nervous system (visceral afferents, sympathetic nervous system, and parasympathetic nervous system) and speculate how each might be related to affective experiences. First, the visceral afferents may be assumed to play a major role in determining "feelings." These mechanisms, which provide us with knowledge of hunger, also may convey a sense of nausea during emotional distress. We frequently hear subjective reports of individuals feeling "sick to their stomach" during periods of severe emotional strain associated with profound negative experiences. Similarly, negative states have been associated with reports of breathlessness or feelings that the heart has stopped. Second, the sympathetic nervous system and adrenal activity are associated with mobilization. Activation of the sympathetic nervous system is usually linked to increased skeletal movement of the major limbs. Thus, consistent with Cannon, the sympathetic nervous system provides the metabolic resources required for fight or flight behaviors. The sympathetic nervous system enhances mobilization by increasing cardiac output and decreasing the metabolic demands of the digestive tract by actively inhibiting gastric motility. Third, as proposed by Darwin and Bernard, the parasympathetic nervous system and specifically the vagus are related to emotional state. Few researchers have investigated the link between parasympathetic activity and affective state. However, over the last decade my laboratory has focused on this issue. We documented that vagal tone, a component of parasympathetic control, is related to affect and affect regulation.[9–11] We presented theoretical models explaining the importance of vagal regulation in the development of appropriate social behavior.[12] The parasympathetic nervous system is generally associated with fostering growth and restoration.[13,14]

Moreover, knowledge of the polyvagal system allows an appreciation of the importance of the brainstem origin of the specific vagal fibers in the determination of affective and behavioral response strategies.[12,15]

Researchers and clinicians have had difficulties in the organization or categorization of intensive affective states that appear to have totally different etiologies or behavioral expressions. For example, intense feelings of terror might result in total immobilization or freezing. By contrast, intense feelings of anger or anxiety might be associated with massive mobilization activity. This problem exists, in part, because of a bias towards explanations of affective states defined in terms of either overt behavior such as facial expression (i.e., following Darwin) or sympathetic activity (i.e., following Cannon). The emphasis on sympathetic activity is based on three historical factors. First, theories regarding emotions have minimized or totally neglected the parasympathetic nervous system. Second, Cannon's focus on the sympathetic efferents and mobilization responses associated with fight and flight as the sole domain of autonomic reactivity during emotional states has not been challenged. Third, the data base of autonomic correlates of affect, collected to identify autonomic "signatures" of specific affective states, is dominated by measures assumed to be related to sympathetic function.[4–7]

EVOLUTION OF THE AUTONOMIC NERVOUS SYSTEM: EMERGENT STRUCTURES FOR THE EXPRESSION OF EMOTIONS IN MAN AND ANIMALS

Although there is an acceptance that the autonomic nervous system and the face play a role in emotional expression, there is great uncertainty regarding the autonomic "signature" of specific or discrete emotions. Most researchers evaluating autonomic responses during affective experiences assumed, as did Cannon, that the sympathetic nervous system was the determinant of emotion or at least the primary physiological covariate of emotion. This, of course, neglects the potential role of the parasympathetic nervous system and its neurophysiological affinity to facial structures including facial muscles, eye movements, pupil dilation, salivation, swallowing, vocalizing, hearing, and breathing. By investigating the evolution of the autonomic nervous system, we may gain insight into the interface between autonomic function and facial expression. In the following sections the phylogenetic development of the autonomic nervous system will be used as an organizing principle to categorize affective experiences.

The polyvagal theory of emotion is derived from investigations of the evolution of the autonomic nervous system. The theory includes several rules and assumptions.

1. Emotion depends on the communication between the autonomic nervous system and the brain; visceral afferents convey information on physiological state to the brain and are critical to the sensory or psychological experience of emotion, and cranial nerves and the sympathetic nervous system are outputs from the brain that provide somatomotor and visceromotor control of the expression of emotion.

2. Evolution has modified the structures of the autonomic nervous system.

3. Emotional experience and expression are functional derivatives of structural changes in the autonomic nervous system due to evolutionary processes.

4. The mammalian autonomic nervous system retains vestiges of phylogenetically older autonomic nervous systems.

TABLE 1. Method of Cardiac Control as a Function of Vertebrate Phylogeny

	CHM	DMX	SNS	ADN	NA
Cyclostomes					
Myxinoids	x+				
Lamproids	x+	x+			
Elasmobranchs	x+	x−			
Teleosts	x+	x−	x+		
Amphibians	x+	x−	x+		
Reptiles	x+	x−	x+	x+	
Mammals	x+	x−	x+	x+	x−

Abbreviations: CHM = chromaffin tissue; DMX = vagal pathways originating in the dorsal motor nucleus of the vagus; SNS = spinal sympathetic nervous system; ADN = adrenal medulla; NA = vagal pathways originating in the nucleus ambiguus; + = increases cardiac output; − = decreases cardiac output.

5. The phylogenetic "level" of the autonomic nervous system determines affective states and the range of social behavior.

6. In mammals, the autonomic nervous system response strategy to challenge follows a phylogenetic hierarchy, starting with the newest structures and, when all else fails, reverting to the most primitive structural system.

This paper focuses on the phylogenetic shift in the neural regulation of the vertebrate heart. The heart has been selected because, in response to environmental challenge, cardiac output must be regulated to mobilize for fight or flight behaviors or to immobilize for death feigning or hiding behaviors. To regulate cardiac output several efferent structures have evolved. These structures represent two opposing systems: one, a sympathetic-catecholamine system including chromaffin tissue and spinal sympathetics; and two, a vagal system (a component of the parasympathetic nervous system) with branches originating in medullary source nuclei (i.e., dorsal motor nucleus of the vagus and nucleus ambiguus). In addition, vertebrates have chromaffin tissue containing high concentrations of catecholamines. Chromaffin tissue is defined as having morphological and histochemical properties similar to those of the adrenal medulla. Classes of vertebrates that do not have an adrenal medulla have relatively more chromaffin tissue, which regulates circulating catecholamines.

TABLE 1 lists the regulatory structures that influence the heart in vertebrates.[16–18] Two phylogenetic principles can be extracted from TABLE 1. First, there is a phylogenetic pattern in the regulation of the heart from endocrine communication, to unmyelinated nerves, and finally to myelinated nerves. Second, there is a development of opposing neural mechanisms of excitation and inhibition to provide rapid regulation of graded metabolic output.

In the most primitive fish, the cyclostomes, the neural control of the heart is very primitive. Some cyclostomes such as the myxinoids (hagfish) use circulating catecholamines from chromaffin tissue to provide the sole excitatory influences on the heart. Other cyclostomes such as the lampetroids (lampreys) have a cardiac vagus. However, in contrast to all other vertebrates that have a cardioinhibitory vagus that acts via muscarinic cholinoceptors, the cyclostome vagal innervation is excitatory and acts via nicotinic cholinoceptors. One striking feature of the cyclostome heart is the location of chromaffin tissue within the heart that stores large quantities of epinephrine and norepinephrine. As in other vertebrates, the circulating catecholamines produced by the chromaffin tissue stimulate beta-adrenergic receptors in the heart. Thus, the cyclostomes appear to have only excitatory mechanisms to regulate the heart.

The elasmobranchs (cartilaginous fish) are the first vertebrates to have a cardioinhibitory vagus. The vagus in these fish is inhibitory and the cholinoceptors on the heart are muscarinic as they are in other vertebrates. The cardioinhibitory vagus is functional in the elasmobranchs as a response to hypoxia. In conditions of hypoxia, metabolic output is adjusted by reducing heart rate. This modification of neural regulation may provide a mechanism to enable the elasmobranchs to increase their territorial range, by providing a neural mechanism that adjusts metabolic output to deal with changes in water temperature and oxygen availability. However, unlike more evolutionarily advanced fish or tetrapods, elasmobranchs do not have direct sympathetic input to the heart. Instead, cardiac acceleration and increases in contractility are mediated via beta-adrenergic receptors stimulated by circulating catecholamines released from chromaffin tissue. Thus, because activation of metabolic output is driven by circulating catecholamines and not by direct neural innervation, once the excitatory system is triggered, the ability to self-soothe or calm is limited.

In vertebrates with sympathetic and vagal neural innervation, vagal influences to the sinoatrial node inhibit or dampen the sympathetic influence and promote rapid decreases in metabolic output[19] that enable almost instantaneous shifts in behavioral state. As a whole, the teleosts may be considered phylogenetically the first class of vertebrates with both sympathetic and parasympathetic neural control of the heart, with innervation similar to that found in tetrapods. This enables rapid transitory changes in metabolic output, permitting changes from mobilization to immobilization. These are observed as "darting" and "freezing" behaviors. Amphibia, similar to the teleosts, have dual innervation of the heart via systems with direct neural components from the spinal cord via the sympathetic chain, producing increases in heart rate and contractility, and direct neural pathways from the brainstem via the vagus, producing cardioinhibitory actions.

True adrenal glands, in which a distinct medulla is formed of chromaffin tissue, are only present in birds, reptiles, and mammals.[16] Neural regulation by the spinal sympathetics of the adrenal medulla provides a neural mechanism for rapid and controlled release of epinephrine and norepinephrine to stimulate cardiovascular function. In teleosts, chromaffin tissue is primarily related to parts of the cardiovascular system, but chromaffin tissue is also associated with the kidney. However, in amphibia, chromaffin tissue is primarily associated with the kidney, and substantial aggregations of chromaffin cells are located along the sympathetic chain ganglia. Thus, we can observe a phylogenetic shift in the location of chromaffin tissue and the concurrent evolution of a distinct adrenal medulla near the kidney.

In mammals the morphology of the vagus changes.[1] Unlike that of all other vertebrates with cardioinhibitory vagi, the mammalian vagus contains two branches. One branch originates in the dorsal motor nucleus of the vagus and provides primary neural regulation of subdiaphragmatic organs such as the digestive tract. However, at the level of the heart, the dorsal motor nucleus of the vagus does not play a major role in normal dynamic regulation of cardiac output. Rather, during embryological development in mammals, cells from the dorsal motor nucleus of the vagus migrate ventrally and laterally to the nucleus ambiguus[20] where they form the cell bodies for visceromotor myelinated axons that provide potent inhibition of the sinoatrial node, the pacemaker for the heart.

By transitory downregulation of the cardioinhibitory vagal tone to the heart (i.e., removal of the vagal brake), the mammal is capable of rapid increases in cardiac output without activating the sympathetic-adrenal system. By engaging this system rather than the sympathetic-adrenal system, mammals have the opportunity to rapidly increase metabolic output for immediate mobilization. Under prolonged challenge, the sympathetic system also may be activated. However, by rapidly reengaging the vagal system, mammals can inhibit sympathetic input on the heart[19] and rapidly decrease metabolic output to self-soothe and calm.

PHYLOGENETIC DEVELOPMENT OF THE AUTONOMIC NERVOUS SYSTEM: AN ORGANIZING PRINCIPLE FOR HUMAN EMOTION

Inspection of TABLE 1, which summarizes the primary regulatory structures of the heart in vertebrates, provides a basis for speculation on the behavioral repertoire of various classes of vertebrates. These speculations support the premise that the phylogenetic development of the autonomic nervous system provides an organizing principle for affective experiences and determines the limits on social behavior and, therefore, the possibility of affiliation. Phylogenetic development generally results in increased neural control of the heart via mechanisms that can rapidly increase or decrease metabolic output. This phylogenetic course results in greater central nervous system regulation of behavior, especially behaviors to engage and disengage with environmental challenges.

To further focus on the impact of phylogenetic development of the neural regulation of the autonomic nervous system, we can observe five phylogenetically dependent response systems: (1) a *chemical excitatory system* via the catecholamine-rich chromaffin tissue to increase cardiac output and to support mobilization; (2) an *inhibitory vagal system* via the dorsal motor nucleus of the vagus to reduce cardiac output when metabolic resources are scarce and to support immobilization in response to danger; (3) a *spinal sympathetic nervous system* to provide neural excitation to promote rapid mobilization for behaviors associated with fight and flight; (4) A neurally regulated *adrenal medulla system* to provide more direct control over the release of circulating catecholamines to support mobilization for the prolonged metabolic requirements of fight or flight behaviors; (5) the specialization of the *mammalian vagal system* into a "tonic" inhibitory system that allows graded withdrawal of the vagal brake, which can promote transitory mobilization and the expression of sympathetic tone without requiring sympathetic or adrenal activation. With this new vagal system, transitory incursions into the environment can be initiated without the severe biological prices of either metabolic shutdown, via primitive vagal inhibition, or metabolic excitation, via sympathetic-adrenal activation.

TABLE 2. Physiological Functions Associated with Each Subsystem of the Autonomic Nervous System

	VVC	SNS	DVC
Heart rate	+/–	+	–
Bronchi	+/–	+	–
Gastrointestinal		–	+
Vasoconstriction		+	
Sweat		+	
Adrenal medulla		+	
Vocalization	+/–		
Facial muscles	+/–		

Abbreviations: VVC = ventral vagal complex; SNS = sympathetic nervous system; DVC = dorsal vagal complex. DVC slows heart rate, constricts bronchi, and stimulates gastrointestinal function. SNS increases heart rate, dilates bronchi, inhibits gastrointestinal function, promotes vasoconstriction, increases sweating, and activates catecholamine release from the adrenal medulla. Depending on the degree of neural tone, VVC either slows or speeds heart rate, constricts or dilates bronchi, lowers or raises vocalization pitch, and increases or decreases facial expressivity.

The five phylogenetically dependent response systems are associated with three neuroanatomical constructs related to affective experience and expression: (1) dorsal vagal complex (DVC), (2) sympathetic nervous system (SNS), and (3) ventral vagal complex (VVC). Each of these three neural constructs is linked to a specific emotion subsystem observable in humans. Each emotion subsystem is manifested via differentiated motor output from the central nervous system to perform specific adaptive functions: to immobilize and conserve metabolic resources, to mobilize in order to obtain metabolic resources, or to signal with minimal energy expense. The constituent responses associated with each subsystem are listed in TABLE 2.

DORSAL VAGAL COMPLEX: A VESTIGIAL IMMOBILIZATION SYSTEM

The dorsal vagal complex (DVC) is primarily associated with digestive, taste, and hypoxic responses in mammals. It includes the nucleus tractus solitarius (NTS) and the interneuronal communication between the NTS and the dorsal motor nucleus of the vagus (DMX). The efferents for the DVC originate in the DMX and primary vagal afferents terminate in the NTS. The DVC provides primary neural control of subdiaphragmatic visceral organs. It provides low tonic influences on the heart and bronchi. This low tonic influence is the vestige from the reptilian vagal control of the heart and lung. In contrast to reptiles, mammals have a great demand for oxygen and are vulnerable to any depletion in oxygen resources. The metabolic demand for mammals is approximately five times greater than that for reptiles of equivalent body weight.[21] Thus, reptilian dependence on this system provides a shutdown of metabolic activity to conserve resources during diving or death feigning. The DVC provides inhibitory input to the sinoatrial node of the heart via unmyelinated fibers and thus is less tightly controlled than the myelinated fibers from the VVC. Hypoxia or perceived loss of oxygen resources appears to be the main stimulus that triggers the DVC. Once triggered, severe bradycardia and apnea are observed, often in the presence of defecation. This response strategy is observed in the hypoxic human fetus. Although adaptive for the reptile, hypoxic triggering of this system may be lethal for mammals. In addition, it is important to note that the DVC has beneficial functions in humans. Under most normal conditions, the DVC maintains tone to the gut and promotes digestive processes. However, if upregulated, the DVC contributes to pathophysiological conditions including the formation of ulcers via excess gastric secretion and colitis. Recent research supports the importance of the unmyelinated vagal fibers in bradycardia[22] and suggests the possibility that massive bradycardia may be determined by the unmyelinated vagal fibers associated with the DVC recruiting myelinated vagal fibers to maximize the final vagal surge on the heart.[23]

THE SYMPATHETIC NERVOUS SYSTEM: ADAPTIVE MOBILIZATION SYSTEM FOR FIGHT OR FLIGHT BEHAVIORS

The sympathetic nervous system is primarily a system of mobilization. It prepares the body for emergency by increasing cardiac output, stimulating sweat glands to protect and lubricate the skin, and inhibiting the metabolically costly gastrointestinal tract. The evolution of the sympathetic nervous system follows the segmentation of the spinal cord, with cell bodies of the preganglionic sympathetic motor neurons located in the lateral horn of the spinal cord. The sympathetic nervous system has long been associated with emotion. The label ''sympathetic'' reflects the historical identity of this system as a nervous system ''with feelings'' and contrasts it with the parasympathetic nervous system, a label that reflects a nervous system that ''guards against feelings.''

VENTRAL VAGAL COMPLEX: THE MAMMALIAN SIGNALING SYSTEM FOR MOTION, EMOTION, AND COMMUNICATION

The primary efferent fibers of the ventral vagal complex (VVC) originate in the nucleus ambiguus. The primary afferent fibers of the VVC terminate in the source nuclei of the facial and trigeminal nerves. The VVC has primary control of supradiaphragmatic visceral organs including the larynx, pharynx, bronchi, esophagus, and heart. Motor pathways from the VVC to visceromotor organs (e.g., heart and bronchi) and somatomotor structures (e.g., larynx, pharynx, and esophagus) are myelinated to provide tight control and speed in responding. In mammals, visceromotor fibers to the heart express high levels of tonic control and are capable of rapid shifts in cardioinhibitory tone to provide dynamic changes in metabolic output to match environmental challenges. This rapid regulation characterizes the qualities of the mammalian vagal brake that enable rapid engagement and disengagement in the environment without mobilizing the sympathetics.

A major characteristic of the VVC is that the neural fibers regulating somatomotor structures are derived from the branchial or primitive gill arches that evolved to form cranial nerves V, VII, IX, X, and XI. Somatomotor fibers originating in these cranial nerves control the branchiomeric muscles including facial muscles, muscles of mastication, neck muscles, larynx, pharynx, esophagus, and middle ear muscles. Visceromotor efferent fibers control salivary and lacrimal glands as well as the heart and bronchi. The primary afferents to the VVC come from facial and oral afferents traveling through the facial and trigeminal nerves and the visceral afferents, terminating in the nucleus tractus solitarius. The VVC is involved in the control and coordination of sucking, swallowing, and vocalizing with breathing.

EVOLUTION AND DISSOLUTION: HIERARCHICAL RESPONSE STRATEGY

The evolution of the autonomic nervous system provides substrates for the emergence of three emotion systems. This phylogenetic adjustment of the autonomic nervous system represents an exaptation (see Crews, this volume) of structures to express emotions that initially evolved in primitive vertebrates to extract oxygen from water, to oxygenate and transport blood, and to adjust metabolic output to match resources. The polyvagal theory of emotion is based on a phylogenetic model. The polyvagal theory of emotion proposes a hierarchical response strategy to challenge, with the most recent modifications employed first and the most primitive last. This phylogenetic strategy can be observed in our day-to-day interactions. Our social behavior follows a strategy that focuses initially on communication via facial expressions and vocalizations. This strategy has low metabolic demand and, if appropriately interpreted, results in contingent social interactions via verbal-facial mechanisms. Often, hand gestures and head movements contribute to increase the mammalian repertoire of communication-related behavior. An important characteristic of these prosocial behaviors is their low metabolic demand and the rapid contingent "switching" of transitory engagement to transitory disengagement strategies (i.e., speaking then switching to listening).

This phylogenetically based hierarchical response strategy is consistent with the concept of dissolution proposed by Jackson[24] to explain diseases of the nervous system. Jackson proposed that "the higher nervous arrangements inhibit (or control) the lower, and thus, when the higher are suddenly rendered functionless, the lower rise in activity." This is observed in the polyvagal theory of emotion, not in terms of disease, but in terms of response strategies to differential challenges to survival. The VVC with its mechanisms of "signaling" and "communication" provides the initial response to the environment. The VVC inhibits, at the level of the heart, the strong mobilization responses of the sympathetic nervous system. Withdrawal of VVC, consistent with Jackson's model, results in a "disinhibition" of the sympathetic control of the heart. Similarly, withdrawal of sympathetic tone results in a "disinhibition" of the DVC control of the gastrointestinal tract and a vulnerability of the bronchi and heart. There are several clinical consequences to unopposed DVC control including defecation, due to relaxation of the sphincter muscles and increased motility of the digestive tract, apnea, due to constriction of the bronchi, and bradycardia, due to stimulation of the sinoatrial node. Thus, when all else fails, the nervous system elects a metabolically conservative course that is adaptive for primitive vertebrates, but lethal to mammals. Consistent with the Jacksonian principle of dissolution, specific psychopathologies defined by affective dysfunction may be associated with autonomic correlates consistent with the three phylogenetic levels of autonomic regulation. The three levels do not function in an all-or-none fashion; rather, they exhibit gradations of control determined by both visceral feedback and higher brain structures.

UNVEILING DARWIN

Contemporary research and theory on emotion owes much to Darwin and his volume, *The Expression of Emotions in Man and Animals.*[8] Through careful and astute observations of facial expressions, Darwin insightfully interpreted emotional expressions within an evolutionary model of adaptation and natural selection. However, Darwin's knowledge of neurophysiology and neuroanatomy was limited. In contrast to Darwin's creative insights into the adaptive function of facial expression, his understanding of underlying physiological mechanisms and the linkage between facial muscles and emotion was synthetic and derivative. He repeatedly referenced the 1844 edition of *Anatomy and Philosophy of Expressions,* written by Sir Charles Bell, for physiological explanations of facial expression. As further support for the importance of facial muscles in emotional expressions, Darwin incorporated the work of Duchenne in his text. Duchenne conducted experiments by electrically stimulating the face of humans. Electrical stimulation of selected facial muscles provided expressions that were readily perceived as different emotional states.

In contrast to the polyvagal theory of emotion, which uses evolution of the autonomic nervous system as the primary organizing principle for the expression and experience of affect, Darwin's writings did not emphasize the importance of the nervous system as a structure involved in the evolution of emotion. Rather he focused on affect as a functional system that responded to the determinants of evolution to produce the facial and vocal expressions of human emotion. Darwin neglected the importance of treating the nervous system as a structure that is vulnerable to the pressures of evolution. A choice between investigating affect as a functional behavioral system or investigating the structural determinants of affect (i.e., nervous system) was clearly made by researchers who followed Darwin. This research tradition followed the observational approach of organizing facial expression into affective categories. Although the physiological correlates of affect and facial expression were investigated,[6,7,25] these investigations were made on a psychophysiological or correlative level and did not emphasize specific neural regulatory processes.

Consistent with the observational approach, Tomkins[26,27] developed a theory of affect that emphasized the importance of the face not only as a structure of communication, but also as a structure of self-feedback. Following Tomkins,[26,27] Ekman[28] and Izard[29] developed detailed coding systems for facial affect and have used these methods to study individual differences, developmental shifts, and the cross-cultural consistency of human facial expression.

Several contemporary theories of emotion have focused on facial expressions in a manner similar to that initially presented by Darwin. Rather than incorporating knowledge of neural regulation of the face or the evolution of neural regulation of autonomic function, researchers and theorists have attempted to organize information in terms of the functional significance of sequences or patterns of facial expressions. This difficult task, modeled on Darwin, often becomes bogged down in semantics, philosophical inconsistencies, and circularity. Darwin in his descriptions of emotions speculated and provided hypothetical examples of natural selection contributing to the uniqueness of species-specific affective response patterns. However, the terms selected to characterize specific emotions often vary from culture to culture. Tomkins and later Ekman and Izard promoted the description of affective experiences in terms of the specific facial muscles or groups of muscles involved in the facial expression. However, they then used subjective reports to label these facial expressions.

We may "unveil" Darwin by investigating the neural regulation that underlies facial expression. Facial expressions are controlled by cranial nerves. Motor pathways from the trigeminal nerve (V) control the muscles of mastication with branches to the temporalis, masseter, medial, and lateral pterygoid muscles. Motor pathways from the facial nerve (VII) control the muscles of facial expression including zygomaticus, frontalis, orbicularis oculi, elevators, orbicularis oris, depressors, and platysma. Nucleus ambiguus serves as the source of cell bodies for motor pathways traveling through several cranial nerves including the glossopharyngeal (IX), vagus (X), and accessory nerves (XI). Pathways from the glossopharyngeal nerve regulate pharyngeal muscles. Pathways from the vagus regulate the muscles of the pharynx and larynx, and pathways of the accessory nerve control the neck muscles, allowing rotation and tilting of the head. These cranial nerves are derivative from primitive gill arches[30,31] and may be collectively described as the ventral vagal complex. Thus, the evolutionary origins (i.e., primitive gill arches) of the somatomotor pathways traveling through these cranial nerves provide us with an organizing principle to understand affective expressions. In addition to the aforedescribed neural regulation of somatomotor structures, these branchiomeric (i.e., derived from the primitive arches) cranial nerves also regulate the visceromotor processes associated with salivation, tearing, breathing, and heart rate.

Other cranial nerves contribute to the expression of emotions. The hypoglossal nerve (XII) innervates the muscles of the tongue. The trochlear (IV), abducens (VI), and oculomotor (III) nerves innervate muscles to provide movements of the eyes and eyelids. Thus, the facial expressions observed by Darwin, detailed by Tomkins, and coded by Ekman and Izard are a direct reflection of the regulation of the face by the cranial nerves.

VOODOO OR VAGUS DEATH?: THE TEST OF THE POLYVAGAL THEORY

The polyvagal theory of emotion provides a theoretical framework to interpret the phenomenon of voodoo or fright death described by Cannon[32] and Richter.[33] Cannon believed that extreme emotional stress, regardless of the specific behavioral manifestation, could be explained in terms of degree of sympathetic-adrenal excitation. In 1942 Cannon described a phenomenon known as voodoo death. Voodoo death was assumed to be directly attributable to emotional stress. Being wed to a sympathico-adrenal model of emotional experience (as just described), Cannon assumed that voodoo death would be the consequence of the state of shock produced by the continuous outpouring of epinephrine via excitation of the sympathetic nervous system. According to the Cannon model, the victim would be expected to breathe very rapidly and have a rapid pulse. The heart would beat fast and gradually lead to a state of constant contraction and, ultimately, to death in systole. Because his speculations were not empirically based, he offered the following challenge to test his model of voodoo death: ''If in the future, however, any observer has opportunity to see an instance of ''voodoo death,'' it is to be hoped that he will conduct the simpler tests before the victim's last gasp.''

Richter responded to Cannon's challenge with an animal model. Rats were prestressed and placed in a closed turbulent water tank, and the latency to drowning was recorded. Most domestic laboratory rats lasted for several hours, whereas unexpectedly all of the wild rats died within 15 minutes. In fact, several wild rats dove to the bottom and, without coming to the surface, died. To test Cannon's hypothesis that stress-induced sudden death was sympathetic, Richter monitored heart rate and determined whether the heart was in systole or diastole after death. He assumed, on the basis of Cannon's speculations, that tachycardia would precede death and that at death the heart would be in a state of systole, reflecting the potent effects of sympathetic excitation on the pacemaker and the myocardium. However, Richter's data contradicted the Cannon model. Heart rate slowed prior to death, and at death the heart was engorged with blood, reflecting a state of diastole. Richter interpreted the data as demonstrating that the rats died a ''vagus'' death, the result of overstimulation of the parasympathetic system rather than the sympathico-adrenal system. However, Richter provided no physiological explanation except the speculation that the lethal vagal effect was related to a psychological state of ''hopelessness.''

The immediate and reliable death of the wild rats in Richter's experiment may represent a more global immobilization strategy. Sudden prolonged immobility or feigned death is an adaptive response exhibited by many mammalian species. Hofer[34] demonstrated that several rodent species, when threatened, exhibited prolonged immobility accompanied by very slow heart rate. For some of the rodents, heart rate during immobility was less than 50% of the basal rate. During prolonged immobility respiration become so shallow that it was difficult to observe, although the rate greatly accelerated. Although physiologically similar, Hofer distinguished between prolonged immobility and feigned death. The onset of feigned death was sudden with an apparent motor collapse during active struggling. Similar to Richter, Hofer interpreted this fear-induced slowing of heart rate as a vagal phenomenon. In support of this interpretation, he noted that of the four species that exhibited prolonged immobility, 71% of the subjects had cardiac arrhythmias of vagal origin; in contrast, in the two species that did not exhibit immobility behaviors, only 17% exhibited cardiac arrhythmias of vagal origin.

The polyvagal theory of emotion places Richter and Hofer's observations in perspective. Following the Jacksonian principle of dissolution, the rodents would exhibit the following sequence of response strategies: (1) removal of VVC tone, (2) increase in sympathetic tone, and (3) a surge in DVC tone. The more docile domestic rats in Richter's experiment apparently progressed from removal of VVC tone, to increased sympathetic tone, and then death from exhaustion. However, the profile of the wild rats was different. Being totally unaccustomed to enclosure, handling, and also having their vibrissae cut, a mobilization strategy driven by increased sympathetic tone was not functional. Instead, these rats reverted to their most primitive system to conserve metabolic resources via DVC. This strategy promoted an immobilization response characterized by reduced motor activity, apnea, and bradycardia. Unfortunately, this mode of responding, although adaptive for reptiles, is lethal for mammals. Similarly, the onset of feigned death, as described by Hofer, illustrates the sudden and rapid transition from an unsuccessful strategy of struggling requiring massive sympathetic activation to the metabolically conservative immobilized state mimicking death associated with the DVC.

These data suggest that the vagus contributes to severe emotional states and may be related to emotional states of "immobilization" such as extreme terror. Application of the polyvagal approach enables the dissection of vagal processes into three strategic programs: (1) when tone of the VVC is high, the ability to communicate via facial expressions, vocalizations, and gestures exists; (2) when tone of the VVC is low, the sympathetic nervous system is unopposed and easily expressed to support mobilization such as fight or flight behaviors; and (3) when tone from DVC is high, immobilization and potentially life-threatening bradycardia, apnea, and cardiac arrhythmias occur.

CONCLUSION

Three important scientific propositions provide the basis for this theory. First, Darwin provided the concept of evolution and the processes that contribute to phylogenetic variation. Second, Jackson provided the concept of dissolution as a viable explanation for diseases of brain function. And, third, MacLean[35] provided the concept that the human brain retains structures associated with phylogenetically more primitive organisms.

The polyvagal theory of emotion focuses on the evolution of the neural and neurochemical regulation of structures involved in the expression and experience of emotion as a theme to organize emotional experience and to understand the role of emotion in social behavior. Over 100 years ago Jackson, intrigued with Darwin's model of evolution, elaborated on how evolution in reverse, termed "dissolution," might be related to disease. According to Jackson, higher nervous system structures inhibit or control lower structures or systems and "thus, when the higher are suddenly rendered functionless, the lower rise in activity." The polyvagal theory of emotion follows this Jacksonian principle.

ACKNOWLEDGMENTS

Special thanks are extended to Sue Carter for encouraging me to formalize the ideas presented in this paper. In addition, I would like to thank Jane Doussard-Roosevelt for commenting on earlier drafts and the students in my graduate seminar who provided a forum for the discussion of the concepts described in the Polyvagal Theory of Emotion.

REFERENCES

1. PORGES, S. W. 1995. Orienting in a defensive world: Mammalian modifications of our evolutionary heritage. A polyvagal theory. Psychophysiology **32:** 301-318.

2. CANNON, W. B. 1927. The James-Lange theory of emotions: A critical examination and an alternative theory. Am. J. Psychol. **39:** 106-124.
3. CANNON, W. B. 1928. The mechanism of emotional disturbance of bodily functions. N. Engl. J. Med. **198:** 877-884.
4. AX, A. F. 1953. The physiological differentiation between fear and anger in humans. Psychosom. Med. **15:** 433-442.
5. SCHACHTER, J. 1957. Pain, fear, and anger in hypertensives and normotensives: A psychophysiological study. Psychosom. Med. **19:** 17-29.
6. EKMAN, P., R. W. LEVENSON & W. V. FRIESEN. 1983. Autonomic nervous system activity distinguishes between emotions. Science **221:** 1208-1210.
7. LEVENSON, R. W., P. EKMAN & W. V. FRIESEN. 1990. Voluntary facial action generates emotion-specific autonomic nervous system activity. Psychophysiology **27:** 363-384.
8. DARWIN, C. 1872. The Expression of Emotions in Man and Animals. D. Appleton. New York.
9. PORGES, S. W. 1991. Vagal tone: An autonomic mediator of affect. *In* The Development of Affect Regulation and Dysregulation. J. A. Garber & K. A. Dodge, Eds.: 111-128. Cambridge University Press. New York.
10. PORGES, S. W., J. A. DOUSSARD-ROOSEVELT & A. K. MAITI. 1994. Vagal tone and the physiological regulation of emotion. *In* Emotion Regulation: Behavioral and Biological Considerations. Monograph of the Society for Research in Child Development. N. A. Fox, Ed. **59:** (2-3, Serial No. 240): 167-186.
11. PORGES, S. W. & J. A. DOUSSARD-ROOSEVELT. The psychophysiology of temperament. *In* The Handbook of Child and Adolescent Psychiatry. J. D. Noshpitz, Ed. Wiley Press. New York. In press.
12. PORGES, S. W., J. A. DOUSSARD-ROOSEVELT, A. L. PORTALES & S. I. GREENSPAN. 1996. Infant regulation of the vagal "brake" predicts child behavior problems: A psychobiological model of social behavior. Dev. Psychobiol. **29:** in press.
13. PORGES, S. W. 1992. Vagal Tone: A physiological marker of stress vulnerability. Pediatrics **90:** 498-504.
14. PORGES, S. W. 1995. Cardiac vagal tone: A physiological index of stress. Neurosci. Biobehav. Rev. **19:** 225-233.
15. PORGES, S. W., J. A. DOUSSARD-ROOSEVELT, A. L. PORTALES & P. E. SUESS. 1994. Cardiac vagal tone: Stability and relation to difficultness in infants and three-year-old children. Dev. Psychobiol. **27:** 289-300.
16. SANTER, R. M. 1994. Chromaffin systems. *In* Comparative Physiology and Evolution of the Autonomic Nervous System. S. Nilsson & S. Holmgren, Eds.: 97-117. Harwood Academic Publishers. Switzerland.
17. MORRIS, J. L. & S. NILSSON. 1994. The Circulatory System. *In* Comparative Physiology and Evolution of the Autonomic Nervous System. S. Nilsson & S. Holmgren, Eds.: 193-246. Harwood Academic Publishers. Switzerland.
18. TAYLOR, E. W. 1992. Nervous control of the heart and cardiorespiratory interactions. *In* Fish Physiology: The Cardiovascular System. W. S. Hoar, D. J. Randall & A. P. Farrell, Eds. **12:** (Part B) 343-387. Academic Press. New York.
19. VANHOUTTE, P. M. & M. N. LEVY. 1979. Cholinergic inhibition of adrenergic neurotransmission in the cardiovascular system. *In* Integrative Functions of the Autonomic Nervous System. C. McC. Brooks, K. Koizumi & A. Sato, Eds.: 159-176. University of Tokyo Press. Tokyo.
20. SCHWABER, J. S. 1986. Neuroanatomical substrates of cardiovascular and emotional-autonomic regulation. *In* Central and Peripheral Mechanisms of Cardiovascular Regulation. A. Magro, W. Osswald, D. Reis & P. Vanhoutte, Eds.: 353-384. Plenum Press. New York.
21. ELSE, P. L. & A. J. HULBERT. 1981. Comparison of the "mammal machine" and the "reptile machine:" Energy production. Am. J. Physiol. **240:** R3-R9.

22. DALY, M. DEBURGH. 1991. Some reflex cardioinhibitory responses in the cat and their modulation by central inspiratory neuronal activity. J. Physiol. **422:** 463-480.
23. JONES, J. F. X., Y. WANG & D. JORDAN. 1995. Heart rate responses to selective stimulation of cardiac vagal C fibres in anesthetized cats, rats and rabbits. J. Physiol. **489:** 203-214.
24. JACKSON, J. H. 1958. Evolution and dissolution of the nervous system. *In* Selected Writings of John Hughlings Jackson. J. Taylor, Ed.: 45-118. Stapes Press. London.
25. STIFTER, C. A., N. A. FOX & S. W. PORGES. 1989. Facial expressivity and vagal tone in five- and ten-month old infants. Infant Behav. **12:** 127-137.
26. TOMKINS, S. S. 1962. Affect, Imagery, Consciousness. Vol. 1. The Positive Affects. Springer. New York.
27. TOMKINS, S. S. 1963. Affect, Imagery, Consciousness. Vol 2. The Negative Affects. Springer. New York.
28. EKMAN, P. 1978. Facial Action Coding System: A Technique for the Measurement of Facial Movement. Consulting Psychologists Press. Palo Alto, CA.
29. IZARD, C. E. 1979. The Maximally Discriminative Facial Movement Coding System (MAX). University of Delaware Instructional Resource Center. Newark, DE.
30. GIBBINS, I. 1994. Comparative anatomy and evolution of the autonomic nervous system. *In* Comparative Physiology and Evolution of the Autonomic Nervous System. S. Nilsson & S. Holmgren, Eds. Harwood Academic Publishers. Singapore.
31. LANGLEY, J. N. 1921. The Autonomic Nervous System. Part I. W. Heffer and Sons. Cambridge.
32. CANNON, W. B. 1957. ''Voodoo'' death. Psychosom. Med. **19:** 182-190. (Reprinted from: 1942. Am. Anthropol. **44:** 169.)
33. RICHTER, C. P. 1957. On the phenomenon of sudden death in animals and man. Psychosom. Med. **19:** 191-198.
34. HOFER, M. A. 1970. Cardiac respiratory function during sudden prolonged immobility in wild rodents. Psychosom. Med. **32:** 633-647.
35. MACLEAN, P. D. 1990. The Triune Brain in Evolution. Plenum Press. New York.

II
Organismic Perspectives on Affiliation and Social Behavior

5
Psychobiological Consequences of Social Relationships

S. Levine, D. M. Lyons, and A. F. Schatzberg

Social psychobiological research, and particularly research on affiliation, has increased dramatically in the last 25 years (FIG. 1). In 1971, fewer than 30 published reference citations in the MEDLINE database were keyword indexed under "affiliation," whereas 516 citations were indexed under "aggression." In 1994, more than 270 citations were indexed under "affiliation" (10-fold increase), whereas 475 citations were indexed under "aggression" (8% decrease). To review this large and diverse literature is impossible to accomplish in this report, so we have taken the following approach. First, we briefly describe social life-span development in squirrel monkeys, a gregarious New World primate that lives in complex groups. Then we discuss social effects on squirrel monkey hypothalamic-pituitary-adrenal (HPA) physiology, focusing on factors that activate or inhibit HPA-axis activity, resulting in increases or decreases in the secretion of cortisol from the adrenal cortex. After characterizing the effects of both social separation and social buffering on stress-induced increases in plasma cortisol, we close with indications for comparative research in human and nonhuman primates.

SOCIAL PSYCHOLOGICAL EFFECTS ON ADRENOCORTICAL ACTIVITY

Squirrel monkeys (*Saimiri sciureus*) are small arboreal primates that live in large groups comprised of males and females in all stages of development. A salient characteristic of these groups is the segregation of males and females into affiliative like-sex subgroups.[1] Around puberty, at 2-3 years of age, subadult males begin to associate with males, and females associate with females. In free-ranging, semi-free ranging, and captive settings, males and females within a group also spend most of

This work was supported by grant MH47573 from the National Institute of Mental Health.

Address for correspondence: David Lyons, Department of Psychiatry and Behavioral Sciences, Stanford University School of Medicine, MSLS P111, Stanford, CA 94305-5485 (tel: 415/725-5931; fax: 415/725-5936; e-mail: david.lyons@forsythe.stanford.edu).

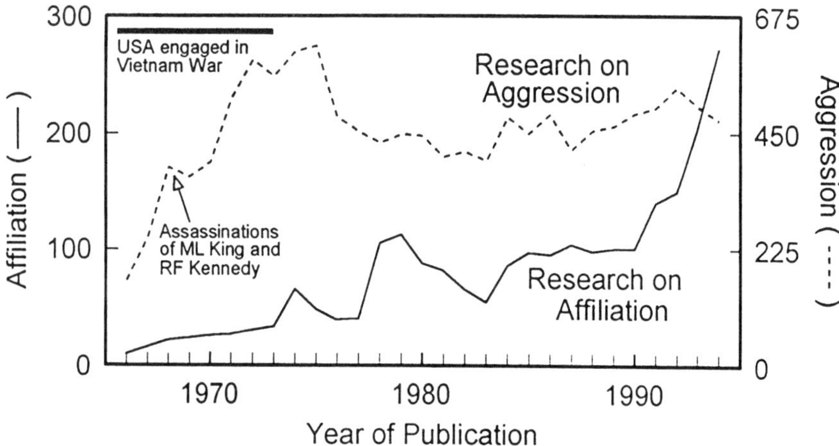

FIGURE 1. Number of published reference citations keyword indexed in the MEDLINE database at yearly intervals from 1966-1994.

their time with like-sex companions in adulthood, and social transactions between the sexes are generally limited to seasonal mating activities. Five months after mating, infants are born and raised by their mothers in groups in which sexual segregation is the norm.

In keeping with reports that emotional arousal plays a causal role in the formation and maintenance of social bonds,[2-4] our initial studies of squirrel monkey adrenocortical activity involved an extensive series of experiments on the psychobiology of mother-infant relationships. This research showed that social separations produce striking increases in cortisol in both mothers and infants.[5,6] Robust adrenocortical responses occur even after multiple separations with little evidence of habituation in infants.[7] We also showed that the magnitude of this physiological effect is at least partly dependent on the degree of social support available to infants.[8] In the company of other mothers and/or familiar peers, social buffering of stress-induced increases in cortisol is apparent.[9] Dramatic increases in cortisol occur during maternal separations when infants are placed in novel environments. Cortisol responses in infants placed in cages adjacent to their mothers are significantly lower than those in isolated infants, but higher than those in maternally separated infants that remain with familiar social companions in their natal group. Although most mother-infant studies are based on maternal separations of short duration (less than 24 hours), we know that social buffering of adrenocortical activity occurs over longer time scales as well. Following maternal separations at weaning, in the absence of familiar social companions cortisol levels in 6-7-month-old juvenile monkeys remain elevated for more than 7 days.[10]

Long-lasting increases in cortisol also occur in subadults and adults. After separation from peers, cortisol levels in subadult males and females housed for 21 days without companions are 18-87% higher than those observed when the same monkeys are housed with like-sex companions in established social groups.[11] Whether this chronic hypersecretion of cortisol is due specifically to the absence of like-sex companionship remains to be determined in subadults, but this is apparently the case in adults. Hypersecretion of cortisol occurs not only when adults are separated from like-sex companions and housed alone,[12] but also when adult males and females are housed without like-sex companions in male-female pairs, and when adult males are housed without male companions in single male, multifemale groups.[13] As generally found in diurnally active animals, plasma cortisol levels are highest just before or just after lights are turned on and lowest just before or just after lights are turned off.[14] Preliminary results suggest this pattern is maintained, but at higher levels across the 24-hour cycle, in singly housed subadults[15] and adults.[16]

BIOLOGICAL BASES OF HYPERCORTISOLISM IN SQUIRREL MONKEYS

One explanation for these findings is that hypersecretion of cortisol reflects a deficiency in glucocorticoid feedback mechanisms that normally inhibit prolonged activation of the adrenal cortex.[11,12,17] We know from earlier research that the squirrel monkey's adrenocortical response to physical restraint is minimally susceptible to the inhibitory effects of dexamethasone,[18] and significantly more dexamethasone is required to suppress baseline cortisol in squirrel monkeys than in humans, titi monkeys, and macaques.[19,20] Similar metabolic clearance rates for cortisol are evident in squirrel monkeys, humans, and macaques,[18,21] but the production rate of cortisol in squirrel monkeys is high,[21,22] and the cortisol-binding capacity of squirrel monkey plasma is low.[23,24] Although the amount of unbound (free) cortisol in squirrel monkeys and other New World primates is greater than that in humans, baboons, or macaques,[20,24] receptor affinities for cortisol in squirrel monkey lymphocytes and skin fibroblasts are strikingly low.[20] In addition to dampening deleterious peripheral effects of hypercortisolism[25] (e.g., during social separations, squirrel monkeys do not develop cushingoid features), low receptor affinities for cortisol in the central nervous system should reduce the effectiveness of cortisol as a negative feedback signal that inhibits biosynthesis and release of pituitary adrenocorticotropic hormone (ACTH). Social separation-induced hypercortisolism might therefore be driven by a long-lasting ACTH response.

To test the hypothesis that hypersecretion of cortisol is due to hypersecretion of ACTH, we collected serial plasma measures of pituitary-adrenal activity from 15 males and 15 females (18-20 months of age) that were housed (1) in established like-sex social groups (*baseline controls*), (2) alone for 21 days in individual cages (*social separations*), and (3) in novel social groups with unfamiliar like-sex companions (*group formations*).[11] Three issues raised by this longitudinal analysis (FIG. 2) deserve comment.

First, we found that when monkeys were separated from groups and housed alone, cortisol levels remained elevated above pre-separation control values, while simultaneous measures of ACTH were significantly reduced. Conversely, during group formations, reductions in cortisol were accompanied by increases in ACTH. These findings suggest that hypersecretion of cortisol does indeed have long-lasting inhibitory effects on ACTH biosynthesis or release and that contrary to expectations, hypersecretion of cortisol is not a consequence of chronic hypersecretion of ACTH.

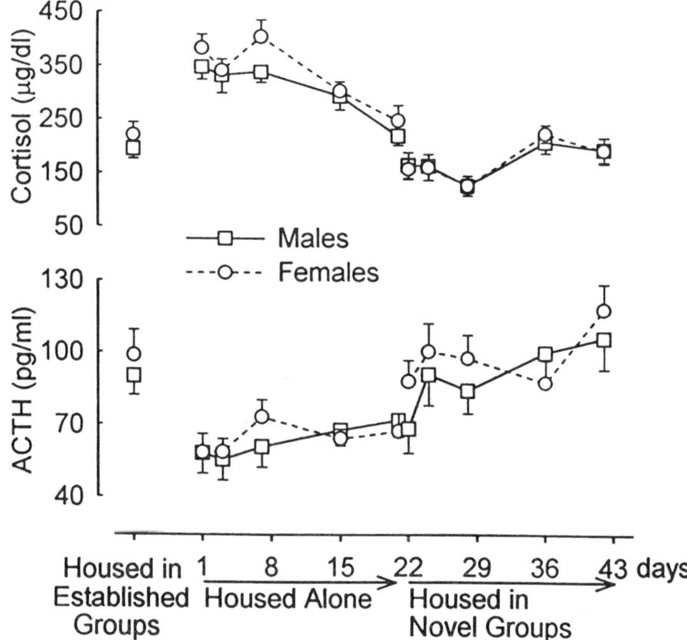

FIGURE 2. Longitudinal changes in plasma cortisol and ACTH (mean ± SEM) in subadult males and females housed in previously established like-sex social groups, housed alone for 21 days in individual cages, and housed in newly formed groups with unfamiliar like-sex social companions. Differences between the sexes are not significant. Based on Lyons & Levine.[11]

Second, we found that in newly formed groups adrenocortical activity was significantly lower than that observed when the same monkeys were housed alone. Apart from low levels of cortisol on the seventh day of group formations, no significant differences were noted in adrenocortical measures collected from monkeys housed with like-sex companions in previously established or newly formed social groups. These results are surprising, because novelty, uncertainty, and lack of predictability are psychogenic factors known to activate HPA-axis activity in a variety of animals, and increased cortisol levels have previously been reported in newly formed squirrel monkey groups.[26,27] Recent evidence suggests, however, that group formation-induced changes in adrenocortical activity probably depend on a monkey's prior social psychobiological state. Apparently, increases in cortisol occur when monkeys from established groups are separated from familiar companions and formed into novel social groups, whereas reductions in cortisol occur when singly housed monkeys with high cortisol levels are provided with like-sex companionship in newly formed pairs[12,28] or small groups.[29,30]

Finally, our observations indicate that hypercortisolism is maintained despite reductions in ACTH, which implies that adrenal responsiveness to ACTH is enhanced. To test this hypothesis, we recently measured adrenal responsiveness in standard

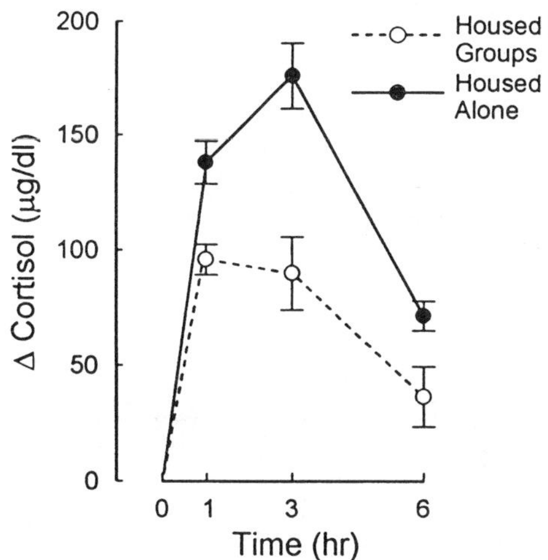

FIGURE 3. Incremental plasma cortisol responses (mean ± SEM) to a morning ACTH stimulation test in dexamethasone-pretreated monkeys that were housed alone (*solid line*) or with like-sex companions in established social groups (*dotted line*). Based on Lyons *et al.*[15]

ACTH stimulation tests administered 7 days after 6 males and 6 females (35-38 months of age) were separated from like-sex social groups and temporarily housed alone.[15] Each monkey was pretreated at 8 PM with a 500 μg/kg body weight im injection of dexamethasone and then challenged the following morning at 8 AM with a 1 μg/kg iv injection of synthetic ACTH. Postdexamethasone blood samples were collected immediately before the ACTH challenge at 8 AM, and additional samples were collected at 1-, 3-, and 6-hour intervals after the ACTH challenge. Adrenocortical response profiles were generated to evaluate the magnitude of change in cortisol after the ACTH challenge by subtracting each monkey's prechallenge cortisol value from each of its three postchallenge values. These quantitative measures of adrenal responsiveness to ACTH were compared with those obtained from 6 males and 6 females housed and tested with like-sex companions in established social groups.

Both group housed and singly housed monkeys responded with significant increases in plasma cortisol when challenged with synthetic ACTH (FIG. 3). Consistently greater, more prolonged responses were apparent in singly housed monkeys, however, whether sample intervals after the challenge were analyzed separately or together as a cumulative integrated response (areas under the curve). Group-housed and singly housed monkeys did not differ in measures of circulating ACTH, and no significant gender-related differences in cortisol or ACTH were noted. We did find significant positive correlations between cortisol responses to synthetic ACTH and postdexamethasone cortisol concentrations in monkeys housed alone (TABLE 1). These relationships were not apparent in monkeys housed in groups. Clinical neuroendocrine research likewise suggests that psychological state-related differences in resistance to the inhibitory effects of dexamethasone may be related to differences in adrenal responsiveness to ACTH during major depressions in humans.[31] Nevertheless, little is known about the development of adrenal hyperresponsiveness to ACTH during either social separations in squirrel monkeys or major depressive disorders in humans.

TABLE 1. Pearson Product-Moment Correlations between Plasma Cortisol Responses to Synthetic ACTH (measured at 1-, 3-, and 6-hour intervals) and Postdexamethasone Cortisol Concentrations in Monkeys Housed Alone or with Like-Sex Companions in Established Social Groups

	Housing	
Interval	In Groups	Alone
1-Hour	−0.37	0.72**
3-Hour	−0.25	0.63*
6-Hour	−0.36	0.61*
Integrated response	−0.38	0.70*

* $p < 0.05$ if $r > 0.55$; ** $p < 0.01$ if $r > 0.68$.

HYPERCORTISOLISM IN HUMAN DEPRESSIONS

The loss or absence of valued social companionship is a well known risk factor in many forms of depression,[32-34] and 40-60% of depressed patients hypersecrete cortisol.[35,36] Some reports suggest this chronic hypersecretion of cortisol is due to hypersecretion of ACTH,[37-39] but more often than not, normal or low ACTH levels have been found.[35,36,40-42] Major depressed patients also show exaggerated cortisol responses to supraphysiological (250 μg), maximal (0.2 μg/kg), and submaximal (0.05 μg/kg) doses of synthetic ACTH,[43] and adrenal hyperresponsiveness to ACTH is a state-dependent outcome that subsides with clinical recovery.[44]

One explanation that may account for these findings is that acute increases in ACTH occur at the onset of depressions, and this subsequently enhances the responsiveness of the adrenal cortex. We know from clinical research that when exogenous synthetic ACTH is administered to healthy humans, the adrenal cortex remains hyperresponsive to subsequent ACTH stimulation for days.[45] This long-lasting "potentiation" effect does not require continuous exposure to high levels of ACTH. Adrenal hyperresponsiveness persists after a single ACTH infusion even when chronic 7-day dexamethasone treatments are used to maintain low circulating levels of endogenous ACTH.[46]

This outcome may reflect well known trophic effects of ACTH on the adrenal cortex[47] or long-lasting stimulatory effects on adrenocortical enzyme systems involved in glucocorticosteroid biosynthesis.[48] In keeping with the former possibility, recent radiographic evidence suggests that adrenal glands in depressed patients are enlarged.[49-51] This almost certainly is due to adrenocortical and not adrenomedullary enlargement, because the medulla comprises a small part of the adrenal gland and, unlike the adrenal cortex, has not shown the capacity to change in size after physiological perturbations such as chronic stress.

An alternative possibility is that state-dependent changes in adrenal responsiveness to ACTH reflect regulatory changes induced by hypothalamic-pituitary hormones other than ACTH, such as corticotropin-releasing hormone,[52] melanotropin,[53] or β-endorphin.[54] Extrapituitary mechanisms might also play a role by altering adrenal glucocorticoid biosynthesis or release.[55-58]

SUMMARY AND CONCLUSIONS

Social separations can induce long-lasting increases in cortisol, whereas companionship can result in social buffering. Preliminary evidence from studies of squirrel monkeys suggests that social separation-induced hypersecretion of cortisol is initially driven by hypersecretion of ACTH. From 1-21 days postseparation, however, cortisol remains elevated above pre-separation controls, while ACTH levels are consistently reduced. Hypercortisolism is maintained despite reductions in ACTH, because adrenal responsiveness to ACTH is enhanced. Low circulating ACTH, in turn, is maintained by robust feedback mechanisms that apparently inhibit biosynthesis or release of pituitary ACTH. These findings are consistent with neuroendocrine interactions known or hypothesized to occur during major depressive disorders in humans and raise unique possibilities for comparative research in human and nonhuman primates.

ACKNOWLEDGMENTS

We thank G. Ha, J. Kim, S. Kim, E. Olson, L. Steffey, D. Woo, and L. Yip for assistance with sample collections and S. Lindley, F. Martel, K. Pakianathon, and P. Patel for constructive comments on this research.

REFERENCES

1. Lyons, D. M., S. P. Mendoza & W. A. Mason. 1992. J. Comp. Psychol. **106:** 323-330.
2. Scott, J. P. 1969. Ann. N.Y. Acad. Sci. **159:** 777-796.
3. Mason, W. A. 1971. *In* Nebraska Symposium on Motivation. W. H. Arnold & M. M. Page, Eds. 35-67. University of Nebraska Press. Lincoln, NE.
4. Lyons, D. M., E. O. Price & G. P. Moberg. 1993. Dev. Psychobiol. **26:** 251-259.
5. Mendoza, S. P., W. P. Smotherman, M. T. Miner, J. Kaplan & S. Levine. 1978. Dev. Psychobiol. **11:** 169-175.
6. Levine, S., C. L. Coe & W. P. Smotherman. 1978. Physiol. Behav. **20:** 7-10.
7. Hennessy, M. B. 1986. Physiol. Behav. **36:** 245-250.
8. Levine, S. 1993. Ann. N.Y. Acad. Sci. **697:** 61-69.
9. Wiener, S. G., F. Bayart, K. F. Faull & S. Levine. 1990. Behav. Neurosci. **104:** 108-115.
10. Wiener, S. G., E. L. Lowe & S. Levine. 1992. Psychobiology **20:** 65-70.
11. Lyons, D. M. & S. Levine. 1994. Psychoneuroendocrinology **19:** 283-291.
12. Mendoza, S. P., M. B. Hennessy & D. M. Lyons. 1992. Psychobiology **20:** 300-306.
13. Mendoza, S. P., W. Saltzman, D. M. Lyons, P. A. Schiml & W. A. Mason. 1991. *In* Primatology Today. A. Ehara, T. Kimura, O. Takenaka & M. Iwamoto, Eds.: 443-446. Elsevier. Amsterdam, the Netherlands.
14. Coe, C. L. & S. Levine. 1995. Am. J. Primatol. **35:** 283-292.
15. Lyons, D. M., C. M. G. Ha & S. Levine. 1995. Horm. Behav. **29:** 177-190.
16. Mendoza, S. P., W. Saltzman, D. M. Lyons & P. A. Schiml. 1991. Am. J. Primatol. **24:** 122.
17. Saltzman, W., S. P. Mendoza & W. A. Mason. 1991. Physiol. Behav. **50:** 271-280.
18. Brown, G. M., L. J. Crota, D. P. Penney & S. Reichlin. 1970. Endocrinology **86:** 519-529.
19. Mendoza, S. P. & G. P. Moberg. 1985. Am. J. Primatol. **8:** 215-224.
20. Chrousos, G. P., D. Renquist, D. Brandon, C. Eil, M. Pugeat, R. Vigersky, G. B. Cutler, D. L. Loriaux & M. B. Lipsett. 1982. Proc. Natl. Acad. Sci. USA **79:** 2036-2040.

21. CASSORLA, F. G., B. D. ALBERTSON, G. P. CHROUSOS, J. D. BOOTH, D. RENQUIST, M. B. LIPSETT & D. L. LORIAUX. 1982. Endocrinology **111:** 448-451.
22. ALBERTSON, B. D., D. D. BRANDON, G. P. CHROUSOS & D. L. LORIAUX. 1988. Steroids **49:** 497-506.
23. PUGEAT, M. M., G. P. CHROUSOS, B. C. NISULA, D. L. LORIAUX, D. BRANDON & M. B. LIPSETT. 1984. Endocrinology **115:** 357-361.
24. KLOSTERMAN, L. L., J. T. MURAI & P. K. SIITERI. 1986. Endocrinology **118:** 424-434.
25. CHROUSOS, G. P., D. L. LORIAUX, D. BRANDON, J. SHULL, D. RENQUIST, W. HOGAN, M. TOMITA & M. B. LIPSETT. 1984. Endocrinology **115:** 25-32.
26. MENDOZA, S. P., C. L. COE & S. LEVINE. 1979. Psychoneuroendocrinology **3:** 221-229.
27. GONZALEZ, C. A., M. B. HENNESSY & S. LEVINE. 1981. Am. J. Primatol. **1:** 439-452.
28. SALTZMAN, W., S. P. MENDOZA & W. A. MASON. 1991. Physiol. Behav. **50:** 271-280.
29. MENDOZA, S. P. & W. A. MASON. 1991. Physiol. Behav. **49:** 471-479.
30. LYONS, D. M., S. P. MENDOZA & W. A. MASON. 1994. Am. J. Primatol. **32:** 109-122.
31. JAECKLE, R. S., R. G. KATHOL, J. F. LOPEZ, W. H. MELLER & S. J. KRUMMEL. 1987. Arch. Gen. Psychiatry **44:** 233-240.
32. PAYKEL, E. S., J. K. MEYERS, M. N. DIENELT, G. L. KLERMAN, J. J. LINDENTHAL, M. P. PEPPER. 1969. Arch. Gen. Psychiatry **21:** 753-760.
33. ANESHENSEL, C. S. & J. D. STONE. 1982. Arch. Gen. Psychiatry **39:** 1392-1396.
34. BILLINGS, A. G., R. C. CRONKITE & R. H. MOOS. 1983. J. Abnorm. Psychol. **92:** 119-133.
35. GOLD, P. W., D. L. LORIAUX, A. ROY, M. A. KLING, J. R. CALABRESE, C. H. KELLNER, L. K. NIEMAN, R. M. POST, D. PICKAR, W. GALLUCCI, P. AVERGINOS, S. PAUL, E. H. OLDFIELD, G. B. CUTLER & G. P. CHROUSOS. 1986. N. Engl. J. Med. **314:** 1329-1335.
36. MURPHY, B. E. P. 1991. J. Steroid Biochem. Molec. Biol. **38:** 537-559.
37. KALIN, N. H., S. J. WEILER & S. E. SHELTON. 1982. Psychiatry Res. **7:** 87-92.
38. REUS, V. I., M. S. JOSEPH & M. F. DALLMAN. 1982. N. Engl. J. Med. **306:** 238-239.
39. PFOHL, B., B. SHERMAN, J. SCHLECTE & G. WINOKUR. 1985. Biol. Psychiatry **20:** 1055-1072.
40. FANG, V. S., B. J. TRICOU, A. ROBERTSON & H. Y. MELTZER. 1981. Life Sci. **29:** 931-938.
41. YEREVANIEN, B. I. & P. D. WOOLF. 1983. Psychiatry Res. **9:** 45-51.
42. SHERMAN, B. M., B. PHOHL & G. WINOKUR. 1985. Psychiatr. Med. **3:** 41-52.
43. AMSTERDAM, J. D., G. MAISLIN, N. BERWISH, J. PHILLIPS & A. WINOKUR. 1989. Arch. Gen. Psychiatry **46:** 550-554.
44. AMSTERDAM, J. D., G. MAISLIN, M. CROBA & A. WINOKUR. 1987. Psychiatry Res. **20:** 325-336.
45. KOLANOWSKI, J., M. JEANJEAN & J. CRABBE. 1969. Ann. d'Endocrinol. **30:** 857-864.
46. KOLANOWSKI, J., M. A. PIZZARRO & J. CRABBE. 1975. J. Clin. Endocrinol. Metab. **41:** 453-465.
47. DALLMAN, M. F. 1984. Endocrine Res. **10:** 213-242.
48. SIMPSON, E. R. & M. R. WATERMAN. 1983. Can. J. Biochem. Cell Biol. **61:** 692-707.
49. AMSTERDAM, J. D., D. L. MARINELLI, P. ARGER & A. WINOKUR. 1987. Psychiatry Res. **21:** 189-197.
50. NEMEROFF, C. B., K. R. R. KRISHNAN, D. REED, R. LEDER, C. BEAM & N. R. DUNNICK. 1992. Arch. Gen. Psychiatry **49:** 384-387.
51. RUBIN, R. T., J. J. PHILLIPS, T. F. SADOW & J. T. MCCRACKEN. 1996. Arch. Gen. Psychiatry **52:** 213-218.
52. DE SOUZA, E. & G. R. VAN LOON. 1984. Experientia **40:** 1004-1006.
53. PEDERSEN, R. C. & A. C. BROWNIE. 1980. Proc. Natl. Acad. Sci. USA **77:** 2239-2243.
54. SHANKER, G. & R. K. SHARMA. 1979. Biochem. Biophys. Res. Comm. **86:** 1-5.

55. OTTENWELLER, J. E. & A. H. MEIER. 1982. Endocrinology **111:** 1334-1338.
56. FEHM, H. L., E. KLEIN, R. HOLL & K. H. VOIGT. 1984. J. Clin. Endocrinol. Metab. **58:** 410-414.
57. HOLZWARTH, M. A., L. A. CUNNINGHAM & N. KLEITMAN. 1987. Ann. N.Y. Acad. Sci. **512:** 449-464.
58. ZHU, Q., A. BATEMAN, A. SINGH & S. SOLOMON. 1989. Endocrine Res. **15:** 129-149.

6
Attachment Relationships in New World Primates

Sally P. Mendoza and William A. Mason

The concept of attachment as elaborated by Bowlby[1] has had a substantial influence on our views of primate social proclivities. In its most simple formulation, attachment is characterized by one individual (usually the infant) striving to maintain proximity with a specific other individual (usually the mother), displaying distress upon separation from or loss of the other, and attempting to restore proximity following separation. Although attachment was identified and defined in behavioral terms, Bowlby and others inferred from the behavior the existence of an emotional bond between individuals that provided the motivational basis for continued association between them. From studies of attachment in nonhuman primates we have learned that infants can develop attachment bonds with individuals or objects other than the mother,[2] that mothers often form a reciprocal attachment bond with their infants,[3] and that relationships other than the mother-infant dyad can be characterized as attachments.[4]

In this essay we consider the extent to which the concept of attachment applies to all affinitive primate social relationships. In a recent review of the animal literature it was suggested that involuntary separation of social companions results in rapid activation of the pituitary-adrenal system only if there is behavioral evidence of an attachment bond between them.[5] The specific question we address is whether relationships exist among primates that cannot be characterized as attachments and yet are expressed in consistent patterns of affinitive interactions among the participants. Such relationships may differ from the attachment bond in intensity or, alternatively, they may be analogous to human friendship, differing qualitatively from the filial bond and requiring a different vocabulary and conceptual scheme for their understanding. Finally, we consider the contribution of the formation of attachment bonds or other relationships to social order in nonhuman primates.

This research focuses on two species of South American primates, squirrel monkeys (*Saimiri sciureus*) and titi monkeys (*Callicebus moloch*). These species are both small arboreal omnivores. Squirrel monkeys are polygynous and live in large social groups consisting of several males and several females in each age and sex category. Other than those between mother and infant, the most frequent interactions occur between squirrel monkeys of the same age and sex.[6] In contrast, titi monkeys are monogamous and live in small family groups consisting of an adult male, an adult female, and up to three offspring.[7] Relations within the family group are highly

Preparation of this manuscript was supported by grant RR00169 from the National Institutes of Health, Bethesda, Maryland.

affiliative, and males contribute substantially to infant care; interactions outside the family unit are generally restricted to ritualized encounters with neighboring groups at the territorial boundaries. Although these species may represent extreme examples within the range of social organizations maintained by nonhuman primates, they are similar in that members of both species are highly social throughout their lives and apparently form long-term relationships with specific others.

SQUIRREL MONKEY MOTHER-INFANT ATTACHMENT

Ainsworth[8] argued that a critical criterion of attachment was unequivocal distress upon sudden and complete separation from the attachment figure. This criterion is clearly met by infant squirrel monkeys when separated from their mothers and by mother squirrel monkeys when separated from their infants. Using the pituitary-adrenal response to separation advocated by Hennessy,[5] for example, a 30-60-minute separation of mother and infant squirrel monkeys leads to increased plasma cortisol levels in both mother and infant, even when the separated individual remains in the home cage with other familiar companions.[9]

Early studies of pituitary-adrenal responses to mother-infant separation in squirrel monkeys illustrate another of Ainsworth's[8] criteria of attachment, that is, alleviation of distress by interaction with the attachment figure. Inasmuch as separation of mother and infant necessarily involves considerable disturbance incidental to separating the animals, identification of a response specific to separation from the attachment figure requires comparison with disturbance-control procedures in which all the steps necessary to establish the separation condition are followed except that both members of the dyad are reunited within a few seconds of separation and returned to the home cage. To our surprise, this disturbance-control condition, although seemingly traumatic to the subjects, failed to elicit an increase in adrenocortical activity when compared to basal, undisturbed conditions. This was all the more surprising when we found that simply capturing an adult female squirrel monkey (without an infant), a much less traumatic procedure, was sufficient to increase cortisol levels.[10] We therefore concluded that stress-buffering was also characteristic of attachment bonds and that the immediate presence of the attachment figure could attenuate or eliminate the pituitary-adrenal response to potentially stressful circumstances.[3]

The finding that squirrel monkey mothers also showed the separation response when their infants were removed and stress-buffering upon reunion indicated that adults as well as infants form attachment bonds. Given the strong positive relations among adult primates that enable them to form and maintain long-term associations with one another, it was reasonable to postulate that adult monkeys develop attachments with one another, similar to the bonds that squirrel monkey mothers form with their infants, and that such attachments were a major source of social cohesion in primate groups.

SEPARATION STUDIES IN JUVENILE AND ADULT SQUIRREL MONKEYS

Aside from the mother-infant relationships, squirrel monkeys typically associate with other individuals of the same age and gender.[6] Females are particularly attracted to one another and spend considerable time in close association.[11] For this reason, and because it was clear from the mother-infant studies that adult female squirrel monkeys were capable of forming attachment bonds, our initial studies of separation among juvenile and adults focused on females.

Juvenile and young adult females housed in unisexual triads were subjected to a 30-minute separation from their cagemates.[12] Behaviorally, animals distinguished the removal of one peer from the home cage from the disturbance-control procedures by an increase in frequency of scent marking. Moreover, females were more active and vocalized more when introduced to a novel environment alone than when they experienced the new surroundings in the company of their cagemates. Cortisol levels were not differentially affected by the experimental conditions, however, and animals showed no evidence that the pituitary-adrenal system was specifically activated by social separation or was buffered by the presence of one or more companions. Thus, whether animals were tested in the home cage or in a novel environment, with all cagemates or alone, cortisol levels were elevated by the disturbance involved in catching the animals but not specifically by separation from one or more companions. Similarly, no evidence existed that the physiological response to the stress of capture and handling was buffered by social companions in either juvenile or young adult female squirrel monkeys.

When housed in large social groups, female squirrel monkeys associate preferentially with some individuals and rarely interact with others.[13] Hennessy[14] examined the possibility that animals who actively affiliate with one another in large stable groups would be likely to buffer one another from the deleterious effects of stress associated with exposure to a novel environment. Adult female squirrel monkeys were removed either individually or in pairs from large breeding groups and placed in a novel environment for 25 hours. Pairs were constituted so that they were (1) highly affiliative members of the same social group, (2) members of the same social group that rarely engaged with one another affiliatively, or (3) members of different social groups and hence strangers to one another. All animals responded to the novel environment with an increase in adrenocortical activity. There was no evidence that familiarity or affiliation buffered the adrenocortical response to a novel environment. In fact, animals tested with familiar partners were more likely to exhibit increased cortisol levels 1 hour after introduction to the test cage than animals tested alone, and they were also more likely to exhibit a further increase in adrenocortical activity by 25 hours than were animals tested with complete strangers. Whether animals had an affiliative relationship with their familiar partner did not alter the adrenocortical response to the novel environment; however, behavioral data indicated that the tendency to affiliate with social partners in the test cage was similar to patterns in the home cage.

Lactating females may be more responsive than nonlactating females to separation from adult cagemates.[15] When two mother-infant dyads were housed together, the adrenocortical response of one pair to removal of the other exceeded their response to their own capture and handling. These animals did not respond to exposure to a novel environment, as long as both dyads were introduced to the test cage together. However, the implications of these results are not altogether clear, inasmuch as the animals also responded to capture of their cagemates even though all animals were immediately returned to the home cage and thus neither separated nor exposed to novelty during the test period.

The adrenocortical response to separation has also been evaluated in male and female squirrel monkeys housed as heterosexual pairs.[16] In this study, adult monkeys were separated from their cagemate for 1 hour. Subjects remained in the home cage during the separation period, and the cagemate was removed to a remote location. Animals in this study were trained to enter a transport cage, so that separation could be accomplished without manually capturing the animals. The results indicated that neither the disturbance-control procedures nor removal of the cagemate (and only companion) increased cortisol levels in comparison with basal conditions for either male or female squirrel monkeys.

Even though we cannot unequivocally conclude that adult squirrel monkeys never respond to separation from their adult companions with increased pituitary-adrenal activity, the preponderance of evidence suggests that adults do not respond specifically to separation from their adult companions and they generally do not provide an effective buffer for one another from the stress engendered by capture and brief manual restraint or exposure to novelty.[17] The relationships formed between adult squirrel monkeys, while generally affiliative, do not resemble the intense emotional attachment bond characteristic of mothers' relationships with their infants.

PATTERNS OF ATTACHMENT WITHIN A MONOGAMOUS SOCIETY

Studies of the monogamous titi monkey clearly show that adults will form an attachment bond with another adult monkey and that disruption of this bond activates the pituitary-adrenal stress response. In two studies, the adrenocortical response of adult male and female titi monkeys was evaluated following removal of their mate. Cortisol levels 1 hour after separation from their heterosexual cagemate were elevated relative to basal levels and disturbance-control procedures.[4,16]

Titi monkeys tend to be extremely responsive to minor changes in their physical environment. In most studies, therefore, exposure to a novel cage maximally elevates adrenocortical activity, and this response is not attenuated by the presence of a cagemate.[4,18] However, cagemates do buffer the response to capture and handling involved in establishing the separation conditions.[4] Moreover, titi monkeys do not respond to minor changes in their physical environment when the cagemate is present, but they do when the cagemate is absent.[19]

By contrast to squirrel monkeys, parenting in titi monkeys is a shared activity. Infant titi monkeys may spend as much as 90% of their time riding on their father's back during the first 2 months of life.[4,20] Typically, infants will transfer from the father to the mother for only brief periods surrounding nursing. Transfer between parents is generally accomplished by the infant without any active assistance by either parent. As the infants mature and their locomotor skills enable them to locomote independently, they retain a preference for their fathers.[4] This pattern of parental-infant behavior suggested that infant titi monkeys may form a stronger attachment bond with their fathers than with their mothers.

Separation studies have supported the suggestion that the infant's bond is stronger to its father than to its mother.[21] Infant titi monkeys respond to 1 hour of separation from their fathers with elevated cortisol levels regardless of whether the mother is present or not. Infants do not respond to separation from their mothers, however, unless their fathers are also absent. That the pituitary-adrenal response to separation is greater when both parents are gone than when only the father is absent suggests that the mother is providing limited buffering for the infant, but cortisol levels are still substantially elevated in this condition. In contrast, the father completely buffers the infant's response to maternal separation, capture, and handling. Thus, in keeping with behavioral data, infant titi monkeys appear to form a stronger attachment bond to their fathers than to their mothers, despite the fact that the mothers are their sole source of food for the first several weeks of life. The response to separation in young titi monkeys wanes somewhat as they mature, but removal of the parents continues to elicit heightened pituitary-adrenal activity even after the offspring reach reproductive age (Valeggia, unpublished data).

The infant titi monkey's attachment to its parents is not reciprocated. Neither mothers nor fathers show an adrenocortical response to separation from their dependent offspring.[4] Moreover, the infant does not attenuate the parents' response to separation from one another. Behaviorally, parents do respond to distress vocalizations emitted by their infant and will retrieve a separated infant, so it would be incorrect to assert that parents are totally unresponsive to infants. They do not, however, appear to differentiate between their own infant and another of comparable age,[22] and when given a choice between their mate and their infant, the choice is generally for their mate.[4]

CONTRIBUTION OF ATTACHMENT BONDS TO SOCIAL STRUCTURE

Both squirrel monkeys and titi monkeys form attachment bonds that we believe contribute to the maintenance of each species' normal grouping pattern. Squirrel monkeys raise their infants in large social groups in which several infants are born within a short period of time.[23] As young develop locomotor independence, they frequently leave their mothers for brief periods to interact with other young monkeys and occasionally other adults. The reciprocal attachment bond that develops between mother and infant probably helps to maintain proximity between them and facilitates reunion during times of danger or when the infant needs supplemental nurturance. There is some indication that these attachment bonds, at least between mothers and daughters, persist into adulthood and may contribute to the apparent cohesion among adult females.[24] Aside from this possibility of filial attachment continuing into adulthood, it does not appear that adult squirrel monkeys form intense emotional bonds with specific other adults; however, we have never examined male-male separation and, although we consider it unlikely, they may form specific attachments with each other.

In titi monkeys, the bond between mates facilitates maintenance of proximity between a specific adult male and female, a common feature of a monogamous social system. The bond that develops between adults also facilitates biparental care, in the sense that if parents are in proximity to one another, they are readily available to their infant for transfer between its source of food and the object of its attachment.[4]

Male titi monkeys are generally very tolerant of infant contact, particularly if they are experienced fathers. Mothers tend to be less tolerant of prolonged contact with their infant and often become agitated and actively attempt to dislodge it. Usually, older siblings are also very intolerant of a clinging infant. As a result, infants quickly learn to avoid clinging to all members of the social group except the father.

Separation studies clearly indicate that attachment bonds are not ubiquitous and many relationships that are characterized by social affinity and high levels of affiliative behavior are not attachment-like. Disrupting these relationships does not elicit an adrenocortical response to separation, and some evidence suggests that individuals of the same age and sex category are essentially interchangeable. Thus, titi monkey parents do not readily discriminate their own infant from another,[22] and squirrel monkey females may interact at least as readily with a stranger as they do with a familiar cagemate with whom they frequently affiliate.[14] Although parent-offspring relations in titi monkeys and same-sex relationships in squirrel monkeys have important organizing effects on social behavior, the relationships seem to lack the individual specificity and emotional intensity of attachment bonds. Rather than viewing these relationships as reflecting weak attachment bonds, it seems more reasonable to consider them to be qualitatively different. In human societies, we readily differentiate between close, romantic, attachment-like relationships and friendships. It seems likely that many highly affiliative relationships among nonhuman primates reflect a condition more closely analogous to friendship than to a mutual attachment bond.

REFERENCES

1. Bowlby, J. 1969. Attachment and Loss. Vol. 1. Attachment. Basic Books, Inc. New York.
2. Mason, W. A. & M. D. Kenny, 1974. Redirection of filial attachments in rhesus monkeys: Dogs as surrogates. Science **183:** 1209-1211.
3. Mendoza, S. P., C. L. Coe, W. P. Smotherman, J. Kaplan & S. Levine. 1980. Functional consequences of attachment: A comparison of two species. *In* Maternal Influences and Early Behavior. R. W. Bell & W. P. Smotherman, Eds.: 235-252 Spectrum Publication. New York.
4. Mendoza, S. P. & W. A. Mason. 1986. Parental division of labour and differentiation of attachments in a monogamous primate (*Callicebus moloch*). Anim. Behav. **34:** 1336-1347.
5. Hennessy, M. B. 1996. Hypothalamic-pituitary-adrenal responses to brief social separation. Neurosci. Biobehav. Rev. In press.
6. Baldwin, J. D. 1985. The behavior of squirrel monkeys (*Saimiri*) in natural environments. *In* Handbook of Squirrel Monkey Research. L. A. Rosenblum & C. L. Coe, Eds. 35-53. Plenum Press. New York.
7. Mason, W. A. 1966. Social organization of the South American monkey, *Callicebus moloch:* A preliminary report. Tulane Studies Zool. **13:** 23-38.
8. Ainsworth, M. D. S. 1972. Attachment and dependency: A comparison. *In* Attachment and Dependency. J. L. Gewirtz, Ed.: 97-137. V. H. Winston and Sons, Washington D.C.
9. Coe, C. L., S. P. Mendoza, W. P. Smotherman & S. Levine. 1978. Mother-infant attachment in the squirrel monkey: Adrenal response to separation. Behav. Biol. **22:** 256-263.
10. Mendoza, S. P., W. P. Smotherman, M. T. Miner, J. Kaplan & S. Levine. 1978. Pituitary-adrenal response to separation in mother and infant squirrel monkeys. Dev. Psychobiol. **11:** 169-175.
11. Mason, W. A. & G. Epple. 1969. Social organization in experimental groups of *Saimiri* and *Callicebus*. Proc. Second Int. Congr. Primatol. **1:** 59-65.

12. Hennessy, M. B., S. P. Mendoza & J. N. Kaplan. 1982. Behavior and plasma cortisol following brief peer separation in juvenile squirrel monkeys. Am. J. Primatol. **3:** 143-151.
13. Leger, D. W., W. A. Mason & D. M. Fragaszy. 1981. Sexual segregation, cliques and social power in squirrel monkey (*Saimiri*) groups. Behaviour **76:** 163-181.
14. Hennessy, M. B. 1986. Effects of social partners on pituitary-adrenal activity during novelty exposure in adult female squirrel monkeys. Physiol. Behav. **38:** 803-807.
15. Jordan, T. C., M. B. Hennessy, C. A. Gonzalez & S. Levine. 1985. Social and environmental factors influencing mother-infant separation-reunion in squirrel monkeys. Physiol. Behav. **34:** 489-493.
16. Mendoza, S. P. & W. A. Mason. 1986. Contrasting responses to intruders and to involuntary separation by monogamous and polygynous New World monkeys. Physiol. Behav. **38:** 795-801.
17. Mendoza, S. P., D. M. Lyons & W. Saltzman. 1991. Sociophysiology of squirrel monkeys. Am. J. Primatol. **23:** 37-54.
18. Cubicciotti, D. D., S. P. Mendoza, W. A. Mason & E. N. Sassenrath. 1986. Differences between *Saimiri sciureus* and *Callicebus moloch* in physiological responsiveness: Implications for behavior. J. Comp. Psychol. **100:** 385-391.
19. Hennessy, M. B., S. P. Mendoza, W. A. Mason & G. P. Moberg. 1995. Endocrine sensitivity to novelty in squirrel monkeys and titi monkeys: Species differences in characteristic modes of responding to the environment. Physiol. Behav. **57:** 331-338.
20. Fragaszy, D. M., S. Schwarz & D. Shimosaka. 1982. Longitudinal observations of care and development of infant titi monkeys (*Callicebus moloch*). Am. J. Primatol. **2:** 191-200.
21. Hoffman, K. A., S. P. Mendoza, M. B. Hennessy & W. A. Mason. 1996. Responses of infant titi monkeys, *Callicebus moloch,* to removal of one or both parents: Evidence for paternal attachment. Dev. Psychobiol. **28:** 399-407.
22. Teskey, N., S. P. Mendoza, D. J. Mayeaux, C. Ruiz & W. A. Mason. 1993. Parental responsiveness in titi monkeys. Am. J. Primatol. **30:** 351.
23. Boinski, S. 1987. Birth synchrony in squirrel monkeys (*Saimiri oerstedi*): A strategy to reduce neonatal predation. Behav. Ecol. Sociobiol. **21:** 383-400.
24. Tabor, B. A. 1986. The development and structure of *Saimiri* social relationships. Doctoral dissertation, University of California, Davis.

7

Hormonal Modulation of Sexual Behavior and Affiliation in Rhesus Monkeys

Kim Wallen and Pamela L. Tannenbaum

Rhesus monkeys are a seasonal breeding species whose society is based principally upon relations between females.[1,2] Females remain in their natal troop, while males emigrate to a new social group, which may occur several times during the male's life. Females, in contrast, become fully integrated into the female-bonded[2,3] structure of the troop, a process that is evident early in life.[4] Males must immigrate into this female-centered social structure to mate with group females. The processes by which male immigration and sexual activity are socially accommodated have not been extensively investigated; however, it has been evident for some time that male immigration occurs almost exclusively during the rhesus monkey breeding season when females are sexually interested in males.[5–7] Here we present evidence suggesting that the hormonal changes associated with ovarian cycles influence female sexual attraction towards males, affecting the occurrence of sexual behavior within the social group and affiliation between males and females and between females. In addition, this same hormonally mediated sexual attraction to males makes the group permeable, allowing the entry of new males. In our view, rhesus monkey society is not only female centered, but female hormonal cycles critically and dramatically influence social relationships and the social structure and character of rhesus monkey groups. Understanding the behavioral endocrinology of female rhesus monkeys is crucial to revealing the mechanisms underlying rhesus monkey sexual behavior and affiliation.

Much has been written about the sexual behavior of male-female pairs of rhesus monkeys tested under controlled laboratory conditions.[8] For almost 30 years, such studies served as the model for investigating the behavioral endocrinology of rhesus monkey sexual behavior. This research produced elaborate models of sexual behavior based upon hormonally mediated female sexual attraction, which in turn resulted in male sexual initiation.[9] In the last 15 years, laboratory research has focused on the sexual behavior of captive groups of rhesus monkeys, a social context that incorporates more

This research was supported in part by grants BNS 81-17627, BNS 84-10860, BNS 86-07295, and BNS 89-19888 from the National Science Foundation, grant RR-00165 from the National Institutes of Health to the Yerkes Regional Primate Research Center, and NIMH award K02-MH01062 to K.W. The Yerkes Regional Primate Research Center is fully accredited by the American Association for the Accreditation of Laboratory Animal Care.

aspects of the complex social environment under which rhesus monkey sexual behavior probably evolved than does the laboratory pair-test.[8,10–15] The results of these studies echo findings from a captive, socially complex population which argued, more than 50 years ago, that rhesus monkey sexual behavior was strongly coupled to the female's ovarian cycle and that females, not males, initiated most sexual interactions.[16]

Modern endocrinological techniques and the development of methods allowing physiological manipulations of rhesus monkeys in intact social groups[11] have resulted in studies that precisely measure both behavior and hormonal changes in a context sharing many social characteristics of free-ranging groups of rhesus monkeys. These studies, in contrast to studies of pairs of rhesus monkeys, uniformly find that sexual behavior in large social groups is limited to a relatively brief period around ovulation,[10,13] with the hormones that produce fertility also stimulating female initiation of sexual behavior.[14] Differences between results from studies of pairs of monkeys and groups of monkeys are partly due to the amount of physical space the animals have for social interactions,[12] but principally result from the effect that social context has on the expression of endocrine influences on female sexual behavior.[8,14,17]

Although we now know a great deal about how ovarian hormones influence female sexual initiation in social groups, less attention has been paid to how social relationships between females and other females and males vary with the ovarian cycle.[17,18] This paper describes the interplay between changes in sexual behavior and affiliative behavior in group-living rhesus monkeys. Our research illustrates how the complex changes in ovarian hormones that occur across the menstrual cycle have a impact on the social environment of both males and females. The hormonal changes that regulate sexual behavior also have a marked effect on the social relations between females, the core of rhesus monkey groupings.

SOCIAL CONTEXT OF MATING

Rhesus monkeys are seasonal breeders who are not pair-bonded and show little evidence of consistent partner preferences when observed in the large multimale, multifemale groups characteristic of this species.[1,19,20] Although the earliest work on sexual behavior in social groups used a free-ranging captive population of rhesus monkeys on the island of Cayo Santiago,[16] there are still no studies of the behavioral endocrinology of free-ranging natural populations of rhesus monkeys. Twenty-five years after Carpenter's work, researchers at the Yerkes Regional Primate Research Center Field Station pioneered techniques to allow the study of daily changes in hormones and sexual behavior in social groups with a known history and stable social structure.[11] Although these groups did not share the complex physical environment of free-ranging populations or even of the captive Cayo Santiago island population, they were multimale, multifemale groups sharing the matrilineal structure and multimale breeding system characteristic of rhesus monkeys.[1,2,19,20] Studies of such groups do not duplicate all aspects of rhesus monkey society, but they do exhibit the same seasonal breeding pattern and cyclical pattern of female mating.[10,11–14]

To investigate the nature of heterosexual pairing during mating we studied a group of more than 75 rhesus monkeys including 20 sexually active females and 7 males housed in a 45 by 45 m outdoor compound at the Yerkes Regional Primate

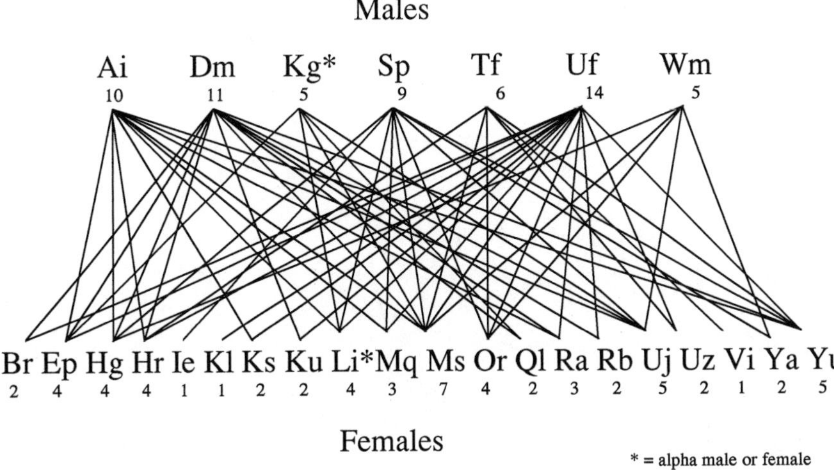

FIGURE 1. Mating relationships among 7 adult male and 20 adult female rhesus monkeys demonstrate substantial evidence of multiple partners. Only three females and none of the males had a single mating partner during the 7 weeks of observation. The highest ranking (alpha) male and female did not have the greatest number of partners.

Research Center Field Station during the breeding season. Three times per week the group was observed for 3 hours with all occurrences of sexual behavior recorded by focusing on the 7 males in the group. Adult males were vasectomized, allowing consecutive ovarian cycles without the confounding effects of pregnant and nonpregnant females. Over a 7-week period we observed 100 copulations with ejaculation. FIGURE 1 illustrates the distribution of these copulations among the 7 males and 20 females. Specific partner preferences were not evident, as 17 of 20 females mated with more than 1 male and all 7 males mated with 5 or more of the females. Interestingly, the highest ranking (alpha) male had the smallest number of sexual partners among the males, tying with the lowest ranking male at 5/20 female partners. Males mated with significantly more partners than did females (mean ± SEM; males: 8.6 ± 1.3; females: 3.0 ± 0.4, $F_{1,25} = 34.2$, $p < 0.001$). However, on any given day males and females mated with a comparable number of partners (males: 2.0 ± 0.3; females: 1.9 ± 0.2, $F_{1,25} = 0.1$, $p > 0.75$). The overall sex difference in total number of sexual partners reflected the fact that female mating was cyclic and limited to a small number of days, whereas males mated on a significantly greater number of the 21 test days (males: 10.1 ± 1.2 days; females: 3.0 ± 0.4 days; $F_{1,25} = 60$, $p < 0.001$). Thus, both males and females mate promiscuously, with the greater number of sexual partners for males reflecting their more continuous mating in comparison with females.

OVARIAN CYCLES AND SEXUAL AND AFFILIATIVE BEHAVIOR

In groups with multiple males and females, mating behavior is characterized by relatively consistent daily mating by males during the breeding season, with females

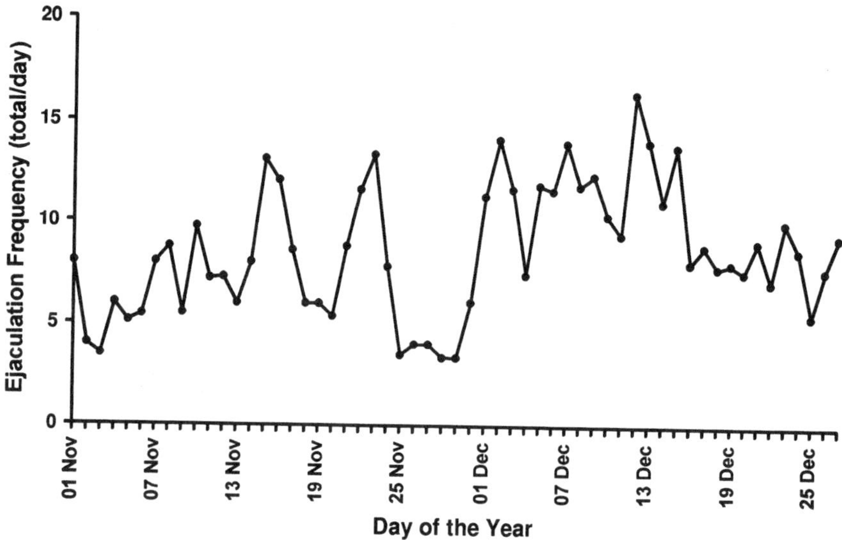

FIGURE 2. Daily total ejaculations in a group of 9 adult female rhesus monkeys observed with each of 4 adult males tested singly in the group for 30–60 minutes each day.

displaying brief intense periods of mating, typically with at least two partners during each ovulatory cycle. When females are not mating, they infrequently interact with males and associate with either other females or their offspring.[1,16,19] To understand the dynamics of female-female interactions in detail we studied daily changes in behavior and ovarian hormones in a social group of nine adult cycling females and each of four vasectomized males introduced into the females' social group for 30-60 minutes each day. This design eliminated male-male competition, allowing a more precise focus on interactions with females. Again, vasectomized males were used to allow the study of the full ovarian cycle without the confound of pregnancy. The methodology for collecting behavioral and blood samples, as well as the group composition, have previously been described.[14]

The daily introduction of nonresident males partially mimics the process by which free-ranging rhesus monkey males enter new groups to become socially integrated. Initially, males copulate with sexually active group females on the group's periphery,[21] who eventually facilitate their entry into the group. Although our acute introductions did not duplicate the gradual familiarization typical of free-ranging groups, they did preclude males establishing stable relationships with group females. This constant reintroduction, combined with the limited time for social interaction each day, probably intensified interactions between males and females. Therefore, it is probably best to interpret our findings as a more extreme expression of naturally occurring processes.

Copulatory Behavior. The group was observed 7 days per week from November 1 through December 27, representing the peak months of the breeding season. When considered on a day-to-day basis, mating behavior occurred seemingly randomly throughout the 57 days (FIG. 2). However, during these 57 days of observation

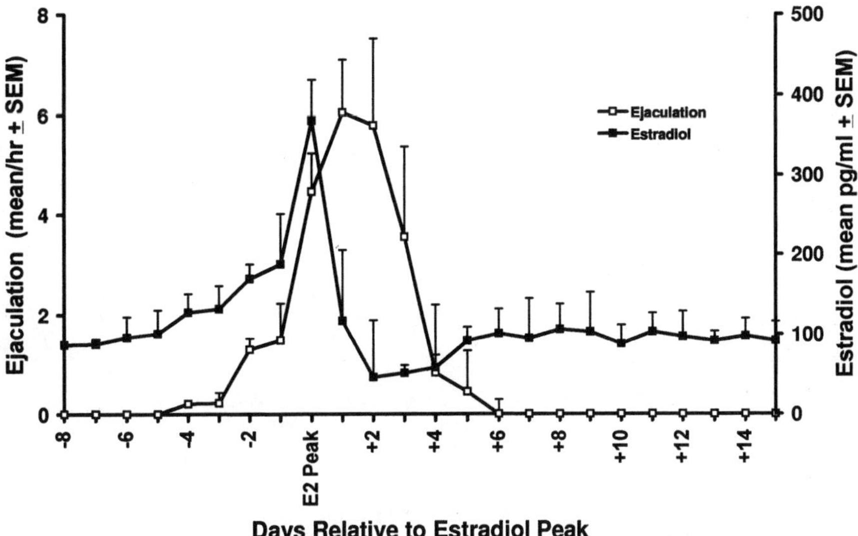

FIGURE 3. Mean rate of ejaculation in relation to peak estradiol level during the ovarian cycles of nine adult female rhesus monkeys.

each female experienced one or more ovarian cycles, and ovarian cycles were not synchronized between females. How behavior varies in relation to the female's ovarian cycle, however, is key to understanding possible effects of hormones on the social dynamics of a rhesus monkey group. For this purpose we investigated the relationship between hormonal changes, sexual behavior, and affiliation in a randomly selected ovarian cycle in each female.[14]

When aligned to the estradiol peak in each female's cycle, sexual behavior is decidedly nonrandom and varies systematically with changes in ovarian steroids. Ejaculation only occurs with females in the periovulatory portion of the female's cycle; mating is not seen during either the early follicular or luteal phases of the cycle. FIGURE 3 illustrates that increases in ovarian estradiol are associated with the first increases in ejaculation, and increased estradiol and ejaculation are strongly correlated.[14] However, after peak estradiol levels have been reached, and while estradiol is declining, ejaculation remains elevated for 3 more days. Therefore, that the hormones leading to ovulation apparently initiate behavioral changes which are then maintained by the social dynamics of the male and female.

Proximity. This effect of ovarian hormones on social relationships is seen in the frequency with which females initiate sitting or standing within 20 cm (proximity) of the male in relation to changes in estradiol (FIG. 4). Female initiation of proximity is strongly correlated with estradiol during the follicular phase,[14] remaining elevated after peak estradiol levels are reached and start to decline. Because increases in female initiation of proximity precede increases in ejaculation (FIG. 5), female initiation of proximity appears to reflect attempts by the female to initiate sexual activity. This

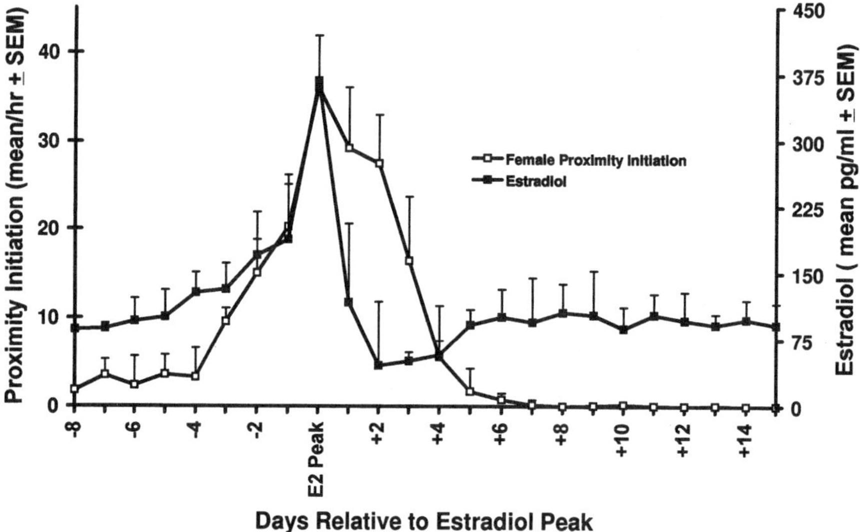

FIGURE 4. Mean rate of female initiation of proximity to the male in relation to peak estradiol level during the ovarian cycles of nine adult female rhesus monkeys.

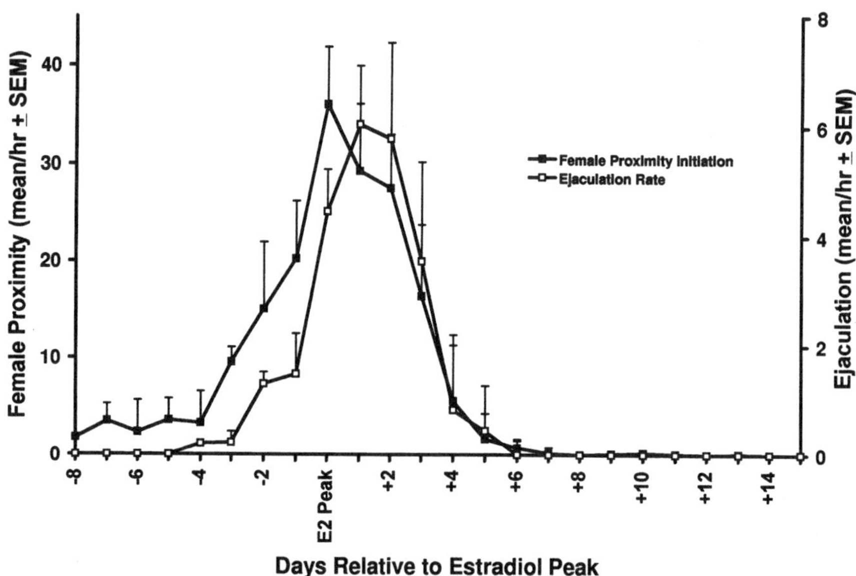

FIGURE 5. Relationship between female initiated proximity rate and ejaculation rate across the ovarian cycles of nine adult female rhesus monkeys aligned by the day of peak estradiol.

persistent courting of males by females at midcycle is an important characteristic of rhesus monkey sexual behavior.[1,16,19]

When approached closely for the first time by a female, a male typically sits momentarily and then moves away. If the female is sexually interested, she pursues the male, following within a meter or less of the male, eventually reestablishing proximity. This courtship ritual may be repeated many times, over a period of minutes or hours, until either the female stops pursuing the male or the male does not leave, but mounts the female instead. Once mounting starts, the mating pair remain in proximity and the male mounts and intromits several times, with pauses of many seconds or several minutes in between, before ejaculating.[14,16,19] Thus, although males may control the timing of intermount intervals to some extent, it is clearly the females who control sexual initiation by manipulating proximity to the male, with more than 90% of proximities initiated by females during the periovulatory portion of the female's cycle.[14] Thus, the events underlying sexual behavior are: (1) ovarian hormones increase the sexual attraction of the female to the male, (2) resulting in increased pursuit of the male and (3) eventually leading to increased copulation as the female nears ovulation.

Grooming. The hormonal changes underlying courtship and mating are also associated with changes in affiliation, both between females and males and among females with each other. Grooming is the primary affiliative behavior in rhesus monkey society.[2,22] Females groom other females, their offspring, and adult males. Males, however, groom others less frequently. In our single-male multiple-female group, for example, less than 1% of all grooming events were by males (25 of 3,248 events or 0.77%). Thus, as with the initiation of heterosexual proximity, grooming is most often done by females. Because of the rarity of male grooming, only grooming by females is considered here. Marked daily fluctuations were seen in the time females spent grooming male or female partners throughout the 57 days of the study. Although grooming appears randomly distributed, a significant correlation occurs between daily grooming by females of male and female partners ($r = 0.55$, $p < 0.01$), suggesting that a common underlying factor influences female grooming.

When female cycles are aligned by peak estradiol levels, grooming of the stimulus male by females is decidedly nonrandom, increasing during the follicular phase with peak grooming durations coinciding almost exactly with peak occurrence of ejaculation (FIG. 6). During portions of the female cycle when there is no sexual activity, females rarely interact with the stimulus male, and grooming of males ceases completely during the luteal phase. This strong correlation between ejaculation and female grooming of males reflects the manner in which grooming is used in the sexual interaction, where it is often the primary activity of the mating pair between mounts.

Rhesus monkey society is built around relationships between females within a matrilineal structure.[2,22,23] Male incorporation in this social structure is not lifelong. Males emigrate from their natal troop around puberty and migrate into an unfamiliar group.[6,24,25] When they successfully enter a new group, they have a relatively limited tenure, changing groups approximately every 5 years. While resident in the group, males' social rank increases with the length of their tenure.[24] Unlike females, whose social position results from the rank of her matriline, males show more social mobility within a group. On the other hand, male position in the group is transitory and they do not have the social alliances from kin that

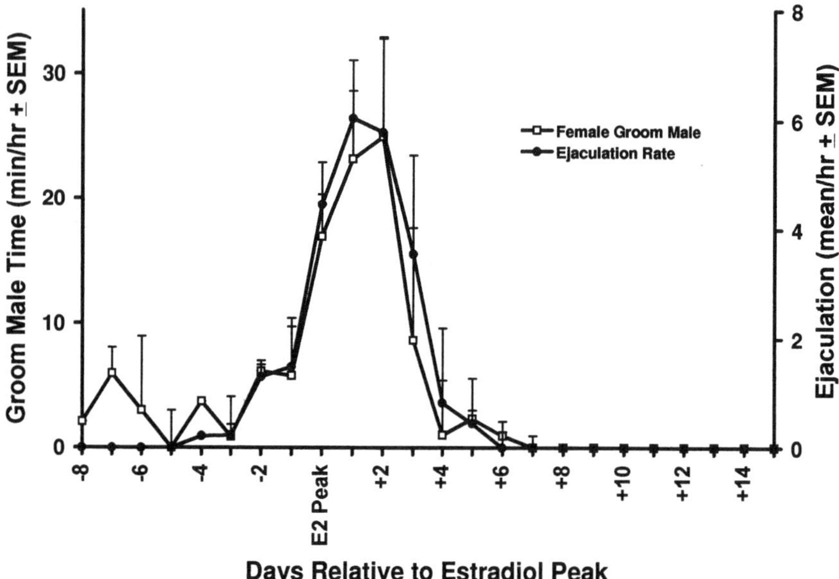

FIGURE 6. Occurrence of female grooming of males in relation to ejaculation rate across the ovarian cycles of nine adult female rhesus monkeys aligned by the day of peak estradiol.

are an integral part of female social life. Perhaps the tenuous nature of male group tenure influences the character of heterosexual relations within rhesus monkey groups. If a male makes a social mistake within a group, it is likely to have serious consequences. Lacking female alliances and male support, a male must be careful how he interacts with the permanent members of the group, the adult matriarchs and their female offspring. Therefore, where mating is concerned, a male probably cannot afford to try to force mating on a female. If unwanted, his mating attempt could result in expulsion from the group and potentially to death. We suspect that the courtship pattern in rhesus monkeys, in which the female initiates proximity and the male moves away, reflects an attempt by the male to reduce or eliminate ambiguity in the female's behavior. Persistent pursuit of the male and reestablishment of proximity by the female could unambiguously communicate to the male her sexual interest and reduce the possibility that the male will attempt to mate with an unwilling female who might use her relatives' aid to remove the male from the group. In this context, female grooming of a male between mounts can communicate the female's nonhostile intentions, maintaining the social interaction. If this is the case, it is not surprising that female grooming almost exactly mirrors the occurrence of sexual activity.

In contrast to grooming of males, grooming of females varies inversely with sexual activity (Fig. 7); therefore, females groom other females significantly less during the period of increased mating than they do at other times in the cycle. After the female stops mating with the male, to be a gradual increase in her

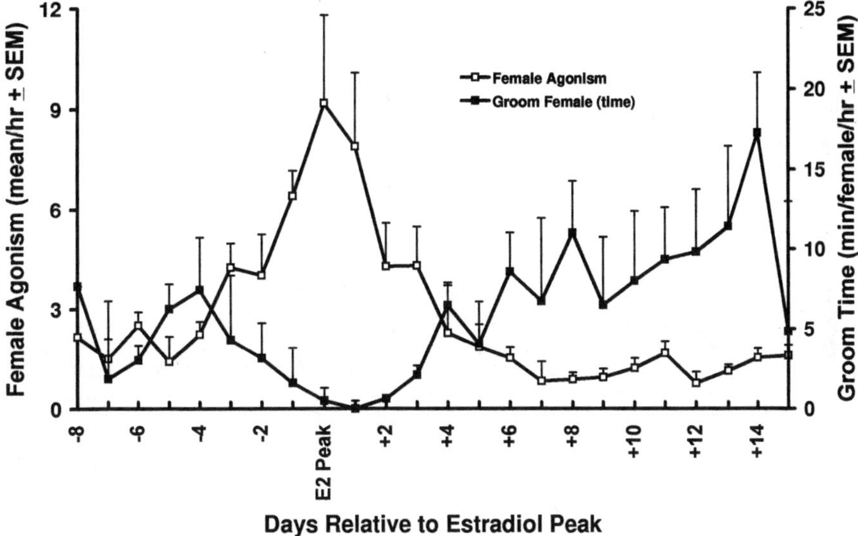

FIGURE 7. Decrease in female grooming of other group females during increases in ejaculation in relation to the peak estradiol level in the ovarian cycles of nine adult female rhesus monkeys.

grooming of other females occurs. As illustrated in FIGURE 8, this variation in grooming probably reflects the changes in female agonism that occur during the ovarian cycle.

Agonism. As females approach ovulation, both submissiveness and aggressiveness to other females increase. Whether it is primarily submissiveness or aggressiveness that increases depends on the social rank of the female. Thus, the highest ranking (alpha) female displays only increased aggression, because she is dominant to all the other females in the group. By contrast, the lowest ranking female (omega) displays only increased submissiveness during the periovulatory period. At midcycle, females who rank between the alpha and omega females are more aggressive to females ranking below them and more submissive to higher ranking females. Across ranks, however, these results suggest that increased sexual activity with the stimulus male disrupts social relationships between females. Thus, as females show increased and persistent affiliation with males at midcycle, they show decreased affiliation and increased agonism, both aggression and submission, to females. This relationship is illustrated in FIGURE 9, which shows female-female agonism in relation to the time spent grooming other females. One striking relationship in this figure is that as female agonism rapidly declines along with declining estradiol, female-female grooming increases. During the luteal phase, as female agonism remains low, grooming appears to increase, raising the possibility that females must actually repair their relations with other females after the disruption caused by sexual interactions with the male.

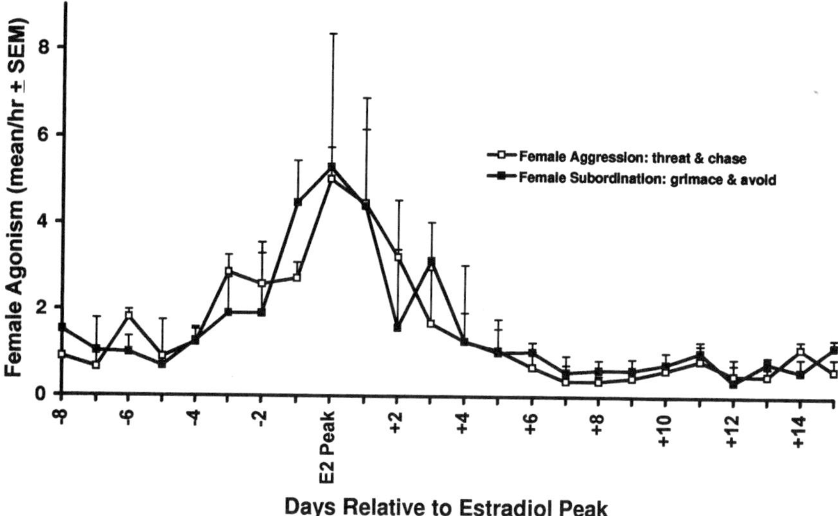

FIGURE 8. Female-directed aggression and submission across the ovarian cycle of nine adult female rhesus monkeys aligned on the day of peak estradiol.

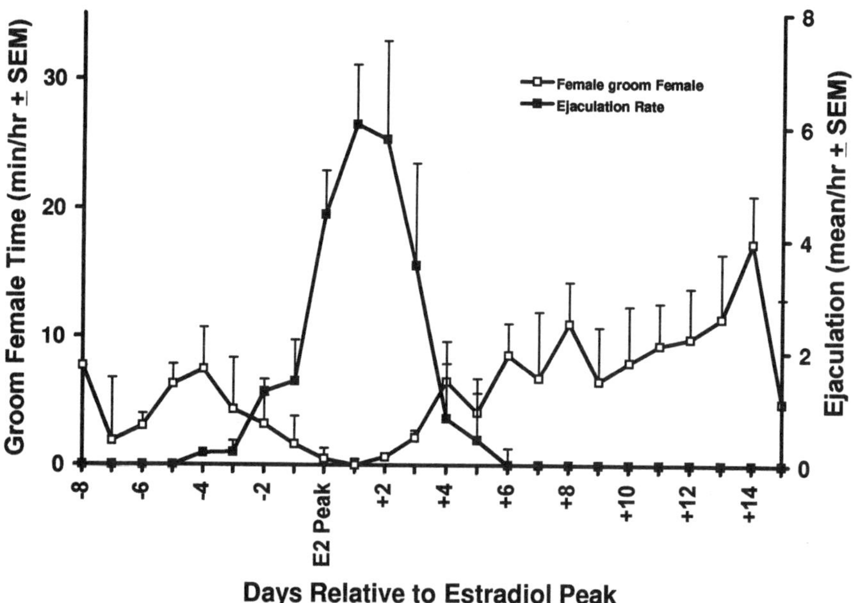

FIGURE 9. Relationship between female-directed agonism and grooming by females of other group females in relation to the peak estradiol level in the ovarian cycles of nine adult female rhesus monkeys.

A MODEL OF HORMONALLY MEDIATED SEXUAL BEHAVIOR AND AFFILIATION

Taken together these social interactions suggest a possible sequence of hormonally mediated events that modulate both male and female behavior. The female under rising levels of ovarian hormones, probably primarily from increases in estradiol,[14,26] becomes sexually interested in the male. This increases her attraction to the male and decreases her affiliative interactions with group females. As she actively courts the male, the female interacts less positively with other group females and, depending upon rank, may receive increased aggression from other females. In addition, as she pursues the male, she may become more aggressive towards other females. Her affiliative interactions switch from females to the male or, more typically in a multimale rhesus monkey troop, to males. Thus, pursuing and grooming the male increases the likelihood that the male will mate with the female, but it may also increase the potential for conflict with other group females. It is unlikely that the increased agonism between females, in our study, reflects competition for the male, because typically only one female or at most two were ever in the periovulatory portion of their cycle simultaneously. Instead, aggression towards a female showing sexual interest in a male probably reflects the potential social threat the sexually active female's association with the male may pose to the group's structure. Thus, the female experiences two opposing motivational forces, her own sexual interest in the male and the negative interactions with other group females.

For alpha females, this is not a particular conflict, but for lower-ranking females it appears to exert a marked effect on when they mate. For these females, sexual motivation must be very high to cause the female to risk aggression from higher-ranking females when she pursues the male. This appears to be exactly the case, as higher ranking females mate earlier in their ovarian cycle (when they would have had a shorter period of stimulation from ovarian hormones) and mate for more days in their cycle than do low-ranking females.[8] These findings suggest that the behavioral effects of ovarian steroids may have evolved to produce the sexual motivation necessary to induce mating in a social context where heterosexual activity is socially disruptive. In this regard it is particularly interesting that the hormonal changes that produce increased sexual interest in the male also switch female affiliative behavior away from group females to the male. Thus, the same hormonal changes that produce fertility also increase the female's sexual and affiliative interest in the male and decrease her affiliative interactions with females. As levels of these ovarian hormones decline, the social pattern reverses itself, and the female no longer courts or affiliates with the male and once again directs her affiliation towards group females. Although this fluctuation in female affiliation is easily detected within a closed social group, it is probable that the increased affiliation towards males associated with fertility is most important in the permeable groups that occur in the wild where unfamiliar males must integrate themselves into a new group. We discovered the potential power of hormonally modulated female affiliation towards males as part of an ongoing developmental study.

HORMONES, AFFILIATION, AND MALE SOCIAL INTEGRATION

As part of a study of the transition to adult sexual behavior, we introduced a group of 10 adolescent males to a group of 6 ovariectomized adult females when the males averaged 3.5 years of age, just prior to full pubertal onset. This female group consisted of females reared together from birth in a larger social group and then removed as an intact unit to a 15 by 15 m outdoor compound. These females were sexually experienced and had lived together as a group for 6 years before the male's introduction. The males and the females came from different social groups at the Yerkes Regional Primate Center Field Station and were unrelated and unfamiliar with each other.

We expected that by being housed together with the females, the two sexes would quickly socially integrate and we would later be able to study their adult sexual behavior by treating the females with estradiol. The group remained housed together for 2.5 years, without the females receiving any hormonal treatment. Contrary to our expectations, and we suspect anyone else's who would have done this manipulation, the males did not integrate with the females. When we formally observed the behavior of these males and females 2.5 years after the male introduction, no evidence of any affiliative interactions between males and females was found during 42 hours of observations over a 4-week period. The only social interactions between the males and females were aggression by the females directed towards the males and submissive behavior by the males towards the females (FIG. 10).

These formal observations corroborated more casual observations that we had made over the 2.5 years of continuous housing, which detected no evidence of positive social interactions between males and females. In reality the behavioral evidence suggested two completely separate social groups living together within a compound with all of the females outranking all of the males. Thus, continuous daily contact with females was not sufficient to socially integrate the males into the female's group. If this had been a free-ranging population, there is little doubt that these males and females would not have associated with each other at all. Only the artificial nature of the walled compound allowed us to see the lack of social integration of these males and females.

To investigate the effect that female hormonal state might have on social integration, all females simultaneously received hormonal treatments that produced periovulatory levels of estradiol.[27] Females received 3 weeks of estradiol treatment followed by 1 week without estradiol, another 3 weeks of estradiol treatment followed by a 4-week break. This treatment/nontreatment cycle was repeated three times, encompassing the spring and summer nonbreeding seasons and the fall breeding season. Behavioral data were collected for 10.5 hours each week for the spring, summer, and fall. After treatments ended, an additional 42 hours of behavioral data were collected during the spring 3 months and the spring 1 year after the last estradiol treatment (*Post Treatment*).

Estradiol treatments were started on a Friday afternoon with behavioral observations commencing the following Monday. The estradiol treatment rapidly and dramatically altered the social organization of these animals. The change was already apparent on Monday morning prior to formal observations as females were found grooming

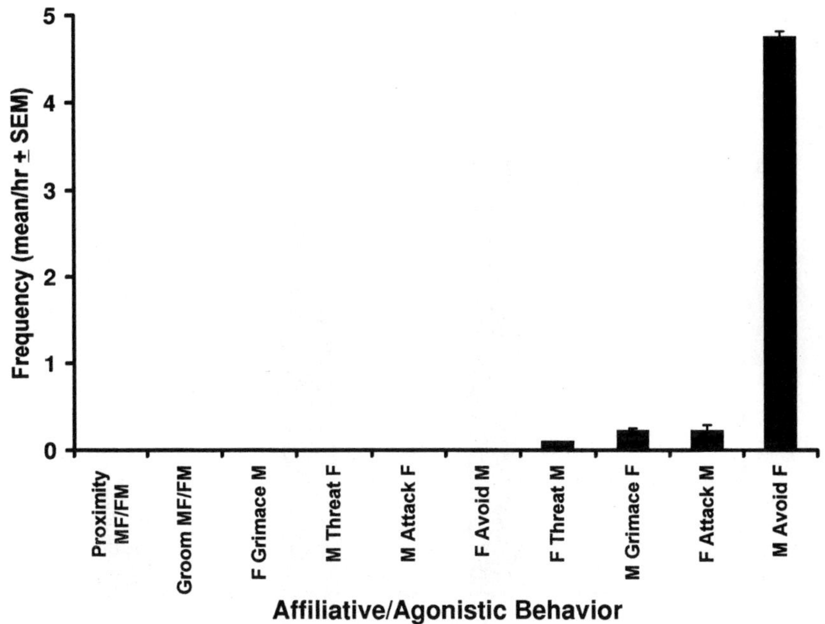

FIGURE 10. Mean rate of affiliative and agonistic behavior observed in a group of 10 adult male and 6 ovariectomized adult female rhesus monkeys after 2.5 years of continuous housing together. (**Key:** *Proximity* = sitting or standing within 20 cm of a partner; *Grimace* = lip-retraction submissive gesture; *Avoid* = active avoidance of an approach by another animal; *Threat* = staring, woofing, or open-mouthed facial gesture with or without vocalization; *Attack* = biting or slapping of another animal; *MF/FM* = male to female or female to male.)

males in the group, something never seen in the previous 2.5 years. This initial impression of rapid social integration was borne out during the formal data collection, as the females mated with and groomed 6 of the 10 group males. Thus, 3 days of exposure to estradiol, and possibly less, had effected what more than 900 days of continuous social contact could not. However, not all males were equally affected by the changed behavior of the females, as only 6 of the 10 males were observed to mate with the 6 ovariectomized estradiol-treated females during the 2 years of observation following the initial estradiol treatment. These mated males integrated into the female's group and showed the most profound change in their social relations with the females. That there were only six mated males may be related to the skewed sex ratio in this group which had more males than females and contrasted to the female-dominated sex ratio seen in free-ranging troops.[1] Although there were six mated males and six estradiol-treated females, there was not a one-one relationship, as the females each mated with several males and none of the males and females mated exclusively with each other.

Given the rhesus monkey proclivity for promiscuity, it is unclear why four males apparently never mated with the females. In none of the males did their developmental

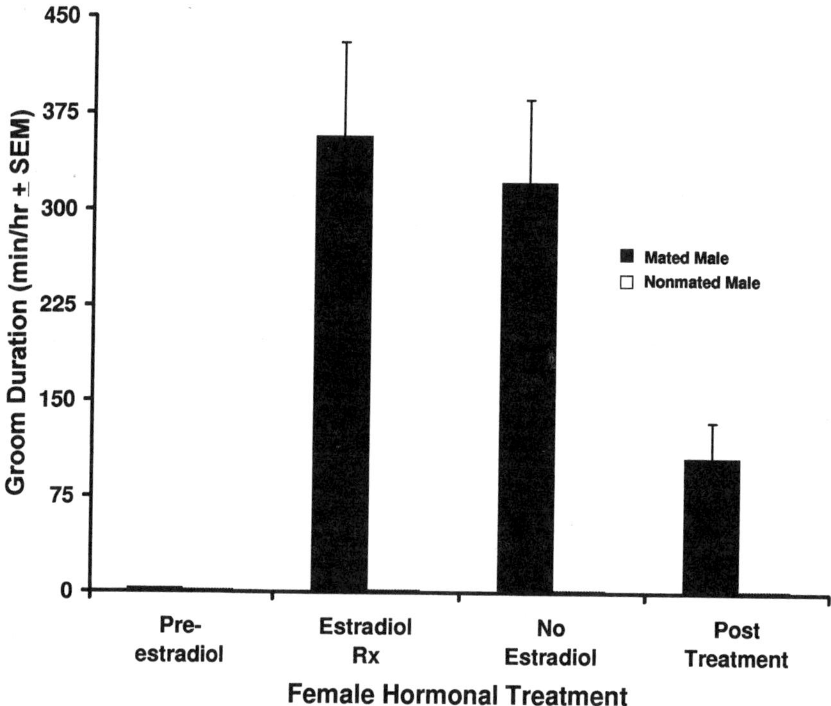

FIGURE 11. Duration of grooming by females towards males who either mated with females (mated) or did not (nonmated) during different female hormonal conditions over a 2-year period. (**Key:** *Pre-estradiol* = prior to any female hormonal treatment; *Estradiol Rx* = during the six 3-week estradiol treatment periods; *No estradiol* = during the three 1-week breaks between estradiol treatments; *Post Treatment* = 3 months and 1 year 3 months after the last estradiol treatment.)

history or social position prior to the female estradiol treatment predict whether they would mate or not. Furthermore, during the third estradiol treatment round (fall breeding season), the nonmated males mated when they received pair tests with one of the group females away from the rest of the group.[27] Thus, these nonmated males were capable of mating. However, this mating experience with the females out of the group setting did not alter their social relations within the group, and they essentially only interacted with other males. Although we have no explanation for the failure of these males to mate in the group, their social relationship with the females clearly did not show comparable changes to those seen in the mated males. FIGURE 11 illustrates the duration of female grooming of the two groups of males before, during, and after estradiol treatment and then 3 months and 1 year and 3 months after the cessation of estradiol treatment. The mated males differed significantly from the nonmated males at all time points except prior to estradiol treatment (*Estradiol Rx:* $F_{1,8} = 14.6$, $p < 0.0001$; *No Estradiol:* $F_{1,8} = 15.4$, $p < 0.0001$; *Post Treatment:*

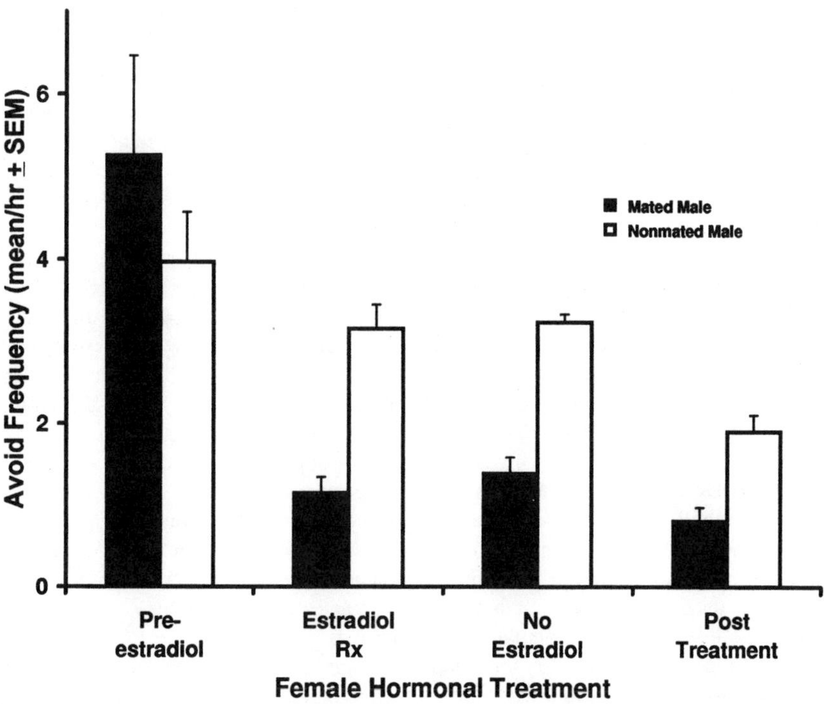

FIGURE 12. Mean frequency with which mated and nonmated males avoided approaches by group females when females were under different hormonal conditions. Key as in FIGURE 11.

$F_{1,8} = 8.1$, $p < 0.008$). Similarly, the mated but not the nonmated males were groomed by females significantly more at every time period after the pre-estradiol period (*Overall:* $F_{3,24} = 24.2$, $p < 0.001$; vs. *Estradiol Rx:* $t_5 = 6.0$, $p < 0.001$; vs. *No Estradiol:* $t_5 = 6.2$, $p < 0.001$; vs. *Post Treatment:* $t_5 = 5.1$, $p < 0.001$).

Not only did estradiol treatment significantly increase affiliation between mated males and females, but this increase was sustained even when the females had not received estradiol treatment for more than a year. Other affiliative behavior, such as female initiation of proximity, showed the same pattern of change during and after estradiol treatment. In contrast, mating behavior, which was stimulated by estradiol treatment, ceased completely once the females stopped estradiol treatment. Thus, hormonal treatment induced both sexual activity and affiliation, but increased affiliation continued after hormonal treatment stopped, whereas sexual behavior did not. This suggests that either the hormonal treatment itself, the act of sexual intercourse, or the affiliative relationships associated with mating permanently altered the associations between the females and those males that mated. Nonmated males did not show this change in affiliation with the females and continued to avoid females (FIG. 12) at rates comparable to those seen before estradiol treatment ($F_{3,24} = 1.8$, $p = 0.18$), whereas mated males showed a significant decrease in avoidance of females which was sustained even after the females no longer received estradiol ($F_{3,24} = 15.8$, $p < 0.001$; all comparisons to *Pre-estradiol* avoid significantly lower *p*s < = 0.002)

Estradiol treatment altered the social rankings of the males. Whereas before the estradiol treatment all males ranked below all females, within 6 weeks after the initial estradiol treatment four of the six mated males increased in rank, with two mated males ranked just below the alpha female and her daughter. The four nonmated males occupied the lowest four ranks within the group, which was a decline in rank for three of the four males. Thus, while initial social rank did not predict which of the 10 males would mate, after mating and affiliating with group females, all mated males outranked all nonmated males.

Thus, estradiol treatment rapidly, profoundly, and apparently permanently transformed the social structure of this captive group. Because both sexual activity and affiliative behavior increased almost simultaneously, it is not possible to say whether the social transformation resulted from increased sexual activity or whether the estradiol treatment simultaneously increased the females' affiliative and sexual interest in the males. However, the changes seen in this group are consistent with the model presented earlier, where changes in ovarian hormones produce social change by first altering the female's sexual attraction and motivation towards males. These motivational changes result in female sexual initiation which alters the social context of the group. In the present case, this sequence of events also permanently altered the character of social relations between the females and some males.

These results also support the notion that it is the sexual interest of females in males that facilitates male entry into a new social group. In the present case, familiarity without estrogen stimulation was insufficient to integrate these males with the females. Free-ranging male rhesus monkeys enter new groups almost exclusively during the breeding season,[5–7] suggesting that female sexual interest induced by ovarian cycles is an effective way to establish affiliations between males and group females allowing male entry into the group.

ROLES OF OVARIAN HORMONES IN SEX AND SOCIETY

These studies illustrate the tremendous power that the female's ovarian cycle exerts over the social character of rhesus monkey groups. As females near ovulation, their sexual and affiliative interest in males increases, affecting their social interactions with both males and females. This sexual interest in males can alter social relationships between females, and, in our studies and others,[18] conflict between group females increases during periods of heightened sexual activity. However, the period of increased conflict between females lasts a few days and then more peaceful relations are rapidly restored. The existence of mechanisms to maintain a balance between affiliating with males to engage in sex and affiliating with females to maintain a stable social structure is crucial to rhesus monkey social organization. The cyclical nature of female reproduction, with the same hormones producing fertility, sexual desire, and sexual affiliation, is one such mechanism that assures each female of mating without producing chronic stress on the social structure of the group. While potentially disruptive to established social relationships within a group, cyclical female sexual interest makes rhesus monkey groups permeable to new male immigrants. Thus, sexual motivation and its behavioral consequences can put stress on some social relationships while simultaneously facilitating the formation of new affiliations. Possibly the seasonal breeding pattern of rhesus monkeys[1,11,13] is an adaptation to limit socially disruptive activity to a small portion of the year.

Zuckerman[28] was partly correct when he argued that sexual activity was the basis of primate social organization. Sexual interest is probably the crucial motivational system, facilitating initial male-female social integration within rhesus monkey and, we suspect, other primate groups. However, it cannot be that rhesus monkey social structure is maintained as a result of continuous sexual activity, because few, if any, primates (including humans) mate continuously. Although most primate species are physically capable of mating at any time, with or without hormonal stimulation,[8,15] mating behavior is cyclic under socially complex conditions, with periods from weeks to years in which no mating occurs. Instead, it is affiliative mechanisms, initiated as a consequence of sexual attraction, that maintain social cohesion when sexual activity ceases completely. In this view, hormonally mediated sexual motivation profoundly transforms social relations within groups and influences the fundamental character of rhesus monkey social organization.

REFERENCES

1. Lindburg, D. G. 1971. The rhesus monkey in North India: An ecological and behavioral study. *In* Primate Behavior: Developments in Field and Laboratory Research L. A. Rosenblum, Ed.: 1-137, Academic Press. New York.
2. Missakian, E. A. 1972. Genealogical and cross-genealogical dominance relations in a group of free-ranging rhesus monkeys (Macaca mulatta) on Cayo Santiago. Primates **13:** 169-180.
3. Wrangham, R. W. 1980. An ecological model of female-bonded primate groups. Behaviour **75:** 262-300.
4. Lovejoy, J. & K. Wallen. 1988. Sexually dimorphic behavior in group-housed rhesus monkeys (*Macaca mulatta*) at 1 year of age. Psychobiology **16**: 348-356.
5. Koford, C. B. 1966. Population changes in rhesus monkeys: Cayo Santiago, 1960-64. Tulane Stud. Zool. **13:** 1-7.
6. Lindburg, D. G. 1969. Rhesus monkeys: Mating season mobility of adult males. Science **166:** 1176-1178.
7. Drickamer, L. C. & S. H. Vessey. 1973. Group changes in free-ranging male rhesus monkeys. Primates **14:** 359-368.
8. Wallen, K. 1990. Desire and ability: Hormones and the regulation of female sexual behavior. Neurosci. Biobehav. Rev. **14:** 233-241.
9. Michael, R. P. & D. Zumpe. 1993. A review of hormonal factors influencing the sexual and aggressive behavior of macaques. Am. J. Primatol. **30:** 213-241.
10. Cochran, C. G. 1979. Proceptive patterns of behavior throughout the menstrual cycle in female rhesus monkeys. Behav. Neurol. Biol. **27:** 342-353.
11. Gordon, T. P. 1981. Reproductive behavior in the rhesus monkey: Social and endocrine variables. Am. Zool. **21:** 185-195.
12. Wallen, K. 1982. Influence of female hormonal state on rhesus sexual behavior varies with space for social interaction. Science **217:** 375-377.
13. Wilson, M. E., T. P. Gordon & D. C. Collins. 1982. Variation in ovarian steroids associated with the annual mating period of female rhesus (*Macaca mulatta*). Biol. Reprod. **27:** 530-539.
14. Wallen, K., L. Winston, S. Gaventa, M. Davis-DaSilva & D. C. Collins. 1984. Periovulatory changes in female sexual behavior and patterns of steroid secretion in group-living rhesus monkeys. Horm. Behav. **18:** 431-450.

15. WALLEN, K. 1995. The evolution of female sexual desire. *In* Sexual Nature Sexual Culture. P. R. Abramson & S. D. Pinkerton, Eds.: 57-79. University of Chicago Press. Chicago.
16. CARPENTER, C. R. 1942. Sexual behavior of free-ranging rhesus monkeys (*Macaca mulatta*). II. Periodicity of estrus, homosexual, autoerotocism and nonconformist behavior. J. Comp. Psychol. **33:** 143-162.
17. WALLEN, K. & L. A. WINSTON. 1984. Social complexity and hormonal influences on sexual behavior in rhesus monkeys (*Macaca mulatta*). Physiol. Behav. **32:** 143-162.
18. WALKER, M. L., M. E. WILSON & T. P. GORDON. 1983. Female rhesus monkey aggression during the menstrual cycle. Anim. Behav. **31:** 1047-1054.
19. ALTMANN, S. A. 1962. A field study of the sociobiology of rhesus monkeys, *Macaca mulatta.* Ann. N.Y. Acad. Sci. **102:** 338-435.
20. HRDY, S. B. & P. L. WHITTEN. 1987. Patterning of sexual activity. *In* Primate Societies. B. B. Smuts, D. L. Cheney, R. M. Seyfarth, R. W. Wrangham & T. T. Struhsaker, Eds.: 370-384. The University of Chicago Press. Chicago.
21. BERARD, J. D., P. NURNBERG, J. T. EPPLEN & J. SCHMIDTKE. 1994. Alternative reproductive tactics and reproductive success in male rhesus macaques. Behaviour **129:** 177-201.
22. GOUZOULES, S. & H. GOUZOULES. 1987. Kinship. *In* Primate Societies. B. B. Smuts, D. L. Cheney, R. M. Seyfarth, R. W. Wrangham & T. T. Struhsaker, Eds.: 299-305. The University of Chicago Press. Chicago.
23. SADE, D. S. 1965. Some aspects of parent-offspring and sibling relationships in a group of rhesus monkeys, with a discussion of grooming. Am. J. Phys. Anthrop. **23:** 1-18.
24. BERARD, J. D. 1990. Life history patterns of male rhesus macaques on Cayo Santiago. Ph.D. Dissertation, University of Oregon.
25. COLVIN, J. 1983. Influences of the social situation on male emigration. *In* Primate Social Relationships. R. A. Hinde, Ed.: 160-170. Sinauer Associates. Sunderland, Massachusetts.
26. LOVEJOY, J. & K. WALLEN. 1990. Adrenal suppression and sexual initiation in group-living female rhesus monkeys. Horm. Behav. **24:** 256-269.
27. EISLER, J. A., P. L. TANNENBAUM, D. R. MANN & K. WALLEN. 1993. Neonatal testicular suppression with a GnRH agonist in rhesus monkeys: Effects on adult endocrine function and behavior. Horm. Behav. **27:** 551-567.
28. ZUCKERMAN, S. 1932 reprinted in 1981. The Social Life of Monkeys and Apes. Routledge & Kegan Paul. Boston.

8

Conflict Resolution and Distress Alleviation in Monkeys and Apes

Frans B. M. de Waal and Filippo Aureli

Many social animals are characterized by permanent associations between individuals with partly overlapping, partly conflicting interests. Whereas the existence of these associations must mean that the parties on balance gain from them, this does not imply that competition has disappeared. Often, animals continue to compete over resources, such as food and mates, despite association and cooperation.

For such an arrangement to work, conflict needs to be regulated so that it does not undermine relationships. Thus, aggressive behavior is subject to strong constraints imposed by the need to preserve cooperative relationships. Realization of these constraints has resulted in a shift in attention from aggression as the expression of an internal state or drive to aggression as the product of social decision-making. This framework is referred to here as the *Relational Model* (FIG. 1) as it concerns the functioning of aggressive behavior within interindividual relationships. It looks at aggressive behavior as only one of several methods to resolve conflict, but one that is problematic as it may endanger the relationship. In other words, winning a fight is one thing, but winning it without harming one's position in a complex support network is quite something else.

One of the discoveries underlying the Relational Model is that nonhuman primates engage in nonaggressive reunions between former opponents not long after an aggressive confrontation. Dependent on the species, these reunions include mouth-to-mouth contact, embracing, sexual contact, grooming, holding hands, clasping the hips of the other, and so on. Opponents thus engage in rather intense mutual contact following conflict. Comparisons between postconflict events and behavior during control observations not preceded by aggression have demonstrated major differences (Section 2). Results from these studies contrast sharply with earlier views of aggression as a dispersive social force (i.e., one causing increased interindividual distance). All monkey and ape species studied thus far, both in captivity and in the field, exhibit a significant tendency towards reunion following aggressive conflict, thus usually reducing interindividual distance. On the assumption that these postconflict reunions serve to protect valuable relationships against the undermining effects of aggression, these reunions are now widely known as *reconciliations.*

The question why aggression sometimes escalates to violence or becomes so frequent as to damage relationships beyond repair achieves special significance within

Address for correspondence: Department of Psychology, Emory University, Atlanta, GA 30322 (tel: 404 727-7898; dewaal@rmy.emory.edu).

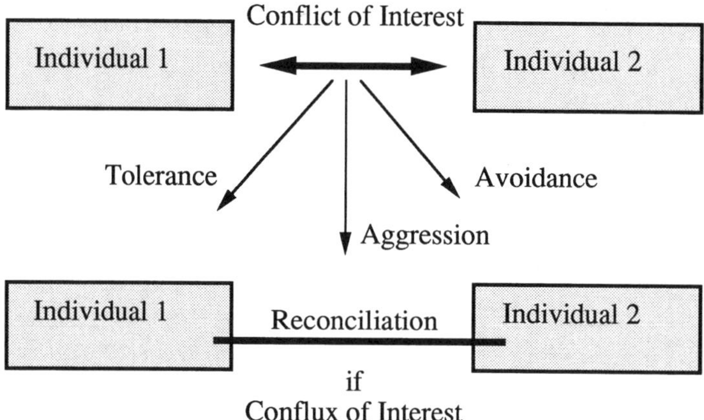

FIGURE 1. According to the Relational Model, aggressive behavior is one of several ways in which conflicts of interest are settled. Other possible ways are tolerance (e.g., sharing of a resource) or avoidance of confrontation. If aggression does occur, the nature of the relationship will determine if repair attempts will be made. If mutual interest in maintenance of the relationship is strong, reconciliation is likely. Parties negotiate the terms of their relationships by going through cycles of conflict and reconciliation.

this model, as it automatically translates into questions about the value individuals attach to their relationships and the social skills required to settle disputes in an alternative manner. The days of a deterministic view of aggressive behavior isolated from other social phenomena seem behind us.[1–3]

Rather than attempting a complete overview of the steadily growing stream of conflict resolution studies in nonhuman primates (an estimated 50 scientific studies on this topic have appeared in the last 15 years), our purpose here is to highlight specific areas that may benefit from the approach to conflict now being developed by students of primate behavior.

PEACEMAKING

After the first descriptive study of postconflict behavior in chimpanzees (*Pan troglodytes*),[4] a strong need was felt for controlled procedures permitting correction for baseline levels of behavior. This led to the so-called PC/MC method introduced by de Waal and Yoshihara[5] in a study of rhesus monkeys (*Macaca mulatta*). The procedure consists of a focal observation on an individual immediately following an aggressive incident in which this individual participated (postconflict observation, PC), and a control observation of the same duration on the same individual during the next possible observation day, starting at exactly the same time of day as had the PC observation (matched-control observation, MC). This paradigm has been applied, amongst others, to patas monkeys (*Erythrocebus patas*),[6] stump-tailed macaques (*M. arctoides*),[7] long-tailed macaques (*M. fascicularis*),[6] and golden monkeys

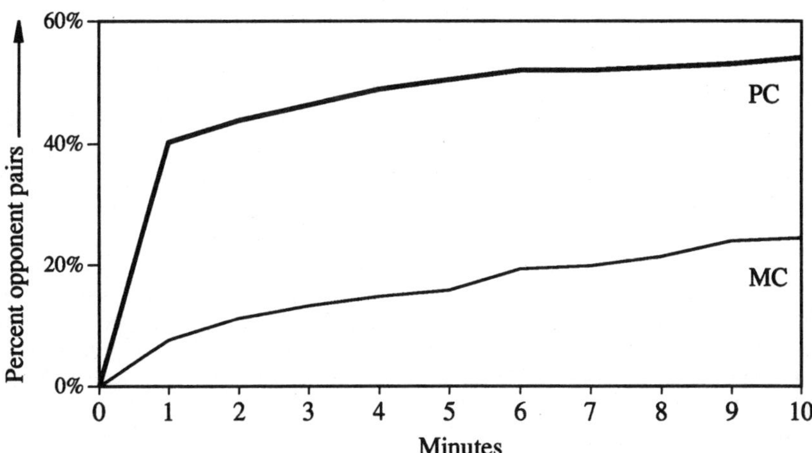

FIGURE 2. Chinese golden monkeys show a dramatic increase in nonagonistic body contact between former opponents during postconflict (PC) as compared to matched-control observations (MC). The graph provides the cumulative percentage of opponent-pairs engaging in contact during a 10-minute time window (after ref. 9).

(*Rhinopithecus roxellanae*).[9] FIG. 2 shows a typical result from such studies, that is, a high probability of contact following conflict.

Apart from increased contact following aggression, the hypothesis that these contacts serve reconciliation is supported by data demonstrating that (a) the contact-increase is selective, that is, it does not indiscriminately involve all possible partners but specifically involves former opponents, and (b) the probability of renewed aggression is reduced and tolerance is restored following postconflict contact.[10–12]

In chimpanzees, the same behavior patterns that characterize reconciliations are also employed to *forestall* aggression. For example, if an animal caretaker arrives with a bucket full of fruits and vegetables, the apes will rush towards each other embracing, kissing, and patting each other on the back before coming forward to collect their share. A more than 100-fold increase in contact behavior was documented upon the sight of food.[13] Based on the speculation that this behavior serves to reduce competition, an experiment was designed with different opportunities for prefeeding affiliation.[14] As predicted, aggressive competition over food was more common in food trials not preceded by such contact. Probably, these buffering mechanisms allow for the characteristic food-sharing of chimpanzees as they help reduce competitive tendencies. Similar mechanisms have been documented in a close relative, the bonobo (*Pan paniscus*).[15]

Finally, although observations of human conflict resolution are scarce and less rigorously controlled than the data available for nonhuman primates, attention to similar phenomena in child behavior is growing. The findings fit the Relational Model: conciliatory behaviors to terminate conflict among young peers are positively associated with peaceful associative outcomes and are used preferentially among friends.[16–19]

VALUABLE RELATIONSHIP HYPOTHESIS

As Kummer[20] was the first to point out, long-term relationships are an investment worth maintaining and defending. This insight has profound consequences for the way we view intragroup competition. It means that if two individuals compete over a particular resource, they need to take into account not only the value of the resource and the risk of bodily harm, but also the value of their relationship. Sometimes the resource may not be worth straining a cooperative relationship.

Even though primates differ dramatically in the behavior used to reconcile conflicts and the general tendency towards this behavior, all species seem to follow one general rule: reconciliation aims at restoring valuable relationships.[21] Thus, in species in which kin relationships are highly cooperative, related individuals reconcile more often than unrelated ones.[8,22–24] In chimpanzees, in which males form alliances that serve both intragroup and intergroup competition, conflicts among males are more often reconciled than among females.[25–26]

One experimental study adds strong support for the Valuable Relationship Hypothesis.[27] These investigators trained monkeys to cooperate during feeding. They induced a dramatic increase in reconciliation following conflict between partners who had learned to rely on each other for food acquisition.

Another way of investigating the relation between conciliatory tendency and social variables is through comparisons at the species level. Closely related species often differ on dimensions such as group cohesion, the strictness of the dominance hierarchy, the symmetry of aggressive encounters, social tolerance, and rates of affiliative behavior. Thus, studies on the genus Macaca have explored conflict resolution and the nature of dominance relationships from the perspective of group cohesion. These studies have demonstrated variation in dominance style, ranging from "despotic" to "tolerant." The first category of species, exemplified by the rhesus monkey, seems to emphasize priority rights in competitive situations, whereas the second category, exemplified by the stumptail macaque, emphasizes amicable social relationships. The evolution of these differences has theoretically been related to ecological factors and reliance of dominants on the cooperation of subordiates.[22,28–30]

AROUSAL REDUCTION

In macaques, displacement activities (e.g., self-scratching, self-grooming, and yawning) appear to reflect arousal due to "anxiety" and social tension. For example, self-scratching increases along with physiological signs of stress induced by anxiogenic drug treatment, but decreases following anxiolytic drug treatment.[31–34] Furthermore, it was demonstrated that being groomed by another monkey reduces a monkey's displacement activities.[35] This concurs with the finding of heart rate reduction in an individual being groomed.[36] It seems, therefore, that displacement activities are correlated with physiological measures of arousal.

Behavioral measures of arousal (just discussed) were investigated to determine their usefulness in relation to postconflict situations.[8,10] This research showed that (a) the rate of self-scratching and other displacement activities increased sharply on receipt of aggression, and (b) the rate declined much more rapidly to baseline levels following interopponent contact than without such contact. The implication is that reconciliation, in addition to affecting the social relationship between former opponents, has an immediate effect on the arousal state of losers.

Studies further indicate that not only the recipients of aggression, but also the aggressors themselves experience anxiety. Thus, in Barbary macaques (*Macaca sylvanus*) both aggressors and recipients of aggression scratch themselves more frequently in the aftermath of a conflict.[37] Furthermore, rhesus monkey aggressors were found to groom third parties who had not been involved in the preceding conflict. This grooming occurred especially after serious conflict between closely bonded partners. It may therefore reflect an internal conflict between continued hostility and attraction towards the opponent.[5]

If aggressors show signs of anxiety following conflict, both opponents may experience uncertainty about their relationship. This may stimulate attempts to restore the relationship. If true, the higher rate of reconciliation found between opponents with high-quality relationships could be due to a higher level of postconflict anxiety in both partners. Individuals with high-quality relationships have more to lose from the disruption of their relationships. This view is supported by data on scratching rates in long-tailed macaques. Recipients of aggression scratched themselves more often after unreconciled conflicts with high-quality partners than after conflicts with low-quality partners.[37] The fact that the same monkey showed a differential increase in scratching depending on the relationship quality with its opponent supports the hypothesis that postconflict anxiety is not a reaction to the mere loss of a confrontation. What matters most, it seems, is the disruption of a high-quality relationship as also expressed in more frequent reconciliation of conflicts in this category of relationships.[8]

SOCIAL LEARNING

Interspecific variability in aggressivity and conciliatory tendency makes it possible to experimentally expose members of a given species to a social environment with dramatically different rates of these behaviors. This can be done by housing them together with another species. If reconciliation is a learned social skill, such a manipulation is expected to have an effect. This problem has been examined by exposing rhesus monkeys, a rather intolerant species with low levels of reconciliation, to a highly conciliatory species, the stumptail macaque.[38]

Juveniles were housed in mixed-species groups of seven monkeys each for 5 months. Following this, they were observed for 6 weeks in groups of conspecifics only. Control rhesus monkeys, matched in age and sex to the experimental subjects, went through the same procedure without contact with the other species (i.e., all-rhesus groups). The main result of this manipulation was a three- to fourfold increase in the proportion of fights that were followed by reconciliation. This difference emerged gradually during the cohousing phase and was sustained following removal of the "tutor" species (FIG. 3). This result shows that reconciliation behavior can be modified through environmental manipulation.

DISTRESS ALLEVIATION AND EMPATHY

Sensitivity to the emotions of others emerges early in humans, such as when a nursery room with infants bursts out crying in response to the cries of one amongst

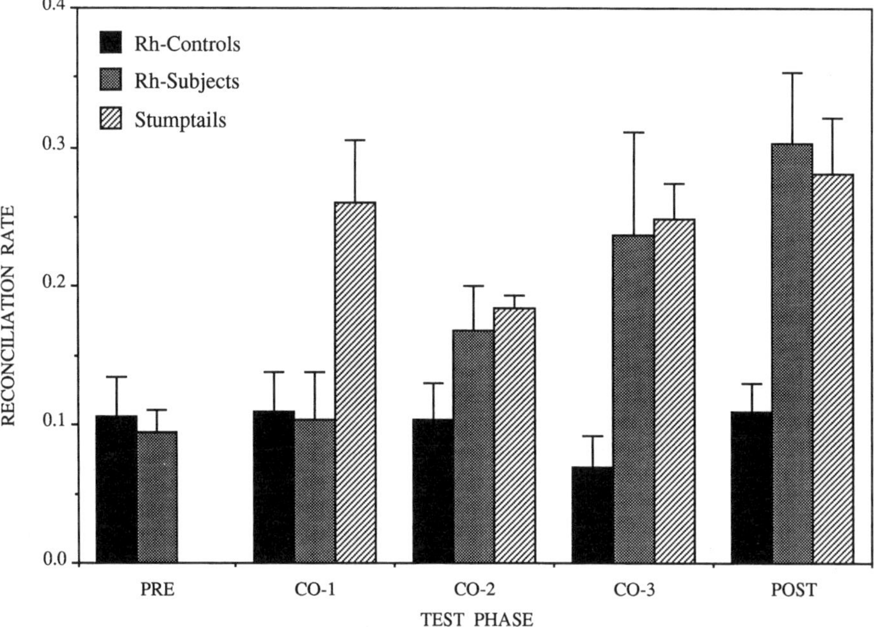

FIGURE 3. Mean (± SEM) proportion of aggressive encounters followed within 3 minutes by a reconciliation initiated by the subject. Data are for rhesus controls (Rh-Controls) housed with conspecifics only; rhesus experimental subjects (Rh-Subjects) exposed to stumptail monkeys; and stumptail monkeys acting as "tutors" for the rhesus subjects. The conciliatory tendency of the rhesus subjects was similar to that of the controls before cohousing (PRE) and during the first cohousing phase (CO-1). It steadily increased during continued cohousing to remain above control levels even after the rhesus subjects had been separated from the tutor species (POST). For the stumptails, no data were available for the prephase period (after ref. 38).

them. This process, known as "empathic distress" or "emotional contagion,"[39,40] provides the ontogenetic basis for cognitively more advanced responses to distress in which the actor understands the other's situation, distinguishes the other's distress from his or her own feelings, and acts out of genuine concern about the other's well-being. Hence, dependent on the precise mechanism involved, *empathy,* or the capacity to be emotionally affected by someone else's feelings, can be cognitively simple or complex. It is generally assumed that in the course of development, empathic distress becomes associated with the emergence of a cognitive sense of self and others.[40,41] In support of this assumption, cognitively mediated empathic responses emerge at approximately the same time during development as mirror self-recognition.[42–44]

The aforementioned developmental perspective is relevant in connection with a comparative one because of possible interspecific variation in self-knowledge. The work of Gallup and others[45,46] on self-recognition in mirrors suggests that humans and apes differ in this regard from most or all monkey species. Even if we accept that passing the mirror test demonstrates self-awareness, however, this does not mean that failing the test proves its absence. The mirror test provides a compelling, yet very limited measure of animal self-knowledge.[47,48] Nevertheless, the noted difference in performance on the mark test is an empirical difference that may bear on expressions of empathy. It is of interest, therefore, that reassuring responses to distress in others are frequently observed in chimpanzees, yet are rare or absent in monkeys studied thus far.

An early study on chimpanzees indicated that affiliative contact between recipients of aggression and nonopponent third parties (bystanders) occurred more often in the first minute following a conflict than in subsequent minutes.[4] Moreover, first-minute contacts included three times more embracing and gentle touching than did contacts during subsequent minutes. The high rate of embracing made interactions with bystanders behaviorally distinct from reconciliation (between opponents), which is typified by kissing. Postconflict contact with bystanders was labeled *consolation.*

Because of the brevity of the observation window and the lack of control data, the study just described was replicated. We analyzed a large data set (based on 345 hours of observation) on a colony of 17 chimpanzees in an outdoor compound at the Field Station of the Yerkes Regional Primate Research Center. Postconflict data were compared with control data to test predictions derived from the hypothesis that postconflict affiliative contact with nonopponents is consolatory, that is, it serves to alleviate stress caused by the previous incident. This hypothesis predicts more contact with recipients of aggression than with the aggressors themselves and more contact with recipients of serious aggression than of mild aggression.

Both predictions were supported by the data. One only needs to watch a group of chimpanzees for a short while to witness acts of consolation and reassurance. This species evolved specific behavior to alleviate distress in others, probably derived from maternal gestures to comfort and calm infants (FIG. 4A).[50,51]

In macaques, in contrast, none of the studies addressing this behavior has thus far produced any evidence for consolation. Despite various measures and statistical methods, the finding has been the same in four different species: affiliative contact between recipients of aggression and bystanders does not occur more often following conflict than during control periods.[10,52–55] Despite this lack of evidence, qualitative observations suggest that macaques do engage in consolation behavior at least when very young. We have regularly seen infant rhesus monkeys being attracted to the screams of one amongst them (e.g., after punishment by an adult or after a fall), approach the vocalizer, and establish contact (FIG. 4B). Occasionally, this resulted in a pile of infants clambering over each other. Given this strong empathic distress response, why is there so little of it left at later ages?

One possible explanation is that association with the recipient of aggression is fraught with risk. In macaques, recipients of aggression continue to attract aggression in the period immediately following the aggressive incident.[5,10,11,53] If this elevated chance of further aggression extends to bystanders approaching recipients of aggression, this is a risk bystanders need to reckon with. Only bystanders able to repel potential aggressors, either alone or together with the original recipient of aggression, do not face this constraint on consolation.

The strict hierarchy and kin-based alliance system typical of macaques do not leave much room for a protective role of bystanders. This may discourage them to associate with recipients of aggression. In chimpanzees, on the other hand, this

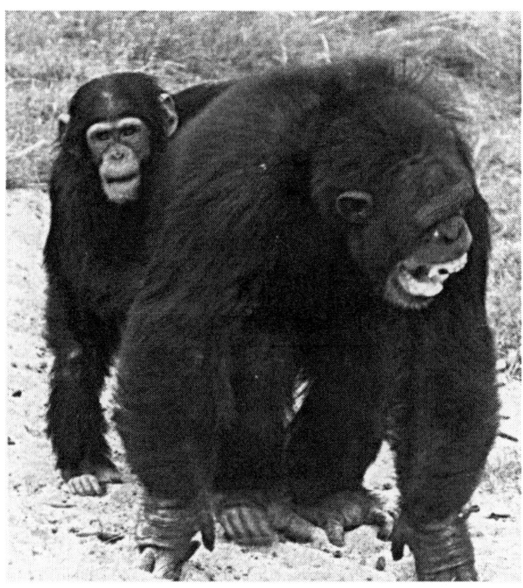

FIGURE 4A. Consolation in chimpanzees. A juvenile embraces a screaming adult male who has lost a confrontation with a rival (photograph by F. de Waal).

constraint may be less important because of the loose hierarchy, high level of social tolerance, and more flexible alliances.[49] This explanation in terms of social constraints, and possible interspecific differences in this regard, serves as an alternative to the foregoing possibility of an interspecific difference in self-other distinction, hence in social cognition.

One way to distinguish between these two hypotheses is through experiments that eliminate the risks associated with approaching a distressed group mate. For example, bystanders could be allowed to approach a recipient of aggression in the absence of the original aggressor. Cues may also be found by studying the response to distress not associated with aggressive incidents, such as distress caused by a fall or fear-inducing stimulus. If macaques still fail to show consolation responses under these circumstances, this would strengthen the case for a cognitive explanation of the difference with chimpanzees.

CONCLUSION

The foregoing results regarding reconciliation behavior and distress alleviation in nonhuman primates have recently been tied to the evolution of morality in our own species. If it is agreed that empathy and a need to get along despite interpersonal conflict are essential ingredients of human moral systems, that moral systems are, in effect, systems of conflict resolution,[56] the observed conciliatory and comforting tendencies of other primates hint at continuity with our behavior even in this domain.[57]

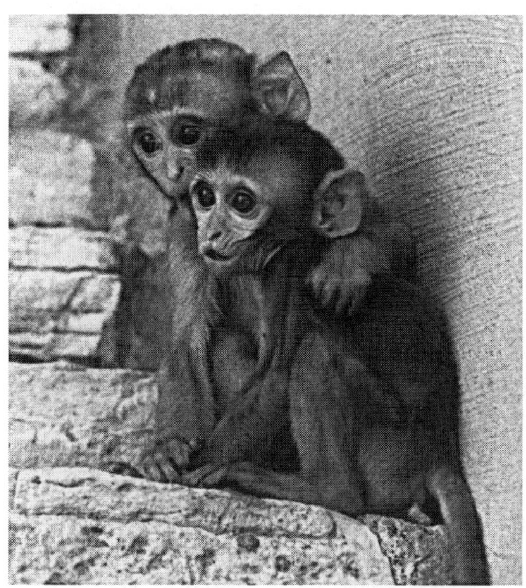

FIGURE 4B. Two 3-month-old infant rhesus monkeys following an incident in which the monkey in the foreground was seriously bitten by a dominant female. The victim is embraced by a peer. At this age, rhesus monkeys do seem to show affiliative responses to distressed conspecifics, but this response almost entirely disappears at later ages (photograph by F. de Waal).

This continuity, if confirmed by further research, will have far-reaching implications for the way we look at human existence. But also at a more concrete level there is ground for a thorough reevaluation of previous assumptions. For example, the reviewed findings indicate that most of the time, aggressive behavior is a well-integrated component of primate social relationships. This view is radically different from the earlier view of aggression as a destructive force; aggressive behavior appears to serve as a tool of negotiation within well-established relationships. Aggression can be used in this way precisely because its deleterious effects are buffered by postconflict interactions that alleviate anxiety and repair valuable relationships. The aftermath of conflict in primate groups thus provides a key to an understanding of the dynamic interplay between conflictual and integrative tendencies.

SUMMARY

Research on nonhuman primates has produced compelling evidence for reconciliation and consolation, that is, postconflict contacts that serve to respectively repair social relationships and reassure distressed individuals, such as victims of attack. This has led to a view of conflict and conflict resolution as an integrated part of social relationships, hence determined by social factors and modifiable by the social environment. Implications of this new model of social conflict are discussed along with evidence for behavioral flexibility, the value of cooperation, and the possibility that distress alleviation rests on empathy, a capacity that may be present in chimpanzees and humans but not in most other animals.

REFERENCES

1. DE WAAL, F. B. M. 1989. Peacemaking among Primates. Harvard University Press. Cambridge, MA.
2. SILVERBERG, J. & J. P. GRAY, EDS. 1992. Aggression and Peacefulness in Humans and Other Primates. Oxford University Press. New York, NY.
3. MASON, W. A. & S. P. MENDOZA, EDS. 1993. Primate Social Conflict. SUNY Press. Albany, NY.
4. DE WAAL, F. B. M. & A. VAN ROOSMALEN. 1979. Reconciliation and consolation among chimpanzees. Behav. Ecol. Sociobiol. **5:** 55-66.
5. DE WAAL, F. B. M. & D. YOSHIHARA. 1983. Reconciliation and redirected affection in rhesus monkeys. Behaviour **85:** 224-241.
6. YORK, A. D. & T. E. ROWELL. 1988. Reconciliation following aggression in patas monkeys, *Erythrocebus patas*. Anim. Behav. **36:** 502-509.
7. DE WAAL, F. B. M. & R. REN. 1988. Comparison of the reconciliation behavior of stumptail and rhesus macaques. Ethology **78:** 129-142.
8. AURELI, F., C. P. VAN SCHAIK & J. A. R. A. M. VAN HOOFF. 1989. Functional aspects of reconciliation among captive long-tailed macaques (*Macaca fascicularis*). Am. J. Primatol. **19:** 39-51.
9. REN, R., K. YAN, Y. SU, H. QI, B. LIANG, W. BAO & F. B. M. DE WAAL. 1991. The reconciliation behavior of golden monkeys (*Rhinopithecus roxellanae roxellanae*) in small breeding groups. Primates **32:** 321-327.
10. AURELI, F. & C. P. VAN SCHAIK. 1991. Post-conflict behaviour in long-tailed macaques (*Macaca fascicularis*): I. The social events. II. Coping with the uncertainty. Ethology **89:** 89-114.
11. CORDS, M. 1992. Post-conflict reunions and reconciliation in long-tailed macaques. Anim. Behav. **44:** 57-61.
12. DE WAAL, F. B. M. 1993. Reconciliation among primates: A review of empirical evidence and unresolved issues. *In* Primate Social Conflict. W. A. Mason & S. P. Mendoza, Eds.: 111-144. SUNY Press. Albany, NY.
13. DE WAAL, F. B. M. 1989. Food sharing and reciprocal obligations among chimpanzees. J. Hum. Evol. **18:** 433-459.
14. DE WAAL, F. B. M. 1992. Appeasement, celebration, and food sharing in the two Pan species. *In* Topics in Primatology: Vol. 1, Human Origins. T. Nishida, W. C. McGrew, P. Marler, M. Pickford & F. B. M. de Waal, Eds.: 37-50. University of Tokyo Press. Tokyo.
15. DE WAAL, F. B. M. 1987. Tension regulation and nonreproductive functions of sex among captive bonobos (*Pan paniscus*). National Geographic Res. **3:** 318-335.
16. SACKIN, S. & E. THELEN. 1984. An ethological study of peaceful associative outcomes to conflict in preschool children. Child Dev. **55:** 1098-1102.
17. HARTUP, W., B. LAURSEN, M. STEWART & A. EASTENSON. 1988. Conflict and the friendship relations of young children. Child Dev. **59:** 1590-1600.
18. VESPO, J. E. & M. CAPLAN. 1993. Preschoolers' differential conflict behavior with friends and acquaintances. Early Ed. Dev. **4:** 45-53.
19. VERBEEK, P. & H. D. CREVELING. 1996. Conflict participation, conflict behavior, and social functioning, in 4-5 yr-old preschoolers. Under revision.
20. KUMMER, H. 1978. On the value of social relationships to nonhuman primates: A heuristic scheme. Soc. Sci. Info. **17:** 687-705.

21. KAPPELER, P. M. & C. P. VAN SCHAIK. 1992. Methodological and evolutionary aspects of reconciliation among primates. Ethology **92:** 51-69.
22. THIERRY, B. 1985. A comparative study of aggression and response to aggression in three species of macaque. *In* Primate Ontogeny, Cognition and Social Behaviour. I. Else & P. Lee, Eds.: 307-313. Cambridge University Press. Cambridge.
23. VEENEMA, H. C., M. DAS & F. AURELI. 1994. Methodological improvements for the study of reconciliation. Behav. Processes **31:** 29-38.
24. DEMARIA, C. & B. THIERRY. 1992. The ability to reconcile in Tonkean and rhesus macaques. The XIVth Congress of the International Primatological Society, Strasbourg, Abstract Book, p. 101.
25. DE WAAL, F. B. M. 1986. Integration of dominance and social bonding in primates. Q. Rev. Biol. **61:** 459-479.
26. GOODALL, J. 1986. The Chimpanzees of Gombe: Patterns of Behavior. Belknap of Harvard University Press. Cambridge, MA.
27. CORDS, M. & S. THURNHEER. 1993. Reconciliation with valuable partners by long-tailed macaques. Ethology **93:** 315-325.
28. DE WAAL, F. B. M. & L. M. LUTTRELL. 1989. Toward a comparative socioecology of the genus Macaca: Different dominance styles in rhesus and stump-tailed macaques. Am. J. Primatol. **19:** 83-109.
29. DE WAAL, F. B. M. 1989. Dominance "style" and primate social organization. *In* Comparative Socioecology. V. Standen & R. Foley, Eds.: 243-263. Blackwell. Oxford.
30. VAN SCHAIK, C. P. 1989. The ecology of social relationships amongst female primates. *In* Comparative Socioecology: The Behavioral Ecology of Humans and Other Mammals. V. Standen & R. Foley, Eds.: 195-218. Blackwell. Oxford.
31. NINAN, P. T., T. M. INSEL, R. M. COHEN, J. M. COOK, P. SKOLNICK & S. M. PAUL. 1982. Benzodiazepine receptor-mediated experimental "anxiety" in primates. Science **218:** 1332-1334.
32. INSEL, T. R., P. T. NINAN, J. ALOI, D. C. JIMERSON, P. SKOLNICK & S. M. PAUL. 1984. A benzodiazepine receptor-mediated model of anxiety. Arch. Gen. Psychiatry **41:** 741-750.
33. CRAWLEY, J. N., P. T. NINAN, D. PICKAR, G. P. CHROUSOS, M. LINNOILA, P. SKOLNICK & S. M. PAUL. 1985. Neuropharmacologic antagonism of the b-carboline induced "anxiety" response in rhesus monkeys. J. Neurosci. **5:** 474-486.
34. MAESTRIPIERI, D., G. SCHINO, F. AURELI & A. TROISI. 1992. A modest proposal: Displacement activities as an indicator of emotions in primates. Anim. Behav. **44:** 967-979.
35. SCHINO, G., S. SCUCCHI, D. MAESTRIPIERI & P. G. TURILLAZZI. 1988. Allogrooming as a tension-reduction mechanism: A behavioral approach. Am. J. Primatol. **16:** 43-50.
36. BOCCIA, M. L., M. REITE & M. LAUDENSLAGER. 1989. On the physiology of grooming in a pigtail macaque. Physiol. Behav. **45:** 667-670.
37. AURELI, F. 1996. Post-conflict anxiety in nonhuman primates: The mediating role of emotion in conflict resolution. Aggressive Behav. In press.
38. DE WAAL, F. B. M. & D. L. JOHANOWICZ. 1993. Modification of reconciliation behavior through social experience: An experiment with two macaque species. Child Dev. **64:** 897-908.
39. HATFIELD, E., J. T. CACIOPPO & L. RAPSON. 1993. Emotional contagion: Curr. Dir. Psychol. Sci. **2:** 96-99.
40. HOFFMAN, M. L. 1987. The contribution of empathy to justice and moral judgment. *In* Empathy and Its Development. N. Eisenberg & J. Strayer, Eds.: 47-80. Cambridge University Press. Cambridge.
41. HOFFMAN, M. L. 1981. Perspectives on the difference between understanding people and understanding things: The role of affect. *In* Social Cognitive Development. J. H. Flavell & L. Ross, Eds.: 67-81. Cambridge University Press. Cambridge.
42. BISCHOF-KÖHLER, D. 1988. Über den Zusammenhang von Empathie und der Fähigkeit sich im Spiegel zu erkennen. Schweiz. Z. Psych. **47:** 147-159.

43. JOHNSON, D. B. 1982. Altruistic behavior and the development of self in infants. Merril-Palmer Q. **28:** 379-388.
44. ZAHN-WAXLER, C. & K. D. SMITH. 1992. The development of prosocial behavior. *In* Handbook of Social Development. V. B. van Hasselt & M. Hersen, Eds.: 229-256. Plenum Press. New York.
45. GALLUP, G. G. 1982. Self-awareness and the emergence of mind in primates. Am. J. Primatol. **2:** 237-248.
46. POVINELLI, D. J. 1987. Monkeys, apes, mirrors and minds: The evolution of self-awareness in primates. Human Evol. **2:** 493-507.
47. MITCHELL, R. W. 1993. Mental models of mirror-self-recognition: Two theories. New Ideas Psychol. **11:** 295-325.
48. CENAMI SPADA, E., F. AURELI, P. VERBEEK & F. B. M. DE WAAL. 1995. The self as reference point: Can animals do without it? *In* The Self in Infancy: Theory and Research. P. Rochat, Ed.: 193-215. Elsevier. Amsterdam.
49. DE WAAL, F. B. M. & F. AURELI. 1996. Consolation, reconciliation, and a possible cognitive difference between macaque and chimpanzee. *In* Reaching into Thought: The Minds of the Great Apes. A. E. Russon, K. A. Bard & S. T. Parker, Eds: 80-110. Cambridge University Press. Cambridge.
50. MASON, W. A. 1964. Sociability and social organization in monkeys and apes. *In* Advances in Experimental Social Psychology. L. Berkowitz, Ed.: 227-305. Academic Press. New York.
51. VAN LAWICK-GOODALL, J. 1968. The behaviour of free-living chimpanzees in the Gombe Stream Reserve. Anim. Behav. Monogr. **1:** 161-311.
52. JUDGE, P. G. 1991. Dyadic and triadic reconciliation in pigtail macaques (*Macaca nemestrina*). Am. J. Primatol. **23:** 225-237.
53. AURELI, F. 1992. Post-conflict behaviour among wild long-tailed macaques (*Macaca fascicularis*). Behav. Ecol. Sociobiol. **31:** 329-337.
54. AURELI, F., H. C. VEENEMA, C. J. VAN PANTHALEON VAN ECK & J. A. R. A. M. VAN HOOFF. 1993. Reconciliation, consolation, and redirection in Japanese macaques (*Macaca fuscata*). Behaviour **124:** 1-21.
55. AURELI, F., M. DAS, D. VERLEUR & J. A. R. A. M. VAN HOOFF. 1994. Post-conflict social interactions among Barbary macaques (*Macaca sylvanus*). Int. J. Primatol. **15:** 471-485.
56. ALEXANDER, R. D. 1987. The Biology of Moral Systems. Aldine. New York.
57. DE WAAL, F. B. M. 1996. Good Natured: The Origins of Right and Wrong in Humans and Other Animals. Harvard University Press. Cambridge, MA.

9

Social Facilitation, Affiliation, and Dominance in the Social Life of Spotted Hyenas

Stephen E. Glickman, Cynthia J. Zabel, Sonja I. Yoerg, Mary L. Weldele, Christine M. Drea, and Laurence G. Frank

Spotted hyenas (*Crocuta crocuta*) are social carnivores, living in multifemale, multimale "clans."[1,2] With female philopatry and male dispersal, separate female and male dominance hierarchies, and female matrilines that constitute the fundamental social core of the clan, the social organization of spotted hyenas approximates that of many common old world monkeys in the broad outline of their sociality.[3,4] Membership in the clan enables hyenas to hunt prey as large as zebra and is essential to defense of kills against lions and of hunting territories against other groups of hyenas.

Spotted hyenas also display some rather unique characteristics. Adult females and their juvenile, or subadult, offspring dominate adult immigrant males in virtually all social interactions.[4–6] In addition, hyenas often spend their days alone at solitary dens, typically reassembling in the late afternoon and socializing at the communal den before forming smaller hunting parties. For many hyenas there is a daily transition from a solitary existence to the intense, highly differentiated social interactions of life within the clan.[1]

All social carnivores display a delicate balance between cooperation and competition. In spotted hyenas, competition may simply be evinced by speed-of-eating at a kill. That is, with a group of hyenas feeding at a dead wildebeest and reducing it to a small pile of horns and hooves in less than 30 minutes, the individual that can eat most rapidly will have an advantage over colleagues that eat more slowly. Overt aggression and the formation of dominance hierarchies also play a role in access to resources, and dominance rank is directly related to ultimate reproductive success.[7]

The present paper focuses on the integration of cooperation and competition, and correlated behavioral mechanisms of aggression, dominance, and affiliation, within the social life of the spotted hyena. Towards that end, we focus on three themes that have emerged from our studies of these animals: (1) the emergence of individually differentiated systems underlying cooperation and competition from a more general tendency of hyenas to do-what-other-hyenas-are-doing; (2) the role of "meeting

This work was supported by a grant from the National Institute of Mental Health (MH-39917).

ceremonies'' in mediating daily transitions between solitary and social existence; and (3) the fact that the most aggressive, dominant animals in our social groups are also, commonly, the most affiliative animals, displaying high levels of prosocial behavior in a variety of contexts. In regard to the last theme, Wingfield and his collaborators provided compelling evidence that in certain social systems, high levels of aggression are incompatible with successful mating and reproduction.[8] That could be operative in hyenas as well, with consistent selection against excessive, undifferentiated aggression. However, there is another side to this issue. As long as aggression, dominance, and affiliation remain appropriately differentiated, they are not incompatible components of individual sociality.

THE BERKELEY HYENA PROJECT

The data cited in this report were drawn from a decade-long study of the morphology and behavior of spotted hyenas in captivity. Our research has focused on the physiological substrates of sexual differentiation and a set of questions raised by the unusual genital masculinization of this species. Female spotted hyenas have no external vagina, as the labia of the external vagina have fused to form a pseudoscrotum. The clitoris is hypertrophied, approximating the size and contour of the male penis, and female hyenas display erections similar to those of the male.[9–11] This clitoris is traversed by a central urogenital canal through which the female spotted hyena urinates, copulates, and gives birth.[10,12] Our investigations have provided a route through which an inactive androgen generated by the maternal ovary (androstenedione) is transformed by the placenta into testosterone and transmitted to developing fetuses of both sexes.[13,14] This maternally derived testosterone could provide at least a partial explanation of the genital masculinization observed in female hyenas. It might also contribute to the neonatal aggression observed in hyenas of both sexes[15] and the persistent aggressiveness of female spotted hyenas. Ongoing studies involving the administration of anti-androgens to pregnant female hyenas, however, suggest that placental T is just one contributory factor, and other nontraditional mechanisms may be involved.[16,17]

Our studies were initiated with two groups of hyenas collected in Kenya as infants and reared in peer groups. In terms of behavior, a striking feature of our investigations was the emergence of the natural characteristics of hyena sociality in our peer-reared animals despite the absence of the many potentially critical aspects of the natural situation, including sustained maternal influence, the need to hunt for food, or danger from predation by lions. These included the gradual development of female dominance[18,19] and the ultimate appearance of female matrilineal organization, with a separate female dominance hierarchy, cubs acquiring their mother's rank, and dominance of all cubs and adult females over adult males.[20] In addition, as will be detailed, many of the specific behavioral mechanisms displayed by hyenas in nature not only have been observed in captivity, but also have followed the same rules of social expression as those found in nature. This has given us confidence that novel phenomena observed in our captive animals also occur in nature, but the frequency of expression is almost surely different in the natural situation.

SOCIAL FACILITATION OF BEHAVIOR

"In many behavior patterns a clear attraction is apparent between individuals which seems to exist regardless of sex or family tie. This is most obvious when one watches communal activities like zebra hunting, fighting between clans, pasting, social defecating, and so on. But with some activities, I had the impression that they were performed with the sole function of 'doing something together,'. . . ."[1,p241].

For the dedicated spotted hyena watcher, one of the most striking characteristics of the spotted hyena is the tendency of individual animals to do what other hyenas are doing, that is, to exhibit social facilitation of behavior.[21] In his work with wolves, Lockwood[22] made a similar set of observations and suggested that behavioral synchrony was required in social hunting groups on the move. It is a characteristic that pervades virtually every aspect of daily life. For example, within our colony, such social facilitation was observed to increase the probability of ingestive behavior, scent marking, meeting ceremonies, olfactory investigation, and play as well as promote the development of coalitions that serve to reinforce the existing dominance hierarchy.

Ingestive Behavior. In the natural setting, the cooperative hunting of spotted hyenas is followed by intensely competitive feeding. Even in our captive animals, for which food is provided on a daily basis and efforts are made to insure that the lowest ranking animal gets its share, the presence of a feeding hyena stimulates others to eat. The powerful facilitatory effects of observing other hyenas eat could be used to overcome an experimentally induced food aversion.[23] In this investigation, an aversion was established by pairing a novel food with lithium chloride in individual hyenas that were members of small social groups. The aversion was clear and inhibited eating as long as these individuals were tested in solitary fashion. However, when exposed to the food in concert with other group members that had not been conditioned, the conditioned animals could not resist joining their colleagues, even as the conditioned animals sometimes illustrated their ambivalence by approach-withdrawal or taking small, dainty bites instead of their preferred gulps of food. It was also possible to demonstrate social facilitation of spontaneous drinking at a spout in straightforward fashion. When two groups of hyenas (n's = 5 and 7) were released into a yard, individuals that watched a comrade drink were much more likely to drink in the minutes immediately following such drinking. The probability of a second animal drinking declined rapidly in the minutes that followed drinking by the first animal. Observation further indicated that social drinking was provoked by visual observation of the act on the part of the second animal (FIG. 1).

Scent-Marking. Hyenas scent-mark within their territories by communal defecating[1] as well as by marking stalks of grass and other objects with "paste" extruded from their anal scent glands.[24] Although we have seen hyenas defecate or strain to defecate when another hyena is defecating, we do not have good numbers in hand to document this aspect of social facilitation. However, Woodmansee and her collaborators[25] were able to quantify the social facilitation of pasting among animals in our colony. The probability of pasting was markedly increased by the prior pasting of another hyena, with the second animal apparently responding to both the visual stimulus of another hyena marking and the olfactory stimulus provided by the soapy odor of paste.

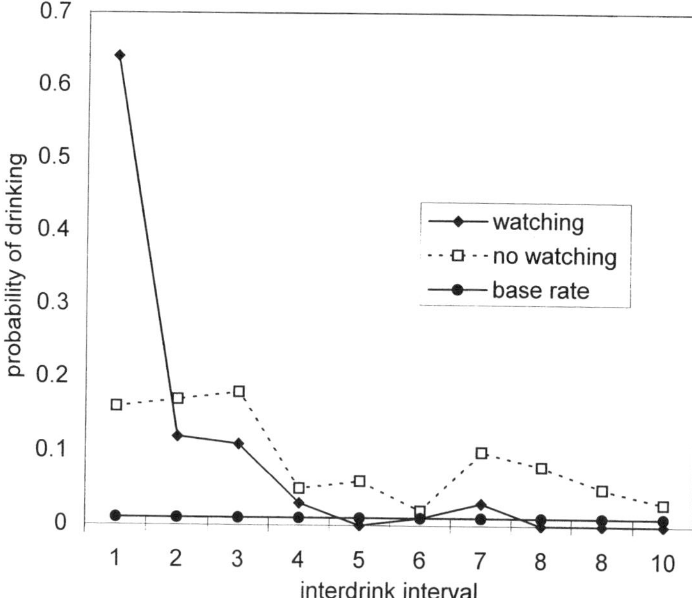

FIGURE 1. Probability of drinking as a function of time elapsed since another hyena drank. Inter-drink intervals (IDIs) represent successive 30-second intervals: ID 1 is comprised of drinking that occurred 0–30 seconds after another hyena drank; ID 2 is comprised of drinking that occurred 31–60 seconds after another hyena drank, etc. Data are presented separately for instances in which hyenas had watched another hyena drink in the preceding 5 minutes and cases in which such observation had not taken place. The base rate is the expected probability if drinking had been distributed randomly in time.

Olfactory stimuli frequently provide the focus for socially facilitated group behavior patterns. "The reaction of any hyenas . . . to the sight and sound of another one regurgitating is to run up, sniff the results of this action, and then immediately roll in it, shoulder first, then with the whole back."[1,p244] We also observed this within our colony and recorded several occasions on which groups of five to eight juvenile hyenas were simultaneously engaged in excited sniffing, with tails elevated, before rolling in the regurgitated product of one of their cohort (FIG. 2). Less dramatic olfactory stimuli often result in "social sniffing." As described by Kruuk,[1,p241] this typically involves a group of hyenas walking ". . . together at a brisk pace, fairly close, several with their tails up. Suddenly, one would stop, sniffing the ground in a place apparently randomly chosen–immediately all the others came rushing up, all starting to sniff the same place or immediately next to it." Mills[2] supports Kruuk's general description, although he suggests the possibility of an identifiable olfactory stimulus.

Coalitions. The preceding cases involve typical prosocial behavior patterns commonly enacted by groups of hyenas. However, affiliation and social facilitation also operate in the service of aggression and dominance. Kruuk,[1,p225 and plates 38&39] first

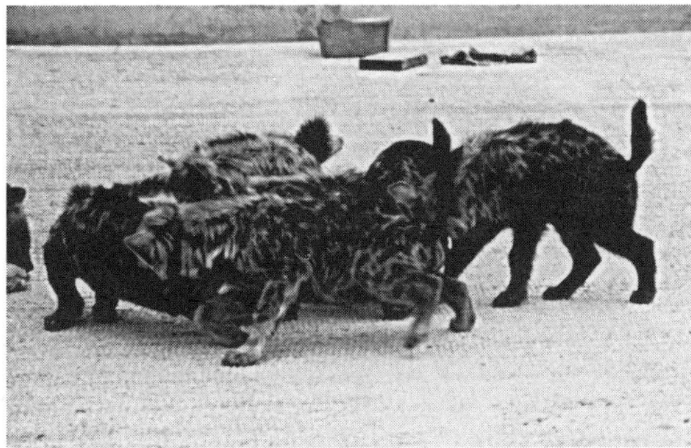

FIGURE 2. An excited group of juvenile spotted hyenas (note the erect tails). One hyena, in the center of the group, has just regurgitated some appropriately odoriferous material and the animals on the periphery were taking turns "rolling" in the substrate.

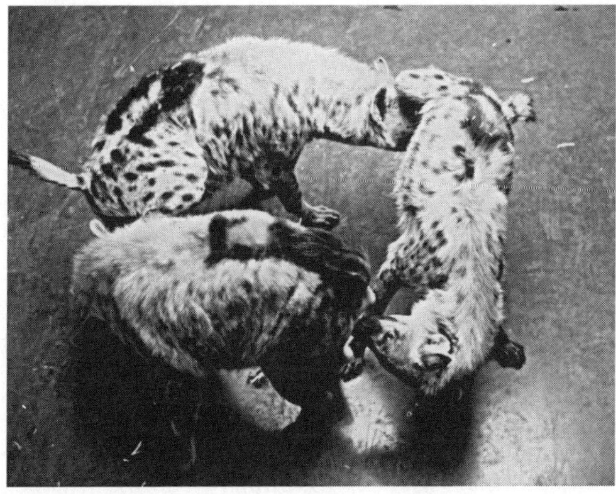

FIGURE 3. The hyena meeting ceremony. It is reasonably common, in the Berkeley colony, for a third hyena to approach and join two hyenas engaged in a meeting ceremony.

described the parallel walk in which two hyenas, walking shoulder to shoulder, threaten a third hyena by approaching the target animal in an attack posture. Mills[2] later described the formation of both transient and permanent coalitions in which groups of animals coordinate threats or attacks on individual hyenas. Such coalitions probably form more frequently in the captive situation because the entire group is in continuous proximity. However, the "rules" of coalition formation are presumably similar to those observed in nature. Within our colony, dyadic aggressive encounters were commonly joined by other hyenas according to a simple rule: join the side of the dominant animal as long as you are also dominant to the animal being threatened or attacked.[26] It is a rule that reinforces the existing dominance hierarchy and reduces social mobility in the group. Hyenas did occasionally aid at risk, that is, join a subordinate animal in attacking a higher ranking animal, but that was a relatively infrequent event. We also observed several small males enlist the aid of a high-ranking female in threatening/attacking a large female who, in a simple dyadic encounter, would have been expected to totally dominate the males. However, these latter cases are memorable precisely because they are exceptions. In general, one or more hyenas are drawn to an ongoing dyadic encounter, and the species-typical tendency to do what other hyenas are doing is activated. But at this point, social history enters as a variable and the animal has to remember her/his relationship to the combatants and adjust behavior accordingly. If our observing hyena is lower in rank than either of the participants, any tendency to join should be inhibited and s/he should discreetly leave the scene, because the subordinate participant in the ongoing encounter may be able to redirect the attack of the dominant animal, forming a new coalition against a lower ranking hyena. Alternatively, if our observing hyena is dominant to the animal being attacked, s/he can safely join in a coalition attack, reinforcing the lower status of the target animal and, perhaps, solidifying his/her own relationship with the higher ranking hyena. In this case, social facilitation appears to drive the tendency to attack, but it is always modulated or differentiated by the prior social history of the individuals involved.

MEETING CEREMONIES

Spotted hyenas have much more elaborate meeting ceremonies than do brown hyenas (*Hyaena brunnea*)[2] or striped hyenas (*Hyaena hyaena*).[28] This might well correlate with the greater complexity of social relationships in spotted hyenas as well as the daily transition from solitary to social existence. In the spotted hyena meeting ceremony, the participants approach one another, stand head to tail, and engage in intense olfactory investigation of the external genitalia, anal scent glands, and surrounding tissues. Data obtained by Kruuk,[1] Mills,[2] and East *et al.*[27] suggest that hyena etiquette has firm rules: the subordinate hyena lifts its hindleg first and offers its erect penis or clitoris for inspection by the dominant animal, which will usually then reciprocate. Many authors have called attention to the potential role of the meeting ceremony in maintaining group cohesion and speculated that the hypertrophied clitoris of the female spotted hyena might have been naturally selected as the result of benefits that accrued from participation in the meeting ceremony.[1,27]

In a study that involved a captive group of 10 subadult hyenas, Krusko and her collaborators[29] found that following a 4-hour period during which the animals were divided into two groups of five hyenas and separated in areas without visual or olfactory contact, a marked increment was noted in frequency of meeting ceremonies at the time of reunion. Moreover, the subjects apparently had kept track of who they had been separated from during the 4-hour interval, for each hyena engaged in a proportionally greater number of meeting ceremonies with the five animals from which they had been separated than the four animals with which they had resided during the interval. Krusko *et al.*[29] also observed that merely releasing the entire group of 10 animals from a semienclosed sleeping area to a somewhat larger outside area resulted in an increment in the number of meeting ceremonies, albeit a much less dramatic increment than that observed accompanying reunion after separation. This appeared to be a simple excitement-induced enhancement of meeting ceremony activity. Finally, as in nature, subordinate animals initiated meetings with dominant animals more frequently than the reverse. If dominance rank (as determined by threats, displacement, and subordinate postures during group competitive feeding[18]) was correlated with proportion of meetings received, there was an inverse correlation (rho = –0.85): high ranking animals received proportionally more meeting ceremonies than subordinate members of the group. Dominant animals also participate in more meeting ceremonies than do subordinates (rho = –0.74). As suggested by Kruuk[1] and substantially amplified by East *et al.*,[27] meeting ceremonies provide a crucial behavioral mechanism facilitating the transition between solitary and social existence, reinforcing dominance relationships that are of critical importance in the daily life of the clan, and adding to the cohesiveness of topranking members of the clan. The more frequent meeting ceremonies observed in situations involving tension or excitement suggest that these ceremonies may also operate as a device promoting reconciliation after, e.g., squabbles over food.

INTEGRATING AFFILIATION AND AGGRESSION

Affiliative and aggressive behavior was recorded in both cohorts of captive hyenas during an extended subadult period (from 11-21 months of age). A critical incident sampling procedure was employed, using a standardized list of behavioral definitions, with trained observers dictating an account of social interactions during evening observation periods. The auditory record from a voice-operated tape recorder was then entered into a computer database and analyzed in 30-second bins by way of an SAS package. The existence of this dataset provides an opportunity for examination of the relation between dominance and various patterns of affiliative behavior among members of the social group. It seemed possible that highly aggressive, dominant hyenas would be unable to surmount their aggressive tendencies and fully participate in the affiliative activities. Alternatively, it was also possible that given the apparent cohesion observed within high-ranking matrilines in nature, high-ranking members of our cohorts would engage in more affiliative behavior than low ranking hyenas.

Data bearing on these hypotheses are presented in TABLE 1. Although substantial variation exists in the magnitude of correlations observed in the two cohorts, results clearly support the second hypothesis. The correlational matrices show a strong tendency for positive correlations among measures of social (olfactory) investigation, participation in meeting ceremonies, scent-marking (''pasting''), and play. Moreover, all of these affiliative behaviors are positively related to dominance rank, as determined in a competitive feeding situation,[18] and dominance in hyenas is transsituational. Within our cohorts, there was a strong positive correlation between dominance rank determined in tests of competitive feeding and relative frequencies of giving (as opposed to receiving) aggression during spontaneous nightly, nonfeeding activities (Zabel, unpublished observations). If the power of statistical evaluation is increased by combining correlation coefficients from the two cohorts,[30,p157-158] only the relationship between play and scent-marking fails to achieve statistical significance. Similar cohesiveness among high-ranking animals recently was described in the field.[31]

TABLE 1. Rank-Order Correlation Coefficients among Measures of Social Behavior[a]

	Social Investigation	Meeting Ceremonies	Scent-Marking	Play	Dominance
		Cohort I (n = 10)			
Social investigation	—	0.40	0.47	0.63*	0.49
Meeting ceremonies	0.65*	. . .	0.71	0.13	0.66*
Scent-marking	0.53	0.60	. . .	0.23	0.60
Play	0.76*	0.86*	0.63*	. . .	0.59
Dominance	0.50	0.85*	0.74*	0.80*	—
		Cohort II (n = 10)			

* $p < 0.05$.

[a] Values for hyenas in cohort I are represented in the upper right portion of the table; Cohort II, the lower left section of the table.

ANDROGENS, DOMINANCE, AND AFFILIATION

It is common to associate the presence of androgens with aggressive behavior and social dominance.[32] However, in the ordinary case, that is obviously not incompatible with the same subjects also exhibiting high levels of affiliative behavior. As long as behavior remains "differentiated," that is, sensitive to the details of the social context and individual relationships, affiliative and aggressive behavior patterns can not only coexist, but also facilitate one another. We suspect that in spotted hyenas, dominance resulting (in part) from aggression and supported by coalition formation both permits and encourages high ranking animals to display affiliative behavior and forge cohesive social bonds.

SOME CONCLUDING THOUGHTS

A century ago, Morgan[33] described a process of social learning in chicks that were stimulated to peck by the presence of an experienced tutor. He referred to the process as *instinctive imitation* and allowed that it was a fundamental characteristic of social behavior. In its modern guise as social facilitation, such behavioral tendencies remain a fundamental substrate of social organization, albeit that they are modulated by a broad array of cognitive mechanisms, including histories of individual social relationships.

ACKNOWLEDGMENTS

The writers are indebted to Kathy Morehouse and the staff of the Office of Laboratory Animal Care of the University of California, Berkeley, for their dedicated work with the hyenas observed in the present report. We also thank the Office of the President and the Ministry of Tourism and Wildlife of the Government of Kenya, and the Narok County Counsel, for permission to collect and assistance in assembling the original cohorts of hyenas.

REFERENCES

1. Kruuk, H. 1972. The Spotted Hyena. University of Chicago Press. Chicago, IL.
2. Mills, M. G. L. 1990. Kalahari Hyaenas: Comparative Behavioral Ecology of Two Species. Unwin Hyman. London, England.
3. Frank, L. G. 1986. Social organization of the spotted hyena (*Crocuta crocuta*). I. Demography. Anim. Behav. **34:** 1500–1509.
4. Frank, L. G. 1986. Social organization of the spotted hyaena *Crocuta crocuta.* II. Dominance and reproduction. Anim. Behav. **34:** 1510–1527.
5. Holekamp, K. E. & L. Smale. 1991. Dominance acquisition during mammalian social development: The "inheritance" of maternal rank. Am. Zool. **31:** 306–317.
6. Smale, L., L. G. Frank & K. E. Holekamp. Ontogeny of dominance in free-living spotted hyaenas: Juvenile rank relations with adults. Anim. Behav. **46:** 467–476.
7. Frank, L. G., K. E. Holekamp & L. Smale. 1995. Demography, dominance and reproductive success in spotted hyenas: A long-term field study. *In* Serengeti II: Research, Management and Conservation of an Ecosystem A. Sinclair & P. Arcese, Eds.: 364–384. University of Chicago Press. Chicago, IL.
8. Wingfield, J. C., R. E. Hegner, A. M. Dufty, Jr. & G. F. Ball. 1990. The "challenge hypothesis": Theoretical implications for patterns of testosterone secretion, mating systems, and breeding strategies. Am. Nat. **136:** 829.
9. Matthews, L. H. 1939. Reproduction in the spotted hyaena *Crocuta crocuta* (Erxleben). Philos. Trans. R. Soc. Lond. B **230:** 1–78.
10. Neaves, W. B., J. E. Griffin & J. D. Wilson. 1980. Sexual dimorphism of the phallus in spotted hyaena (*Crocuta crocuta*). J. Reprod. Fertil. **59:** 506–512.
11. Frank, L. G., S. E. Glickman & I. Powch. 1990. Sexual dimorphism in the spotted hyaena. J. Zool. Lond. **221:** 308–313.
12. Frank, L. G. & S. E. Glickman. 1994. Giving birth through a penile clitoris: Parturition and dystocia in the spotted hyaena (*Crocuta crocuta*). J. Zool. Lond. **234:** 659–665.
13. Licht, P., L. G. Frank, S. Pavgi, T. Yalcinkaya, P. K. Siiteri & S. E. Glickman. 1992. Hormonal correlates of "masculinization" in female spotted hyaenas (*Crocuta crocuta*). II. Maternal and fetal steroids. J. Reprod. Fertil. **95:** 463–474.
14. Yalcinkaya, T. M., P. K. Siiteri, J.-L. Vigne, P. Licht, S. Pavgi, L. G. Frank & S. E. Glickman. 1993. A mechanism for virilization of female spotted hyenas *in utero.* Science **260:** 1929–1931.
15. Frank, L. G., S. E. Glickman & P. Licht. 1991. Fatal sibling aggression, precocial development, and androgens in neonatal spotted hyenas. Science **252:** 702–704.
16. Forger, N. G., L. G. Frank, S. M. Breedlove & S. E. Glickman. 1996. Sexual dimorphism of perineal muscles and motoneurons in spotted hyenas. J. Comp. Neurol. **374:** 1–11.
17. Drea, C. M., M. Weldele, L. G. Frank, P. Licht & S. E. Glickman. 1996. Effects of prenatal anti-androgen treatment on genital development in spotted hyenas (*Crocuta crocuta*). Paper presented at the Western Regional Conference on Comparative Endocrinology, Berkeley, California.
18. Frank, L. G., S. E. Glickman & C. J. Zabel. 1989. Ontogeny of female dominance in the spotted hyaena. Symp. Zool. Soc. Lond. **61:** 127–146.
19. Baker, M. G. 1990. Effects of ovariectomy on dyadic aggression and submission in a colony of peripubertal spotted hyenas (*Crocuta crocuta*). M. A. Thesis, University of California, Berkeley.

20. JENKS, S. M., M. WELDELE, L. G. FRANK & S. E. GLICKMAN. 1995. Acquisition of matrilineal rank in captive spotted hyaenas (*Crocuta crocuta*): Emergence of a natural social system in peer-reared animals and their offspring. Anim. Behav. **50:** 893-904.
21. ZAJONC, R. B. 1965. Social facilitation. Science **149:** 269-274.
22. LOCKWOOD, R. 1976. An ethological analysis of social structure and affiliation in captive wolves (*Canis lupus*). Ph.D Thesis, Washington University, St. Louis.
23. YOERG, S. I. 1991. Social feeding reverses learned flavor aversions in spotted hyenas. J. Comp. Psychol. **105:** 185-189.
24. GORMAN, M. L. & M. G. L. MILLS. 1984. Scent-marking strategies in hyaenas (Mammalia). J. Zool. **202:** 535-547.
25. WOODMANSEE, K., C. J. ZABEL, S. E. GLICKMAN, L. G. FRANK & G. KEPPEL, 1991. Scent-marking (''pasting'') in a colony of immature spotted hyenas (*Crocuta crocuta*): A developmental study. J. Comp. Psychol. **105:** 10-14.
26. ZABEL, C. J., S. E. GLICKMAN, L. G. FRANK, K. B. WOODMANSEE & G. KEPPEL. 1992. Coalition formation in a colony of prepubertal spotted hyenas. *In* Coalitions and Alliances in Humans and Other Animals. A. H. Harcourt & F. B. M. De Waal, Eds.: 113-136. Oxford University Press. Oxford.
27. EAST, M. L., H. HOFER & W. WICKLER. 1993. The erect 'penis' is a flag of submission in a female-dominated society: Greetings in Serengeti spotted hyenas. Behav. Ecol. Sociobiol. **33:** 355-370.
28. RIEGER, I. 1978. Social behavior of striped hyenas at the Zurich zoo. Carnivore **1:** 49-60.
29. KRUSKO, N. A., M. L. WELDELE & S. E. GLICKMAN. 1988. Meeting ceremonies in a colony of juvenile spotted hyenas. Paper presented at the annual meeting of the Animal Behavior Society, Missoula, Montana.
30. MCNEMAR, Q. 1969. Psychological Statistics, 4th Ed. John Wiley. New York.
31. HOLEKAMP, K. E., S. M. COOPER, C. I. KATONA, N. A. BERRY, L. G. FRANK & L. SMALE. 1997. Patterns of association among female spotted hyenas (*Crocuta crocuta*). J. Mammal. **78:** in press.
32. MONAGHAN, E. P. & S. E. GLICKMAN. 1992. Hormones and aggressive behavior. *In* Behavioral Endocrinology. J. B. Becker, S. M. Breedlove & D. Crews, Eds.: 261-286. MIT Press. Cambridge. MA.
33. MORGAN, C. L. 1896. Habit and Instinct. E. Arnold. London.

10
Affiliative Processes and Vocal Development

Charles T. Snowdon

The vocal communication system of many nonhuman primate species is richly complex with threat calls, alarm calls that in some species refer to specific predators, intergroup spacing calls, food associated calls, and others.[1,2] Relatively few studies have focused on vocalizations mediating affiliative relationships, in part because affiliative vocalizations are softer and more cryptic and therefore difficult to observe except in captive or highly habituated wild populations. In addition, affiliative relationships generally occur when animals are in close proximity and therefore other modalities such as facial expressions or chemical signals can be used in affiliative interactions.

In this chapter, I review briefly some of the studies on affiliative vocalizations in nonhuman primates and then move on to a topic I think is potentially more important: how affiliative processes mediate the ontogeny of vocal communication. Although my examples are drawn from nonhuman primates, the basic findings parallel recent studies on birds, cetaceans, and human children[3] and suggest that affiliative interactions during development are critical for acquiring communication skills in a wide range of species.

AFFILIATIVE VOCALIZATIONS

Rhesus macaques (*Macaca mulatta*) have been the subject of most research on affiliative vocalizations with the primary focus being the vocalizations used by infants when separated from their mothers. The calls given by separated infants have been classified as affiliative by several authors.[4–6] The coo structure of macaques varies with social contexts, and monkeys separated from mothers and out of their sight give different variants of coo vocalizations than they do when separated but in sight of the mother.[7] The rate of coo vocalizations is different as well, with more calls being given when infants and mother are in sight of each other. In a naturalistic study of stumptail macaques (*Macaca arctoides*), Lillehei and Snowdon[8] described two different forms of coo vocalizations, one used by infants seeking contact with mothers and another variant when they were seeking contact with other group members. Newman[9] used the separation paradigm to study vocal development in several species:

This research was supported by United States Public Health Service grants MH 29,775 and MH 00,177 and the University of Wisconsin Graduate School Research Committee.

rhesus macaques, squirrel monkeys (*Saimiri sciureus*), and common marmosets (*Callithrix jacchus*).

However, it is difficult to know whether to interpret the calls of separated infant monkeys as affiliative calls, distress calls, or fearful vocalizations. Because cortisol levels and other measures of stress often increase with separation, the vocalizations that are given might be more appropriately identified as stress or fear vocalizations. An alternative paradigm is to separate monkeys and then reunite them with their mothers, and monitor the vocalizations given during reunion. These vocalizations are more likely to reflect affiliative processes than are those given during separation. Kalin *et al.*[10] studied vocalizations produced by infant rhesus macaques during separation, during reunion with the mother, or during social interactions with an adult male. High levels of coos were recorded during both separation and interactions with the male, especially after the male rejected contact with the infant, but coos were rarely observed during reunion with the mother, suggesting that they do not function as affiliative calls. However, another vocalization, the girn, was found at high rates with the mother and during the first few minutes of interaction with males when infants attempted to attain contact with the male. After males rejected an infant, the rate of girns declined. Thus, the girn vocalization is probably the best candidate for an affiliative vocalization in infant rhesus macaques, and affiliative processes may be better studied during reunion rather than separation conditions.

A structurally similar vocalization was described for female Japanese macaques (*Macaca fuscata*).[11,12] These calls are used by females approaching other females with infants, by lower ranked females approaching a higher ranked female, and by groomers and recipients of grooming. In squirrel monkeys, the "chuck" vocalization serves as an affiliative call and is exchanged between females who have a preferential social relationship with each other ("friendship").[13] Thus, in polygynous species vocalizations appear to be used in affiliative interactions between females and between infants and mothers.

We studied the trill vocalizations of cooperative breeding pygmy marmosets (*Cebuella pygmaea*) in both captive and field environments. We observed a complex of four trill types, one variant was used prior to agonistic interactions, but the remaining three appear to be used primarily to promote contact among group members and to inform animals of the location of other group members. We found that trills are produced within a group antiphonally with each group member calling in turn.[14] Thus, in a group of three monkeys, sequences of each animal calling in turn occurred much more often than predicted by random production, and one particular sequence of turn-taking (1, 3, 2) occurred much more often than the other possible sequence (1, 2, 3). This turn-taking provides each animal with the opportunity to monitor the location of each other group member. In a field study in the Peruvian Amazon, we found that we could rank the three trill types according to how easily they could be localized and then observed that trills that were easy to localize were used by monkeys when they were relatively far away from other group members, and the most cryptic trill was used only when animals were in close proximity.[15] Thus, pygmy marmosets alter trill structure according to how close or how far they are from other group members. The trills were commonly given late in the day as animals moved to a sleeping site and appeared to have a clear affiliative function. The trills constitute the most frequent vocalization heard within a group of pygmy marmosets.

AFFILIATIVE PROCESSES AND VOCAL DEVELOPMENT

Modification of Trill Structure

Because of our extensive work with the trill vocalizations and the importance that they have for intragroup cohesion in pygmy marmosets, we have been interested in determining how the structure and usage of trills develop. We completed a longitudinal study of trill development in five litters of pygmy marmosets, recording at systematic intervals over the first 2 years of life.[16] We measured several variables of trills and evaluated four models of vocal development. We rejected the idea that trills were innately structured, because although trills were produced early in life, change in vocal structure was evident in each of our infants over time. We also rejected a model of maturational change because the changes that we observed over development were not completely consistent with predictions about maturation. Although several monkeys showed decreased pitch and increased duration of vocalizations with increasing age, other monkeys changed structures towards higher pitches and shorter durations. We also rejected a model of closed learning (equivalent to a sensitive period model) because we found that calls did not become stereotyped with age. Rather, the variability of call parameters for each individual as measured by coefficients of variability remained high throughout the study. This last finding was puzzling and appears to contradict results from language development and birdsong development studies.

In our attempts to find explanations for the developmental patterns of pygmy marmoset trills, we looked at literature on the modifiability of non-song calls in birds, in which changes in social composition lead to changes in call structure, even in adult birds. For example, Nowicki[17] reported that black-capped chickadees changed the structure of the "chick-a-dee" call within a week after a winter flock was formed, with all birds converging towards a common structure. Mundinger[18] reported that the American goldfinch changes its call notes with pair formation. After pair formation, males and females each drop some of their individual-specific call notes and acquire notes used by their mate.

Do similar results occur in mammals? We have two experiments that illustrate how changes in social companions affect the trill structure of pygmy marmosets. In the first study we utilized the arrival of two groups of pygmy marmosets donated by Dr. John Newman of the Laboratory of Comparative Ethology at the National Institutes of Health. We recorded trill vocalizations from these monkeys while they were in quarantine and at the same time recorded calls from monkeys in our own colony. After several weeks, we housed both populations in the same colony room. Each group was kept separate from the other and was visually isolated, but each group from our original colony and from the NIH groups could hear the calls of all other groups. Within the first 10 weeks after groups were housed in the same environment, significant changes were noted in the peak frequency and bandwidth of all monkeys for which we had an adequate sample size of trills. Changes were not restricted to the Madison or NIH population. All animals changed call structure in a similar direction regardless of their age or reproductive status.[19] Thus, mere exposure to the calls of novel social groups led to a change in trill structure.

In the second study, we recorded trills from four males and four females while they were postpubertal and living in their natal families. We paired each animal with an unfamiliar animal of the opposite sex and recorded trills over the first 6 weeks after pairing. We subsequently recorded several of the animals 3 years after pairing. We found little change in trill structure during the 2 months before pair formation, but within 3-6 weeks after being paired all individuals showed significant changes in some aspects of trill structure. We measured four variables in the trills of each individual, and of the 16 possible variables (four for each pair) we found significant change in structure in 13 variables. Although many pairs showed convergence towards similar call features, there was also evidence of both individuals shifting a parameter in the same direction, but maintaining a difference, or animals diverging from each other for a parameter that by chance had overlapped in the pre-pairing condition. When we recorded the same animals 3 years after pairing, we found the same trill parameters as we found 6 weeks after pairing. Thus, trill structure was stable for a few months before pairing and was stable for up to 3 years after pairing, but structure changed dramatically within a few weeks after animals were paired with a new mate.

Although relatively little attention has been paid to these subtle changes in vocal structure in mammals, several other studies reported similar findings. Tyack and Sayigh[20] report that male dolphins use each other's signature whistles when they are coalition partners. Stanger[21] reported that dwarf lemurs changed the pitch of their whistle vocalizations when groups were rearranged and animals placed in contact with new social companions. Randall[22] found that kangaroo rats changed the pattern of foot-drumming patterns to avoid overlap with the patterns of new neighbors. Hausberger *et al.*[23] reported that both male and female starlings change the song types they use when the structure of social groups was changed. Each bird typically had another bird in the flock with which it had the closest associations, and these birds shared many of the same song types. Starlings could produce totally new song types that they had not been heard to produce before to match the songs of a new companion.

All of these examples illustrate a phenomenon of human speech called "optimal convergence."[24] We frequently adjust our communication to speak with children in a different way than we do with each other, but because speech style provides cues of group membership, adults also shift aspects of speech to "fit in" with a new social group. We can signal our interest in staying with the new group by adjusting some aspects of our speech, but we risk being viewed as patronizing or insincere if we imitate another's speech patterns too closely. Thus, it is valuable to show solidarity by changing speech style while maintaining individual distinctiveness. Each of the examples described from pygmy marmosets to dwarf lemurs to dolphins to kangaroo rats to starlings illustrates a similar sort of "optimal convergence." This phenomenon is another example of how affiliation patterns affect communication.

Babbling

Babbling is ubiquitous in human infants and is hypothesized to play an important role for an infant to practice the sounds of language and the combination of sounds into words and phrases.[25] Babbling is also a highly social act. Caretakers interact with infants more when they are babbling, and this provides social reinforcement of babbling. Even deaf infants show manual babbling.[26]

The major nonhuman animal model for babbling has been the song bird. Marler[27] argued that birdsong was a good model for speech development in humans, and he identified two periods: subsong and plastic song which appeared similar to the babbling of human infants. During these phases of song development, birds produce a variety of calls and notes that over time become organized into the species-typical adult song. Recently, it was shown that social interactions with breeding males during the subsong and plastic song phases influence the final adult song structure of an individual bird.[28]

There have been no mammalian models for infant babbling, creating the impression of an evolutionary gap between birds and humans. We noted that pygmy marmoset infants produced long sequences of vocalizations that appeared early in development. We define a bout of babbling as consisting of at least four different types of vocalizations included in a sequence with at least 1 s separating adjacent bouts. This definition is similar to that of "variegated" babbling in human infants, a later developmental stage than "canonical" babbling. Thus, our definition for pygmy marmoset babbling is a conservative one.

We completed a longitudinal study of eight infant pygmy marmosets in which we recorded babbling and social behavior in systematic observations over the first 20 weeks of life. We found seven aspects of pygmy marmoset babbling that parallel babbling in human infants.

1. Babbling is universal: All human infants babble, and we have found that it occurred in each of the 78 pygmy marmosets born in our colony over the last 20 years.

2. Babbling is rhythmical and repetitive: The same call type is repeated several times in succession before the infant switches to a different call type. The rate of vocalization is constant within and between individuals at about 3 calls per second.

3. Babbling occurs early in life: Human infants start babbling by 7 months of age, and half of our sample of monkeys babbled in the first 2 weeks of life and all were showing regular babbling by the fourth week.

4. The sounds of babbling are subsets of adult speech sounds. We documented 20 different vocalizations in adult pygmy marmosets,[29] but only 16 different call types were used by infant marmosets. Of these, 10 call types were identical to those used by adults, 4 types were similar to those of adults, and 2 types were unique to infant monkeys.

5. Sounds are well formed and recognizable as speech. Of the 20,500 calls we analyzed, 71% were identifiable as adult-like, and 19% were variants on adult vocalizations. Only 10% of the calls could not be classified.

6. Babbling has no obvious referent. When human infants babble, the sounds are functionally meaningless. Several different consonant-vowel combinations are produced in close juxtaposition. In pygmy marmosets, infants produce a mean of 10 different call types per bout, and these range from threat vocalizations to fear to alarm to affiliative vocalizations, all juxtaposed closely with no relationship to the adult usage of these calls.

7. Babbling is a social act. Just as caretakers of human infants approach and interact more with infants when they babble, so do pygmy marmoset caretakers approach and interact more with babbling infants. We found significant differences

with babbling infants being approached significantly more often, being picked up, being carried, being groomed by or huddling with other group members than when these same infants were not babbling.[30]

We found what we would label "babbling" in reports of infant vocalizations in other species of marmosets, suggesting that this genus provides a good nonhuman primate model of infant babbling. The nonhuman primate model has several advantages over the birdsong model. First, nonhuman primates have greater phylogenetic affinities with humans. Second, birdsong in the north temperate zone is generally restricted to males and is under the control of testosterone. The plastic and subsong phases occur around the age of puberty. In contrast, pygmy marmoset babbling is found in both sexes and occurs well before puberty. In fact, the babbling is no longer present by the time monkeys reach puberty. Third, song represents just one of many types of vocalizations given by birds, whereas the babbling of pygmy marmosets involves nearly 70% of the call types of the adult repertoire.

We are currently examining the timing of caretaker social interactions during a babbling bout to determine if social reinforcement of specific call types or particularly well-formed calls is occurring, and we will be examining babbling beyond 20 weeks to determine if it serves as a form of practice, leading to increasingly well-formed vocalizations. Babbling in pygmy marmosets can be an important phenomenon for understanding how affiliative interactions shape vocal development.

Ontogeny of Food-Associated Calls

In many species of birds and primates there are vocalizations that appear to be used specifically when animals are feeding. We have documented that both pygmy marmosets and cotton-top tamarins (*Saguinus oedipus*) have calls that are used exclusively in feeding contexts. In adult cotton-top tamarins, two types of short frequency modulated vocalizations (C-chirps and D-chirps) are used in feeding contexts. We have shown that more than 97% of these calls are produced in the presence of food, with C-chirps being given when animals approach and sort through food items in a dish and D-chirps being produced when animals pick up and eat food. Tamarins were presented with small, manipulable nonfood objects such as pen caps and paper clips, and the chirps were rarely heard in the presence of these nonfood items or in other nonfeeding contexts. We tested each individual adult to determine its preference hierarchy for different foods and found a significant correlation with the rate of calls produced and the animal's preference scores. Thus, these food-associated calls are both referential, signifying the presence of food, and motivational, conveying honest information about the caller's preference for food.[31]

Subsequently, we studied the development of both the structure and usage of food-associated calls in cotton-top tamarins.[32] We tested animals ranging in age from 4-28 months using the same methods we had with adults. Individuals were presented with food and nonfood items and individual preference ranks were determined through a series of two-choice feeding tests. Several differences were found between juvenile and subadult tamarins versus adults. First, young tamarins tended to overgeneralize the use of C-chirps and D-chirps by giving chirps to nonfood manipulable objects at a significantly higher rate than baseline, but at a significantly lower rate than the chirp rate to food items.

Second, whereas C-chirps and D-chirps were virtually the only calls given by adults in feeding contexts, young tamarins produced a high proportion of other types of calls, unrelated to food-associated calls and also produced a high proportion of chirp-like calls that were similar to those of adults but more than 1 SD beyond the mean of adult parameters. We expected that the youngest animals in our sample might produce more imperfect versions of chirps and more "other" vocalizations with a progression towards adult forms with increasing age. To our surprise, we found no age-related changes in the quality of vocal production. Older animals were as likely to produce imperfect forms of chirps and to produce "other" vocalizations as were younger animals.

Third, none of the juvenile and subadult animals showed the correlations with food preference and rate of vocalization that we found in adults, and there were many violations of transitivity in food preferences. When we separated the animals into prepuberal (before 18 months) and postpubertal groups (over 18 months), we still found no differences on any aspect of structure or usage of food-associated calls. This parallels our earlier results[33] that juvenile and subadult animals do not produce the vocalizations used by adults to defend territories against intruders.

Because tamarins and marmosets are cooperatively breeding species in which typically only one pair reproduces while other group members remain reproductively inhibited and help care for infants,[34] it appears likely that a relationship exists between social status and vocal production and usage. The failure of nonreproductive helpers to use territorial vocalizations in response to intruders makes sense, because it is the reproductive pair whose status is most threatened by intruders and because in many birds and primates the use of territorial calls was shown to be under the control of gonadal steroids.

However, it is more difficult to account for the immature structure and usage of food-associated calls over such a broad age range. One hypothesis we proposed was that the use of immature vocalizations even by postpubertal animals might be a way of signaling subordinate status. Thus, by giving imperfect forms of C-chirps and D-chirps and by adding many other vocalizations not used by adults in feeding contexts, the nonreproductive helpers are communicating that they are still immature and therefore not a threat to adults. A strong test of this hypothesis is to test subadult animals while still helpers in the family and then continue to test them after they have been removed from the group, paired with a mate, and allowed to be reproductively active.

We carried out this experiment with nine subadult tamarins.[35] Each monkey was tested for 3 successive weeks prior to pairing with three different food types, and both food preferences and the types of vocalizations were recorded. The monkeys were then removed from the family group, paired with a new mate, and tested weekly for 10 weeks with the same three foods. Behavioral data were collected on the amount of time the pair spent in contact, grooming, and sexual behavior.

The results supported our hypothesis. There was a rapid reduction in the number of "other" vocalizations given in food contexts after pairing compared to the family condition. Furthermore, a significant positive correlation was noted between the affiliative relationships expressed by a pair and how quickly the "other" calls were reduced in feeding contexts. By the third week, all tamarins reached adult levels of "other" vocalizations. There was a slower decline in the number of C-like and D-like chirps with adult levels being reached 6-7 weeks after pairing. No correlation was evident between affiliative behavior and the rate at which C-chirps and D-chirps reached adult forms.

These results provide evidence of two types of affiliative influences on vocal production and usage. First, social interactions can inhibit the adult expression of vocalizations. All animals tested did produce adult forms of both territorial calls and food-associated calls while they were reproductively inhibited helpers, but they produced these adult forms rarely and instead gave imperfect forms of food-associated calls or produced other call types not usually found in feeding or territorial contexts. This appears to be a true inhibition of responding because these tamarins produced adult-like calls in adult-like contexts within a very short period of time after their social status was changed.

Second, the finding that the quality of the affiliative relationship with a new mate had a direct effect on the rate of change of at least one vocalization type suggests that positive affiliative processes can induce a rapid change in vocal structure. Thus, affiliative social interactions can have both inhibitory and stimulatory influences on vocal development.

MECHANISMS OF SOCIAL INFLUENCE

I have described several studies not only in marmosets and tamarins but also in other species that indicate that vocal communication skills are shaped by affiliative social interactions. A variety of species adjust the fine structure of songs, calls, or speech to adjust to new social companions while maintaining individual specific features. This accommodation provides a social "badge" or signifies membership in a group or solidarity between individuals. Subsong in birds and babbling in marmosets and humans provide a mechanism for vocal practice that, in turn, is influenced by social companions. And social influences in cooperatively breeding monkeys can both inhibit and facilitate the acquisition and usage of adult vocalizations.

However, ultimately the mechanisms by which affiliative processes affect vocal development must be identified and specified. Once affiliative processes are demonstrated to be of importance, the next step is to determine how they are important. At least three mechanisms of social influences might operate. First, social influences are generally multimodal. When we interact with social companions, we not only hear their voices but often also see facial expressions and gestures, feel tactile sensations, and even smell them. Many studies of vocal development have tried to identify the minimal stimulation needed to acquire vocal production by presenting animals with tape or video recorded stimuli alone. Yet natural social companions provide multiple inputs, and these multiple stimulus channels may facilitate the acquisition of information and may allow the extension of learning beyond a critical or sensitive period. Second, social companions provide an attentional focus. If the subject responds to a social companion, its attention is focused on the behavior of that companion, so sounds or gestures made by a companion may become more relevant to the subject. This attentional focus allows a companion to make connections for the learner, say a particular vocalization coupled with a particular object. If I repeat the word "dog" while pointing to a dog. I am helping the learner attend to the relationship between the word and the object. Third, social companions provide reinforcement for responses made by the learner. Often social reinforcement may be as effective as physical reinforcement, but whatever the form of reinforcement interactions with a companion can lead to improved acquisition.

There are two examples of how these three mechanisms can work in vocal development. Pepperberg[36] has trained parrots to produce a variety of words as labels for objects, and the birds can indicate the number, substance, or color of various objects. Pepperberg used a Model-Rival technique in which one human trainer offers an object to another in the presence of the parrot and names the object as it is presented. The human learner repeats the word and is offered the object. The roles are exchanged and eventually the parrot is included. The human trainers provide multimodal stimulation using postures, gestures, and voices as well as presenting a concrete object. They provide an attentional focus for the parrot through their interaction and they provide reinforcement when the parrot produces the appropriate label by offering the object and by giving verbal praise and occasionally food. Thus, all three components of social interaction are present. Pepperberg has shown that each of these components must be present. Parrots do not learn object labels through audiotapes, through videotapes, or watching noninteractive humans. The process of acquiring labels for objects or attributes requires a complex form of social interaction.

We observed a natural parallel to this in cotton-top tamarins. During the process of weaning, adult tamarins offer to share pieces of solid food with infants, and when they offer solid food to infants, the adults frequently emit a sequence of several D-chirps. Frequently other group members will stop their activities and orient towards the adult offering food, and these other animals also emit D-chirps. The combination of intensified vocalizations coupled with visual orientation towards a piece of food provides multimodal stimulation for the infant. The animal offering food and the other group members provide a close contingency between food and the appropriate vocalizations for food, creating an attentional focus for the young infant. Finally, we observed that infants can only obtain solid food from adults after the adults have vocalized. Food sharing almost never occurs in the absence of appropriate vocalizations. So a reinforcement contingency is established as well. As with parrots learning English labels from human tutors, cotton-top tamarins appear to receive similar input as they learn about solid food and the appropriate vocalizations to use in feeding contexts from adults in their family.

SUMMARY

Affiliative behavior is often expressed through communication, and the nature of affiliative interactions affects the ontogeny of communication. I presented three phenomena that demonstrate the importance of affiliation in vocal development in marmosets and tamarins, but the results have parallels in many other species including birds, dolphins, and humans. Pygmy marmosets use trill-like vocalizations to maintain contact with other group members. Individuals change subtle aspects of call structure when they encounter new social groups or acquire a new mate. This process of vocal accommodation is common in many other species. Infant pygmy marmosets go through a stage of "babbling," producing long sequences of vocalizations that have several similarities to the babbling of human infants. Babbling infants receive more social attention than nonbabbling infants, and these social interactions may shape vocalizations towards more adult forms. In adult cotton-top tamarins, food-associated vocalizations communicate the presence and quality of food. However, reproductively inhibited juveniles and subadults use many other types of calls in feeding situations and display a high proportion of imperfect forms of adult food-associated calls. When subadult monkeys are paired with new mates and change their reproductive status, they rapidly (within 3-6 weeks) display both adult structure and adult usage of food-associated calls, suggesting that affiliative processes can both facilitate and inhibit vocal ontogeny. Three mechanisms of how social interactions affect communication (multimodal stimulation, attentional focus, and reinforcement) were proposed and illustrated through examples of parrots learning English labels for objects and attributes and infant cotton-top tamarins acquiring food-associated vocalizations.

ACKNOWLEDGMENTS

I am grateful to A. Margaret Elowson, Rebecca S. Roush, and Cristina Lazaro-Perea for their collaboration in the research reported here.

REFERENCES

1. Cheney, D. L. & R. M. Seyfarth. 1990. How Monkeys See the World. University of Chicago Press. Chicago, IL.
2. Snowdon, C. T. 1990. Language capacities of nonhuman animals. Yearb. Phys. Anthropol. **33:** 215-243.
3. Snowdon, C. T. & M. Hausberger, Eds. 1997. Social Influences on Vocal Development. Cambridge University Press. Cambridge, UK.
4. Rowell, T. E. & R. A. Hinde. 1962. Vocal communication by the rhesus monkey (*Macaca mulatta*). Proc. Zool. Soc. Lond. **138:** 279-294.
5. Levine, S. E., D. Franklin & C. A. Gonzalez. 1984. Influence of social variables on biobehavioral response to separation in rhesus monkey infants. Child Dev. **55:** 1386-1393.
6. Levine, S., S. G. Wiener, C. L. Coe, F. E. S. Bayart & K. T. Hayashi. 1987. Primate vocalization: A psychobiological approach. Child Dev. **58:** 1408-1419.
7. Bayart, F., K. T. Hayashi, K. F. Faull, J. D. Barchas & S. Levine. 1990. Influence of maternal proximity on behavioral and physiological responses to separation in infant rhesus monkeys (*Macaca mulatta*). Behav. Neurosci. **104:** 98-107.
8. Lillehei, R. A. & C. T. Snowdon. 1978. Individual and situational differences in the vocalizations of young stumptail macaques (*Macaca arctoides*). Behaviour **65:** 270-281.
9. Newman, J. D. 1995. Vocal ontogeny in macaques and marmosets: Convergent and divergent lines of development. *In* Recent Advances in Primate Vocal Communication. E. Zimmermann, J. D. Newman & U. Jurgens, Eds. Plenum Publishing. New York, NY.
10. Kalin, N. H., S. E. Shelton & C. T. Snowdon. 1992. Affiliative vocalizations in infant rhesus macaques (*Macaca mulatta*). J. Comp. Psychol., **106:** 254-261.
11. Blount, B. G. 1985. "Girney" vocalizations among Japanese macaque females: Context and function. Primates **26:** 424-435.
12. Masataka, N. 1989. Motivational referents of contact calls in Japanese monkeys. Ethology **80:** 265-273.

13. SMITH, H. J., J. D. NEWMAN & D. SYMMES. 1982. Vocal concomitants of affiliative behavior in squirrel monkeys. *In* Primate Communication. C. T. Snowdon, C. H. Brown & M. R. Petersen, Eds.: 30-49. Cambridge University Press. New York, NY.
14. SNOWDON, C. T. & J. CLEVELAND. 1984. "Conversations" among pygmy marmosets. Am. J. Primatol. **7:** 15-20.
15. SNOWDON, C. T. & A. HODUN. 1981. Acoustic adaptations in pygmy marmoset contact calls: Locational cues vary with distances between conspecifics. Behav. Ecol. Sociobiol. **9:** 295-300.
16. ELOWSON, A. M., C. S. SWEET & C. T. SNOWDON. 1992. Ontogeny of trill and J-call vocalizations in the pygmy marmoset (*Cebuella pygmaea*). Anim. Behav. **42:** 703-715.
17. NOWICKI, S. 1989. Vocal plasticity in captive black-capped chickadees: The acoustic basis of call convergence. Anim. Behav. **37:** 64-73.
18. MUNDINGER, P. 1970. Vocal imitation and recognition of finch calls. Science **168:** 480-482.
19. ELOWSON, A. M. & C. T. SNOWDON. 1994. Pygmy marmosets, *Cebuella pygmaea,* modify vocal structure in response to changed social environment. Anim. Behav. **47:** 1267-1277.
20. TYACK, P. L. & L. S. SAYIGH. 1997. Vocal learning in cetaceans. *In* Social Influences on Vocal Development. C. T. Snowdon & M. Hausberger, Eds.: 208-233. Cambridge University Press. Cambridge, England.
21. STANGER, K. F. 1993. Structure and Function of the Vocalizations of Nocturnal Prosimians (Cheirogaleidae). Unpublished Ph.D. dissertation. Eberhard-Karls-Universtaet, Tubingen, Germany.
22. RANDALL, J. A. 1995. Modification of foot-drumming signatures by kangaroo rats: Changing territories and gaining new neighbours. Anim. Behav. **49:** 1227-1237.
23. HAUSBERGER, M., M.-A. RICHARD-YRIS, L. HENRY, L. LEPAGE & I. SCHMIDT. 1995. Song sharing reflects the social organization in a captive group of European starlings (*Sturnus vulgaris*). J. Comp. Psychol. **109:** 222-241.
24. GILES, H. & P. SMITH. 1979. Accommodation theory: Optimal levels of convergence. *In* Language and Social Psychology. H. Giles & R. N. St. Clair, Eds.: 45-65. Basil Blackwell. Oxford, UK.
25. LOCKE, J. L. 1993. The Child's Path to Spoken Language. Harvard University Press. Cambridge, MA.
26. PETITTO, L. A., & P. F. MARENTETTE. 1991. Babbling in the manual mode: Evidence for the ontogeny of language. Science **251:** 1493-1496.
27. MARLER, P. Birdsong and human speech: Could there be parallels? Am. Scientist **58:** 669-674.
28. NELSON, D. A. 1997. Social interaction and sensitive phases for song learning: A critical review. *In* Social Influences on Vocal Development. C. T. Snowdon & M. Hausberger, Eds.: 7-22. Cambridge University Press. Cambridge, UK.
29. POLA, Y. V. & C. T. SNOWDON. 1975. The vocalizations of pygmy marmosets, *Cebuella pygmaea,* Anim. Behav. **23:** 823-826.
30. ELOWSON, A. M., C. T. SNOWDON & C. LAZARO-PEREA. "Babbling" in infant monkeys: Parallel to human babbling. In preparation.
31. ELOWSON, A. M., P. L. TANNENBAUM & C. T. SNOWDON. 1991. Food associated calls correlate with food preferences in cotton-top tamarins. Anim. Behav. **42:** 931-937.
32. ROUSH, R. S. & C. T. SNOWDON. 1994. Ontogeny of food-associated calls in cotton-top tamarins. Anim. Behav. **47:** 263-273.
33. MCCONNELL, P. B. & C. T. SNOWDON. 1986. Vocal interactions among unfamiliar groups of cotton-top tamarins. Behaviour **97:** 273-296.
34. SNOWDON, C. T. 1996. Infant care in cooperatively breeding animals. *In* Advances in the Study of Behavior: Vol. 25. Parental Care. J. S. Rosenblatt & C. T. Snowdon, Eds.: 643-689. Academic Press. San Diego, CA.

35. R. S. Roush & C. T. Snowdon. 1996. The effects of social status on food associated calling behavior in captive cotton-top tamarins. In preparation.
36. Pepperberg, I. M. 1997. Social influences on the acquisition of human-based codes in parrots and nonhuman primates. *In* Social Influences on Vocal Development. C. T. Snowdon & M. Hausberger. Eds.: 157-177. Cambridge University Press. Cambridge, UK.

III

Monogamous Mammals as Models for Understanding Affiliation and Social Bonds

11

Brain Sexual Dimorphism and Sex Differences in Parental and Other Social Behaviors

Geert J. DeVries and Constanza Villalba

In most mammalian species, males and females assume very different roles in rearing young, with females typically taking the lion's share; in some species, males as well as females take part in parental care.[1] For example, male gerbils, California mice, and prairie voles stay with their mates throughout gestation and engage in parental activities such as grooming, crouching over, and retrieving pups.[2–6] This variability in rearing patterns among species can be exploited to study how sex and species differences in neural structure contribute to differences in reproductive strategies. To discuss this approach, we first describe some landmark findings in the study on the physiological basis of parental behavior, made mostly in rats. For recent, more comprehensive reviews on the physiological basis of parental behavior or on sex differences in the brain, see references 7 and 8.

CONTROL OF MATERNAL BEHAVIOR

In addition to nursing, mothers display an elaborate set of behaviors such as retrieving and grooming the young, building and maintaining a nest, and defending the nest against intruders.[8,9] These behaviors are under multisensory control. In rats, auditory, olfactory, visual, and tactile stimuli can all generate parental behavior, but none of these stimuli appears to be crucial for the behavior, with the possible exception of tactile stimuli in the perioral region, which are important for retrieval.[10–13] Olfactory stimuli from both the primary olfactory epithelium and the vomeronasal organ may play a decisive role in the induction of maternal behavior. In virgin female rats, these stimuli appear to inhibit maternal behavior. Virgin females with severed vomeronasal nerves will start showing maternal behavior with shorter latencies than females without such lesions.[14] The same is true for lesions of the olfactory and accessory olfactory bulb, which receives vomeronasal input, and with lesions of the bed nucleus of the accessory olfactory tract, the medial amygdaloid nucleus (MA), which receives input from the accessory olfactory bulb.[14–16] The impact of olfactory and accessory olfactory input appears to change during pregnancy, because for lactating rats pup odors may actually be attractive.[17]

This work was supported by National Science Foundation grant IBN 9421658 to G. J. de V.

These changes in maternal responsiveness during pregnancy are caused by hormones. When a virgin female rat is presented with pups for the first time, she typically does not show responsiveness towards them. During pregnancy, responsiveness towards pups increases gradually until about 1-1.5 days before parturition at which point females show all aspects of maternal behavior.[18–20] This increase is apparently caused by hormonal changes during pregnancy, the most noteworthy being a rise in estrogen and prolactin levels in the later stages of pregnancy and the sudden drop in progesterone levels after birth.[21,22] Once maternal behavior has been induced, these hormones need not be present to maintain the behavior;[23] but they appear to enhance the quality of the behavior.[22] This suggests that the regulation of maternal behavior should be subdivided into at least two different phases, induction and maintenance.

In rats, the brain area most crucial for the regulation of maternal behavior appears to be the medial preoptic area (MPOA). Electrolytic, radiofrequency, and axon-sparing neurochemical lesions of the MPOA as well as knifecuts that sever inputs and outputs of the MPOA severely disrupt induction as well as maintenance of maternal behavior.[8] In addition, implants of estradiol into the MPOA, the area with the highest concentration of estradiol-concentrating neurons in the brain,[24] facilitate maternal behavior.[25] It is not yet known which particular neural systems mediate the actions of progesterone and prolactin on parental behavior. Lesion studies have implicated several other areas that project directly or indirectly to the MPOA in maternal behavior, such as the cingulate cortex,[26] hippocampus,[27] septum,[28] lateral habenular nucleus,[29] bed nucleus of the stria terminalis (BST),[30] and the areas involved in olfaction just mentioned. Similar studies have also implicated several output areas of the MPOA in maternal behavior, that is, the ventral and lateral tegmental area.[31,32] Lesions in these different areas tend to impair maternal behavior in a site-specific way. For example, lesions in the midline cortical and hippocampal areas predominantly affect pup retrieval, whereas lesions in lateral midbrain areas predominantly affect the defense of the nest.[8]

SEX DIFFERENCES IN THE CONTROL OF PARENTAL BEHAVIOR

Male rats are not naturally responsive to pups, and once they become 3 months old, most of them have lost the ability to become parentally responsive even after prolonged exposure to pups, which induces parental responsiveness in virgin female rats.[33,34] This sex difference in parental responsiveness may be caused by sex differences found in most of the aforementioned sensory processes, hormones, and neural structures. For example, the processing of accessory olfactory information may be sexually dimorphic.[35] The accessory olfactory bulbs, which receive vomeronasal input, are larger in males than in females.[36] The same is true for several areas that receive direct input from the accessory olfactory bulb, such as the bed nucleus of the olfactory tract,[37] the MA,[38,39] and the posteromedial division of the BST.[39,40] Lesions within this pathway facilitate parental behavior in male[41,42] as well as in female rats.[14–16] Therefore, the larger size of these structures appears to correlate with greater inhibition of parental responsiveness in males than in females.

Although the aforementioned differences in the accessory olfactory system result from sex differences in gonadal hormones around birth,[38–40] qualitative and quantitative sex differences in gonadal hormone levels in sexually inexperienced animals may further contribute to sex differences in parental responsiveness. Whether sex differences in gonadal hormone levels play a significant role in sex differences in parental responsiveness has not been studied as systematically as has been done for reproductive behavior in rats, in which sex reversal of gonadal hormone levels in adulthood does not lead to sex reversal of behavioral patterns, presumably because the underlying brain structure is sexually differentiated during development.[43] However, the abundance of androgen and estrogen receptors in the aforementioned areas that were implicated in the control of maternal behavior[24,44] suggests that different levels of gonadal hormones may lead to differences in the physiology of the cells in these areas.

Although almost all of the aforementioned areas implicated in the regulation of parental behavior are sexually dimorphic,[7] perhaps the most striking sex differences are found in the area most central to the control of maternal behavior, the MPOA. This area contains a cluster of cells that in Nissl-stained sections is five times larger in males than in females, that is, the sexually dimorphic area of the preoptic area.[45] Various studies have suggested that the size of this area correlates with the quantity and quality of male sexual behavior.[43] Such a size correlation of a sexually dimorphic area with competence in a function controlled by that area is commonly found in sex differences in the brain. For example, in songbirds, brain areas that control song are larger in males, which sing, than in females, which do not sing.[46] This correlation also holds for the neural circuit that relays vomeronasal information and its presumed inhibitory influence on parental behavior. It does not hold for the MPOA, which despite its ability to facilitate maternal behavior, is generally smaller in females than in males. Yet, the extent of dimorphism in the MPOA correlates with the extent of dimorphism in parental behavior. In the California mouse, *Peromyscus californicus,* in which males as well as females take care of the offspring, the sex difference in the size of the MPOA is greater between virgin males and females than between fathers and mothers.[47] In addition, the sex difference in the size of the MPOA is greater in montane voles, in which only females display parental care, than in prairie voles, in which males and females display parental care.[48]

SEXUALLY DIMORPHIC NEUROTRANSMITTER SYSTEMS IMPLICATED IN PARENTAL BEHAVIOR

To better understand the nature of sex differences in the areas that control parental behavior, their connections and neurochemical makeup must be known.[49,50] This knowledge would allow better assessment of the impact of a particular sex difference on other brain areas. In addition, it would expand the number of tools with which to test the function of a sexually dimorphic area by allowing such manipulations as local injections of specific agonists and antagonists or antisense oligonucleotide to block the synthesis of neurotransmitters or their receptors.[51,52] Two sets of neuropeptides that have so been studied may serve as an example.

Endogenous Opioid Peptides

The MPOA contains a number of neurotransmitter systems that are distinctly sexually dimorphic.[50] Of these, the endogenous opioid peptide innervation has been implicated in maternal behavior. Injections of the opioid analog morphine into the MPOA inhibited maternal behavior in lactating rats.[53] It is not clear with which particular opioid system morphine may interfere. The MPOA contains various fiber systems that contain opioid peptides that belong to the proenkephalin, opiomelanocortin, or prodynorphin families of peptides.[54] Each of these fiber systems show sex differences. For example, in the preoptic part of the periventricular nucleus, the innervation of methionine-enkephalin-immunoreactive (met-enkephalin) fibers is denser in females than in males.[55] In addition, the medial preoptic nucleus contains more leucine-enkephalin-immunoreactive cells in males than in females, and the areas covered by a dense plexus of β-endorphin fibers is larger in the MPOA of males than of females.[54] In addition, the μ opioid receptors, which would respond to endorphins and enkaphalins, are denser in females than in males.[56] A clear picture of the role of sex differences in the opioid peptide innervation of the MPOA does not easily emerge. Although the larger area covered by the β-endorphin fiber plexus in males suggests greater inhibition of maternal behavior, the sex difference in the density of the μ opioid receptor runs counter to this notion. Changes in the content of opioid peptides and their receptors over the reproductive cycle are more suggestive. In addition, β-endorphin content and opioid binding sites are increased during pregnancy and decreased during lactation,[57] which suggests that maternal behavior coincides with a decrease in the activity and efficiency of the β-endorphin system.

Oxytocin and Vasopressin

The literature on the rat offers many indications that oxytocin acts within the brain to induce maternal responsiveness. An initial experiment showed that intraventricular injections of oxytocin reduced the latency with which ovariectomized, estrogen-primed, sexually naive female rats begin to show parental behavior when exposed to pups.[58] Although follow-up experiments indicated that this effect critically depends on test conditions, experiments with oxytocin antagonists and antisera confirmed the role of oxytocin in parental behavior.[8,59] It is not clear where oxytocin may act. For example, oxytocin comes mainly from the paraventricular nucleus and cells scattered throughout the hypothalamus.[60] Lesioning this nucleus during pregnancy impairs subsequent maternal behavior,[61] but lesioning the paraventricular nucleus in maternal animals does not interfere with maternal behavior,[62] which suggests that oxytocin is more important for induction than for maintenance of maternal behavior. Oxytocin binding studies have suggested an increase in oxytocin receptors in the lateral division of the BST during pregnancy.[59] It is not known if there are sex differences in the ability of rats to increase the number of oxytocin binding sites in the BST. Such a difference could contribute to a sex difference in paternal responsiveness.

Intraventricular injections of vasopressin (AVP) also reduce the latency with which sexually naive female rats begin to show parental responsiveness.[58] In addition, Brattleboro rats, which are genetically unable to produce AVP, show inferior parental care.[63] It is not known if their parental behavior is inferior because of the absence of AVP or the diabetic state of Brattleboro rats. Intraventricularly injected AVP can interact with a number of different AVP systems. Most AVP in the brain is derived from neurons in the suprachiasmatic nucleus, paraventricular nucleus, MA, and BST,

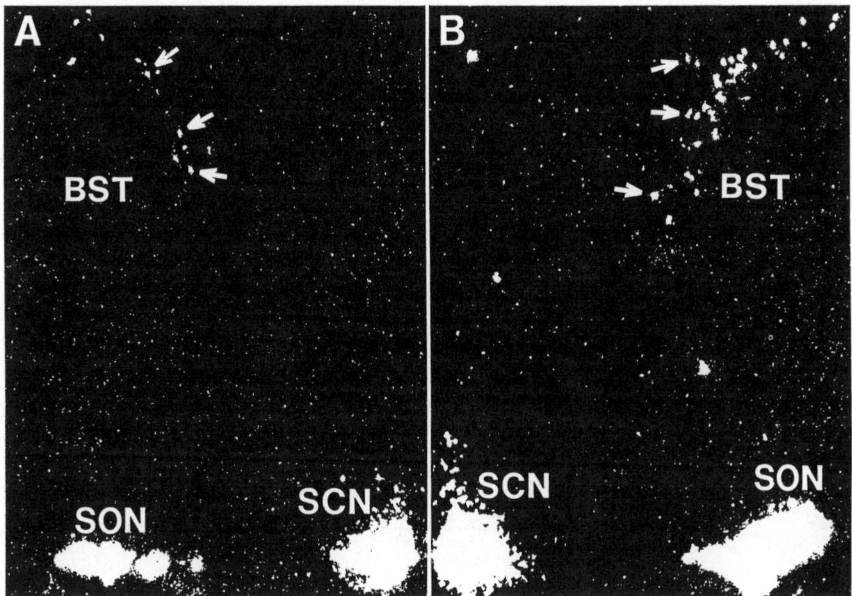

FIGURE 1. Dark-field-illuminated sections with cells labeled for vasopressin mRNA in the bed nucleus of the stria terminalis (BST, *white arrows*) of a female (**A**) and a male rat (**B**). Labeled cells are also found in the supraoptic nucleus (SON) and the suprachiasmatic nucleus (SCN).

the projections of which do not extensively overlap.[60] Of these areas, the AVP-immunoreactive (AVP-ir) cells of the BST and MA project to most of the aforementioned areas that were implicated in parental behavior. They are, therefore, in a very strategic position to regulate parental behavior. In fact, AVP-ir projections of the BST and MA show reproduction-related changes. For example, AVP-ir fibers in the lateral septum are more intensely stained in pregnant than in nonpregnant guinea pigs.[65] In addition, the lateral habenular nucleus contains higher levels of radioimmunoassayable AVP in lactating than in pregnant rats,[66] and the release of AVP from the septum is markedly greater in pregnant and parturient than in sexually naive female rats.[67] These reproduction-related changes suggest that AVP-ir projections of the BST and MA are implicated in behaviors or functions that change in pregnant and parturient rats. These changes may be due to the extreme steroid responsiveness of the AVP-ir projections of the BST and MA. After gonadectomy, BST and MA cells and their projections lose their AVP immunoreactivity and can no longer be labeled for AVP mRNA.[68–70] If these projections are involved in parental behavior, they may mediate some of the effect of gonadal hormones on this behavior. The AVP-ir cells may also contribute to the sexually dimorphic nature of the control of parental behavior, because there are about twice as many AVP-ir cells in the BST and MA in males than in females, and the projections of these cells are accordingly denser in males than in females (FIG. 1).[69,71–73]

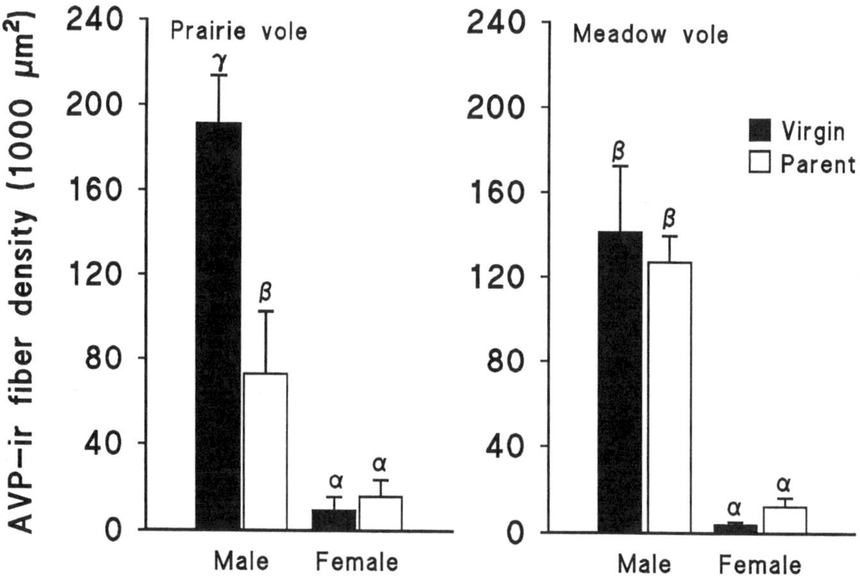

FIGURE 2. Vasopressin-immunoreactive (AVP-ir) fiber density in the lateral septum of prairie and meadow voles that were either sexually naive (*closed bars*) or parental (*open bars*). Greek letters indicate significant differences among groups (ANOVA, $p < 0.001$). Bars: means ± SEM.

COMPARATIVE ASPECTS IN THE CONTROL OF PARENTAL BEHAVIOR

Voles are an attractive subject for the study of the role of AVP in parental behavior, because closely related vole species show dramatically different patterns of social behavior, which appears to be reflected in differences in the AVP-ir projections of the BST and MA. For example, prairie voles (*Microtus ochrogaster*) and pine voles (*Microtus pinetorum*) are monogamous species in which fathers as well as mothers provide parental care; montane voles (*Microtus montanus*) and meadow voles (*Microtus pennsylvanicus*) are promiscuous species in which only mothers provide parental care.[74,75] In comparing sexually naive prairie and meadow voles with voles 6 days after the birth of their first litter, we found that in prairie vole males, the density of the AVP-ir innervation of the lateral septum and lateral habenular nucleus was lower in parental males than in sexually naive males (FIG. 2).[76] A follow-up experiment showed that the density of AVP-ir projections in prairie vole males decreases initially after mating, then increases only to decrease again once the pups are born.[77] The initial drop in AVP-ir fiber density appears to reflect an increase in AVP release, because it coincides with an increase in AVP mRNA in the BST, the most probable source of these fibers (FIG. 3).[78]

Because mating-induced changes in AVP projections were not seen in meadow vole males or in females of either species,[76,78] they may contribute specifically to the changes in social behavior in male prairie voles. In prairie voles, mating induces

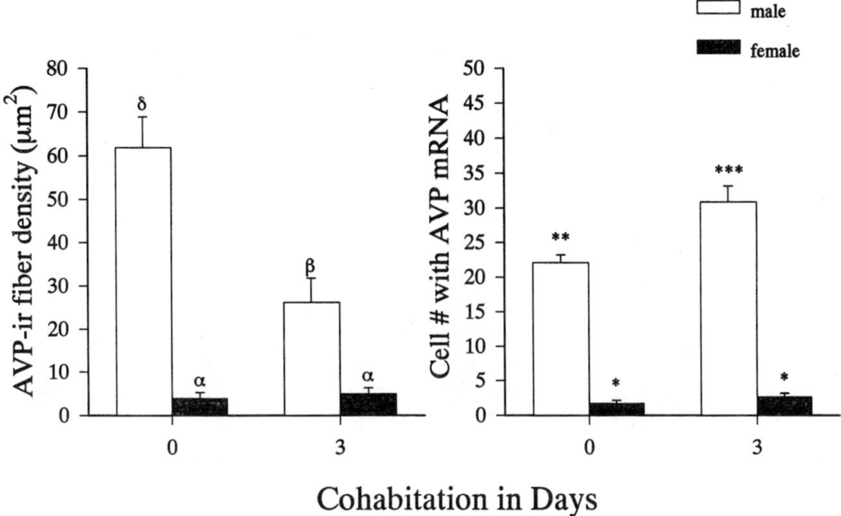

FIGURE 3. Changes in vasopressin-immunoreactive (AVP-ir) fiber density in the lateral septum (μm^2 covered with AVP immunoreactivity per 1,000 μm^2 test area) and in the number of cells of the bed nucleus of the stria terminalis (BST) labeled for vasopressin mRNA in sexually naive male and female prairie voles and in prairie voles 3 days after mating. Greek letters and symbols indicate significant differences among groups (ANOVA $p < 0.01$ and $p < 0.05$ for the interaction between sex and reproductive state for AVP fiber density and the number of AVP mRNA-labeled cells, respectively).

pair-bonding and increases aggressive behavior directed to unfamiliar prairie voles in males as well as females.[79] Mating also increases paternal responsiveness in prairie voles.[77] Injections of AVP into the lateral septum of sexually naive male prairie voles indeed stimulated grooming, crouching over, and contacting pups, whereas injections of a $V1_a$ receptor antagonist blocked these behaviors (FIG. 4).[80] These effects appeared to be site-specific, because injections of AVP into other areas or into the ventricles did not stimulate paternal behavior.

Vasopressin may also play a role in pair-bonding and the changes in aggressive behavior in males, because intraventricular injections of a $V1_a$ receptor antagonist prior to mating blocked the increase in aggression and pair-bonding seen after mating.[81] Although this study did not identify the septum as the site where the antagonist blocked the action of AVP, injections of the same antagonist have implicated the AVP innervation of the lateral septum and the amygdala in intermale aggression in rats.[82]

The relatively low levels of AVP immunoreactivity and AVP mRNA in female compared to male prairie voles (FIG. 3) suggest that AVP does not play an equally important role in the changes in female social behavior. In female prairie voles, however, oxytocin rather than AVP appears to influence pair-bonding.[81,83] Whether oxytocin influences mating-induced aggression in female prairie voles is unknown.

If activation of the AVP innervation is indeed important for the changes in social behavior in prairie voles, including changes in paternal behavior, the question remains

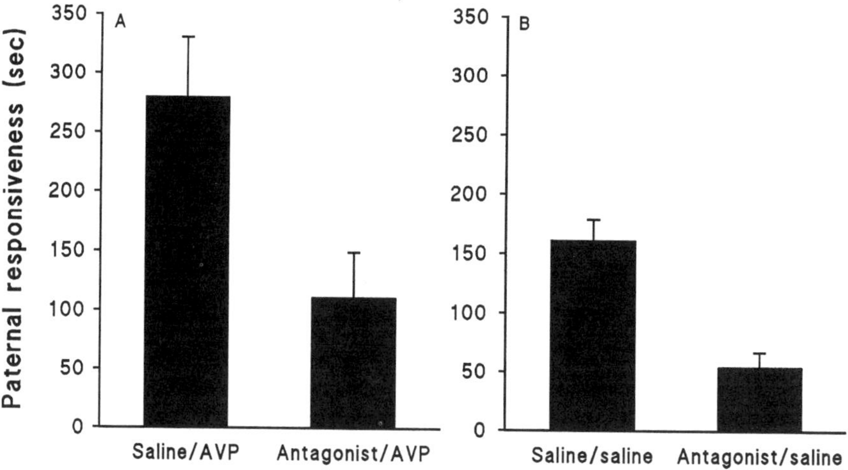

FIGURE 4. Time spent on paternal behavior during a 10-minute testing period of prairie vole males injected into the septum with saline solution followed by vasopressin (Saline/AVP) or by a $V1_a$ antagonist followed by vasopressin (Antagonist/AVP, *t* test, $p < 0.05$) and by prairie voles injected twice with saline (Saline/saline) or by a $V1_a$ antagonist followed by saline (Antagonist/saline, *t* test $p < 0.001$). Bars: means ± SEM.

as to why the same innervation does not change social behavior in meadow voles or rats as it does in prairie voles. These differences may involve differences in the neural or hormonal input of AVP cells, which cause these cells to change after mating in prairie voles but not in meadow voles. For example, mating increases testosterone levels in prairie but not meadow vole males.[78] These differences may also involve differences in the cells innervated by the AVP projections from the BST and MA. The monogamous prairie and pine voles have indeed fewer AVP binding sites in the lateral septum than do the promiscuous montane and meadow voles.[84] This suggests that a similar release of AVP in the lateral septum would have different consequences for monogamous and promiscuous voles.

RECONSIDERING THE ROLE OF SEXUAL DIMORPHISM IN PARENTAL AND OTHER SOCIAL BEHAVIORS

Although our discussion of sex differences in systems that control parental behavior initially focused on how those differences contribute to sex differences in parental behavior, our discussion of parental behavior in prairie voles suggests an opposite role for sex differences in brain structure. The effects of oxytocin and AVP on social behavior in prairie voles suggest that sex differences in the brain may not always generate sex differences in physiology and behavior, but may just as well enable males and females to display similar behaviors despite their exposure to different hormonal and physiological conditions. Parental behavior in monogamous species appears to need such a solution. In most mammals, maternal behavior is believed to

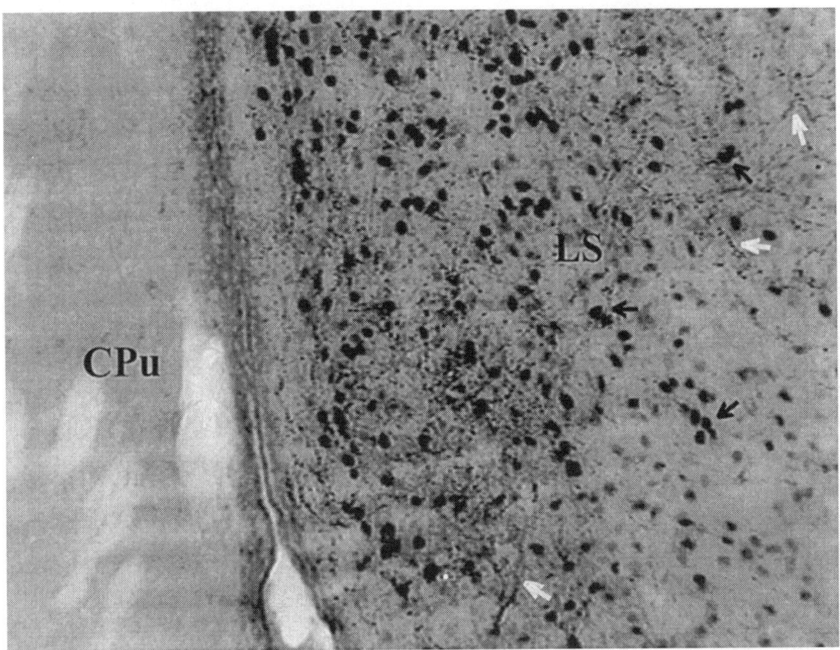

FIGURE 5. Distribution of androgen receptor and vasopressin immunoreactivity in the lateral septum (LS). *Black and white arrows* point at isolated androgen receptor-immunoreactive nuclei and vasopressin-immunoreactive fibers, respectively. Note that the density of immunoreactive structures increases towards the lining of the lateral ventricles. CPu: striatum.

be induced through hormonal changes associated with pregnancy.[9] In monogamous male rodents, however, in the absence of pregnancy and its associated hormonal changes, paternal behavior must be induced through different mechanisms. This may very well translate in sexual dimorphism in brain function and therefore in brain structure, which may allow males and females to show similar levels of parental behavior. For prairie voles, changes in the AVP projections of the BST and MA may well induce changes in the processing of vomeronasal information mentioned in the beginning of this chapter, because AVP projections from the BST and MA to the lateral septum mediate vomeronasal influences on recognition of conspecifics in rats.[85]

Even though the lifestyle of prairie voles is uncommon among mammals, solutions to the problem of generating similar behaviors despite physiological and hormonal sex differences are not necessarily unique to monogamous animals. Many behaviors and functions are not ostensibly different between males and females, even though the neural circuitry generating them is continuously exposed to a different set of hormones. Areas such as the septum have been implicated in many functions ranging from sexually dimorphic functions, such as female sexual behavior, to functions such as the regulation of autonomic processes[86] that do not show spectacular sex differences. Yet, in the lateral septum, virtually all neurons have androgen receptors (FIG. 5), leading almost certainly to a spectacular sex difference in the occupation of these receptors by androgens. Perhaps a sexually dimorphic involvement of neuropeptides in certain functions controlled by the septum shelters these functions from sex differences that could have been caused by sex differences in the physiology of septal cells. Learning to recognize conspecifics may be such a function. In rats, social recognition memory, which is not very different between males and females, is controlled by septal AVP in male but not in female rats.[87,88]

A sexually dimorphic involvement of neuropeptides in functions and behaviors has many important clinical implications. For example, it would offer an additional explanation for sex differences in the etiology of certain behavioral disorders such as schizophrenia, which in males has earlier onset and fewer positive symptoms than it has in females.[89] If such disorders depend on the malfunction of certain neural circuits, and if those neural circuits are involved in these behaviors to a different extent in males and females, it would lead to different vulnerabilities in males and females. Furthermore, if indeed social behaviors have a sexually dimorphic neurochemical basis, then novel therapies to treat disorders in social behavior based on altering neurotransmission in the brain should be developed independently for men and women.

REFERENCES

1. Kleiman, D. 1977. Monogamy in mammals. Q. Rev. Biol. **52:** 39-69.
2. Dudley, D. 1974. Paternal behavior in the California mouse *Peromyscus californicus.* Behav. Biol. **11:** 247-252.
3. Årgen, G. 1976. Social and territorial behaviour in the Mongolian gerbil (*Meriones unguiculatus*) under seminatural conditions. Biol. Behav. **1:** 267-285.
4. Elwood, R. W. 1977. Changes in the responses of male and female gerbils (*Meriones unguiculatus*) towards test pups during the pregnancy of the female. Anim. Behav. **25:** 46-51.
5. Gubernick, D. J. & J. R. Albers. 1987. The biparental care system of the California mouse, *Peromyscus californicus.* J. Comp. Psychol. **101:** 169-177.
6. Getz, L. L. & J. E. Hofmann. 1986. Social organization in free-living prairie voles, *Microtus ochrogaster.* Behav. Ecol. Sociobiol. **18:** 275-282.
7. Dulce Madeira, M., & A. R. Lieberman. 1995. Sexual dimorphism in the mammalian limbic system. Progr. Neurobiol. **45:** 257-333.
8. Numan M. 1988. Maternal behavior. *In* The Physiology of Reproduction. E. Knobil & J. Neill, Eds.: 1569-1645. Raven Press. New York.
9. Rosenblatt, J. S. & H. I. Siegel. 1981. Factors governing the onset and maintenance of maternal behavior among nonprimate mammals. *In* Parental Care in Mammals. D. J. Gubernick & P. H. Klopfer, Eds.: 13-76. Wiley. New York.
10. Beach, F. A. & J. Jayens. 1956. Studies of maternal retrieving in rats: III. Sensory cues involved in the lactating female's response to her young. Behaviour **10:** 104-125.
11. Benuck, I. & F. A. Rowe. 1975. Centrally and peripherally induced anosmia: Influences on maternal behavior in lactating female rats. Physiol. Behav. **14:** 439-447.
12. Herrenkohl, L. R. & P. A. Rosenberg. 1972. Exteroceptive stimulation of maternal behavior in the naive rat. Physiol. Behav. **8:** 595-598.
13. Kenyon, P., P. Cronin & S. Keeble. 1981. Disruption of maternal behavior by perioral anesthesia. Physiol. Behav. **27:** 313-321.
14. Fleming, A. S., F. Vaccarino, L. Tambosso & P. Chee. 1979. Vomeronasal and olfactory system modulation of maternal behavior in the rat. Science **203:** 372-374.

15. FLEMING, A. S., F. VACCARINO & C. LUEBKE. 1980. Amygdaloid inhibition of maternal behavior in the nulliparous female rat. Physiol. Behav. **25:** 731-743.
16. DEL CERRO, M. C. R., M. A. P. IZQUIERDO, P. COLLADO, S. SEGOVIA & A. GUILLAMON. 1991. Bilateral lesions of the bed nucleus of the accessory olfactory tract facilitate maternal behavior in virgin female rats. Physiol. Behav. **50:** 67-71.
17. SMOTHERMAN, W. P., R. W. BELL, J. STARZEC, J. ELIAS & T. A. ZACHMAN. 1974. Maternal responses to infant vocalizations and olfactory cues in rats and mice. Behav. Biol. **12:** 55-66.
18. ROSENBLATT, J. S. & H. I. SIEGEL. 1975. Hysterectomy-induced maternal behavior during pregnancy in the rat. J. Comp. Physiol. Psychol. **89:** 685-700.
19. BRIDGES, R. S., H. H. FEDER & J. S. ROSENBLATT. 1977. Induction of maternal behaviors in primigravid rats by ovariectomy, hysterectomy, or ovariectomy, plus hysterectomy: Effect of length of gestation. Horm. Behav. **9:** 156-169.
20. MAYER, A. D. & J. S. ROSENBLATT. 1984. Prepartum changes in maternal responsiveness and nest defense in *Rattus norwegicus.* J. Comp. Psychol. **98:** 177-188.
21. ROSENBLATT, J. S., A. D. MAYER & A. L. GIORDANO. 1988. Hormonal basis during pregnancy for the onset of maternal behavior in the rat. Psychoneuroendocrinology **13:** 29-46.
22. BRIDGES, R. S. 1990. Endocrine regulation of parental behavior in rodents. *In* Mammalian Parenting. Biochemical Neurobiological, and Behavioral Determinants. N. A. Krasnegor & R. S. Bridges, Eds.: 93-117. Oxford University Press. New York.
23. ROSENBLATT, J. S. 1967. Nonhormonal basis of maternal behavior in the rat. Science **156:** 1512-1514.
24. PFAFF, D. W. & M. KEINER. 1973. Atlas of estradiol-concentrating cells in the central nervous system of the female rat. J. Comp. Neurol. **151:** 121-158.
25. NUMAN, M., J. S. ROSENBLATT & B. R. KOMISARUK. 1977. Medial preoptic area and onset of maternal behavior in the rat. J. Comp. Physiol. Psychol. **91:** 146-164.
26. SLOTNICK, B. M. 1967. Disturbances of maternal behavior in the rat following lesions of the cingulate cortex. Behaviour **29:** 204-236.
27. KIMBLE, D. P., L. ROGERS & L. HENDRICKSON. 1967. Hippocampal lesions disrupt maternal, not sexual, behavior in the albino rat. J. Comp. Physiol. Psychol. **63:** 401-407.
28. FLEISCHER, S. & B. M. SLOTNICK. 1978. Disruption of maternal behavior in rats with lesions of the septal area. Physiol. Behav. **21:** 189-200.
29. CORODIMAS, K. P., J. S. ROSENBLATT, M. E. CANFIELD & J. I. MORRELL. 1993. Neurons in the lateral subdivision of the habenular complex mediate the hormonal onset of maternal behavior in rats. Behav. Neurosci. **107:** 827-843.
30. NUMAN, M. & M. NUMAN. 1996. A lesion and neuroanatomical tract-tracing analysis of the role of the bed nucleus of the stria terminalis in retrieval behavior and other aspects of maternal responsiveness in rats. Dev. Psychobiol. **29:** 23-51.
31. NUMAN, M. & H. G. SMITH. 1984. Maternal behavior in rats: Evidence for the involvement of preoptic projections to the ventral tegmental area. Behav. Neurosci. **98:** 712-727.
32. HANSEN, S. & A. FERREIRA. 1986. Food intake, aggression, and fear behavior in the mother rat: Control by neural systems concerned with milk ejection and maternal behavior. Behav. Neurosci. **100:** 64-70.
33. MAYER, A. D., N. C. G. FREEMAN & J. S. ROSENBLATT. 1979. Ontogeny of maternal behavior in the laboratory rat: Factors underlying changes in responsiveness from 30 to 90 days. Dev. Psychobiol. **12:** 425-439.
34. BROWN, R. E. 1986. Paternal behavior in the male Long-Evans rat (*Rattus norvegicus*). J. Comp. Psychol. **100:** 162-172.
35. SEGOVIA, S. & A. GUILLAMON. 1993. Sexual dimorphism in the vomeronasal pathway and sex differences in reproductive behaviors. Brain Res. Rev. **18:** 51-74.
36. SEGOVIA, S., L. M. ORENSANZ, A. VALENCIA & A GUILLAMON. 1984. Effects of sex steroids on the development of the accessory olfactory bulb in the rat: A volumetric study. Dev. Brain Res. **16:** 312-314.

37. Collado, P., A. Guillamon, A. Valencia & S. Segovia. 1990. Sexual dimorphism in the bed nucleus of the accessory olfactory tract in the rat. Dev. Brain Res. **56:** 263-268.
38. Mizukami, S., M. Nishizyka & Y. Arai. 1983. Sexual difference in nuclear volume and its ontogeny in the rat amygdala. Exp. Neurol. **79:** 569-575.
39. Hines, M., L. S. Allen & R. A. Gorski. 1992. Sex differences in subregions of the medial nucleus of the amygdala and the bed nucleus of the stria terminalis of the rat. Brain Res. **579:** 321-326.
40. Del Abril, A., S. Segovia & A. Guillamon. 1987. The bed nucleus of the stria terminalis in the rat: Regional sex differences controlled by gonadal steroids early after birth. Dev. Brain Res. **32:** 295-300.
41. Menella, J. A. & H. Moltz. 1988. Infanticide in the male rats: The role of the vomeronasal organ. Physiol. Behav. **42:** 303-306.
42. Izquierdo, P., P. Collado, S. Segovia, A. Guillamon & M. A. P. Del Cerro. 1992. Maternal behavior induced in male rats by bilateral lesions of the bed nucleus of the accessory olfactory tract. Physiol. Behav. **52:** 707-712.
43. Yahr, P. 1988. Sexual differentiation of behavior in the context of developmental psychobiology. *In* Handbook of Behavioral Neurobiology. Vol. 9. E. M. Blass, Ed.: 197-243. Plenum. New York.
44. Sar, M. & W. E. Stumpf. 1977. Distribution of androgen target cells in rat forebrain and pituitary after [^{3}H]-dihydrotestosterone administration. J. Steroid Biochem. **8:** 1131-1135.
45. Gorski, R. A., J. H. Gordan, J. E. Shryne & A. M. Southam. 1978. Evidence for a morphological sex difference within the medial preoptic area of the rat brain. Brain Res. **148:** 333-346.
46. Nottebohm, F. & A. P. Arnold. 1976. Sexual dimorphism in vocal control areas of the songbird brain. Science **194:** 211-213.
47. Gubernick, D. J., D. R. Sengelaub & E. M. Kurz. 1993. A neuroanatomical correlate of paternal and maternal behavior in the biparental California mouse (*Peromyscys californicus*). Behav. Neurosci. **107:** 194-201.
48. Shapiro, L. E., C. M. Leonard, C. E. Sessions, D. A. Dewsbury & T. R. Insel. 1991. Comparative neuroanatomy of the sexually dimorphic hypothalamus in monogamous and polygamous vole. Brain Res. **541:** 232-240.
49. Simerly, R. B., R. A. Gorski & L. W. Swanson. 1986. Neurotransmitter specificity of cells and fibers in the medial preoptic nucleus: An immunohistochemical study in the rat. J. Comp. Neurol. **246:** 343-363.
50. De Vries, G. J. 1990. Sex differences in neurotransmitter systems. J. Neuroendocrinol. **2:** 1-13.
51. Popper, P., C. A. Priest & P. E. Micevych. 1995. Effects of sex steroids on the cholecystokinin circuit modulating reproductive behavior. *In* Neurobiological Effects of Sex Steroid Hormones. P. E. Micevych & R. P. Hammer, Jr., Eds.: 160-183. Cambridge University Press. Cambridge.
52. McCarthy, M. M., P. J. Brooks, J. G. Pfaus, H. E. Brown, L. M. Flanagan, S. Schwartz-Giblin & D. W. Pfaff. 1993. Antisense oligodeoxynucleotides in behavioral neuroscience. Neuroprotocols **2:** 67-74.
53. Rubin, B. S. & R. S. Bridges. 1984. Disruption of ongoing maternal responsiveness in rats by central administration of morphine sulfate. Brain Res. **307:** 91-97.
54. Simerly, R. B., L. D. McCall & S. J. Watson. 1988. Distribution of opioid peptides in the preoptic region: Immunohistochemical evidence for a steroid-sensitive enkephalin sexual dimorphism. J. Comp. Neurol. **276:** 442-459.
55. Watson, R. E., Jr., G. E. Hoffman & S. J. Wiegand. 1986. Sexually dimorphic opioid distribution in the preoptic area: Manipulation by gonadal steroids. Brain Res. **398:** 157-163.
56. Hammer, R. P., Jr. 1984. The sexually dimorphic region of the preoptic area in rats contains denser opiate receptor binding sites in females. Brain Res. **308:** 172-176.

57. Hammer, R. P., & R. S. Bridges. 1987. Preoptic area opioids and opiate receptors increase during pregnancy and decrease during lactation. Brain Res. **420:** 48-56.
58. Pedersen, C. A., J. A. Asche, Y. L. Monroe & A. J. Prange. 1982. Oxytocin induces maternal behavior in virgin female rats. Science **216:** 648-649.
59. Insel, T. R. & L. E. Shapiro. 1992. Oxytocin receptors and maternal behavior. Ann. N.Y. Acad. Sci. **652:** 122-141.
60. De Vries, G. J. & R. M. Buijs. 1983. The origin of the vasopressinergic and oxytocinergic innervation of the rat brain with special reference to the lateral septum. Brain Res. **273:** 307-317.
61. Insel, T. R. & C. R. Harbaugh. 1989. Lesions of the hypothalamic paraventriuclar nucleus disrupt the initiation of maternal behavior. Physiol. Behav. **45:** 1033-1041.
62. Numan, M. & K. P. Corodimas. 1985. The effects of paraventricular hypothalamic lesions on maternal behavior in rats. Physiol. Behav. **35:** 417-425.
63. Wideman, C. H. & H. M. Murphy. 1990. Vasopressin, maternal behavior and pup well-being. Curr. Psychol. Res. Rev. **9:** 285-295.
64. De Vries, G. J., R. M. Buijs, F. W. Van Leeuwen, A. R. Caffé & D. F. Swaab. 1985. The vasopressinergic innervation of the brain in normal and castrated rats. J. Comp. Neurol. **233:** 236-254.
65. Merker, G. S., S. Blahser & E. Zeisberger. 1980. Reactivity patterns of vasopressin containing neurons and its relation to the antipyretic reaction in guinea pig. Cell Tiss. Res. **212:** 47-61.
66. Caldwell, J. D., E. R. Greer, M. F. Johnson, A. J. Prange, Jr. & C. A. Pedersen. 1987. Oxytocin and vasopressin immunoreactivity in hypothalamic and extrahypothalamic sites in late pregnant and postpartum rats. Neuroendocrinology **46:** 39-47.
67. Landgraf, R., I. Neumann & Q. J. Pittman. 1991. Septal and hippocampal release of vasopressin and oxytocin during late pregnancy and parturition in the rat. Neuroendocrinology **54:** 378-383.
68. De Vries, G. J., R. M. Buijs & A. A. Sluiter. 1984. Gonadal hormone actions on the morphology of the vasopressinergic innervation of the adult rat brain. Brain Res. **298:** 141-145.
69. Van Leeuwen, F. W., A. R. Caffé & G. J. De Vries. 1985. Vasopressin cells in the bed nucleus of the stria terminalis of the rat: Sex differences and the influence of androgens. Brain Res. **325:** 391-394.
70. Miller, M. A., G. J. De Vries, H. A. Al-Shamma & D. M. Dorsa. 1992. Rate of decline of vasopressin immunoreactivity and messenger RNA levels in the bed nucleus of the stria terminalis. J. Neurosci. **12:** 2881-2887.
71. De Vries, G. J., R. M. Buijs & D. F. Swaab. 1981. Ontogeny of the vasopressinergic neurons of the suprachiasmatic nucleus and their extrahypothalamic projections in the rat brain: Presence of a sex difference in the lateral septum. Brain Res. **218:** 67-78.
72. Miller, M. A., L. Vician, D. K. Clifton & D. M. Dorsa. 1989. Sex differences in vasopressin neurons in the bed nucleus of the stria terminalis by in situ hybridization. Peptides **10:** 615-619.
73. Al-Shamma, H. A. & G. J. De Vries. 1996. Neurogenesis of the sexually dimorphic vasopressin cells of the bed nucleus of the stria terminalis and amygdala of rats. J. Neurobiol. **29:** 91-98.
74. McGuire, B. & M. Novak. 1984. A comparison of maternal behaviour in the meadow vole (*Microtus pennsylvanicus*), prairie vole (*M. ochrogaster*) and pine vole (*M. pinetorum*). Anim. Behav. **32:** 1132-1141.
75. Oliveras, D. & M. Novak. 1986. A comparison of paternal behaviour in the meadow vole, *Microtus pennsylvanicus,* the pine vole, *M. pinetorum* and the prairie vole, *M. ochrogaster.* Anim Behav. **34:** 519-526.
76. Bamshad, M., M. A. Novak & G. J. De Vries. 1993. Sex and species differences in the vasopressin innervation of sexually naive and parental prairie voles, *Microtus ochrogaster* and meadow voles, *Microtus pennsylvanicus.* J. Neuroendocrinol. **5:** 247-255.

77. Bamshad, M., M. A. Novak & G. J. De Vries. 1994. Cohabitation alters vasopressin innervation and paternal behavior in prairie voles, *Microtus ochrogaster*. Physiol. Behav. **56:** 751-758.
78. Wang, Z. X., W. Smith, D. E. Major & G. J. De Vries. 1994. Sex and species differences in the effects of cohabitation on vasopressin messenger RNA expression in the bed nucleus of the stria terminalis in prairie voles (*Microtus ochrogaster*) and meadow voles (*Microtus pennsylvanicus*). Brain Res. **650:** 212-218.
79. Getz, L. L., C. S. Carter & L. Gavish. 1981. The mating system of prairie vole, *Microtus ochrogaster:* Field and laboratory evidence for pair-bonding. Behav. Ecol. Sociobiol. **8:** 189-194.
80. Wang, Z. X., C. F. Ferris & G. J. De Vries. 1994. The role of septal vasopressin innervation in paternal behavior in prairie voles (*Microtus ochrogaster*). Proc. Natl. Acad. Sci. USA **91:** 400-404.
81. Winslow, J. T., N. Hastings, C. S. Carter, C. R. Harbaugh & T. R. Insel. 1993. A role for central vasopressin in pair bonding in monogamous prairie voles. Nature **365:** 545-547.
82. Koolhaas, J. M., E. Moor, Y. Hiemstra & B. Bohus. 1991. The testosterone-dependent vasopressinergic neurons in the medial amygdala and lateral septum: Involvement in social behaviour of male rats. *In* Vasopressin Colloque INSERM. Vol. 208. S. Jard & R. Jamison, Eds.: 213-219. John Libbey Eurotext Ltd. London.
83. Williams, J. R., T. R. Insel, C. R. Harbaugh & C. S. Carter. 1994. Oxytocin administered centrally facilitates formation of a partner preference in female prairie voles (*Mocrotus ochrogaster*). J. Neuroendocrinol. **6:** 247-250.
84. Insel, T. R., C. F. Ferris & Z. X. Wang. 1994. Pattern of brain vasopressin receptor distribution associated with social organization in microtine rodents. J. Neurosci. **14:** 5381-5392.
85. Bluthe, R.-M. & R. Dantzer. 1992. Role of the vomeronasal system in the vasopressinergic modulation of social recognition in rats. Brain Res. **604:** 205-210.
86. Jakab, R. L. & C. Leranth. 1991. Convergent vasopressinergic and hippocampal input onto somatospiny neurons of the rat lateral septal area. Neuroscience **2:** 413-421.
87. Dantzer, R., G. F. Koob, R. M. Bluthé & M. Le Moal. 1988. Septal vasopressin modulates social memory in male rats. Brain Res. **457:** 143-147.
88. Bluthe, R. M. & R. Dantzer. 1990. Social recognition does not involve vasopressinergic neurotransmission in female rats. Brain Res. **535:** 301-304.
89. Iacono, W. G. & M. Beiser. 1992. Are males more likely than females to develop schizophrenia? Am. J. Psychiatry **149:** 1070-1074.

12

Peptides, Steroids, and Pair Bonding

C. Sue Carter, A. Courtney DeVries, Susan E. Taymans, R. Lucille Roberts, Jessie R. Williams, and Lowell L. Getz

Social bonds are essential components of mammalian social systems. Of particular importance are selective social attachments between males and females, sometimes known as pair bonds. Monogamy in mammals is characterized by heterosexual pair bonds, which provide a social matrix for reproductive behaviors including sexual behavior and parenting. The present paper describes the natural history and behavioral characteristics of a rodent model, *Microtus ochrogaster* (prairie voles). Prairie voles exhibit many features of monogamy including pair bond formation, biparental care, reduced sexual dimorphism, incest avoidance, and reproduction which is regulated by social stimuli.[1]

Studies in prairie voles are used here to examine evidence for an effect on pair bonding of two general classes of hormones: neuropeptides, with emphasis on oxytocin and vasopressin, and steroids, including hormones produced by the gonads and the adrenal cortex. Although mechanisms underlying adult social attachments are emphasized, developmental processes including hormonal and social history, which may influence the subsequent tendency to form pair bonds, also will be considered.

UNIQUE FEATURES OF PRAIRIE VOLE BIOLOGY

Natural History. Voles are small arvicoline rodents found in the northern hemisphere. Voles, and related lemmings, sometimes show dramatic fluctuations or ''cycles'' in population density and for this reason have been studied extensively by ecologists in the 20th century.[2] Prairie voles, which are found in grasslands throughout

This work was supported by the National Science Foundation (BNS 7925713, 8506727, and 8719748 to C.S.C. and DFB 7825713 to L.L.G.), the National Institutes of Health, including the Institute of Child Health and Human Development (HD 16679 to C.S.C. and HD 09328 to L.L.G.), and the National Institute of Mental Health (MH 45836).

midwestern North America, have attracted particular interest because they can be studied under both field and laboratory conditions and because they are monogamous.

Field studies begun in the 1960s provided the first hint that prairie voles were highly social and probably monogamous.[13] Male and female pairs of prairie voles maintain a common nest and territory and tend to enter live traps together as long as both members of a pair are alive. By contrast, in less social, nonmonogamous meadow voles (*M. pennsylvanicus*)[3] and montane voles (*M. montanus*),[4] males and females have separate nests and territories and are usually trapped alone.

Based on a database from populations in Eastern Illinois, it was determined that prairie voles live in communal family groups comprised primarily of a male and female breeder pair and their offspring.[5,6] About 70-75% of young voles do not leave their natal family.[5] The original breeding pair within a family has a reproductive advantage; most other members of the communal group are reproductively inactive offspring that serve as "helpers at the nest," presumably gaining reproductive advantages through inclusive fitness. Familiarity inhibits reproduction in young prairie voles, and incest avoidance is strong. However, some young females may reproduce within the family, probably as a result of matings with nonfamily members. Young males, in contrast, probably remain sexually suppressed within the family nest and must leave the family group to reproduce. New pairs are most likely to form when previously naive males and females leave their group, meet an unfamiliar member of the opposite sex, develop new pair bonds, mate, and generate their own families.

Prairie vole life is treacherous. Most infants do not live to weaning, and the average life span of those that survive is about 2 months. Major life events are compressed in time, and voles must maximize their breeding opportunities.[6] The time course of the reproductive events described here is variable. However, pair bond formation, as defined below, can occur within hours, and reproductive activation and estrus induction, which are initiated by hormonal events associated with meeting a novel stranger of the opposite sex, can occur within a day or two. In new couples, intermittent mating bouts continue for about 24-48 hours followed by a 21-day gestation. After an initial mating, prairie vole females experience a postpartum estrus, allowing females to breed again and nurse one litter while they are pregnant with a second. In most, but not all cases, pair-bonded females exhibit a sexual preference for the familiar male.[7] Pair-bonded males become highly aggressive following mating and may patrol the runways that lead to their nest. Although detailed information on paternity is not yet available, preliminary data suggest that the male partner of an established pair probably fathers most of the offspring that his partner delivers.[6] In nature, when one member of the pair abandons the nest, usually because of mortality, the remaining partner rarely forms a new pair bond. Thus, for prairie voles the first pair bond that young animals form may last until "death do them part" (TABLE 1).

LABORATORY EVIDENCE FOR PAIR BONDING

Partner Preferences. Although field data support the assumption that pair bonds are an essential component of the monogamous social system of the prairie vole, interactions among individual rodents are rarely observed in nature. However, prairie voles adapt easily to the laboratory and therefore it has been possible to investigate various aspects of the behavioral and neuroendocrine control of pair bonding.[7]

TABLE 1. Mating, Peptides, and Partner Preferences in Prairie Voles

	Prairie Voles		
	Male	Female	References
Mating	Facilitation	Facilitation	3,7-9
Oxytocin	No change	Facilitation	22,23
Vasopressin	Facilitation	No change	11

The study of physiological determinants of pair bonding requires the development of an operational definition for this hypothetical construct. In prairie voles we originally attempted to use sexual preferences as an index of pair bonding. However, sexual preferences can only be studied in reproductively active animals, and despite several attempts we found no evidence that sexual preferences existed between female and male prairie voles that had become ''familiar'' through cohabitation or following approximately 1 day of mating.[7] Females in postpartum estrus generally prefer to mate with their established partner, but a substantial number of these animals respond with sexual postures (lordosis) to mating attempts by unfamiliar males.[3]

In subsequent studies a new paradigm was developed to study social or partner preferences. In this paradigm voles were placed in a larger three-chambered apparatus that allowed the experimental animal to spend time with either a stimulus animal designated by familiarity as the ''partner'' or with a comparable ''stranger'' or to elect to be alone in a neutral cage.[8] Both stimulus animals were tethered loosely so that they could move only within their own chamber, whereas the experimental animal was free to explore the entire test apparatus. Tests were extended to 3 hours to take into account reactions to novelty and to provide a more reliable index of social preferences. Time-lapse videotaping provided an efficient index of contact with the stimulus animals, time spent in each chamber, and physical activity measured by movement among the three chambers. Sexual or agonistic behaviors were recorded if these occurred. This paradigm yields reliable social preferences which can be studied as a function of various experiential or physiological manipulations.[8]

Using this procedure, significant preferences for the familiar partner were established in prairie voles of both sexes after prolonged periods of sexual or nonsexual cohabitation. In female prairie voles, preferences for the familiar partner were established more quickly if mating occurred; however, nonsexual cohabitation also was followed by a significant partner preference.[8] Differences in both the amount of physical contact and the choice of a preferred partner exist between polygynous and monogamous species of voles. For example, in contrast to prairie voles, when montane voles are tested under comparable conditions, they usually do not show a significant preference for the familiar partner, but the total amount of time in physical contact is about 20% that seen in prairie voles. Montane voles tend to spend much more time alone in the neutral chamber.[9]

Selective Aggression. Sexual activity involves reflexive behaviors that may be elicited by physical contact. Although social preferences may bias reproduction to favor a familiar or resident male, laboratory studies thus far do not suggest a strong sexual preference for familiar or unfamiliar males in female prairie voles.[7] Thus, in male prairie voles, mate guarding probably plays a role in protecting the female partner from sexual advances by other males. Aggression, which can be indexed in the laboratory by simple dyadic encounters, is easily measured and highly selective in prairie voles.[3,7]

Sexually naive prairie voles of either sex are not aggressive towards conspecifics. By contrast, after approximately 12–24 hours of sexual experience, male prairie voles become extremely aggressive toward unfamiliar males.[10,11] Sexually experienced "breeder" males are socially dominant and drive away or, if necessary, kill male strangers. However, they are usually not aggressive to familiar animals, and breeder males will allow their own offspring to remain in the family, at least as long as these offspring are sexually naive.[6,7] Cohabitation even for several days does not produce a reliable increase in aggression; however, nonsexual cohabitation does cause hormonal changes associated with reproductive activation.[12,13]

Females also become aggressive after mating, but postcopulatory aggression develops more slowly in females than in males, and in females the onset and intensity of aggression are variable.[14,15] If two unrelated females are placed with a male, both may mate with the male. Under these conditions one female becomes socially dominant, and the nondominant female is blocked from social contact with the male. During the postmating period and before either female can deliver young, the nondominant female usually dies. Maternal aggression is common in the postnatal period and is directed towards both unfamiliar females and unfamiliar males.[3] Female prairie voles do not express aggression towards their own offspring. In addition, sibling females successfully share a single male partner, and both reproduce without experiencing the mortality seen in trios composed of one male and two unrelated females.[14,15] The adaptive significance of female aggression is less obvious than that in males, and it may be related to territoriality or offspring defense and/or female-female competition.

GONADAL HORMONES

Partner Preferences. The finding that reliable social preferences between males and females would form in the absence of mating made it possible to examine the role of gonadal hormones in pair bonding. Partner preferences were formed in gonadectomized males and females.[8,16] In addition, when gonadally intact experimental animals were allowed to chose between two unfamiliar stimulus animals of the opposite sex, they did not differentiate between a gonadally intact versus a gonadectomized animal. No evidence currently exists that gonadal hormones play a role in the partner preference component of pair bonding (TABLE 2).

Aggression. The role of gonadal hormones in prairie vole aggression is complicated by the fact in both sexes aggression follows sexual experience.[3,11] Gonadectomy typically is used to eliminate gonadal hormones, but gonadectomy also inhibits sexual behavior. Therefore, it is difficult to examine the role of gonadal hormones in mating-induced aggression.

In naive female prairie voles, female-female aggression is infrequent either before or after ovariectomy. Estrogen treatment alone produces only small increments in

TABLE 2. Steroid Hormones and Partner Preference Development in Prairie Voles

	Prairie Voles		
	Male	Female	References
Gonadal steroids	No change	No change	8,16
Corticosterone	Facilitation	Inhibition	13,20
Stress (3-minute swim)	Facilitation	Inhibition	20

aggressive behavior, whereas females that have received both estrogen and mating experience become slightly more aggressive (Carter, unpublished observations). However, in none of these cases is the level of aggression as intense as that seen in sexually experienced pregnant or postpartum females. Evidence thus far suggests that intense aggression, such as that seen in gonadally intact, sexually experienced females, depends on hormonal changes other than those necessary for estrus induction or sexual behavior. The effects of the hormones associated with pregnancy and/or lactation on aggression remain to be described in female prairie voles.

In summary, partner preferences and selective aggression characterize pair bonding in prairie voles. Sexual and social experiences regulate the expression of pair bonding. However, partner preferences can develop in the absence of gonadal hormones. The initial development of a partner preference may occur prior to mating when levels of gonadal hormones are comparative low.[17] Subsequent sexual experience can affect and perhaps even redirect the pair-bonding process. Attempts to implicate testicular or ovarian hormones in aggression during adulthood have not produced clear results, at least in prairie voles from a stock captured in Illinois, leading us to hypothesize that other hormonal events associated with social interactions and mating might be primarily responsible for pair bond formation.

ADRENAL STEROID HORMONES

Between Species Comparisons and Domestication. The notion that "stress" mediated by the adrenal glands might influence social behavior and reproduction became popular at least 30 years ago and was based in part on observations on voles.[18] However, direct evidence on the validity of this hypothesis has been slow to accumulate. In the decades that followed, studies with laboratory rodents have provided a better appreciation for the complex neuroendocrinology of the hypothalamic-pituitary-adrenal (HPA) axis. However, most research on the HPA axis is done in domestic rats or mice, in which interactions between the HPA axis and the hypothalamic-pituitary-gonadal (HPG) axis may be minimized by artificial selection.

Rats (*Rattus norvegicus*) have experienced "natural" selection for their ability to inhabit, in commensal association with humans, very diverse ecological conditions. Unlike most "wild" animals, rats continue to reproduce in virtually every terrestrial habitat on earth. This ecological diversity would not be possible if the HPA and HPG axes in rats were very sensitive to environmental or social constraints. Domestic rats, in turn, have been selected for their ability to reproduce under diverse laboratory conditions. Domestication may have provided an additional genetic filter that further reduced the capacity of the HPA axis and thus environmental influences to inhibit reproduction.

Adrenal to body weight ratios and adrenocorticoid hormone production are low in domestic rats when compared to prairie voles.[12,19] For example, serum corticosterone levels in male Sprague-Dawley rats that were not deliberately stressed were about 30 ng/ml, while exposure to an ether stress was followed by approximately a doubling of corticosterone levels. Under comparable conditions and in the same assay, corticosterone levels in unstressed male prairie voles averaged 600-1,000 ng/ml (FIG. 1).

Despite a highly active HPA axis, domestication is not necessary for successful breeding of prairie voles, perhaps in part because pair bonding provides a relevant social environment for their reproduction. Adrenocorticoid levels actually declined when naive prairie voles were placed with a novel stranger of the opposite sex.[13] The time course of the decline differs somewhat in the two sexes (FIG. 1); males showed a significant change from baseline in less than 15 minutes, while corticosterone levels in females required approximately 60 minutes to show a significant decline.

Pair Bonding and the Adrenal Response to Separation, Reunion, or Social Novelty. In male and female prairie voles paired by cohabitation, corticosterone responses were examined as a function of separation for 24 hours,[12] (Williams *et al.*, unpublished data). Some animals also were reunited with either the familiar partner or a stranger. Separation was associated with an elevation in corticosterone levels, and reunion with the familiar partner was followed by a return to the unseparated level. Previously paired males also showed low levels of corticosterone in the presence of a novel female, whereas paired females responded to the introduction of a novel male with an increase in corticosterone.

In a separate study[13] (DeVries *et al.*, this volume) in previously paired animals, the time course of corticosterone changes was measured as a function of housing with an unfamiliar animal of the opposite sex. As before, males that had previously been housed with a female partner then housed with an unfamiliar female showed a decline in corticosterone levels (FIG. 1) identical to that seen in unpaired males; in contrast, when a previously paired female was housed with a novel male, corticosterone levels tended to rise. In both sexes, corticosterone levels in socially naive animals did not change significantly in response to exposure to a novel stranger of the same sex.

In many species, elevations in adrenocorticoid production are used as an index of stress. Viewed from this perspective, socially naive prairie voles are not "stressed" by the presence of a stranger of the opposite sex and in fact have reduced adrenal output under these conditions. In contrast, previously paired females, but not paired males (FIG. 1), may find the presence of a novel animal of the opposite sex "stressful" as defined by increased glucocorticoid secretion.

BEHAVIORAL EFFECTS OF CORTICOSTERONE

The unanticipated finding that socially naive prairie voles respond to exposure to a novel stranger of the opposite sex with a decline in corticosterone (FIG. 1) suggested the hypothesis that pair bonding in prairie voles might be inhibited by

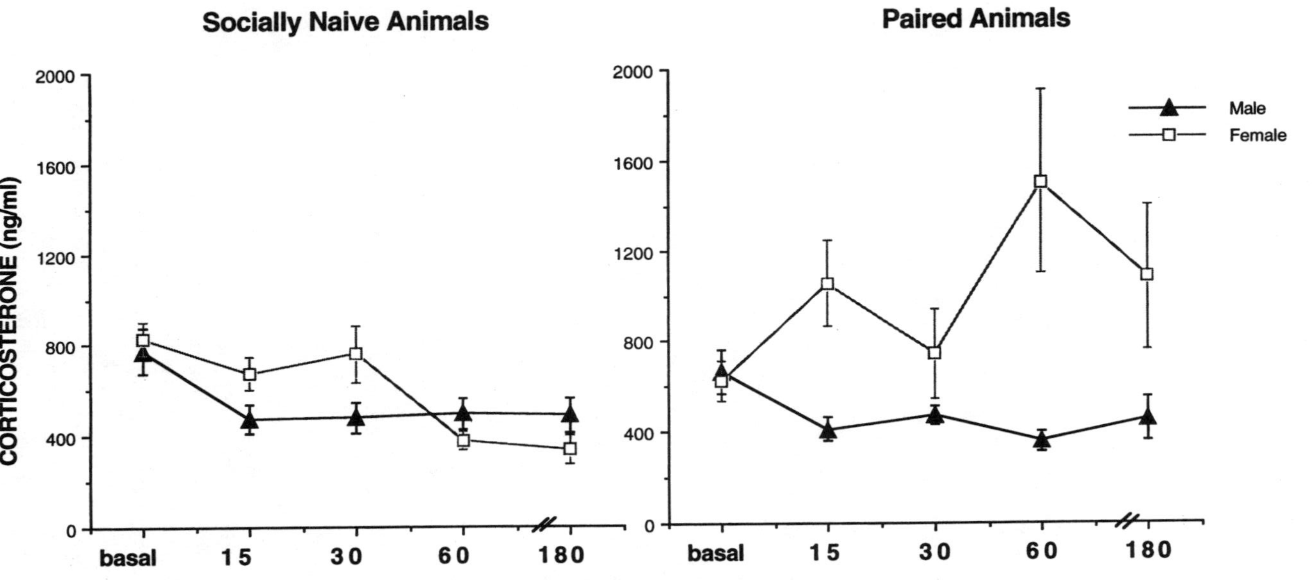

FIGURE 1. Sex differences in patterns of corticosterone change in response to exposure to a novel stranger and as a function of social experience. ''Naive'' animals were exposed only to family members and were housed with same-sex siblings prior to testing. ''Paired'' animals had a similar experience, but they were then pair housed for 3 days with a member of the opposite sex. Immediately following these experiences each animal was placed in a cage with an unfamiliar, socially naive member of the opposite sex (stranger). Serum samples were collected before exposure to the stranger or at 15, 30, 60, or 180 minutes after exposure to the stranger. Each sample was collected from a separate individual, frozen, and later assayed for corticosterone by radioimmunoassay.[13] Data are presented as mean ± SEM. Data points are connected to facilitate comparisons. Females tended to have higher basal corticosterone levels than males. Naive and paired males and naive females showed time-dependent declines from baseline following exposure to a stranger, with significant changes from baseline ($p < 0.05$) measured after 15 minutes in males and 60 minutes in females. By contrast, paired females showed elevations in corticosterone when housed with a stranger.

hormones of the HPA axis. In naive female prairie voles, removal of the adrenal gland facilitated the development of a partner preference. Adrenalectomized females formed a significant preference for the familiar male within 1 hour or less of cohabitation. The facilitatory effect of adrenalectomy was reversed by corticosterone replacement prior to male exposure. In addition, in females, increases in corticosterone levels by exogenous intraperitoneal (ip) injection produced a dose-dependent inhibition of the preference formation.[13] An endogenous increase in corticosterone production (an approximate doubling induced by a 3-minute swim stress) also inhibited pair bond formation in female prairie voles, an effect that was reversed by adrenalectomy.[20]

In socially naive male prairie voles the behavioral effects of corticosterone were examined in experiments that paralleled those in females, but with strikingly different results. Injections of corticosterone[21] or the stress of swimming[20] facilitated the development of partner preferences in males. By contrast, removal of the adrenal gland was followed by failure to form a partner preference,[21] which was restored by corticosterone.

In females, exposure to stress elicits physiological changes that inhibit the formation of new pair bonds. As just described, female prairie voles may be capable of breeding within their natal group, probably from mating with intruder males.[6] Therefore, remaining within the family during stressful periods could provide the female with protection, does not preclude subsequent reproduction, and might enhance fitness both directly and indirectly through contributions to the family. By contrast, in males, stress facilitates pair bonding. Male prairie voles must leave the family to breed and must be capable of forming new pair bonds and mating under stressful conditions. Thus, sex differences in the response to stress or hormones of the HPA axis may reflect or support a sex difference in reproductive strategies.

BEHAVIORAL EFFECTS OF OXYTOCIN AND VASOPRESSIN

Sexual experience facilitates partner preference formation and is necessary to induce selective aggression.[3,8,9] This observation suggested the hypothesis that hormones, such as the neuropeptides oxytocin and vasopressin, which are released during mating, could facilitate social bonding. Of these, oxytocin has been implicated in maternal behavior and filial bonding in female sheep.[21] Oxytocin infusions, when centrally administered, also facilitated the onset of partner preferences in sexually naive female prairie voles. Oxytocin antagonists reduced the behavioral effects of exogenous oxytocin[22] and also blocked partner preference formation during prolonged cohabitation. Oxytocin administered under comparable conditions (and in comparatively low doses) did not facilitate pair bonding in male prairie voles.[23]

In male prairie voles, vasopressin stimulates both partner preference formation and the onset of stranger-directed aggression. Further evidence for a role of vasopressin in pair bonding in males comes from the fact that low doses of a V1a vasopressin antagonist inhibited the effects on pair bonding of either exogenous vasopressin or sexual experience.[11] Again when tested under comparable conditions, infusions of vasopressin were not effective in facilitating partner preference formation in females. (The effects of vasopressin on female-female aggression remain to be studied.) Although, both sexually experienced males and females become aggressive, the timing

of the onset of aggression, stimuli that elicit aggression, and the hormonal modulation of aggression are probably sexually dimorphic.

Sex differences in the presence and behavioral effects of oxytocin and vasopressin are consistent with a larger literature which implicates oxytocin in various aspects of female reproduction and vasopressin in territoriality and defensive behaviors.[24] Vasopressin is more abundant in males and frequently is associated with a male reproductive strategy. Hypothalamic-limbic system vasopressin content, but not receptors, are higher in male versus female prairie voles.[25] Although oxytocin content and hypothalamic oxytocin receptors apparently are not sexually dimorphic in voles,[22] the receptor density in the anterior olfactory nucleus is estrogen dependent in the female prairie vole.[26]

SEX DIFFERENCES IN PAIR BOND FORMATION

Among the characteristics of monogamous mammals is a pattern of reduced sexual dimorphism in both anatomy and behavior.[1,4] For example, male and female prairie voles are similar in body size and lack the physical dimorphisms, including certain sex differences in central nervous system anatomy, that characterized nonmonogamous voles and other polygynous species.[27,28] Both male and female prairie voles engage in parental behavior. Consistent with this pattern of an absence of sex differences is the fact that conditions and behaviors associated with the development of partner preferences in male and female prairie voles are superficially similar. However, striking male-female differences have emerged from studies of the physiological substrates of monogamy.[7]

Recent studies indicate that hormones of the HPA axis can modulate pair bonding in prairie voles. However, males and females respond differently to corticosterone or the stress of swimming. Stress or corticosterone treatments[13,20] facilitate the formation of new pair bonds in males and inhibit the development of preferences for a familiar male in females.

In male prairie voles, either stress, corticosterone, or vasopressin can facilitate pair bonding. In rats, vasopressin is released by stress and is capable of acting as a secretogogue for ACTH, which in turn releases corticosterone. The effects of stress on pair bonding in male prairie voles could be mediated through the behavioral effects of corticosterone directly or indirectly through actions on other neurochemical systems. For example, stress or acute corticosterone treatments might release vasopressin, which in turn could facilitate pair bonding.[11]

In females, stress or corticosterone can inhibit the formation of heterosexual pair bonds. It is known that oxytocin can stimulate partner preference formation in female prairie voles.[22] These treatments may inhibit pair bonding because they interfere with the release or action of oxytocin. The influence of stress on oxytocin release is complex and has not yet been examined in voles. However, under some conditions, stress inhibits the release of oxytocin. Alternatively, oxytocin and corticosterone and/or stress may act independently to influence pair bonding in females. Experiments examining possible effects on pair bonding of interactions among vasopressin, oxytocin, and steroids of the adrenal axis are in progress.

DEVELOPMENTAL INFLUENCES ON PAIR BONDING

Although the behaviors associated with pair bonding appear superficially similar, the mechanisms responsible for pair bonding are apparently different in males and females. However, at least the partner preference component of pair bonding can occur in the absence of gonadal hormones. Sex differences in mammalian anatomy, biochemistry, and behavior are typically attributed to genetically regulated developmental processes that are mediated by hormonal events during the prenatal or perinatal period.[23,28] In laboratory rodents the presence of testicular hormones produces long-lasting anatomical changes necessary for masculine patterns of behavior.

Several features of monogamy in prairie voles appear similar to the changes in behavior that follow exposure to perinatal stress in rats. For example, a relative absence of sex differences in body size and appearance, high levels of male parental behavior, and a vulnerability to reproductive suppression are associated with both monogamy and perinatal stress.[12] In addition, the fact that the HPA axis is exceptionally active in prairie voles led to the hypothesis that developmental changes related to the presence or absence of adrenal and gonadal hormones or interactions between the HPA and HPG systems might account for the characteristics of monogamous behavior.

To test this hypothesis, prairie voles were exposed to various hormonal manipulations during the last trimester of pregnancy and the first 6 days postnatally. The results of these studies support the assumption that postnatal hormonal and social events can alter at least some of the characteristics of monogamy and that the effects of manipulations of postnatal hormonal and social experiences are sexually dimorphic.[29,30] Pair bonding between unfamiliar adults was not investigated in that study; however, sibling social preferences were measured. When given a choice between spending time with a familiar sibling or spending time with a stranger, females, but not males, that were exposed postnatally to exogenous testosterone or corticosterone spent more time with the stranger, whereas females that were exposed prenatally to testosterone or corticosterone were more likely than control animals to select a sibling over a stranger. Alloparental behavior, defined here as care of infants by young adults, which is characteristic of cooperative breeding, was inhibited in males, but not females, by postnatal exposure to androgens. By contrast, in females, but not males, postnatal exposure to exogenous corticosterone inhibited alloparenting. Study of the effects of social rearing conditions on subsequent alloparenting indicated that removal of the father, which is probably a form of mild stress even in the laboratory, was followed by a decrease in alloparenting behavior in females and by a much smaller drop in alloparenting by males.[30] In females, increases in corticosterone and being reared by a single parent, which may be "stressful," were both associated with a decline in alloparenting, whereas postnatal treatment with androgens in males was associated with a pattern of behavior more typical of polygyny. Although rearing without a father inhibited alloparenting in prairie voles of stock from Illinois, which has a resource-rich habitat, prairie voles from a separate stock captured in Kansas, where resources are less abundant, showed a different pattern of response. Female prairie voles from Kansas showed lower levels of alloparenting when reared by two parents, and increased levels when reared only by their mother.[30] Thus, early experiences may modify various social behaviors, including those associated with monogamy or cooperative breeding. In addition, experience can affect intraspecific variation, probably adapting animals to different habitats.

WHAT CAN WE LEARN FROM PRAIRIE VOLES?

Compared to most other rodents, the ecology of prairie voles is well known, providing an opportunity to interpret findings from the laboratory in the context of natural history. Field and laboratory research supports the assumption that prairie voles exhibit the characteristics of monogamy. The finding in rodents of the unusual physical and behavioral traits of monogamy has allowed investigation of the physiological substrates of these traits and supports the assumption that monogamous behaviors, including pair bonding, are influenced by hormones throughout life.

Pair bonding, which is essential to monogamy, includes both the development of social attachments and selective aggression. Most studies of behavioral endocrinology have focused on gonadal steroids, but these hormones apparently are not major determinants of pair bonding in adulthood. Attempts in prairie voles to understand pair bonding, as well as another monogamous trait, male parental care,[25,30–33] have drawn attention to the behavioral effects of oxytocin and vasopressin. Oxytocin and vasopressin have been implicated in various reproductive and homeostatic processes and appear to play a major regulatory role in prairie vole monogamy. Hormones of the HPA axis are very sensitive to social stimuli, and involvement of HPA axis hormones, including corticosterone, in the expression of pair bonding suggests additional mechanisms through which social experiences can modulate social attachments. Although the absence of sexual dimorphism characterizes mammalian monogamy, there is abundant evidence that male and female prairie voles can use different mechanisms to produce phenotypically similar behaviors. Sex differences and similarities in features of monogamy may reflect developmental processes. These processes currently are incompletely understood, but preliminary data suggest the testable hypothesis that expression of monogamous traits can be modified by interactions between the HPA and HPG axes.

Because of the short life span that typifies small mammal natural history, animals must be able to sense resource availability and accommodate their social and reproductive behaviors to the environment. The HPA axis is sensitive to the social and physical environmental and is exceptionally active in prairie voles. Hormones of the HPA axis may influence both the organization and the activation of reproductive and social behaviors including pair bonding. Modifications in steroids and peptides allow individuals to adjust the expression of social behaviors, including the formation of pair bonds, to environmental demands.

ACKNOWLEDGMENTS

We wish to acknowledge the contributions of many investigators including Leah Gavish, Diane Witt, Jim Winslow, and Tom Insel.

REFERENCES

1. KLEIMAN, D. 1977. Monogamy in mammals. Q. Rev. Biol. **52:** 39-69.
2. TAMARIN, R. H., Ed. 1985. Biology of New World *Microtus.* American Society of Mammalogy. Special Publ. **8:** Shippensburg, PA.
3. GETZ, L. L., C. S. CARTER & L. L. GAVISH. 1981. Social organization in *free living prairie voles, Microtus ochrogaster.* Behav. Ecol. Sociobiol. **8:** 189-194.
4. DEWSBURY, D. A. 1987. The comparative psychology of monogamy. Nebr. Symp. Motiv. Pap. **35:** 1-50.
5. MCGUIRE, B., L. L. GETZ, J. E. HOFMANN, T. PIZZUTO & B. FRASE. 1993. Natal dispersal and philopatry in prairie voles (*Microtus ochrogaster*) in relation to population density, season, and natal social environment. Behav. Ecol. Sociobiol. **32:** 293-302.
6. GETZ, L. L. & C. S. CARTER. 1996. Prairie-vole partnerships. Am. Sci. **84:** 56-62.
7. CARTER, C. S., A. C. DEVRIES & L. L. GETZ. 1995. Physiological substrates of mammalian monogamy: The prairie vole model. Neurosci. Biobehav. Rev. **19:** 303-314.
8. WILLIAMS, J. R., K. C. CATANIA & C. S. CARTER. 1992. Development of partner preferences in female prairie voles (*Microtus ochrogaster*): The role of social and sexual experience. Horm. Behav. **26:** 339-349.
9. SHAPIRO, L. R., D. AUSTIN, S. E. WARD & D. A. DEWSBURY. 1986. Familiarity and female mate choice in two species of voles (*Microtus ochrogaster* and *Microtus montanus*). Anim. Behav. **34:** 90-97.
10. GAVISH, L., C. S. CARTER & L. L. GETZ. 1983. Male-female interactions in prairie voles. Anim. Behav. **31:** 511-517.
11. WINSLOW, J. T., N. HASTINGS, C. S. CARTER, C. R. HARBAUGH & T. R. INSEL. 1993. A role for central vasopressin in pair bonding monogamous prairie voles. Nature **365:** 545-548.
12. CARTER, C. S., A. C. DEVRIES, S. E. TAYMANS, R. L. ROBERTS, J. R. WILLIAMS & G. P. CHROUSOS. 1995. Adrenocorticoid hormones and the development and expression of mammalian monogamy. Ann. N.Y. Acad. Sci. **771:** 82-91.
13. DEVRIES, A. C., M. B. DEVRIES, S. E. TAYMANS & C. S. CARTER. 1995. The modulation of pair bonding by corticosterone in female prairie voles (*Microtus ochrogaster*). Proc. Natl. Acad. Sci. USA **92:** 7744-7748.
14. FIRESTONE, K. B., K. V. THOMPSON & C. S. CARTER. 1991. Behavioral correlates of intra-female reproductive suppression in prairie voles, *Microtus ochrogaster.* Behav. Neural Biol. **55:** 31-41.
15. GAVISH, L., C. S. CARTER & L. L. GETZ. 1981. Further evidences for monogamy in the prairie vole. Anim. Behav. **29:** 955-957.
16. DEVRIES, A. C., C. L. JOHNSON & C. S. CARTER. 1996. Characterization of partner preference in male and female prairie voles (*Microtus ochrogaster*). Can. J. Zool., in press.
17. CARTER, C. S., D. M. WITT, S. R. MANOCK, K. A. ADAMS, J. M. BAHR & K. CARLSTEAD. 1989. Hormonal correlates of sexual behavior and ovulation in male-induced and postpartum estrus in female prairie vole. Physiol. Behav. **46:** 941-948.
18. CHRISTIAN, J. J. & D. E. DAVIS. 1966. Adrenal glands in female voles (*Microtus pennsylvanicus*) as related to reproduction and population size. J. Mammal. **47:** 1-18.
19. TAYMANS, S. E., A. C. DEVRIES, M. B. DEVRIES, R. J. NELSON, T. C. FRIEDMAN, M. CASTRO, S. DETERA-WADLEIGH, C. S. CARTER & G. P. CHROUSOS. 1996. Glucocorticoid resistance in prairie voles (*Microtus ochrogaster*). Submitted.
20. DEVRIES, A. C., M. B. DEVRIES, S. E. TAYMANS & C. S. CARTER. 1996. The effects of stress on social preferences are sexually dimorphic in prairie voles. Proc. Natl. Acad. Sci. USA. **93:** 11980-11984.
21. KEVERNE, E. B. & K. M. KENDRICK. 1992. Oxytocin facilitation of maternal behavior in sheep. Ann. N.Y. Acad. Sci. **652:** 83-101.

22. WILLIAMS, J. R., T. R. INSEL, C. R. HARBAUGH & C. S. CARTER 1994. Oxytocin centrally administered facilitates formation of a partner preference in female prairie voles (*Microtus ochrogaster*). J. Neuroendocrinol. **6:** 247-250.
23. INSEL, T. R. & T. J. HULIHAN. 1995. A gender-specific mechanism for pair bonding: Oxytocin and partner preference formation in monogamous voles. Behav. Neurosci. **109:** 782-789.
24. FERRIS, C. 1992. Role of vasopressin in aggressive and dominant/subordinate behaviors. Ann. N.Y. Acad. Sci. **652:** 212-226.
25. BAMSHAD, M., M. A. NOVAK & G. J. DEVRIES. 1993. Species and sex differences in vasopressin innervation of sexually naive and parental prairie voles, *Microtus ochrogaster* and meadow voles, *Microtus pennsylvanicus.* J. Neuroendocrinol. **5:** 247-255.
26. WITT, D. M., C. S. CARTER & T. R. INSEL. 1991. Oxytocin receptor binding in female prairie voles: Endogenous and exogenous oestradiol stimulation. J. Neuroendocrinol. **3:** 155-161.
27. SHAPIRO, L. R., C. M. LEONARD, C. E. SESSIONS, D. A. DEWSBURY & T. R. INSEL. 1991. Comparative neuroanatomy of the sexually dimorphic hypothalamus in monogamous and polygamous voles. Brain Res. **541:** 232-240.
28. GORSKI, R. A. 1990. Structural and sexual dimorphisms in the brain. *In* Mammalian Parenting: Biochemical, Neurobiological and Behavioral Determinants. N. A. Krasnegor & R. S. Bridges, Eds.: 61-92. Oxford University Press. New York, NY.
29. ROBERTS, R. L., E. A. GUSTAFSEN & C. S. CARTER. Perinatal hormone exposure alters the expression of traits associated with cooperative breeding in prairie voles. Ann. N.Y. Acad. Sci., this volume.
30. ROBERTS, R. L. & C. S. CARTER. Intraspecific variation and the presence of a father can influence the expression of monogamous and communal traits in prairie voles. Ann. N.Y. Acad. Sci., this volume.
31. HARTUNG, T. G. & D. A. DEWSBURY. 1979. Paternal behavior in six species of muroid rodents. Behav. Neural Biol. **26:** 466-478.
32. OLIVERAS, D. & M. A. NOVAK. 1986. A comparison of paternal behaviour in the meadow vole *Microtus pennsylvanicus,* the pine vole, *M. pinetorum,* and the prairie vole, *M. ochrogaster.* Anim. Behav. **34:** 519-526.
33. WANG, Z. X., C. F. FERRIS & G. J. DEVRIES. 1994. The role of septal vasopressin innervation in paternal behavior in prairie voles (*Microtus ochrogaster*). Proc. Natl. Acad. Sci. USA **91:** 400-404.

13
Molecular Aspects of Monogamy

Thomas R. Insel, Larry Young, and Zuoxin Wang

First, a note about what this chapter is not. We are not suggesting that monogamy is dictated by a specific gene or are we suggesting that genes will explain why some individuals are monogamous and others are polygynous. The research described here focuses on molecular and cellular differences in the brains of monogamous and nonmonogamous species. This approach, which compares closely related species, provides, at best, correlational data. It may demonstrate an association between a pathway or a gene and monogamous social organization, but it does not explain why a species is monogamous and it does not yield information about individual differences within a species. In our studies, correlations from comparative studies have led to experimental approaches that provide a stronger inference about the molecular basis of monogamy, but the reader is cautioned about extrapolating these results across species. At this point, we have no evidence that the same molecular mechanisms found in rodents are relevant to monogamy in primates.

Monogamy as a form of social organization is found in roughly 3% of mammals, with a somewhat higher percentage in primates.[1] Although definitions differ somewhat across sources, characteristics of monogamy include a male and female pair sharing a nest and home range, preferential (although not exclusive) copulation with the mate, males participating in parental care, and defense of the nest from intruders.[2] Increasingly, with the advent of genotyping of offspring, monogamous pairs that were believed to be sexually exclusive have been found to be raising young from extra-pair copulations. This discovery suggests that either monogamy exists far less frequently than heretofore believed or that monogamy is best viewed as a social rather than a sexual strategy. Here we have adopted the perspective of monogamy as a cluster of social behaviors, including pair bonding (with selective affiliation), paternal care, and nest defense. Monogamy can thus be distinguished from polygyny and promiscuity, two more common forms of social organization in mammals. Polygynous species may live in a harem with one male or female associated with several reproductively active members of the opposite sex. Promiscuous species, which show no evidence of selective social bonds, may live as a loosely organized large social group or may inhabit isolated nests. In every case, social organization is considered a predictable feature of a species, recognizing that individuals may vary from population norms.

Address for correspondence: Thomas R. Insel, MD, Yerkes Primate Center, Emory University, Atlanta, GA 30322 (tel: 404/727-7707; fax: 404/727-0623; e-mail: insel@rmy.emory.edu).

TABLE 1. Behavioral Differences between Prairie Voles and Montane Voles

	Prairie Vole	Montane Vole
Shared nest	+++	−
Maternal care	+++	+
Paternal care	+++	−
Side-by-side time	+++	−
Infant separation distress	+++	−
Monogamy	+++	−

To study the molecular basis of monogamy, one needs a comparative model (closely related monogamous and nonmonogamous species), a candidate gene, and considerable luck. In the following review, we briefly describe the microtine model of monogamy (described more fully by Carter *et al.*[3]), summarize evidence implicating the oxytocin receptor gene as a "candidate gene" for monogamy, and finally discuss molecular differences in the promoter sequences of the oxytocin receptor gene that may underlie species differences in gene expression. Current studies use a transgenic approach to test the role of the oxytocin receptor in monogamy (Young *et al.,* this volume).

VOLES AS A COMPARATIVE MODEL

Among monogamous rodents, the prairie vole, *Microtus ochrogaster,* offers several advantages for laboratory study. Elegant field studies have demonstrated that the prairie vole is monogamous, sharing a nest and home range throughout the breeding season.[4] These animals are found in communal or multigenerational burrows throughout the midwestern part of the United States. These burrows generally contain a single breeding pair with males actively involved in parental care. If the male or the female of this breeding pair is removed, the remaining vole generally does not accept a new mate.[5] These animals breed well under laboratory conditions, and in captivity, adults generally sit side by side and young show high levels of distress responses to social isolation.[3,6,7]

In addition to preserving their field behaviors in the laboratory, prairie voles are attractive as experimental animals because they are closely related to another arvicoline species, the montane vole, *Microtus montanus,* which has an opposite pattern of social organization[2] (TABLE 1). The montane vole, found in the Rocky Mountains, is promiscuous, minimally parental, spends little time in contact with cospecifics, and has offspring that show little if any behavioral or physiologic response to social isolation.[6–8] In contrast to prairie voles, montane voles do not form pair bonds. The genus *Microtus* includes several other species, including pine voles, which like prairie voles appear monogamous, and meadow voles, which like montane voles, appear nonmonogamous in both field and laboratory settings.[2]

A comparison of prairie and montane voles is not exclusively a comparison of a monogamous and a promiscuous species. Prairie voles are more affiliative (in the sense that they spend more time in side-by-side contact) and are more parental. On several measures of nonsocial behavior, the two species cannot be reliably distinguished.[9,10]

THE OXYTOCIN RECEPTOR AS A CANDIDATE GENE

Oxytocin is a nine amino acid peptide that evolved with the emergence of mammals.[11] It is perhaps no coincidence that oxytocin's best known functions, milk ejection and uterine contraction for viviparity, are two prototypic mammalian traits. Oxytocin is synthesized primarily in two hypothalamic nuclei, paraventricular (PVN) and supraoptic (SON) nuclei, where it is cleaved from a precursor molecule, neurophysin.[12] The traditional description of oxytocin focuses on its synthesis in magnocellular secretory neurons of the PVN and SON which project to the posterior pituitary from which oxytocin is released into the general circulation. Increasingly, this view has been extended to include a dense network of nonpituitary projections.[13–15] Oxytocin fibers, arising principally from small cells (parvocellular neurons) in the PVN, have been found in many areas of the limbic system as well as in several autonomic centers in the brainstem. Ultrastructural studies have demonstrated that these "extra-hypothalamic" oxytocin projections make classical synaptic contacts[16] from which oxytocin is released following potassium or veratridine induced depolarization.[17] This central oxytocin pool may be considered independent of neurohypophyseal oxytocin release, at least in the sense that cerebrospinal fluid and plasma oxytocin responses to various stimuli are not correlated.[18–20]

Not only are there oxytocin (OT) projections within the CNS, but also specific receptors for OT are widely distributed in the brain. These receptors appear biochemically identical to receptors found in uterine myometrium and mammary myoepithelium. The recent cloning of this receptor from human uterus[21] and rat uterus[22] and its chromosomal localization[23] have provided the tools for molecular studies of this system. Two remarkable aspects of this receptor deserve special note. First, as in peripheral tissues, the OT receptor in the rat brain is under exquisite control by gonadal steroids, increasing by 300% with either testosterone or estrogen administration following gonadectomy.[24,25] Second, this receptor shows surprising variability in the pattern of its expression in the brain across species. Regions with high levels of expression in the rat brain show little evidence of OT receptors in the mouse brain, and even the pattern of steroid regulation differs between rats and mice.[26]

Given a network of OT projections and an array of OT receptors in the brain, what is OT's role within the CNS? Considerable literature on the effects of central administration of OT agonists or antagonists implicate this neuropeptide in the onset of maternal, reproductive, and infant attachment behaviors in rodents. As we reviewed this literature elsewhere,[27] only a few summary points will be noted here. In maternal and female sexual behavior, increasing central OT facilitates and decreasing central OT (via antagonist, antibodies, antisense, or lesions) inhibits the onset of the behavior. These effects are not observed with peripheral administration, they are dependent on gonadal steroid priming, and they appear to be conferred conspicuously on the initiation and not the maintenance of the behavior. That is, once maternal behavior or estrus is established, OT blockade has no effect. Beyond these pharmacologic effects of exogenous OT or OT antagonist administration, it is clear that parturition and estrus are associated with increases in OT mRNA and increases in OT receptors.[28,29] Changes in OT receptors are particularly notable because of the magnitude of the induction, the anatomically discrete pattern of induction, and the considerable evidence that this induction ultimately depends on gonadal steroids.[25,30] The model that we have described elsewhere, based on studies in rats, posits changes in the brain that mimic those observed in the uterus.[27] Essentially, physiologic changes in gonadal steroids induce OT receptors just prior to parturition, so that critical limbic pathways become increasingly responsive to endogenous peptide with attendant changes in behavior coinciding with changes in uterine contraction.

These data from rat studies suggest that OT or its receptor might be important for the behavioral differences observed between prairie voles and montane voles. Given that these species differ so conspicuously in their affiliative, parental, and infant attachment behaviors and that all of these behaviors appear to be heavily influenced by OT, what is the evidence that brain OT neurotransmission differs between prairie voles and montane voles?

OXYTOCIN RECEPTORS AND THE VOLE BRAIN

In immunocytochemical mapping studies, we found relatively few species differences in the location of OT cell bodies across monogamous and nonmonogamous voles.[31] However, *in vitro* autoradiographic studies indicate that prairie and montane voles show markedly different patterns of binding the selective OT receptor radioligand $^{125}I\text{-}d(CH_2)_5[Tyr(Me)_2,Tyr\text{-}NH_2^9]OVT$ (^{125}I-OTA).[32] This iodinated radioligand possesses high specificity for the OT receptor in the rat brain.[33] Pharmacologic characterization of the binding in voles indicates that the radioligand binds to a similar if not identical receptor in the prairie and montane vole. The species differ not so much in the total number of receptors but in their distribution[32] (FIG. 1).

These anatomic differences may relate to behavioral differences, because (a) other vole species selected as monogamous (pine voles) and nonmonogamous (meadow voles) show many of the same contrasts in binding, (b) monogamous and nonmonogamous voles do not differ in their patterns of benzodiazepine and mu opiate receptor distribution[32] (although see also AVP receptors in ref. 34), and (c) when the montane vole female becomes parental during the postpartum period, the pattern of OT receptor binding shifts to resemble that of the prairie vole.[32] In addition, similar differences in the brain distribution of OT receptor binding were observed in monogamous and nonmonogamous mice (*Peromyscus californicus* vs *P. maniculatus*).[35]

OXYTOCIN AND PRAIRIE VOLE PAIR BONDING

But is OT involved in pair bonding in the prairie vole? Pair bonding usually emerges after a series of intense mating bouts with multiple ejaculations over a 24-hour period.[36] Following mating, females demonstrate selective affiliation (preference for the familiar partner) which persists for at least 2 weeks even in the absence of further exposure to the mate.[37] This behavioral change clearly is facilitated by mating,

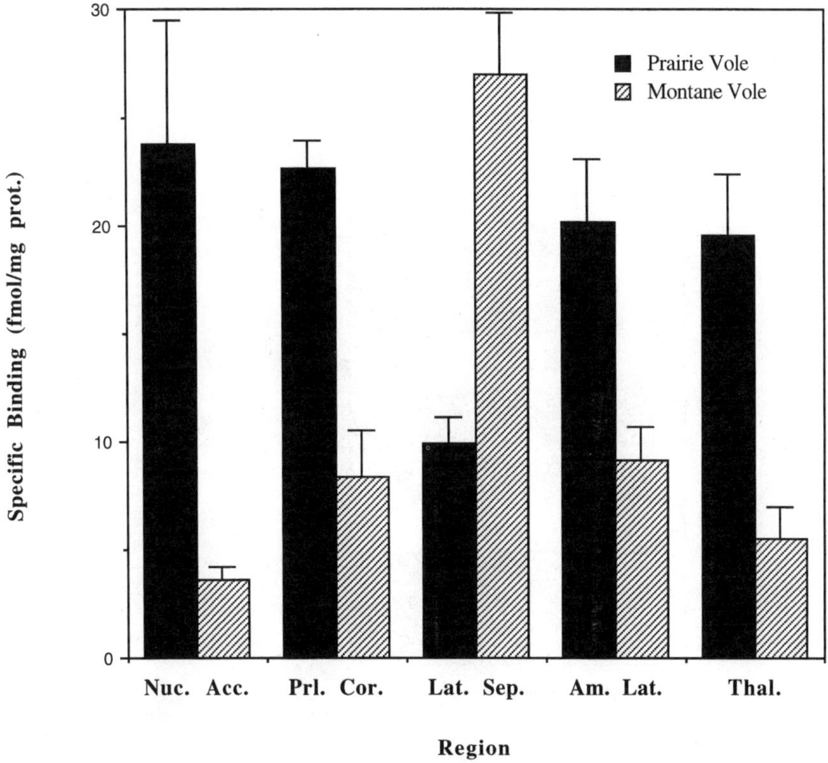

FIGURE 1. Binding of ^{125}I-oxytocin antagonist (OTA) (50 pM) to slide mounted sections from prairie and montane vole brains. Values are taken from computer densitometry measurements of autoradiograms with standards permitting the conversion of optical density to fmol/mg protein equivalents. Values are corrected for nonspecific binding, defined as binding in the presence of a 1,000-fold excess of Thr4-Gly7-OT. Results demonstrate species differences (t test yields $p < 0.05$ in each case) in binding for nucleus accumbens (Nuc. Acc.), prelimbic cortex (Prl. Cor.), lateral septum (Lat. Sep.), lateral nucleus of the amygdala (Am. Lat.), and midline nuclei of the thalamus (Thal.). (Adapted from ref. 32.)

as females with social but not sexual contact with a male fail to develop a partner preference unless they are given much longer periods of male exposure.[38] Mating does not induce a partner preference in the promiscuous montane vole, but montane voles exhibit similar patterns of sexual behavior.[37] Although mating-induced release of central OT has not been demonstrated, mating is associated with an increase in OT mRNA in the prairie vole female, which may be secondary to release (author's unpublished data).

Given that OT is released both peripherally and centrally with sexual behavior in other mammals (reviewed in ref. 39), it might be presumed that OT released with mating influences pair bonding in the prairie vole. Indeed, OT given icv to female prairie voles facilitated partner preference formation when administered by minipump

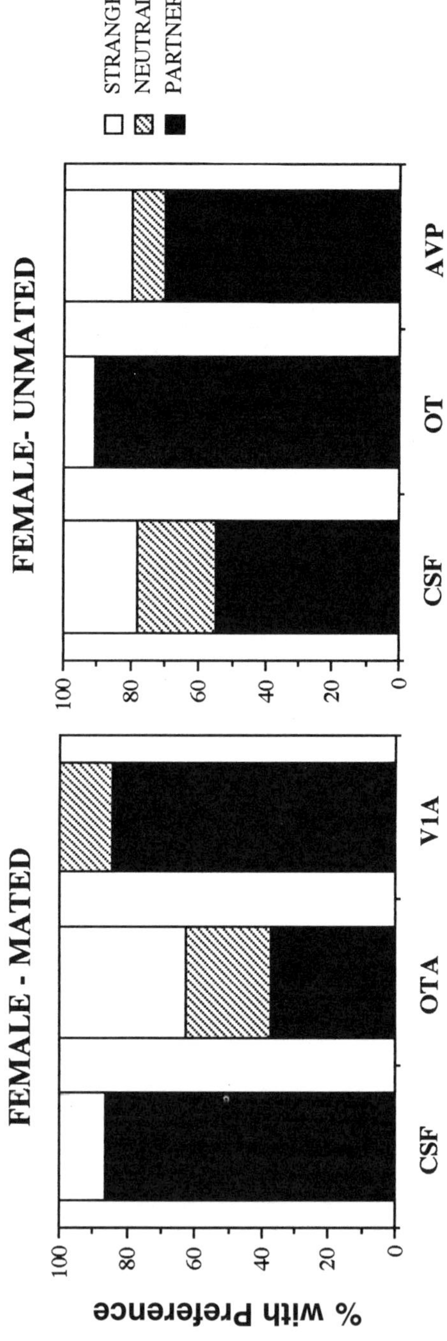

FIGURE 2. Behavior following intracerebroventricular (icv) administration of cerebrospinal fluid (CSF), a selective OT receptor antagonist (OTA), a selective V1a receptor antagonist (VIA), oxytocin (OT), or vasopressin (AVP) to female prairie voles. (**Left**) Estrous females were injected with CSF, OTA (5.0 ng), or V1A (5.0 ng) just before being housed with a conspecific male. After 14 hours of male exposure, females were tested for a partner preference in a three-way testing apparatus with a choice between the mate, a novel male, or a neutral, empty cage. Both mate and novel male were tethered to restrict them to their respective cages while the female could choose to sit in any of the three cages. Following CSF or V1A injection, females chose the familiar mate, but after OTA there was no evidence of a preference. (**Right**) CSF, OT, or AVP was adminstered by minipump for 6 hours at a rate of 1.0 ng/h. Females in this case were not sexually receptive. These conditions were not sufficient to induce a partner preference in females receiving CSF or AVP, but in nonmating females receiving OT a partner preference was evident. These results suggest that OT is necessary and sufficient for partner preference formation in female prairie voles. (Adapted from ref. 37.)

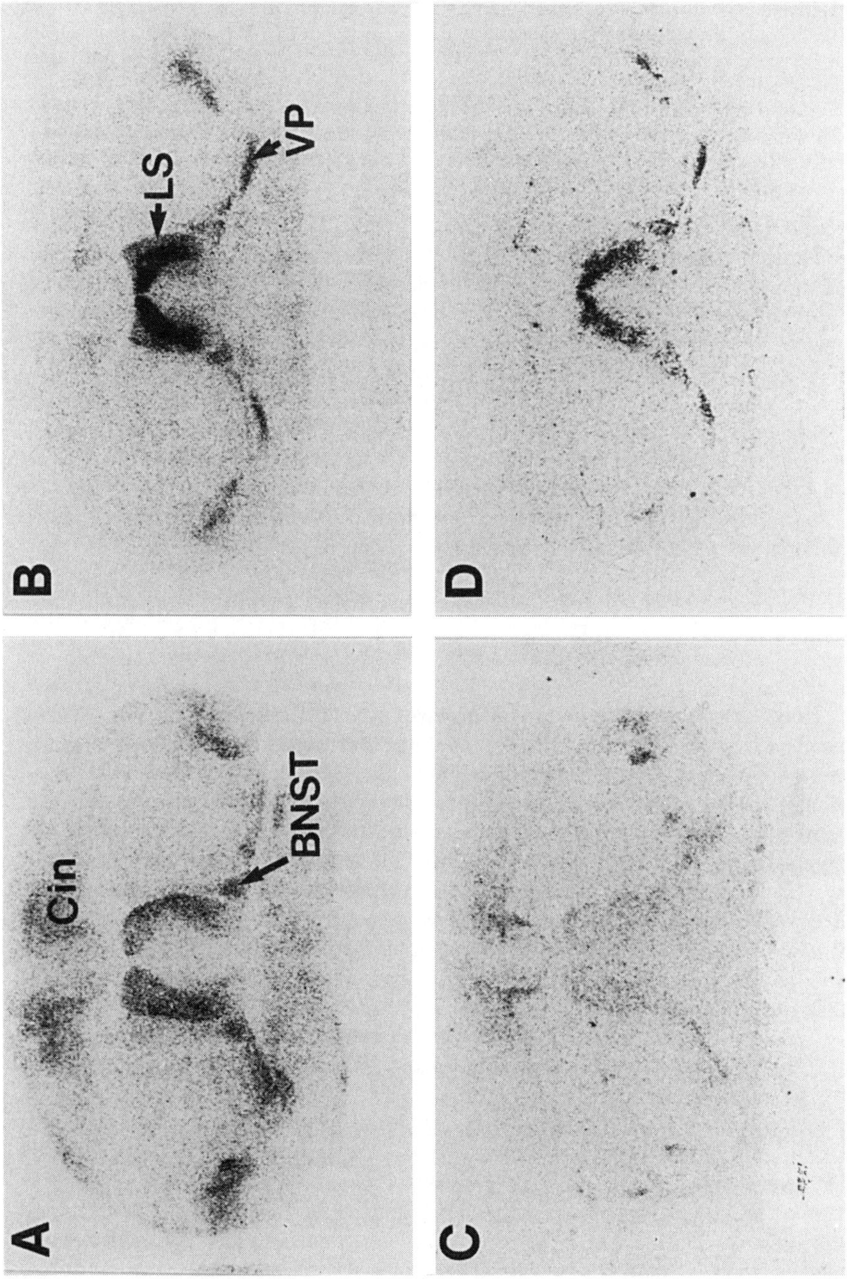

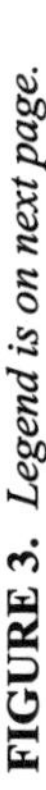

FIGURE 3. *Legend is on next page.*

FIGURE 3. Oxytocin (OT) receptor binding and *in situ* hybridization in coronal brain sections at the level of the crossing of the anterior commissure in prairie (**A** and **C**) and montane (**B** and **D**) voles. Images in **A** and **B** are ^{125}I-oxytocin antagonist (OTA) binding with dark areas demonstrating regions of presumed OT receptors: cing = cingulate cortex; BNST = bed nucleus of the stria terminalis; LS = lateral septum; and VP = ventral pallidum. Images in **C** and **D** are from adjacent sections used for *in situ* hybridization with a 328-bp probe for the montane vole uterine OT receptor. In general, regions with dense binding show hybridization of labeled probe.

(0.5-50.0 ng/h) for 6 hours in the absence of mating (FIG. 2). AVP or CSF given in an identical fashion was ineffective, and the OT effects were blocked by coadministration of a selective antagonist. Conversely, the selective OT antagonist d$(CH_2)_5$[Tyr(-Me)$_2$,Tyr-NH_2^9]OVT (OTA) given icv (5.0 ng) to mating females blocked the emergence of a partner preference without any apparent effects on mating behavior (FIG. 2). A V1A antagonist did not influence partner preference formation.

Oxytocin has little effect on social behavior in the montane vole (Winslow and Insel, unpublished data). Exogenous OT administered icv results in different behavioral outcomes in prairie and montane voles.[40] Taken together, these results suggest that OT is both necessary and sufficient for the mating-induced partner preference in prairie vole females and that the species-typical pattern of OT receptors may be important for activating the neural circuits relevant to pair bonding.

MOLECULAR MECHANISMS FOR SPECIES DIFFERENCES IN OT RECEPTOR DISTRIBUTION

How can prairie voles and montane voles have OT receptors in such different neural pathways? There are three potential answers to this question, each of which can be approached experimentally. First, the radioligand may be binding to different receptors in the two species. That is, there may be structurally different receptors in prairie voles and montane voles, both of which bind ^{125}I-OTA. Second, these species may share the same OT receptor, but differ in the transcriptional regulation of its expression. For instance, promoter elements controlling regional expression may differ between species, so that the OT receptor gene in one species responds to estrogen or corticosterone, whereas the gene in the other species does not. Finally, there may be epigenetic factors that regulate tissue-specific expression differentially in the two species. If the two species have identical OT receptor genes, then differences in *trans*-activating factors (such as levels of estrogen or corticosterone) could account for different patterns of OT receptor expression in the brain. We have investigated each of these possibilities.

Different Receptors? We recently sequenced the OT receptor genes from parturient uteri in both prairie voles and montane voles. The receptors are virtually identical in structure with the coding regions showing complete amino acid homology between the two species (2 synonymous base substitutions in the first 780 bp). We then used a 328-bp fragment for *in situ* hybridization to determine if OT receptor mRNA was expressed in the patterns observed for OT receptor binding.[41] A single probe hybridized to the identical regions where we had observed ^{125}I-OTA binding in both species (FIG. 3).

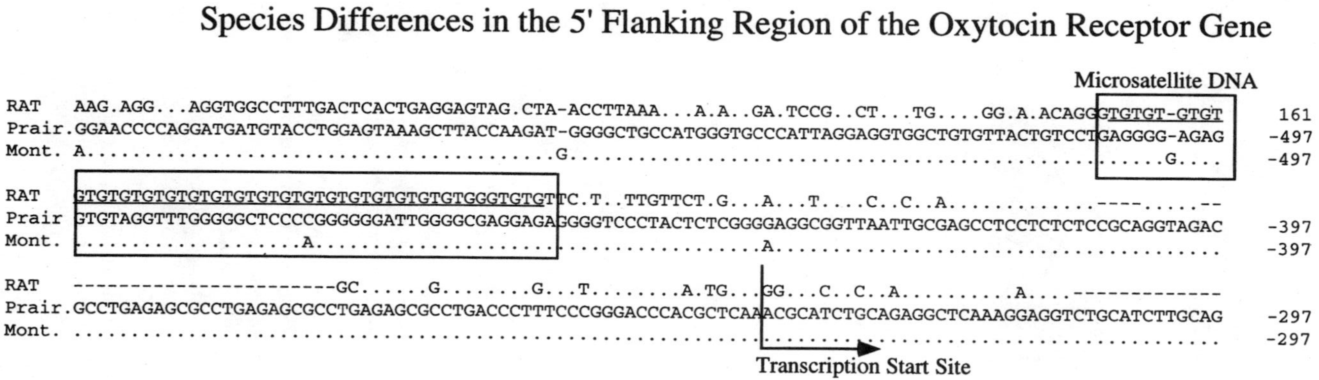

Species Differences in the 5' Flanking Region of the Oxytocin Receptor Gene

```
                                                                                              Microsatellite DNA
RAT   AAG.AGG...AGGTGGCCTTTGACTCACTGAGGAGTAG.CTA-ACCTTAAA...A.A..GA.TCCG..CT...TG....GG.A.ACAGGGTGTGT-GTGT    161
Prair.GGAACCCCAGGATGATGTACCTGGAGTAAAGCTTACCAAGAT-GGGGCTGCCATGGGTGCCCATTAGGAGGTGGCTGTGTTACTGTCCTGAGGGG-AGAG   -497
Mont. A.........................................G....................................................G....   -497

RAT   GTGTGTGTGTGTGTGTGTGTGTGTGTGTGTGTGTGTGGGTGTGTTC.T..TTGTTCT.G...A...T....C..C..A..............----.....--
Prair GTGTAGGTTTGGGGGCTCCCCGGGGGGATTGGGGCGAGGAGAGGGGTCCCTACTCTCGGGGAGGCGGTTAATTGCGAGCCTCCTCTCTCCGCAGGTAGAC   -397
Mont. ....................A.......................................A.......................................   -397

RAT   ----------------------GC......G........G...T........A.TG...GG...C..C..A..........A....-------------
Prair.GCCTGAGAGCGCCTGAGAGCGCCTGAGAGCGCCTGACCCTTTCCCGGACCCACGCTCAAACGCATCTGCAGAGGCTCAAAGGAGGTCTGCATCTTGCAG   -297
Mont. ...................................................................................................   -297
                                                            Transcription Start Site
```

FIGURE 4. Sequences upstream from the coding region in the rat, prairie vole, and montane vole oxytocin (OT) receptor genes. Nearly complete homology is evident between prairie and montane voles throughout this region (shown as . . . .), but there is increasing divergence between vole and rat with little homology above the microsatellite DNA of TG repeats. These repeats have been associated with hypermutability in DNA structure and may explain the great species variability in promoter sequences as well as binding patterns of OT receptors.

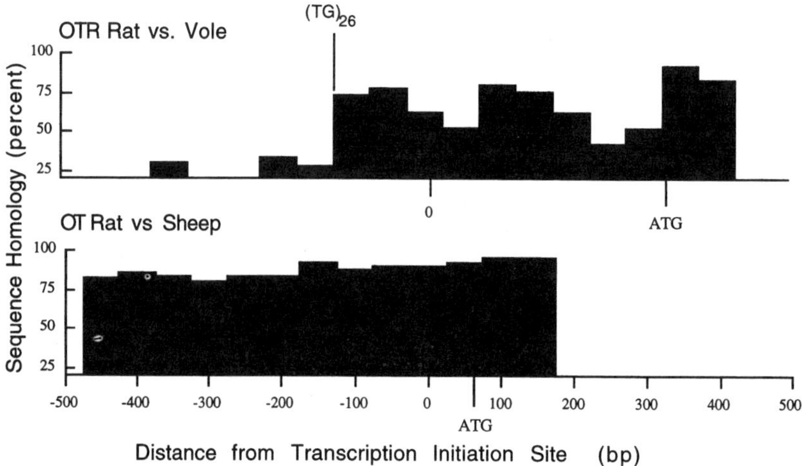

FIGURE 5. Histograms showing the percent of homology of 5′ flanking sequences in the oxytocin (OT) receptor and OT genes. **Upper graph** shows the loss of homology above the microsatellite TG repeats comparing vole and rat. **Lower graph** shows that a phylogenetically more distant comparison of rat and sheep reveals little variation in the promoter sequences controlling OT gene expression. On the basis of such comparisons, more conservation of the OT gene than of the OT receptor gene is apparent.

These *in situ* hybridization results demonstrate that: (a) the binding patterns are an accurate reflection of OT receptor distribution, (b) binding sites are also sites of receptor synthesis (i.e., the receptor is not transported from a distant cell body), and (c) radioligand binding reflects a single class of OT receptors in both species.

Same Receptor–Different Promoters? If the OT receptor is identical in both species, then its regulation may differ because of variability in the promoter regions. We sequenced 1500 bp upstream from the start site in both species to map various promoter elements. In this 5′ flanking region, the two species again show a high level of homology (FIG. 4). They differ in the placement of the response element for an acute-phase response factor (APRF) which is a cytokine sensitive *trans*-activating factor. In addition, a dinucleotide repeat (AG)27 sequence located approximately 1500 bp upstream of the translation start site in the prairie vole is two repeats shorter in the montane vole. These ostensibly subtle differences may be sufficient to account for differences in expression, as only a single base change in the promoter region has been shown to completely alter transcription of other genes.[42]

Of perhaps greater significance is the variability observed between vole and rat sequences (FIG. 5). Although differences in the coding regions between these rodents are few, a comparison of vole and rat promoter sequences reveals an abupt divergence of homology just above a (TG)26 microsatellite repeat found 100 bp upstream from the transcription initiation site of the rat OT receptor gene. This striking lack of homology between vole and rat OT receptor promoters suggests that the OT receptor gene is under different transcriptional control in these species and may account for the marked differences in regional expression and steroid responsiveness of OT receptors in voles and rats. The microsatellite repeats found in the OT receptor promoter are often associated with DNA hypermutability and recombination. The presence of these microsatellite repeat sequences in the 5′ flanking region of the OT receptor gene may contribute to the remarkable species variability in regional OT receptor expression across mammals. By contrast, the promoter regions for the OT gene show relatively few species differences. Evolution of OT function in the brain as well as the uterus may therefore be most rapid at the receptor, with more modest differences observed in the structure of the OT gene.

What does this mean for the molecular basis of monogamy? The nearly identical sequences in prairie vole and montane vole OT receptor genes demonstrate that both species have the same receptor. The small species differences in promoter sequences may be sufficient for the different patterns observed in prairie and montane voles, but relative to the marked species differences between vole and rat or vole and human; differences between vole species appear very subtle. To determine if this minor lack of homology between voles contributes to the ultimate difference in regional receptor expression, we have begun to develop transgenic mice with a recombinant minigene consisting of the prairie vole promoter sequences linked to a reporter gene to determine if this sequence will direct tissue-specific expression in the pattern observed in the prairie vole (Young *et al.,* this volume).

The transgenic approach provides the ultimate tool for testing the role of the OT receptor in vole social behavior. If a montane vole could be induced to express OT receptors in the prairie vole pathways, would it behave like a monogamous vole? The availability of an active prairie vole promoter provides an opportunity to manipulate functional OT receptor expression in the montane vole. We have not yet attempted to transfect the entire OT receptor gene from one vole species to another, but preliminary feasibility studies support the use of this approach.

Same Receptor–Same Promoter–Different Regulators? In fact, much of the data just described argues against species differences in OT receptor expression resulting from species differences in the OT receptor gene. Species differences are mostly quantitative, not qualitative; the coding sequences do not differ between species; and the promoter sequences are virtually (although not completely) identical. These observations suggest that differences in receptor expression may be due to species differences in the amount of various regulatory factors. For instance, because OT receptor expression in other rodents was shown to be regulated by gonadal steroids, perhaps the differences observed in vole species result from species differences in the pattern of gonadal steroid receptors in the brain. This explanation cannot be completely excluded at this time,[43] but studies of estrogen regulation of OT receptor expression in adult prairie voles demonstrate surprisingly weak effects, suggesting that steroids are unlikely to account for species differences among voles.[44] Of course, it is entirely possible that some other transcription factor differs between prairie and montane voles and that brain OT receptor expression varies as a result.

One approach to investigating regulatory factors controlling receptor distribution is to compare the ontogeny of the receptor in the two species. If receptor distribution were found to be identical in the two species during development, then some ontogenetic factor such as neuronal loss or steroid effects might be critical for the differences

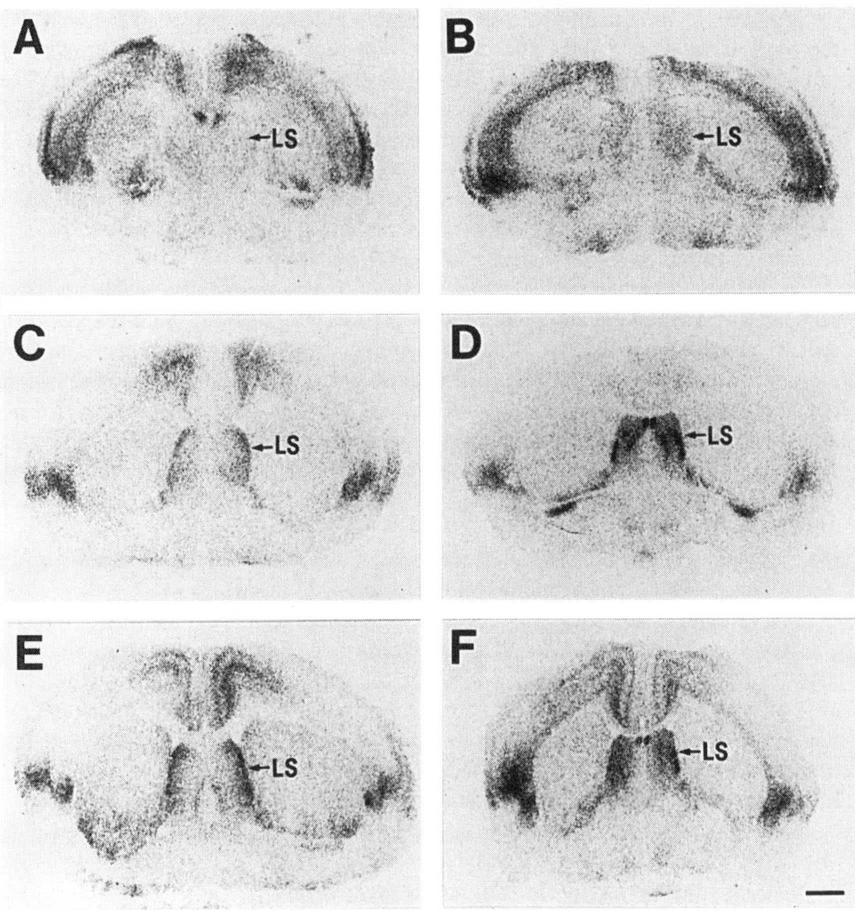

FIGURE 6. Ontogeny of binding of ^{125}I-oxytocin antagonist (OTA) to coronal sections of prairie (**A,C,E**) and montane (**B,D,F**) vole brains at the level of the crossing of the anterior commissure. Little binding is evident on the day of birth (**A** and **B**) in either species. By 1 week postnatal, binding is evident in the lateral septum of the montane vole (**D**) but not the prairie vole (**C**). This pattern is even more evident at 3 months of age in the prairie vole (**E**) and montane vole (**F**). These results suggest that differences in the pattern of ^{125}I-OTA binding shown in FIGURE 1 are evident early in development.

we observe in adulthood. Studies of the development of OT receptors in both species discourage this explanation. From the time OT receptors are detectable in early postnatal life, prairie and montane voles exhibit different patterns of binding (FIG. 6). Some regions show less marked differences in juveniles, but overall, the differences observed in adults can be detected throughout development.

The presence of differences in OT receptor distribution throughout development does not rule out the importance of an epigenetic factor. It merely suggests that whatever regulatory influence controls tissue-specific expression in the vole brain must be active throughout development. The identity of this factor is currently a focus of investigation.

SUMMARY

Comparative studies of monogamous and nonmonogamous voles demonstrate species differences in the regional expression of oxytocin (OT) receptors in the brain. These species differences have not been observed with other neurotransmitter receptors (except vasopressin). Species differences for OT receptor distribution were also observed in other microtine and murine species selected as monogamous or promiscuous. These chemical neuroanatomic differences appear to be functionally relevant, as treatments with selective OT agonists and antagonists influence those behaviors that appear critical to pair bonding in the monogamous prairie vole. To investigate the mechanism controlling tissue-specific expression of OT receptors, we sequenced the OT receptor gene in both prairie voles and montane voles. The findings are inconclusive. Although both species differ markedly from rat and human in their regulatory (but not their coding) sequences, the species show very subtle differences from each other. Ongoing studies are investigating the consequences of these subtle differences between prairie and montane voles. At the same time, several trans-activating factors that might influence OT receptor expression need to be explored.

Note added in proof: The rat oxytocin receptor gene sequence, cited in FIGURES 4 and 5, was based on an error published in ref. 22. The corrected sequence has now been published (Rosen *et al.* 1996. Proc. Natl. Acad. Sci USA **93:** 12501). The correct sequence shows greater homology with the vole oxytocin receptor gene sequences, but the remaining differences support the argument made herein for species differences in regional receptor expression.

REFERENCES

1. KLEIMAN, D. G. 1977. Monogamy in mammals. Q. Rev. Biol. **52:** 39-69.
2. DEWSBURY, D. A. 1981. An exercise in the prediction of monogamy in the field from laboratory data on 42 species of muroid rodents. The Biologist **63:** 138-162.
3. CARTER, C., A. DEVRIES & L. GETZ. 1995. Physiological substrates of mammalian monogamy: The prairie vole model. Neurosci. Biobeh. Rev. **19:** 303-314.
4. GETZ, L. L. & J. E. HOFMAN. 1986. Social organization in free living prairie voles, *Microtus ochrogaster.* Behav. Ecol. Sociobiol. **18:** 275-282.
5. GETZ, L., B. MCGUIRE, T. PIZZUTO, J. HOFFMAN & B. FRASE. 1993. Social organization of the prairie vole (*Microtus ochrogaster*). J. Mammal. **74:** 44-58.
6. SHAPIRO, L. E. & T. R. INSEL. 1990. Infant's response to social separation reflects adult differences in affiliative behavior: A comparative developmental study in prairie and montane voles. Dev. Psychobiol. **23:** 375-394.
7. SHAPIRO, L. E. & D. A. DEWSBURY. 1990. Differences in affiliative behavior, pair bonding, and vaginal cytology in two species of vole. J. Comp. Psychol. **104:** 268-274.
8. JANNETT, F. J. 1980. Social dynamics in the montane vole *Microtus montanus* as a paradigm. The Biologist. **62:** 3-19.
9. DEWSBURY, D. A. 1988. The Comparative Psychology of Monogamy. D. W. Leger, Ed. Nebraska Symposium on Motivation. Vol. **35.** Comparative Perspectives in Modern Psychology: 1-50. University of Nebraska Press. Lincoln, NE.

10. Insel, T., S. Preston & J. Winslow. 1995. Mating in the monogamous male: Behavioral consequences. Physiol. Behav. **57:** 615-627.
11. Archer, R. 1974. Chemistry of the neurohypophyseal hormones: An example of molecular evolution. Handb. Physiol. **4:** 119-130.
12. Brownstein, M. J., J. T. Russell & H. Gainer. 1980. Synthesis, transport, and release of posterior pituitary hormones. Science **207:** 373-378.
13. Swanson, L. W. & H. G. J. M. Kuypers. 1980. The paraventricular nucleus of the hypothalamus: Cytoarchitectonic subdivisions and organization of projections to the pituitary, dorsal vagal complex, and spinal cord as demonstrated by retrograde fluorescence double-labeling methods. J. Comp. Neurol. **194:** 555-570.
14. Buijs, R. 1978. Intra- and extrahypothalamic vasopressin and oxytocin pathways in the rat: Pathways to the limbic system, medulla oblongata and spinal cord. Cell Tissue Res. **252:** 355-365.
15. Sofroniew, M. V. & A. Weindl. 1981. Central nervous system distribution of vasopressin, oxytocin, and neurophysin. Endog. Pept. Learn. Mem. Processes 327-369.
16. Voorn, P. & R. M. Buijs. 1983. An immuno-electronmicroscopical study comparing vasopressin, oxytocin, substance P and enkephalin containing nerve terminals in the nucleus of the solitary tract of the rat. Brain Res. **270:** 169-173.
17. Buijs, R. M. & J. J. van Heerikhuize. 1982. Vasopressin and oxytocin release in the brain—A synaptic event. Brain Res. **252:** 71-76.
18. Jones, P. M., I. C. A. F. Robinson & M. C. Harris. 1983. Release of oxytocin into blood and cerebrospinal fluid by electrical stimulation of the hypothalamus or neural lobe in the rat. Neuroendocrinology. **37:** 454-458.
19. Kendrick, K. M., E. B. Keverne, B. A. Baldwin & D. F. Sharman. 1986. Cerebrospinal fluid levels of acetylcholinesterase, monoamines and oxytocin during labor, parturition, vaginocervical stimulation, lamb separation and suckling in sheep. Neuroendocrinology. **44:** 149-156.
20. Perlow, M. J., S. M. Reppert, H. A. Artman, D. A. Fisher, S. M. Self & A. G. Robinson. 1982. Oxytocin, vasopressin, and estrogen-stimulated neurophysin: daily patterns of concentration in cerebrospinal fluid. Science **216:** 1416-1418.
21. Kimura, T., O. Tanizawa, K. Mori, M. Brownstein & H. Okyama. 1992. Structure and expression of a human oxytocin receptor. Nature **356:** 526-529.
22. Rozen, F., C. Russo, D. Banville & H. Zingg. 1995. Structure, characterization, and expression of the rat oxytocin receptor gene. Proc. Natl. Acad. Sci. USA **92:** 200-204.
23. Simmons, C. F., Jr., T. E. Clancy, R. Quan & J. H. M. Knoll. 1995. The oxytocin receptor gene (OXTR) localizes to human chromosome 3_p25 by fluorescence *in situ* hybridization and PCR analysis of somatic cell hybrids. Genomics **26:** 623-625.
24. Johnson, A. E., H. Coirini, T. R. Insel & B. S. McEwen. 1990. The regulation of oxytocin receptor binding in the ventromedial hypothalamic nucleus by testosterone and its metabolites. Endocrinology **128:** 891-896.
25. Johnson, A. E., G. F. Ball, H. Coirini, C. R. Harbaugh, B. S. McEwen & T. R. Insel. 1989. Time course of the estradiol-dependent induction of oxytocin receptor binding in the ventromedial hypothalamic nucleus of the rat. Endocrinology **125:** 1414-1419.
26. Insel, T., L. J. Young, D. Witt & D. Crews, 1993. Gonadal steroids have paradoxical effects on brain oxytocin receptors. J. Neuroendocrinol **5:** 619-628.
27. Insel, T. R. 1992. Oxytocin: A neuropeptide for affiliation-evidence from behavioral, receptor autoradiographic, and comparative studies. Psychoneuroendocrinology **17:** 3-33.
28. van Tol, H. H. M., E. L. M. Bolwerk, B. Liu & J. P. H. Burbach. 1988. Oxytocin and vasopressin gene expression in the hypothalamo-neurohypophyseal system of the rat during the estrous cycle, pregnancy, and lactation. Endocrinology **123:** 945-951.
29. Insel, T. R. 1990. Regional changes in brain oxytocin receptors post-partum: Time-course and relationship to maternal behavior. J. Neuroendocrinol. **2:** 1-7.

30. Tribollet, E., S. Audigier, M. Dubois-Dauphin & J. J. Dreifuss. 1990. Gonadal steroids regulate oxytocin receptors but not vasopressin receptors in the brain of male and female rats. An autoradiographical study. Brain Res. **511:** 129-140.
31. Wang, Z., L. Zhou, T. Hulihan & T. Insel. 1996. Immunoreactivity of central vasopressin and oxytocin pathways in microtine rodents: A quantitative comparative study. J. Comp. Neurol. **366:** 726-757.
32. Insel, T. & L. Shapiro. 1992. Oxytocin receptor distribution reflects social organization in monogamous and polygamous voles. Proc. Natl. Acad. Sci. USA **89:** 5981-5985.
33. Elands, J., C. Barberis, S. Jard, E. Tribollet, J. Dreifuss, K. Bankowski, M. Manning & W. Sawyer. 1987. ^{125}I-labelled d(CH_2)$_5$[Tyr(Me)^2, Thr^4, Tyr-NH_2^{9}] OVT: A selective oxytocin receptor ligand. Eur. J. Pharmacol. **147:** 197-207.
34. Insel, T. R., Z. Wang & C. F. Ferris 1994. Patterns of brain vasopressin receptor distribution associated with social organization in microtine rodents. J. Neurosci. **14:** 5381-5392.
35. Insel, T. R., R. E. Gelhard & L. E. Shapiro. 1991. The comparative distribution of neurohypophyseal peptide receptors in monogamous and polygamous mice. Neuroscience **43:** 623-630.
36. Witt, D. M., C. S. Carter, K. Carlstead & L. D. Read. 1988. Sexual and social interactions preceding and during male-induced oestrus in prairie voles, *Microtus ochrogaster.* Anim. Behav. **36:** 1465-1471.
37. Insel, T. R. & T. J. Hulihan. 1995. A gender specific mechanism for pair bonding: Oxytocin and partner preference formation in monogamous voles. Behav. Neurosci. **109:** 782-789.
38. Williams, J., K. Catania & C. Carter. 1992. Development of partner preferences in female prairie voles (*Microtus ochrogaster*): The role of social and sexual experience. Horm. Behav. **26:** 339-349.
39. Carter, C. 1992. Oxytocin and sexual behavior. Neurosci. Biobehav. Rev. **16:** 131-144.
40. Winslow, J., L. Shapiro, C. Carter & T. R. Insel. 1993. Oxytocin and complex social behaviors: Species comparisons. Psychopharmacol. Bull. **29:** 409-414.
41. Young, L. & T. R. Insel. 1995. Species differences in the 5′ flanking region of the rodent oxytocin receptor gene. Soc. Neurosci. **21:** Abstr. 332.9.
42. Holmberg, M., G. Leonardsson & T. Ny. 1995. The species-specific differences in the cAMP regulation of the tissue-type plasminogen activator gene between rat, mouse and human is caused by a one-nucleotide substitution in the cAMP-responsive element of the promoters. Eur. J. Biochem. **231:** 466-474.
43. Hnatczuk, O., C. Lisciotto, L. DonCarlos, C. Carter & J. Morrell. 1994. Estrogen receptor immunoreactivity in specific brain areas of the prairie vole is altered by sexual receptivity and genetic sex. J. Neuroendocrinol. **6:** 89-100.
44. Witt, D. M., C. S. Carter & T. R. Insel. 1991. Oxytocin receptor binding in female prairie voles: Endogenous and exogenous estradiol stimulation. J. Neuroendocrinol. **3:** 155-161.

14

Specific Neuroendocrine Mechanisms Not Involving Generalized Stress Mediate Social Regulation of Female Reproduction in Cooperatively Breeding Marmoset Monkeys

David H. Abbott, Wendy Saltzman, Nancy J. Schultz-Darken, and Tessa E. Smith

Competition within a social group can have dramatic consequences for an individual's fertility and fecundity. Social competition is certainly one of the major environmental selection pressures determining individual reproductive success.[1] Recently, increasing numbers of studies employing genetic criteria have supported the principle that reproductive benefits accrue to socially dominant individuals.[2,3] At the proximate level, dominant females have traditionally been thought to gain reproductive advantages over subordinate females as a result of (1) harassment-induced stress inhibiting ovulation in subordinate females (e.g., cynomolgus monkeys, *Macaca fascicularis*),[4] (2) harassment-related pregnancy loss or infant loss suffered by subordinates (e.g., yellow baboons, *Papio cynocephalus*),[5,6] or (3) exclusion of subordinate females from resources crucial for successful reproduction, such as food (e.g., red deer, *Cervus elephas*)[7] or 'helpers' to raise offspring (e.g., saddle back tamarins, *Saguinus fuscicollis*).[8] Such dominance-driven harassment or exclusion exploits the generalized inhibitory reproductive responses that most vertebrate species show to chronic physiological stress, whether it is derived psychologically (i.e., harassment) or environmen-

This research was supported by grants from the National Institutes of Health (RR00167 and HD 07678), National Science Foundation (IBN 92-21771), Wellcome Trust, and an MRC/AFRC Programme Grant. This is publication number 36-039 of the Wisconsin Regional Primate Research Center (WRPRC).

tally (i.e., food deprivation).[1] In addition to these three behavioral tactics exploiting the basic reproductive consequence of physiological stress, a fourth possible mechanism of rank-related reproductive suppression has been suggested: specialized neuroendocrine and behavioral responses by females to subordinate status may directly result in inhibition of sexual behavior (e.g., common marmoset, *Callithrix jacchus*),[9] ovulation (e.g., naked mole-rat, *Heterocephalus glaber*),[10] and implantation (e.g., white-footed mouse, *Peromyscus leucopus*)[11] without the engagement of generalized stress as a physiological mediator of reproductive inhibition.[12] Such specialized social mechanisms regulating reproductive success may well be the products of kin selection and therefore would be expected to be prevalent in highly cohesive societies with an extreme degree of female reproductive suppression and a high likelihood of genetic relatedness within groups (e.g., singular cooperatively breeding species).[13–15]

This paper is particularly concerned with the physiological, behavioral, and sensory mechanisms mediating such social contraception[16] and the specialized reproductive adaptations displayed by certain female mammals encountering inappropriate or suboptimal social environments in which to successfully rear offspring. We previously conceptualized inhibitory neuroendocrine mechanisms in cooperatively breeding species as "a controlled amount of . . . social stress" mediating anovulation in subordinate females (e.g., common marmosets and naked mole-rats).[17–19] However, specialized neuroendocrine responses inhibiting reproduction in subordinate females are manifest in a different fashion from those responses mediating stress-induced reproductive suppression. As exemplified in Table 1, studies of yellow and gelada baboons (*Theropithecus gelada*) exhibited findings consistent with the hypothesis that harassment-induced stress mediated reproductive suppression in subordinate females in established groups, whereas studies of cooperatively breeding common marmosets did not. Overt harassment of female subordinates in the former two species was associated with elevated circulating or urinary cortisol concentrations, and both were particularly pronounced during the subordinates' follicular phase of the ovarian cycle, perhaps reflecting concerted attempts by dominant females to disrupt or inhibit impending ovulation in subordinates[12,22] (Table 1). Decreased frequency of ovulation in subordinate females, as compared to dominant females, accompanied these behavioral and physiological events. In common marmosets, on the other hand, overt harassment of subordinate females and elevations in their circulating cortisol concentrations were not found in established groups (Table 1, Figs. 1 and 4). Nevertheless, subordinate female marmosets exhibited far more extreme forms of reproductive inhibition than did subordinate female baboons, typically manifesting anovulation (Fig. 2) and absence of births. Clearly, the more pervasive inhibition of reproduction operative among subordinate female marmosets was not dependent on behavioral harassment and heightened adrenocortical activity. Interestingly, when subordinate female marmosets in wild and captive groups did occasionally give birth, the likelihood of infant survival was just as poor for subordinate female marmosets as for subordinate female baboons and was similarly linked to brutal intervention by dominant females.[24,25]

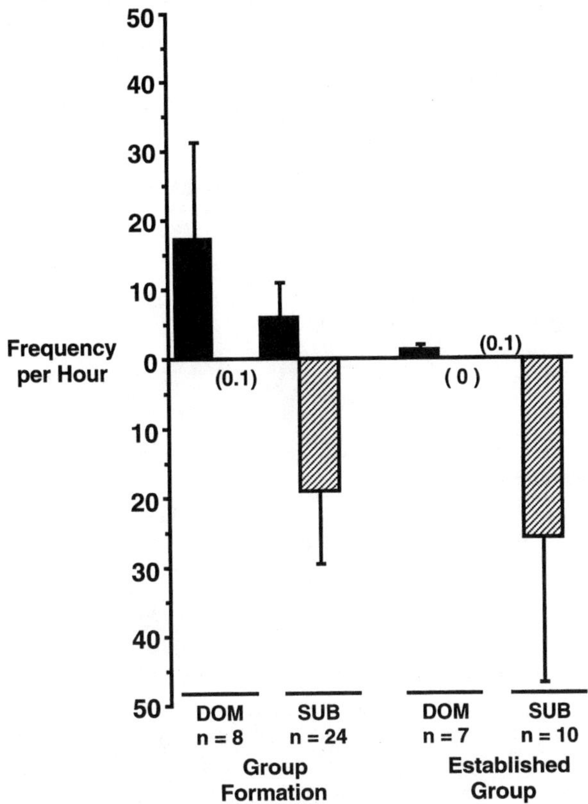

FIGURE 1. Mean (± 95% confidence interval) frequency of aggressive (*solid columns*) and submissive (*shaded columns*) behavior performed by dominant (rank 1) and subordinate (ranks 2 and below) female marmosets during the first 3 days after group formation and during an additional 3-day period, 5 weeks later (established groups). Data adapted from ref. 39.

STRESS-INDUCED REPRODUCTIVE SUPPRESSION

Harassment-induced stress is commonly invoked as the key psychological and physiological mediator of reproductive suppression in socially subordinate mammals.[1,4,12,17,23,26,27] Certainly, prolonged social strife induces persistent, pathological changes.[26,28–30] Glucocorticoid hormones, particularly cortisol or corticosterone, released from the adrenal cortex during stress, specifically inhibit reproductive function at the neuroendocrine hypothalamus, anterior pituitary gland, and gonad.[31–34] Other stress-related physiological changes may similarly inhibit reproductive function. However, the present consideration of physiological mechanisms mediating socially induced reproductive suppression focuses primarily on increased glucocorticoid levels. Elevated blood levels of glucocorticoids are commonly found in dominant and subordinate individuals during periods of social instability or hierarchy formation.[35–39] In

TABLE 1. Summarized Observations from Yellow Baboons, Gelada Baboons, and Common Marmosets Which Suggest That Social Subordination Inhibits Female Reproduction As a Result of Harassment-Induced Stress in Subordinate Females in the Former Two Species, But not in the Latter.

Observations	Yellow Baboons[6,5,20,21]	Gelada Baboons[22,23]	Common Marmoset
(1) Overt aggression towards subordinate females in established groups	+	+	–
(2) Intense harassment of subordinate females during follicular phase of the subordinates' ovarian cycle	+	+	–
(3) Elevated cortisol levels in subordinate females	+	+	–
(4) Inhibited ovarian function in subordinate females	+	+	++
(5) Births and successful infant rearing less frequent in subordinate females	+	+	++

stable, well-established social groups, measures of adrenocortical activity can be greater in subordinates than in dominants,[22,26,27,40–42] but reliable associations of elevated cortisol levels with stable low rank *per se,* rather than with aggression or wounding, are not always found, particularly among nonhuman primates.[26,38,39,43,44] In primates, differences in the dynamic physiological responses of dominant and subordinate individuals to stressful situations may also have physiologically relevant consequences for reproductive suppression (e.g., free-living subordinate male olive baboons, *Papio anubis*).[26] Together, such associations between glucocorticoid levels and social status have been taken to imply that the establishment or disruption of dominance relationships is frequently stressful and that socially subordinate individuals can experience greater psychosocial stress than can dominant ones. This would be consistent with the many studies linking reproductive impairments in subordinate females with the physical or psychosocial stress of subordination.[12] Cooperatively breeding species, however, present an exception to this pattern, because in such species, subordinate female status is not associated with elevated glucocorticoid levels.[10,39,45–48]

REPRODUCTIVE SUPPRESSION IN COOPERATIVELY BREEDING SPECIES

The most extreme examples of social suppression of reproduction in subordinate individuals are found in singular cooperatively breeding species, in which only the dominant female in a social group usually breeds and group members other than the genetic parents are needed to aid in the successful rearing of offspring.[49,50] In such cooperative breeding systems, the social environment provides the predominant proximate cues for timing reproductive effort.[10] This principle is exemplified by the rapid onset of functionally effective reproductive neuroendocrinology, gonadal physiology,

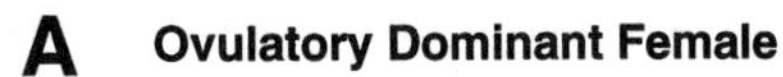

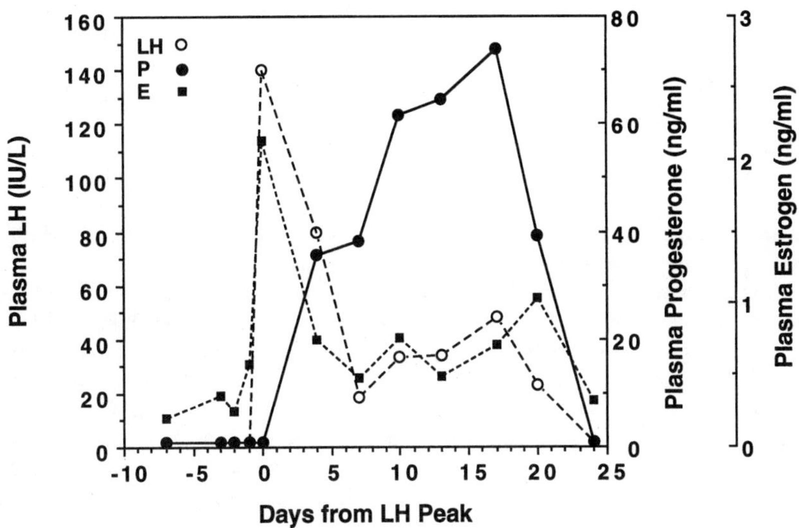

B **Anovulatory Subordinate Female**

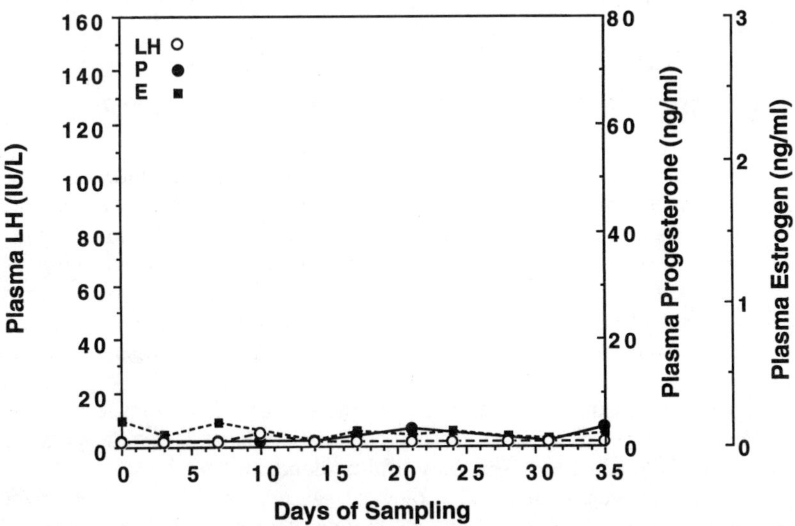

FIGURE 2. Plasma progesterone (*solid circles*), estrogen (*solid squares*), and luteinizing hormone (LH) (*open circles*) concentrations in (**A**) a typical ovarian cycle in a dominant female marmoset and (**B**) an anovulatory subordinate female.

and sexual behavior in individuals that were previously nonreproductive subordinates (originating from within the group or rapidly immigrating from outside the group) after the death or disappearance of the same-sexed dominant breeder (e.g., white-browed sparrow weaver, *Plocopasser mahali;*[45] naked mole-rat;[51,52] or common marmoset).[18] Such precise timing of reproductive effort enables subordinates to engage expeditiously in the intense, intrasexual competition for vacant breeding positions.

Singular cooperative breeders are most readily distinguished from ''competitive'' breeders, species in which competing females can raise their infants unaided (e.g., yellow baboons,[20] red deer,[53] and gelada baboons)[23] by (1) the frequent exclusion of all but one dominant female and one to two dominant males from successfully producing or raising offspring, (2) the critical role of individuals other than the breeding pair in rearing the young of a single breeding female, and (3) the prolonged retention of mature, but nonbreeding offspring in their natal groups.[12,49,54,55] On an ultimate level, reproductive failure among subordinate animals in cooperatively breeding species appears to occur because of competition for resources that limit subordinates' breeding opportunities and because their retention within a group increases the likelihood of their survival and the survival of the breeding female's offspring.[12,49,54,56,57] Nevertheless, there is no evidence to support the notion that harassment-induced elevations in glucocorticoid activity mediate social contraception in cooperatively breeding animals (e.g., (a) free-living groups: white-browed sparrow,[45] Florida scrub jay, *Aphelocoma c. coerulescens,*[56] dwarf mongoose, *Helogale parvula,*[47] and wild dog, *Lycaon pictus;*[47] (b) captive groups: common marmoset,[39] cotton-top tamarin, *Saguinus oedipus,*[48] and naked mole-rat).[10] The common marmoset, in particular, provides an excellent laboratory model in which to examine the mechanisms of socially induced reproductive inhibition in subordinate females of a cooperatively breeding species.

SOCIAL GROUPS OF COMMON MARMOSETS

Common marmosets and other members of the family Callitrichidae are small-bodied New World primates. In the wild, groups of common marmosets comprise 3-15 individuals and typically include 2-4 adults of each sex.[58,59] Groups seem to consist primarily of extended families, but they may also include unrelated immigrants. Offspring remain with their natal families into adulthood, and all group members contribute to infant care.[24,60] Both field[58,61,62] and laboratory[16,63,64] studies of common marmosets typically report that only a single, dominant female breeds in each social group. While infanticide by the dominant female and lack of ''helpers'' to raise offspring may partly explain the ineffective breeding of subordinate female marmosets in free-living groups,[23,65,66] field data as yet do not further address the proximate mechanisms of reproductive sovereignty held by dominant females.

To characterize the proximate (physiological, sensory, and behavioral) regulation of female reproductive success in common marmosets, we established a total of 66 standardized, mixed-sex groups of 4-7 unrelated adults or postpubertal animals at the Wisconsin Regional Primate Research Center in Madison, Wisconsin[39] or at the Institute of Zoology in London, UK,[67] with each group remaining together for 2 months to over 2 years, during an 11-year period. The social structure formed by such groupings was typical for common marmosets. Clear, intrasexual hierarchies that were either linear or despotic were usually quantifiable within 3 days of group formation from the directionality of agonism displayed, and the dominant (rank 1) male and female developed the strongest affiliative relationship within each social group.[16,68] Although little overt aggression was exhibited within social groups established for 6 weeks or more (FIG. 1),[39] subordinate females were clearly distinguishable from the frequency and directionality of their submissive behavior. Infrequent overt aggression among females in established groups of common marmosets is fairly typical of cooperatively breeding societies (e.g., naked mole-rat,[69] *Saguinus* species of tamarins,[70] and dwarf mongoose)[71] and stands in marked contrast to the more frequent aggressive displays and interactions among females in established groups of "competitive" breeders (e.g., yellow baboons).[16]

To sustain unchanging composition of marmoset groups, we gave dominant females intramuscular injections of a synthetic prostaglandin F2α analog, cloprostenol, 14-30 days after each ovulation to terminate the luteal phase of the ovarian cycle or possible early pregnancies.[72] As female marmosets neither menstruate nor exhibit visually obvious cues indicative of ovarian function, blood samples were collected twice weekly from all females (a 4-5-minute procedure not involving anesthesia) to permit endocrine monitoring of ovarian activity.[39,67] Enzymeimmunoassay determination of plasma progesterone concentrations identified the follicular phase (≤ 10 ng/ml for 13 consecutive days or less: mean ± 1 standard deviation) and luteal phase (> 10 ng/ml for 11 consecutive days or more) of the ovarian cycle, ovulation (the day prior to plasma progesterone exceeding 10 ng/ml), and anovulation (≤ 10 ng/ml).[39,73] There were no indications that blood collection procedures resulted in obvious physiological disturbances. Radioimmunoassay of plasma cortisol concentrations in blood samples obtained at 11:45AM were not significantly altered by prior blood sampling at 9 AM on the same day,[39] suggesting that our routine handling and blood sampling did not disrupt the normal diurnal rhythm of plasma cortisol in the female marmosets under study. All plasma cortisol determinations were made from blood samples collected within 3 minutes of cage entry.

REPRODUCTIVE CONSEQUENCES OF SOCIAL SUBORDINATION FOR FEMALE MARMOSETS

While subordinate females occasionally received mounts from dominant and subordinate males, only dominant females sexually solicited males, and only dominant females received ejaculations.[74] When removed from the group for 15-minute behavioral tests with unfamiliar males, however, subordinate females solicited and accepted mounts, illustrating that rapid onset of sexual behavior could be achieved in subordinate females in the absence of their dominant female and that inhibition of their sexual behavior might depend on the presence of their dominant female groupmate. Although reduced circulating levels of ovarian hormones in anovulatory subordinate female marmosets could, on their own, explain the reduced expression of sexual behavior shown by these females, comparable hormonal deficits in ovariectomized female marmosets did not abolish either proceptive or receptive behavior.[75]

Dominant female marmosets continued to undergo regular ovulatory cycles in established social groups, but subordinate females were commonly found to manifest hypogonadotropic anovulation (FIG. 2). Determinations of bioactive luteinizing hormone (LH) levels in serial blood samples taken every 15 minutes for 4 hours from five dominant and five subordinate female marmosets revealed episodic fluctuations in LH values in the dominants in the midfollicular phase of the ovarian cycle, but only nonepisodic and low LH values in anovulatory subordinates.[76] This hypogonadotropic anovulatory condition of subordinates was rapidly reversible by removal of all higher ranking females or removal of the subordinate from her social group followed by subsequent single housing or pairing with a male.[18,67] Following the resumption of ovulatory cycles, reimposition of hypogonadotropic anovulation was readily achieved by returning females to subordinate status in their original group[77] or in a new social group.[67] Such reliable, repeatable, reversible, and rapid social manipulation of gonadotropic control of ovulation is displayed perhaps to a unique extent in female common marmosets and may belie adaptations to changeable ecological conditions, variable group composition, and an opportunistic lifestyle.[78–81]

The remainder of this paper concentrates on the mechanisms underlying reproductive suppression in anovulatory subordinate female common marmosets. It should be noted, however, that subordinate female marmosets exhibit marked variability in the degree and duration of hypogonadotropic anovulation related to rank, age, and group composition[18,82] which may provide important clues about the salient cues from the social environment that impinge on reproductive function in female marmosets.

PHYSICAL AND PHYSIOLOGICAL CORRELATES OF REPRODUCTIVE SUPPRESSION IN SOCIALLY SUBORDINATE FEMALE MARMOSETS

Reduced body weight, altered diurnal rhythms, hyperprolactinemia, and hypercortisolemia have all been associated with impaired ovarian function;[83] the latter two have also been linked with social stress and subordinate social status in females.[4,84] However, as FIGURE 3 illustrates, anovulatory subordinate female marmosets did not exhibit any of these changes. Body weight was not significantly lower in anovulatory subordinates than in dominants undergoing ovulatory cycles (FIG. 3A). Subordinates exhibited no perturbations in circulating levels, circadian patterning, or total exposure to melatonin over 24 hours (melatonin index; FIG. 3B).[85] Moreover, subordinates showed no evidence of hyperprolactinemia (FIG. 3C) or hypercortisolemia (FIG. 3D) in subordinates. Thus, female marmosets clearly showed no signs of a chronic, generalized stress response to established subordinate status, and elevated glucocorticoid levels could not be invoked as a key physiological mediator of anovulation. Even during the first 2 days after group formation, circulating cortisol concentrations failed to show any rise in subordinate females that were not wounded during hierarchy formation, in contrast to the elevated levels of plasma cortisol exhibited by dominant and subordinate females wounded during this time.[39] In both newly formed and established groups, subordinate status *per se* did not appear to increase glucocorticoid levels in female marmosets.

In further contrast to expectations based on a stress-related model, plasma cortisol concentrations in anovulatory subordinate female marmosets not only failed to exceed values in ovulatory dominant females, but also were significantly lower than those in

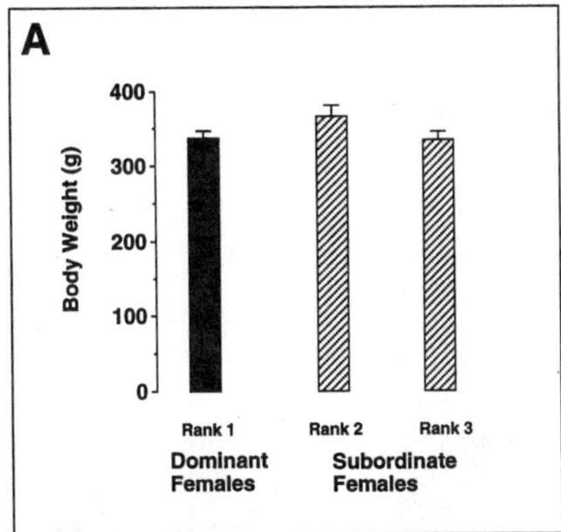

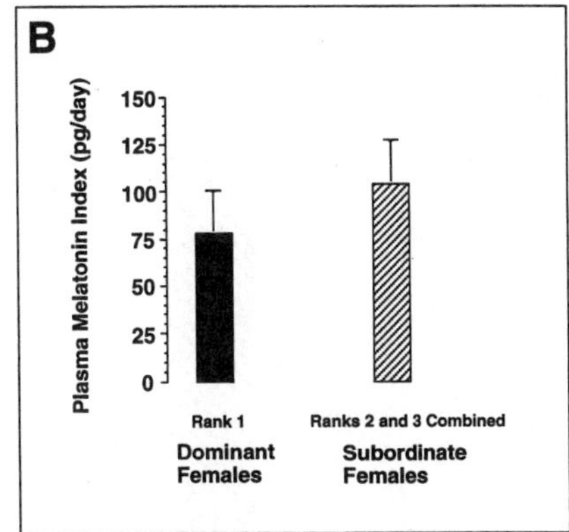

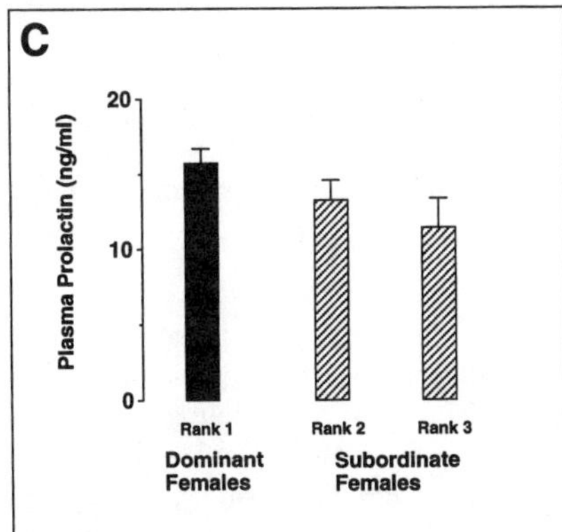

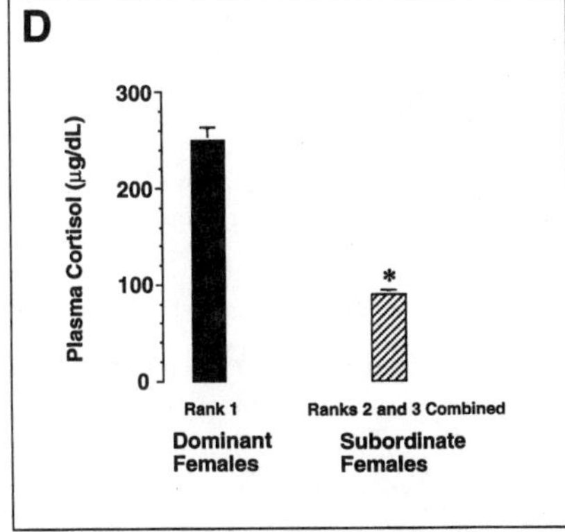

FIGURE 3. Mean ± SEM (**A**) body weight, (**B**) plasma melatonin index, (**C**) plasma prolactin concentrations, and (**D**) plasma cortisol concentrations in dominant (*solid columns*) and subordinate (*shaded columns*) female marmosets. Data for (**B**) adapted from ref. 85. **p* <0.05 vs dominant females.

dominant females (FIG. 3D). Similarly, cortisol values were also lower in anovulatory subordinate female cotton top tamarins than in ovulating dominants, using noninvasive urinary measurements.[48] In marmosets, the difference in plasma cortisol levels between dominant and subordinate females reflected a decrease in cortisol values due to social subordination. As illustrated in FIGURE 4, plasma cortisol concentrations were only significantly altered, following group formation, in females that became anovulatory subordinates. The subordinates' cortisol values were significantly lower than those in the same females before group formation (when they were housed only with males and were undergoing regular ovarian cycles) and were also significantly lower than those in females that had become dominant. Interestingly, bilateral ovariectomy also resulted in a significant reduction in circulating cortisol concentrations in female marmosets 4 or more months after ovariectomy (FIG. 4). Ovariectomized females

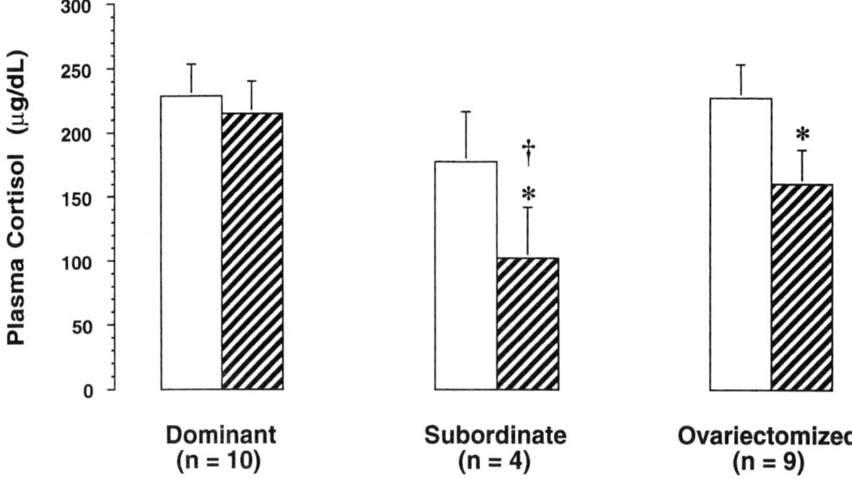

FIGURE 4. Mean ± SEM plasma cortisol concentrations in dominant, subordinate, and ovariectomized female marmosets before (*open columns*) and after (*shaded bars*) group formation or ovariectomy, respectively.* $p < 0.02$ vs before group formation/ovariectomy. †$p < 0.03$ vs dominant females after group formation.

were pair housed with males throughout. These results suggest that ovarian hormones may play as significant a role as subordinate social status in regulating circulating cortisol concentrations in female marmosets. The additional reduction in plasma cortisol levels in ovary-intact, anovulatory subordinate female marmosets compared to ovariectomized females (Fig. 4) might suggest a particular impairment of adrenocortical function due to social subordination *per se,* but this possibility remains to be clarified. Also unclear is the mechanism mediating the hypocortisolemic condition of subordinate female marmosets. In a preliminary study, we have not detected reduced circulating levels of adrenocorticortropic hormone (ACTH) in anovulatory subordinate female marmosets,[25] suggesting instead that alterations in ACTH-mediated cortisol secretion, inhibition of other glucocorticoid secretagogues (such as vasopressin), or increased metabolic clearance of cortisol may be causally involved in the reduction of circulating levels of cortisol. As plasma cortisol binding globulin levels are extremely low in this species and almost all plasma cortisol circulates unbound or loosely bound to albumin,[86–88] it is unlikely that alterations in plasma cortisol binding globulin levels play an important role in mediating the changes found in plasma cortisol in subordinate female marmosets.

SPECIFIC NEUROENDOCRINE INHIBITION OF OVULATION IN SUBORDINATE FEMALE MARMOSETS

To determine whether inhibited or disrupted release of hypothalamic gonadotropin-releasing hormone (GnRH) was implicated in the neuroendocrine imposition

of hypogonadotropic anovulation, we administered GnRH replacement therapy to subordinate females living in their social groups.[17,89] Subordinates were fitted with a lightweight backpack housing a miniaturized infusion pump, programmed to infuse 1 μg GnRH hourly (in approximately 35 μl of saline solution) through an indwelling subcutaneous catheter. This treatment produced a rapid increase in plasma LH levels, and ovulation was induced within 2 weeks in six previously anovulatory subordinate female marmosets remaining in their social groups. Subordinate females quickly reverted to their hypogonadotropic anovulatory condition on removal of the GnRH pumps.[55] These findings did implicate inhibited or disrupted release of hypothalamic GnRH in the neuroendocrine imposition of hypogonadotropic anovulation in subordinate female marmosets.

To confirm this implied inhibition or disruption of hypothalamic GnRH release, we developed a push-pull perfusion method for direct measurement of dynamic GnRH release from the hypothalamus of conscious subordinate female marmosets. It is not possible to accurately determine hypothalamic GnRH release from measurements in the peripheral circulation.[90,91] Modifying a method employed to characterize the neuroendocrine control of GnRH release in female rhesus monkeys,[90] we implanted a cranial pedestal in five anovulatory subordinate and three ovulatory female marmosets.[92] At least 6 weeks later, a micromanipulator was attached to the pedestal and was used to lower a push-pull cannula (outer cannula: 20 ga; inner cannula: 28 ga) into the pituitary stalk-median eminence (S-ME), a hypothalamic area rich in GnRH-containing neuronal terminals.[93] Each female was then placed in a jacket/sling restraint beside its social group. Two days later we perfused the S-ME with artificial cerebrospinal fluid (aCSF, modified Krebs-Ringer phosphate buffer) at 23 μl/min and continually collected perfusate samples in 10-minute fractions for 3–7 hours. Concentrations of GnRH in aCSF perfusate samples were measured by RIA, and GnRH pulses were identified by the computer algorithm PULSAR.[90] Following perfusion, the cannula and micromanipulator were removed and each marmoset was returned to its social group.

In complete contrast to our expectations, GnRH release did not differ markedly between females in the midfollicular phase of the ovarian cycle and those that were anovulatory subordinates.[92] This is particularly well illustrated in FIGURE 5, which shows GnRH measurements in the S-ME over a 7-hour period from one female marmoset in the midfollicular phase of the ovarian cycle (FIG. 5A) and over a second 7-hour period, when the same female was an anovulatory subordinate (FIG. 5B). The GnRH concentrations and dynamic pattern of release were highly similar, while effective ovarian function was strikingly different during the two sampling periods. Considering data from all the females, baseline aCSF concentrations of GnRH were not significantly different between females in the midfollicular phase of the ovarian cycle (4.5 ± 3.3 ng/ml; mean ± sem) and anovulatory subordinates (2.0 ± 0.9 ng/ml). Cycling or subordinate females also demonstrated similar peak concentrations of GnRH (6.4 ± 4.7 vs 3.8 ± 1.8 ng/ml, respectively) and similar interpulse intervals of GnRH (40.9 ± 5.6 vs 38.6 ± 3.5 minutes, respectively).[92] These results suggested that GnRH release in the S-ME of anovulatory subordinate female marmosets was not notably altered from that in the midfollicular phase of the ovarian cycle of regularly ovulating females. Instead, other factors, such as reduced pituitary gonadotropic responsiveness to GnRH[67] or impaired ability to generate an ovulatory LH surge,[94]

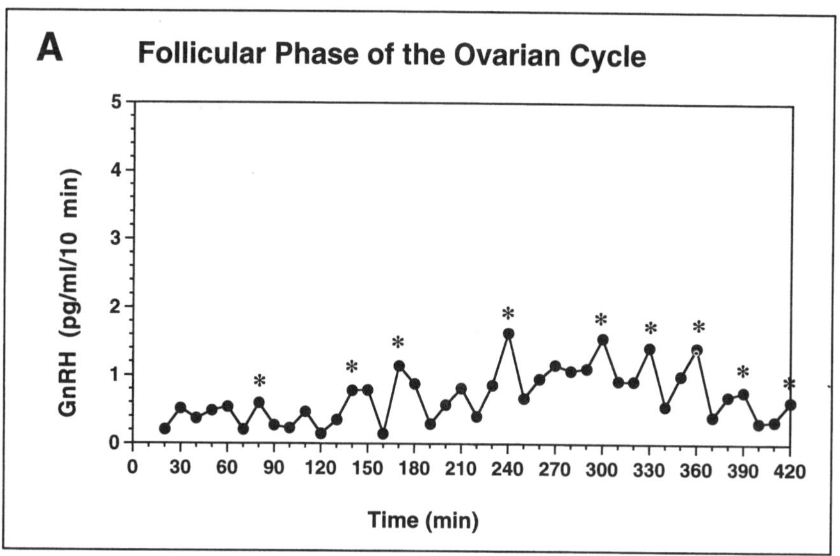

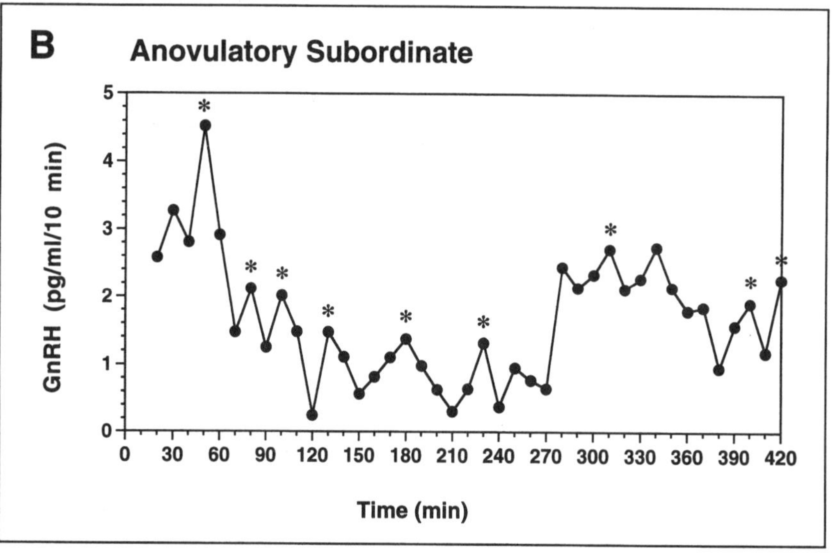

FIGURE 5. Push-pull perfusate concentrations of GnRH obtained from the hypothalamus of the same female marmoset (CJ0086) collected in 10-minute fractions over two separate 7-hour periods when (**A**) in the midfollicular phase of the ovarian cycle and (**B**) as an anovulatory subordinate. *GnRH pulse peak identified by PULSAR computer algorithm.

may be responsible for the hypogonadotropic anovulatory condition of subordinates. Certainly, minimal disruption of hypothalamic GnRH-pituitary gonadotropic function in long-term, anovulatory female marmosets would be consistent with the rapid ability of these females to ovulate within approximately the normal duration of a follicular phase, following removal from subordinate social status.[18,67]

Nevertheless, manipulation of social status and circulating levels of estradiol in subordinate female marmosets has produced clear evidence of specific ovarian hormone-dependent and ovarian hormone-independent mechanisms of LH suppression.[95] With respect to the former, subordinate female marmosets have been shown to exhibit an exquisite gonadotropic sensitivity to the inhibitory influences of estrogen feedback. With respect to the latter, an inhibitory influence of the endogenous opioid peptides on LH release was suggested from the elevated LH responses of ovariectomized subordinate females to the administration of the opiate receptor antagonist naloxone as compared to ovariectomized dominant females.[55] Intact subordinate females, in contrast, showed no such LH response to naloxone treatment. While the specific neuroendocrine nature of these ovarian hormone-dependent and hormone-independent mechanisms remains to be determined in the anovulatory subordinate female marmoset, a similar dichotomy of inhibitory neuroendocrine mechanisms has been implicated in the imposition of anovulation in seasonally anestrus ewes[96,97] and in lactational infertility in rats.[98,99] It is intriguing to speculate that in species that encounter environmentally determined reproductive constraints, there has been convergent evolution of adaptive neuroendocrine responses.

ASSOCIATIVE LEARNING OF CUES FROM FAMILIAR DOMINANT FEMALES MAY FORM AN IMPORTANT COMPONENT OF THE SPECIFIC MECHANISMS INHIBITING OVULATION IN SUBORDINATE FEMALE MARMOSETS

Olfactory, visual, and behavioral cues from dominant female marmosets have all been implicated in maintaining ovarian inhibition in subordinate female marmosets (FIG. 6).[100] Such redundancy in maintenance cues may partly explain the lack of overt aggressive maintenance of ovarian inhibition in subordinates by dominant female marmosets. Marmosets have developed a complex olfactory communication system, they have highly specialized sternal, suprapubic, and anogenital scent glands, and they have a fully functional vomeronasal organ (an accessory olfactory system) in addition to the main olfactory epithelium.[100–102] When anovulatory subordinate females were removed from their social groups to single housing, maintaining them in scent contact with their dominant female delayed the onset of ovulation from 10.8 ± 1.3 days in controls to 31 ± 6.4 days in the scent transfer females (FIG. 6).[77] Similar results, implicating olfactory cues from dominant females in the maintenance of ovarian inhibition in subordinate females, have been achieved using the closely related cotton top and saddleback tamarins.[103,104] Visual cues from dominant female marmosets also extended the period of ovulation suppression in subordinate females removed from their groups, suggesting that cues from the dominant female other than odor may play a role in maintaining anovulation in subordinates (FIG. 6).

However, in all instances the effectiveness of the olfactory or visual cues in inhibiting ovulation in subordinate females expired within a few weeks. Furthermore,

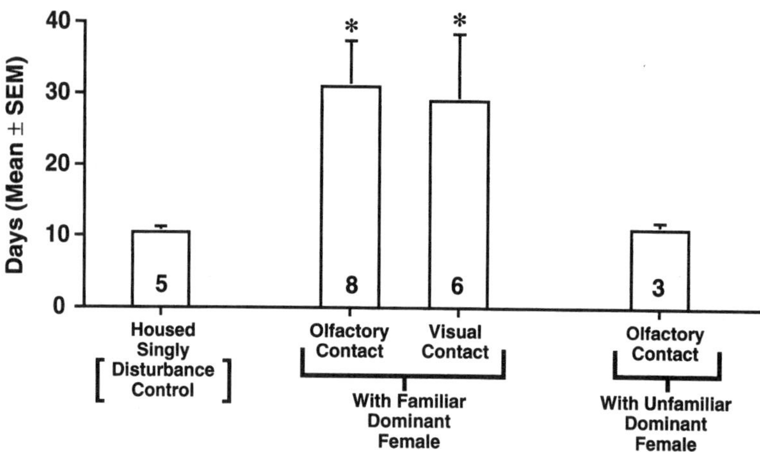

FIGURE 6. Mean ± SEM days until the onset of first ovulation following removal of subordinate female marmosets from their social groups and their subsequent single housing. Numbers of females are shown in each column. $*p < 0.05$ vs disturbance control. Data partially adapted from refs. 77 and 100.

in the marmoset experiments, the length of time a subordinate female remained in her group tended to be positively associated with the latency to ovulate during scent transfer.[77] A similar association was not found in controls. These results implied that an element of associative learning of olfactory cues (and possibly visual cues) from dominant females might play an important role in the neuroendocrine maintenance of anovulation. This hypothesis was supported by recent scent transfer experiments employing odor from unfamiliar dominant females outside the subordinates' groups. In these scent transfer experiments, odor from unfamiliar dominant females failed to produce the delayed onset of ovulation achieved by using the odor from familiar dominant females (FIG. 6).[105] Thus, classical conditioning rather than pheromonal induction might provide the neural basis for reproductive inhibition in subordinate female marmosets. Such a mechanism, founded on recognition of cues from known individuals, is certainly a viable possibility as individual females could readily be identified from extracts of their naturally deposited anogenital scent marks during either behavioral bioassays or quantified chemical analyses.[106] This type of mechanism would mean that cues from only the dominant female groupmate and not those from dominant females in surrounding groups would carry reproductive salience for subordinates and that changes in the social environment, such as disappearance of the dominant female, emigration of the subordinate to a new group, or immigration of new animals to the group could readily extinguish the conditioned reproductive inhibition. A diagrammatic form of our present conceptualization of the conditioning process in subordinate female marmosets is illustrated in FIGURE 7. Initial harassment and intimidation by the dominant female (unconditioned stimulus) result in anovulation (unconditioned response). The association of the dominant female's individualistic olfactory and visual cues with her harassment and intimidation may then result

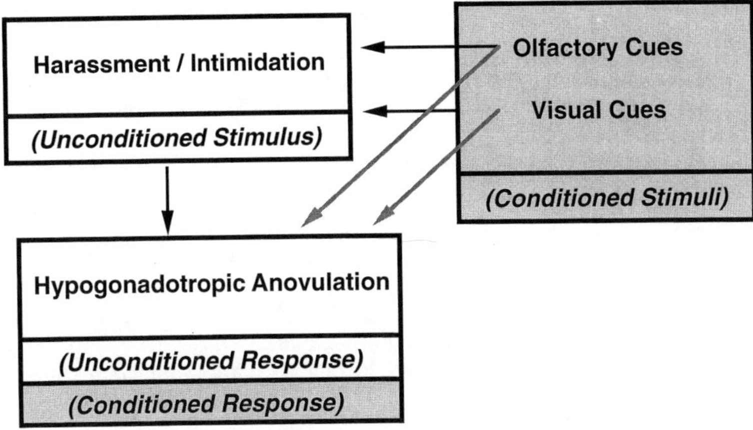

FIGURE 7. Diagrammatic representation of proposed classical conditioning of anovulation in subordinate female marmosets.

in the olfactory and visual cues becoming conditioned stimuli. Such cues would then effectively maintain anovulation as a conditioned response in subordinate female marmosets in established groups.

BEHAVIORAL PREDICTORS OF DOMINANCE IN FEMALE COMMON MARMOSETS

Attainment of dominant or subordinate status by female marmosets in our captive groups was closely related to preexisting individual differences in their agonistic behavior.[68] Prior to group formation, 32 females underwent stranger-encounter testing in which individual females were confronted with female strangers in controlled 15-minute tests, and their agonistic responses were recorded. In six of eight groups, the pre-group formation agonistic behavioral patterns predicted whether a female would subsequently become dominant or subordinate. Once the groups were established, either the behavioral patterns of individual females during the stranger-encounter tests did not change or the females became less responsive.[68] Thus, a female marmoset's likelihood of attaining dominance in a group could be accurately assessed from her agonistic behavior displayed prior to group formation. What was particularly surprising, given that dominance is especially important for female reproductive success in marmosets, was that almost half the females tested before group formation showed submissive responses during stranger-encounter tests and that many of these submissive females did not appear to contend for dominance in their newly formed groups, submitting freely to their female groupmates.[68] It is interesting to speculate on an ultimate level that such interindividual behavioral differences reflect different social/reproductive strategies among female marmosets, with a large proportion of females opting to curtail reproduction until more favorable conditions prevail.[12,68]

SUMMARY

1. Specific neuroendocrine, behavioral, and sensory mechanisms not mediated by generalized stress inhibited ovulation in subordinate female common marmosets.

2. Increased sensitivity to estradiol negative feedback and ovarian hormone-independent mechanisms were identified as the neuroendocrine mediators of hypogonadotropic anovulation in subordinate female marmosets.

3. Direct hypothalamic measurement of GnRH in anovulatory subordinate females provided no clear evidence of reduced or disrupted GnRH release from the hypothalamus.

4. Associative learning of olfactory (and visual) cues from dominant females may provide a psychological conditioning component to the neural mechanisms regulating the anovulatory response to social subordination in female marmosets.

5. Behavioral characteristics of individual female marmosets may play important roles in the attainment of social and reproductive status by each individual.

6. Such specialized behavioral and physiological responses to the social environment contribute to the common marmoset's adaptation to a cooperative breeding strategy.

ACKNOWLEDGMENTS

We thank the animal care and veterinary staff of the Institute of Zoology, London and of WRPRC for their care and maintenance of the marmosets, L.M. George, G.R. Scheffler, F.M. Wegner, and D.W. Wittwer for technical assistance with the hormone assays, and E. Terasawa for assistance with the push-pull perfusion procedure.

REFERENCES

1. Bronson, F. H. 1989. Mammalian Reproductive Biology. The University of Chicago Press. Chicago, IL & London, UK.
2. Martin, R. D., A. F. Dixson & E. J. Wickings, Eds. 1992. Paternity in Primates: Genetic Tests and Theories. Karger. Basel.
3. Pemberton, J. M., S. D. Albon, F. E. Guinness, T. H. Clutton-Brock & G. A. Denver. 1992. Behavioral estimates of male mating success tested by DNA fingerprinting. *In* Behavioral Ecology. J. R. Krebs & N. B. Davies, Eds. Vol. **3:** 66-75. Blackwell Scientific Publications, Oxford, England.
4. Kaplan, J. R., M. R. Adams, D. R. Koritnik, J. C. Rose & S. B. Nanuck. 1986. Am. J. Primatol. **11:** 181-193.
5. Rhine, R. J., S. Wasser & G. W. Norton. 1988. Am. J. Primatol. **16:** 199-212.
6. Wasser, S. K. & A. K. Starling. 1988. Am. J. Primatol. **16:** 97-121.
7. Clutton-Brock, T. H., S. D. Albon & F. E. Guinness. 1986. Anim. Behav. **34:** 460-471.
8. Sussman, R. W. & P. A. Garber. 1987. Int. J. Primatol. **8:** 73-92.
9. Abbott, D. H. 1986. A Primatologia No Brasil **2:** 1-16.
10. Faulkes, C. G. & D. H. Abbott. 1996. Proximate mechanisms regulating a reproductive dictatorship: A single dominant female controls male and female reproduction in colonies of naked mole-rats. *In* Cooperative Breeding in Mammals. N. J. Solomon & J. A. French, Eds.:302-334. Cambridge University Press. Cambridge.
11. Haigh, G., B. S. Cushing & F. H. Bronson. 1988. Biol. Reprod. **38:** 623-626.
12. Wasser, S. K. & D. P. Barash. 1983. Q. Rev. Biol. **58:** 513-538.

13. Faulkes, C. G., D. H. Abbott & A. L. Mellor. 1990. J. Zool. Lond. **221:** 87-97.
14. Sherman, P. W., J. U. M. Jarvis. & S. H. Braude. 1992. Sci. Am. **267:** 72-78.
15. Ferrari, S. F. & L. J. Digby. 1996. Am. J. Primatol. **38:** 19-27.
16. Abbott, D. H. 1984. Am. J Primatol. **6:** 169-186.
17. Abbott, D. H. 1987. J. Zool. Lond. **213:** 455-470.
18. Abbott, D. H. & L. M. George. 1991. Reproductive consequences of changing social status in female common marmosets. *In* Primate Responses to Environmental Change. H. O. Box, Ed.: 294-309. Chapman and Hall. London.
19. Abbott, D. H., J. Barrett, C. G. Faulkes & L. M. George. 1989. J. Zool. Lond. **219:** 703-710.
20. Altmann, J., G. Hausfater & S. A. Altmann. 1988. Determinants of reproductive success in savannah baboons, *Papio cynocephalus*. *In* Reproductive Success: Studies of Individual Variation in Contrasting Breeding Systems. T. H. Clutton-Brock, Ed. University of Chicago Press. Chicago, IL.
21. Sapolsky, R. M. Personal Communication.
22. McCann, C. M. 1995. Social factors affecting reproductive success in female gelada baboons. Ph.D. thesis. CUNY, New York.
23. Dunbar, R. I. M. 1989. Reproductive strategies of female gelada baboons. *In* The Socio-Biology of Sexual and Reproductive Strategies. A. E. Rasa, C. Vogel & E. Voland, Eds.: 74-92. University Press. Cambridge.
24. Digby, L. J. 1995. Behav. Ecol. Sociobiol. **36:** 51-61.
25. Abbott, D. H., W. Saltzman & N. J. Schultz-Darken. Unpublished results.
26. Sapolsky, R. M. 1993. The physiology of dominance in stable versus unstable social hierarchies. *In* Primate Social Conflict. W. A. Mason & S. P. Mendoza, Eds. State University of New York Press. Albany, NY.
27. Keverne, E. B., R. E. Meller & J. A. Eberhardt. 1982. Dominance and subordination: Concepts or physiological states? *In* Advanced Views on Primate Biology. O. Chiarelli, Ed.: 81-94. Springer-Verlag. NY.
28. Weiss, J. M. 1972. Influence of psychological variables on stress-induced pathology. *In* Physiology, Emotion and Psychosomatics Illness.: 253-265. Ciba Foundation Symposium 8. Elsevier. Amsterdam, Netherlands.
29. Kaplan, J. R., S. B. Manuck, T. B. Clarkson, F. M. Lusso, D. M. Taub & E. W. Miller. 1983. Science **220:** 733-734.
30. Mason, W. A. & S. P. Mendoza. 1993. Primate social conflict: An overview of sources, forms, and consequences. *In* Primate Social Conflict. W. A. Mason & S. P. Mendoza, Eds.: 1-11. State University of New York Press. Albany, NY.
31. Dubey, A. K. & T. M. Plant. 1985. Biol. Reprod. **33:** 423-431.
32. Sapolsky, R. M. & L. C. Krey. 1988. J. Clin. Endocrinol. Metab. **66:** 722-726.
33. Gindoff, P. R. & M. Ferin. 1987. Endocrinology **121:** 837-842.
34. Moberg, G. P., J. G. Watson & K. T. Hayashi. 1982. J. Med. Primatol. **11:** 235-241.
35. Louch, C. D. & M. Higginbotham. 1967. Gen. Comp. Endocrinol. **8:** 441-444.
36. Mendoza, S. P., C. L. Coe, E. L. Lowe & S. Levine. 1979. Psychoneuroendocrinology **3:** 221-229.
37. Sapolsky, R. M. 1983. Am. J. Primatol. **5:** 365-379.
38. Martensz, N. D., S. V. Velluci, L. M. Fuller, B. J. Gueritt, E. B. Keverne & J. Herbert. 1987. J. Endocrinol. **115:** 107-320.
39. Saltzman, W., N. J. Schultz-Darken, G. Scheffler, F. H. Wegner & D. H. Abbott. 1994. Physiol. Behav. **56:** 801-810.
40. Barnett, S. A. 1955. Nature **175:** 126-127.
41. Davis, D. E. & J. J. Christian. 1957. Proc. Soc. Exp. Biol. Med. **94:** 728-731.
42. Shively, C. & J. Kaplan. 1984. Physiol. Behav. **33:** 777-782.
43. Coe, C. L., S. P. Mendoza & S. Levine. 1979. Physiol. Behav. **23:** 633-638.
44. Batty, R. A., J. Herbert, E. B. Keverne & S. V. Velluci. 1986. Neuroendocrinology **44:** 347-354.

45. WINGFIELD, J. C., R. E. HEGNER & D. M. LEWIS. 1992. Horm. Behav. **26:** 145-155.
46. SCHOECH, S. J., R. L. MUMME & M. C. MOORE. 1991. The Condor **93:** 354-364.
47. CREEL S., N. M. CREEL & S. L. MONFORT. 1996. Nature **379:** 212.
48. ZIEGLER, T. E., G. SCHEFFLER & C. T. SNOWDON. 1995. Horm. Behav. **29:** 407-424.
49. EMLEN, S. T. 1991. The evolution of cooperative breeding in birds and mammals. *In* Behavioural Ecology: An Evolutionary Approach. 3rd Ed. J. R. Krebs & N. B. Davies, Eds.: 301-337. Blackwell Scientific Publications. Oxford.
50. JENNIONS, M. D. & D. W. MACDONALD. 1994. Trends. Ecol. Evol. **9:** 89-93.
51. FAULKES, C. G., D. H. ABBOTT & J. U. M. JARVIS. 1990. J. Reprod. Fertil. **88:** 559-568.
52. MARGULIS, S. W., W. SALTZMAN & D. H. ABBOTT. 1995. Horm. Behav. **29:** 227-247.
53. CLUTTON-BROCK, T. H., F. E. GUINNESS & S. D. ALBON. 1982. Red Deer: Behavioral Ecology of Two Sexes. University of Chicago Press. Chicago, IL.
54. MACDONALD, D. W. & G. M. CARR. 1989. Food security and the rewards of tolerance. *In* Comparative Socioecology. The Behavioural Ecology of Humans and Other Mammals. V. Standen & R. A. Foley, Eds.: 75-97. Blackwell Scientific Publications. Oxford.
55. ABBOTT, D. H., J. BARRETT & L. M. GEORGE. 1993. Comparative aspects of social suppression of reproduction in female marmosets and tamarins. *In* Marmosets and Tamarins: Systematics, Behaviour and Ecology. A. B. Rylands, Ed.: 152-163. Oxford University Press. Oxford, UK.
56. WASER, P. M., S. R. CREEL & J. R. LUCAS. 1994. Behav. Ecol. **5:** 135-141.
57. SUSSMAN, R. W. & P. A. GARBER. 1987. Int. J. Primatol. **8:** 73-92.
58. DIGBY, L. J. & S. F. FERRARI. 1994. Int. J. Primatol. **15:** 389-397.
59. FERRARI, S. F. & M. A. LOPES FERRARI. 1989. Folia Primatol. **52:** 132-147.
60. PRYCE, C. R., T. MUTSCHLER, M. DOBELI, C. NIEVERGELT & R. D. MARTIN. 1995. Prepartum sex steroid hormones and infant-directed behaviour in primiparous marmoset mothers (*Callithrix jacchus*). *In* Motherhood in Human and Nonhuman Primates, 3rd Schultz-Biegert Symposium. C. R. Pryce, R. D. Martin & D. Skuse, Eds.: 78-86. Basel. Karger.
61. STEVENSON, M. F. & A. B. RYLANDS. 1988. The marmosets, genus Callithrix. *In* Ecology and Behavior of Neotropical Primates. R. A. Mittermeier, A. B. Rylands & A. Coimbra-Filho, Eds.: 131-222. World Wildlife Fund. Washington, DC.
62. HUBRECHT, R. C. 1984. Primates **25:** 13-21.
63. EPPLE, G. 1967. Folia Primatol. **7:** 37-65.
64. ROTHE, H. 1975. Z. Tierpsychol. **37:** 255-273.
65. ALONSO, C. 1986. A Primatologia no Brasil. **2:** 203.
66. RODA S. A. & S. RODA. 1987. Int. J. Primatol. **8:** 497.
67. ABBOTT, D. H., J. K. HODGES & L. M. GEORGE. 1988. J. Endocrinol. **117:** 329-339.
68. SALTZMAN, W., N. J. SCHULTZ-DARKEN & D. H. ABBOTT. 1996. Anim. Behav. **51:** 657-674.
69. REEVE, H. K., & SHERMAN, P. W. 1991. Intracolony aggression and nepotism by the breeding female naked mole-rat. *In* The Biology of the Naked Mole-Rat. P. W. Sherman, J. U. M. Jarvis & R. D. Alexander, Eds.: 384-425. Princeton University Press. New York, NY.
70. CAINE, N. G. 1993. Flexibility and co-operation as unifying themes in *Saguinas* social organization and behaviour: The role of predation pressures. *In* Marmosets and Tamarins: Systematics, Behaviour and Ecology. A. B. Rylands, Ed.: 200-219. Oxford University Press. Oxford, UK.
71. CREEL, S. R., N. CREEL, D. E. WILDT & S. L. MONTFORT. 1992. Anim. Behav. **43:** 231-246.
72. SUMMERS, P. M., C. J. WENNINK & J. K. HODGES. 1985. Reprod. Fertil. **73:** 133-138.
73. HARLOW, C. R., S. GEMS, J. K. HODGES & J. P. HEARN. 1983. J. Zool. Lond. **201:** 273-282.

74. ABBOTT, D. H. 1993. Social conflict and reproductive suppression in marmosets and tamarin monkeys. *In* Primate Social Conflict. W. A. Mason & S. P. Mendoza, Eds.: 331-372. State University of New York Press. Albany, NY.
75. KENDRICK, K. M. & A. F. DIXSON. 1985. Physiol. Behav. **34:** 123-128.
76. ABBOTT, D. H., L. M. GEORGE, J. BARRETT, K. T. HODGES, K. T. O'BYRNE, J. W. SHEFFIELD, I. A. SUTHERLAND, G. R. CHAMBERS, S. F. LUNN & M-C. RUIZ DE ELVIRA. 1990. Social control of ovulation in marmoset monkeys: A neuroendocrine basis for the study of infertility. *In* Socioendocrinology of Primate Reproduction.: 135-158. Wiley-Liss, Inc. New York, NY.
77. BARRETT, J., D. H. ABBOTT & L. M. GEORGE. 1990. J. Reprod. Fertil. **90:** 411-418.
78. RYLANDS, A. B. 1996. Am. J. Primatol. **38:** 5-18.
79. SCANLON, C. E., N. R. CHALMERS & M. A. MONTEIRO DA CRUZ. 1988. Primates **29:** 295-305.
80. PONTES, A. R. M. & M. A. O. MONTEIRO DA CRUZ. 1995. Primates **36:** 335-347.
81. SANTEE, D. Personal Communication.
82. SALTZMAN, W., N. J. SCHULTZ-DARKEN, J. M. SEVERIN & D. H. ABBOTT. 1996. Ann. N.Y. Acad. Sci., this volume.
83. YEN, S. S. C. 1991. Chronic anovulation due to CNS-hypothalamic pituitary dysfunction. *In* Reproductive Endocrinology. 3rd Ed. S. S. C. Yen & R. B. Jaffe, Eds.: 631-688. W. B. Saunders Co. Philadelphia, PA.
84. BOWMAN, L. A., S. R. DILLEY & E. B. KEVERNE. 1978. Nature **275:** 56-58.
85. WEBLEY, G. E., D. H. ABBOTT, L. M. GEORGE, J. P. HEARN & H. MEHL. 1989. Am. J. Primatol. **17:** 73-79.
86. KLOSTERMAN, L. L., J. T. MURAI & P. K. SIITERI. 1986. Endocrinology **118:** 424-434.
87. PUGEAT, M. M., G. P. CHROUSOS, B. C. NISULA, D. L. LORIAUX, D. BRANDON & M. B. LIPSETT. 1984. Endocrinology **115:** 357-361.
88. ROBINSON, P. A., C. HAWKEY & G. L. HAMMOND. 1985. J. Endocrinol. **104:** 251-257.
89. ABBOTT, D. H. 1989. Social suppression of reproduction in primates. *In* Comparative Socioecology. The Behavioural Ecology of Humans and Other Mammals. V. Standen & R. A. Foley, Eds.: 285-304. Blackwell Scientific Publications. Oxford, UK.
90. TERASAWA, E. & M. GEARING. 1988. Brain Res. Bull. **21:** 117-121.
91. CLARKE, I. J. & J. T. CUMMINS. 1982. Endocrinol. **3:** 1737-1739.
92. SALTZMAN, W., N. J. SCHULTZ-DARKEN, E. TERASAWA & D. H. ABBOTT. 1995. *In vivo* release of gonadotropin-releasing hormone (GnRH) in socially subordinate female marmoset monkeys. Abstract No. 112.8, 25th Annual Meeting of the Society for Neuroscience. San Diego, CA.
93. COEN, C. W. Personal Communication.
94. ABBOTT, D. H., A. S. MCNEILLY, S. F. LUNN, M. J. HULME & F. J. BURDEN. 1981. J. Reprod. Fertil. **63:** 335-345.
95. ABBOTT, D. H. 1988. Natural suppression of fertility. *In* Symposia of the Zoological Society of London Number 60. G. R. Smith & J. P. Hearn, Eds.: 7-28. Oxford University Press. New York, NY.
96. KARSCH, F. J., E. L. BITTMAN, D. L. FOSTER, R. L. GOODMAN, S. J. LEGAN & J. E. ROBINSON. 1984. Recent Progr. Horm. Res. **40:** 185-232.
97. MEYER, S. L. & R. L. GOODMAN. 1986. Biol. Reprod. **35:** 562-571.
98. MAEDA, K.-I., H. TSUKAMARA, E. UCHIDA, N. OKHURA, S. OKHURA & A. YOKOYAMA. 1989. J. Endocrinol. **121:** 227-283.
99. SMITH, M. S. & J. D. NEILL. 1977. Biol. Repro. **17:** 255-261.
100. BARRETT, J., D. H. ABBOTT & L. M. GEORGE. 1993. J. Repro. Fertil. **97:** 301-310.
101. EPPLE, G., A. M. BELCHER, I. KUDERLING, U. ZELLER, L. SCOLNICK, K. L. GREENFIELD & A. B. SMITH III. 1993. Making sense out of scents: Species differences in scent glands, scent-marking behaviour, and scent-mark composition in the Callitrichidae. *In* Marmosets and Tamarins: Systematics, Behaviour and Ecology. A. B. Rylands, Eds.: 123-151. Oxford University Press. Oxford, UK.

102. Hunter, A. J., D. Fleming & A. F. Dixson. 1984. J. Anat. **138:** 217-225.
103. Epple, G. & Y. Katz. 1984. Am. J. Primatol. **6:** 215-227.
104. Savage, A., T. E. Ziegler & C. T. Snowdon. 1988. Am. J. Primatol. **14:** 345-359.
105. Smith, T. E. & D. H. Abbott. 1995. Am. J. Primatol. **36:** 156.
106. Smith, T. E. 1994. Role of odour in the suppression of reproduction in female naked mole-rats and common marmosets and the social organisation of these two species. Unpublished doctoral dissertation, University of London.

IV

Neuroendocrine Perspectives on Social Behavior

15

Brain Systems for the Mediation of Social Separation-Distress and Social-Reward: Evolutionary Antecedents and Neuropeptide Intermediaries

Jaak Panksepp, Eric Nelson, and Marni Bekkedal

During the first year of life, human infants display affiliative behaviors and form ''attachment bonds'' with their caregivers. These bonds are manifested through selective approach and interaction with certain individuals who provide a ''secure base'' for other life activities, and various signs of separation-distress along with an emerging fear of strangers when isolation from such sources of support is perceived. Social reunion rapidly dissipates this type of emotional distress. The only way to understand the deep neural nature of such emotional systems is through appropriate animal models which can be employed to unravel the underlying brain substrates that are shared, to some extent, by all mammals.

Research precedents for the existence of attachment systems in the brain, such as those proposed by Kraemer[1] and Panksepp,[2] were established by the well known behavioral research programs of Harlow[3] and Scott,[4] who demonstrated that social motivation and social bonding could arise independently of the reinforcing effects of basic rewards such as food and, by inference, all other conventional regulatory sources of gratification. Social bonding was argued to rely more critically on ''social'' stimuli (namely, stimuli that emanate from living beings) such as bodily warmth, the comforts of touch, and various dynamic movements and odors of social interaction. Although the potential modulatory role of conventional rewards in the elaboration of social attachments remains to be fully evaluated and hence may still be of demonstrable importance, the prevailing wisdom is that social bonding can proceed independently of those factors. Accordingly, Bowlby[5] commandingly argued that mother-infant attachment bonds, based as they are on a sense of security and emotional trust as well as satisfaction arising from social contact, provide the foundation for all subse-

This work was supported by National Institutes of Health grant 1 R15 HD 30387 and Wright-Patterson Contract F336019 MU146 and MT702. We dedicate this work to John Paul Scott.

Address for correspondence: Department of Psychology, Bowling Green State University, Bowling Green, Ohio 43402 (tel: 419 372-2819; fax: 419 3720-6013; e-mail: jpankse@bgnet.bgsu.edu).

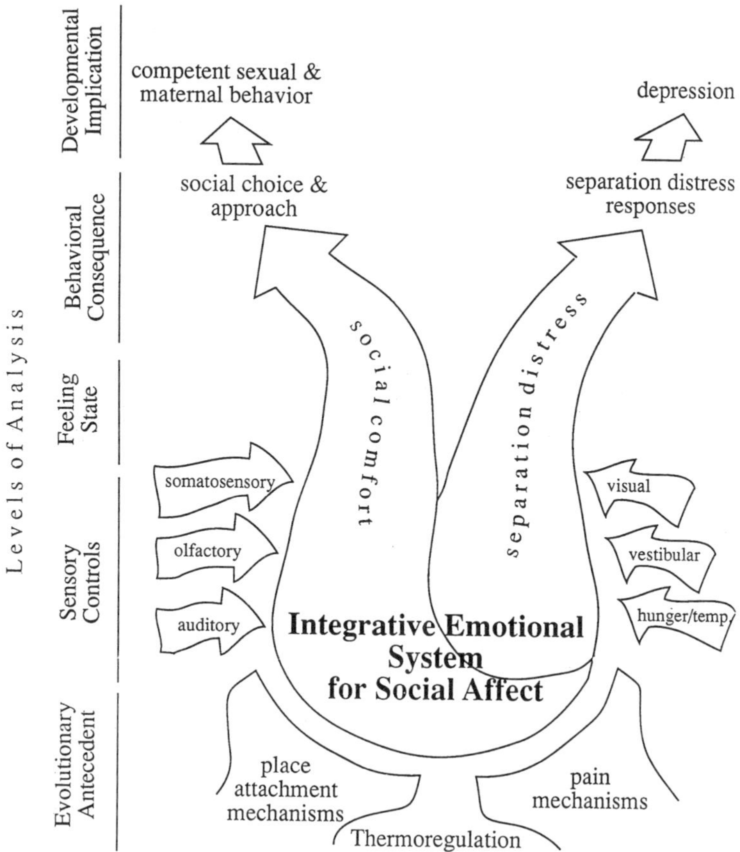

FIGURE 1. A conceptual scheme summarizing the putative nature of a bidimensional integrative emotional system for social affect and the various levels of analysis that can be interfaced with neuroscience approaches. The system mediates separation distress and social reward (e.g., contact comfort) via interaction with various sensory and perceptual inputs. It is suggested that the neural roots of this system go back to brain mechanisms that elaborated pain and temperature perception and place attachment during early phases of evolution. Figure drawn by Brian Knutson.

quent social relationships. The severe behavioral and psychological consequences that result from the severance of such bonds are now well established.[5,6]

The critical conceptual question that will be used to frame the present discussion of these affiliative system(s) of the brain is whether there is a single or multiple evolutionary antecedents for social attachments. If there is no single source process, but rather the converging influences of multiple processes (FIG. 1), such as the contributory effects of contact comfort, energy, and thermoregulatory effects, as well as alleviation and modulation of other forms of emotional distress, then we may have to deal with patterns of control that vary substantially from species to species. Indeed, on the basis of behavioral data it has been argued that, in primates, attachments to peers and parents reflect the existence of independent motivational systems;[7] however, this does not necessarily mean that a variety of seemingly "distinct" behavioral mechanisms may not share underlying controls, such as common neurochemistries. Thus, even as we accept the existence of a diversity of modulatory controls for social homeostasis, we shall argue that important general principles underlie the integrative aspects of affiliative behaviors in all mammalian species.

In somewhat different terms, although the basic urges to indulge in social behaviors arise from neural systems that remain poorly distinguished conceptually and even more poorly understood empirically, we can, on the one hand, be confident that various underlying neural components for social behavior can be usefully distinguished and, on the other, that there will also be many shared controls for these behaviors. For instance, brain circuits for social aggression and dominance are surely distinct from those promoting maternal motivation and social bonding. Those that mediate sexuality are also distinct but certainly interactive with the previously mentioned ones. However, neuropharmacological work suggests that all of these social control systems share important regulatory controls. Thus, even as we can enumerate many distinct types of prosocial behaviors, the existence of an equally large number of distinct motivational substrates for social intent seems unlikely.

Indeed, behavioral neuroscience research has revealed that all prosocial behaviors such as sexuality, maternal nurturance, separation-distress, gregarious-friendliness, social bonding, play, and social-memory systems share neurochemical controls, including prominently oxytocin and endogenous opioids, not to mention the even more generalized state control systems such as the various ascending norepinephrine and serotonin systems.[8] Although such shared neurochemical influences seem to contribute to all social behaviors, existing empirical data are beginning to allow the conclusion that special-purpose sociomotivational systems also exist within the mammalian brain. Even as existing neurobiological data are affirming that distinct brain circuits exist for the behavioral expressions of sexuality, maternal behavior, play, and perhaps other forms of social affiliation, all of these systems appear to derive much of their motivational urgency from some shared substrates. These neurochemical foundations can probably be expressed in diverse ways during the ontogenetic development of each organism. Thus, it is now appropriate to entertain the existence of a generalized socioemotional system that we provisionally conceptualize as a coherently operating bidimensional brain system for the generation of social affect. At the very least, such a concept serves as a useful heuristic for promoting and guiding research into the brain substrates of social affiliation.

The shared neurochemical controls of various social behaviors support the existence of a fundamental bidimensional system for the governance of social affect. We suggest that this system generates painful feelings of separation when social support is lost and satisfying feelings of social gratification when an animal is in the presence of socially supportive cues (FIG. 1). Clearly, the negative emotional side of this system is psychologically and behaviorally more compelling, whereas the outward manifestations of social satisfaction are generally less evident (resembling the air around us that we commonly take for granted). As the behavioral manifestations of distress are more evident than are those of satisfaction, we originally labeled this the "panic" system, because of the theoretical assumption that arousal of this system contributed to that clinical disorder.[9] We envision such a central-state system to be a generalized regulator of social affiliation shared homologously by all mammals. We assume that such an underlying system exists to channel various discrete social behaviors by governing the quality and intensity of internally experienced social emotions which provide feedback to the organism concerning its moment-to-moment interconnectedness to its social community. Depending on this socioemotional barometer, animals presumably choose to spend more time with those in whose presence they feel social gratification and less with those who engender feelings of isolation and stress and thereby provide less social satisfaction. Although such a hypothesis of the probable neuroemotional structure of the mammalian brain is rife with troublesome conceptual problems, the biggest involving the ontology of brain feelings,[10] the tools of the neuroscience revolution are beginning to permit empirical access to such conceptual sticking-points with a rigor that was unimaginable just a few years ago.

EVOLUTIONARY CONSIDERATIONS AND SPECIES DIFFERENCES

Considering the multiple input-determinants for social attachments (FIG. 1), the degree of influence of these components can vary among different species. Such divergent evolutionary trends may help explain a variety of interesting species differences as described in the literature,[11] but we believe that further empirical attempts to explicate the nature of the central processor should help provide insight into key neural mechanisms for social motivation and attachment. So far, the best behavioral index of the functional status of this system has been achieved through the systematic study of the brain control of separation-distress vocalizations.

Although it is an understatement to say that the nature of this central processor remains only provisionally understood, we presently entertain the idea that at its core lies an evolutionary synthesis of more ancient mechanisms which originated to subserve basic needs such as pain perception, thermoregulation, and the establishment of place attachments. These evolutionary antecedents, along with emerging sexual abilities, ultimately led to the evolution of a variety of distinct behavioral action patterns indicative of social affiliation, such as grooming, hugging, huddling, and the urge to move in prosocial union as occurs in playful and courting activities. In many species these behaviors also include distinct facial and vocal patterns. Preexisting thermoregulatory and place-attachment mechanisms presumably contributed substantially to the evolution of brain mechanisms that monitor social presence, whereas ancient pain mechanisms presumably contributed to subcomponents of the attachment system, arousing emotional distress related to social absence. If the basic social-attachment mechanisms reflect elaborations of such multiple antecedents, it is easy to envision that the degree of ontogenetic development (or evolutionary emergence) of the social-affect system may also vary substantially in different species. Thus, the young of precocious species that are especially vulnerable to predation may exhibit unambiguous and rapid social attachments (e.g., herd animals), whereas the bonds of many altricial animals may be closely linked to the more ancient place-attachment mechanisms (e.g., nesting animals such as rats and altricial birds that disperse soon after the development of motor competence). Many species may exhibit intermixtures of the two, with some subspecies being more gregarious than others.[12] Presumably predators, being at the top of the food chain, can exhibit a slower and more complex development of social attachments because of the comparative safety of their life circumstances.

Such issues are bound to complicate a cross-species analysis of social-attachment mechanisms, especially because we know little about those antecedent mechanisms with any level of precision. For instance, little direct data currently exist on the nature of place-attachment mechanisms, even though the vast literature on place-preference conditioning in animals[13] could be used to generate credible hypotheses. Indeed, place preference is easily established by pairing specific environments with opiate administration, and those chemistries are also central not only to the experience of pain but also to various homeostatic pleasures such as feeding.[14] Thus, even though the original brain opioid hypothesis of social attachment was considered to be wildly speculative when it was first proposed,[15] its role in the modulation of social affiliative processes now seems certain.[16]

In sum, a social motivation/attachment system, long postulated by theorists, can now be supported by animal brain research, with substantial implications for understanding human bonding, human friendships, and more complex social motivations as well as the genesis of many psychiatric disorders. Considerably more work has been conducted on the separation-distress dimension of the system than on the social reward aspects. Indeed, the existence of the latter, at least as brain entities independent of the former, should currently remain a matter of considerable doubt. We would like to believe that a form of social reward exists that is independent of separation distress as well as other forms of reward (e.g., gustatory, thermal, and sexual), but we cannot point to unambiguous data that would bear out such a conclusion. In any event, here we will share the most recent lines of inquiry that we have followed in pursuit of a coherent psychobiological view of social affiliation in mammals. We first briefly summarize our past work on separation distress and then cover more recent work on social reward and gregariousness. Although the final word is not in on most matters, a substantial body of work now exists suggesting that brain opioids, oxytocin, and prolactin systems are key contributors to social affect and attachment processes.

THE OPIOID-DEPENDENCE THEORY OF ATTACHMENT

Our own work in the field started a quarter century ago with the simple idea that among the satisfactions obtained from the recently discovered brain opioid systems were the emotional gratifications of social connectedness. In more formal theoretical terms, it was suggested that the main characteristics of narcotic addiction, namely, the development of dependence, tolerance, and withdrawal, represented the main attributes of social affect, specifically the feelings of attachment, alienation/weaning, and separation-distress arising from the disengagement of social bonds. The apparent congruence between the dynamics of opiate addiction and the basic social processes of the brain also led to the heuristic supposition that the emotions associated with social motivation were an evolutionary outgrowth of more primitive motivational systems of the brain such as those that subserve the perception of pain. Inasmuch as pain had already been established as an opioid modulated affect, it did not require an enormous stretch of the imagination to hypothesize that brain opioid systems also participated in the neurobiology of social affiliation.

Research during the ensuing years amply supported that supposition, but obviously many complexities emerged that remain to be empirically resolved.[11,16] Clearly, the social affect system is more complex than we initially envisioned, with multiple inputs and outputs (Fig. 1), but the strategy still serves as a productive empirical path in this murky area of brain research. For instance, among the more striking findings, it was demonstrated that brain opioids are released during social grooming,[17] that benign social interaction among relatives can reduce pain via such opioid release,[18] and when we block opioid receptors, animals as well as humans become more eager to seek social interactions.[19,20] However, as already mentioned, we now envision the social affect system of the brain to have multiple evolutionary roots.

In addition to those related to feelings of pain, we believe that the system is also evolutionarily linked to ancient thermoregulatory and place-attachment mechanisms of the brain. Considering such multiple evolutionary antecedents as well as the many sensory inputs and higher cognitive mechanisms that control social affiliations, there are bound to be many other neurochemical influences that serve as subcomponents within this widely ramifying emotional system. Unfortunately, we do not yet adequately understand the operation of any of these components; for instance, even though oxytocin and prolactin are powerful modulators of separation distress, we do not yet know which social stimuli release them in the brain. For instance, do opioids respond more to touch and oxytocin more to sight and sound, or vice versa? These are important questions for future research. All we can be confident of at present is that there are multiple synaptic neurochemistries that control separation distress and gregariousness and, by inference, social affiliation and bonding.

Until recently, the overriding premise of our work was that neurochemical inputs that alleviate separation distress are those that mediate social attachments, whereas those promoting behavioral indices of separation distress are ones that create the basic motivation for social reunion. Thus, the experience of separation distress provides a primal motivational system which optimizes the salience of social rewards. Here we will more fully consider the possibility that the brain elaborates processes of ''social reward'' that are, in part, independent of the mechanisms of separation distress. The following brief overview of research that we have conducted over the years will be divided into two corresponding parts; a brief summary of our work on separation-distress calls will be followed by more recent work that attempts to evaluate the role of such systems in the mediation of social reward in rodents as analyzed by a variety of techniques. A more detailed summary of some of the earlier work can be found elsewhere.[21,22]

THE NEUROCHEMISTRIES OF SEPARATION-DISTRESS CIRCUITRY

Within the conceptual framework of a bidimensional social-affect system, we certainly have much more evidence on the neurobiological vectors that control separa-

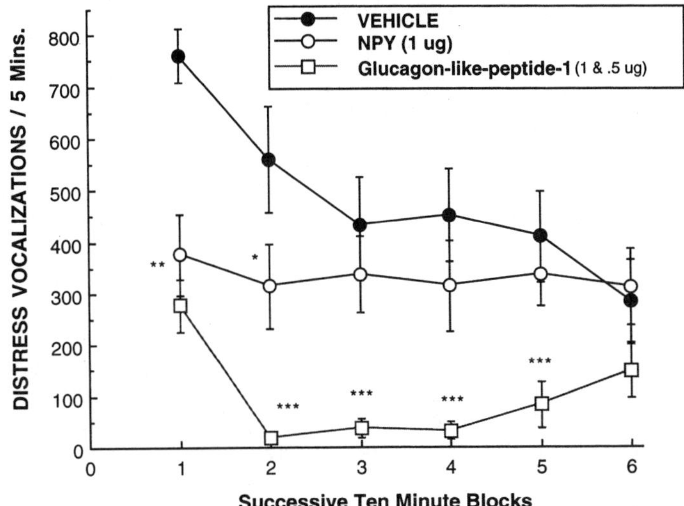

FIGURE 2. Mean (± SEM) distress calls of 2-day-old domestic chicks during a 1-hour period of social separation, which was preceded immediately by central 3-μl injections of saline vehicle into the fourth ventricle region (n = 10), 1 μg of neuropeptide Y (NPY) (n = 14), or 1-0.5 μg of glucagon-like peptide-1 (GLP-1) (7-36) amide (n = 20). Both doses of GLP-1 had similar effects; hence the data are combined. $*p < 0.05$; $**p < 0.01$; $***p < 0.0001$.

tion-distress than those that mediate social-reward, partially, because the distress process is much easier to measure. Young animals that exhibit social bonding exhibit intense and persistent distress vocalizations (DVs) when isolated from their sources of social support. These calls emerge from subcortical systems (e.g., centromedial mesencephalon, dorsomedial thalamus ventral septum, bed nucleus of the stria terminalis, preoptic area, and cingulate cortex) that were provisionally identified using the technique of localized electrical stimulation of the brain.[22] Although there are many pharmacological ways to change the frequency and intensity of these calls, there are only a handful of ways to dramatically reduce or elevate them using brain neurochemical manipulations. Besides localized electrical stimulation of various brain sites, these systems can be activated by administering several distinct substances into the brain; including most prominently various glutamate receptor agonists (NMDA and kainate), corticotrophin releasing hormone (CRH), and curare (which we presently assume increases many forms of emotionality by interacting with glutamate receptors).[23] Agents that are especially efficacious in reducing DVs include oxytocin/vasotocin,[24] opioids that stimulate mu receptors,[25] prolactin,[26] and clonidine.[27] Of course glutamate receptor antagonists also reduce DVs very powerfully,[28] even though we have not yet observed CRH antagonists do the same. Many other neurochemistries no doubt also participate in the specific control of separation distress. The latest one we identified is glucagon-like peptide-I (GLP-1) which has recently emerged as another candidate as a feeding satiety transmitter in the brain.[29] As can be seen in FIGURE 2, GLP-1 is effective in reducing separation-induced DVs. Because hunger is known to promote such DVs, perhaps this effect reflects the emotionally soothing consequences of feeding.

Our most extensive pharmacological and neuropeptide work has been done in young domestic chicks,[21,22,25–27] but much of the work has been replicated in other species.[11,30] The corroborative work in primates is especially suggestive of the possibility that the foregoing findings may translate to the human condition,[31] whereas some of the inconsistencies observed in studies of infant rats may suggest evolutionary divergence in the underlying substrates.[32] Although a variety of control issues still need to be addressed, especially the degree of behavioral specificity of the various manipulations, we do presently assume that this type of work has implications for the understanding and treatment of socioaffective dimensions of human psychiatric disorders ranging from early childhood autism[20,33] and loss-induced depression[34] to the despair of everyday loneliness. For instance, the development of an orally effective ligand for oxytocin receptors in the brain should prove to be a powerful alleviator of loneliness and other forms of separation-distress, just as opiates are effective, but without the clinically problematic addictive features of narcotics.[35]

IMPLICATIONS FOR UNDERSTANDING SOCIAL AFFILIATIONS AND ATTACHMENTS

As mentioned, the general heuristic that we have derived from the preceding lines of thought is that any neurochemical factor that dramatically reduces separation-distress may be a vector for promoting the development of social attachments by creating a "secure emotional base" in the brain. Indeed, we have obtained some evidence that brain opioids can mediate discriminative aspects of social imprinting,[36] even though the results have generally been rather modest and less robust than we originally anticipated. For instance, in naturalistic imprinting experiments with newborn chicks measuring the tendency of chicks to develop a following-response to humans, high doses of naloxone (e.g., up to 5 mg/kg) have not impeded the development of the following response.[37] Therefore, it does not seem that brain opioids are essential for mediating the basic tendency to become imprinted in newborn domestic chicks, but they may be important in the choices animals make among the available social objects.

At the same time, we have entertained the possibility that neurochemistries that alleviate separation distress would be candidates for promoting social confidence and independence. Hence, animals that have high synaptic levels of opioids, oxytocin, and prolactin might be expected to exhibit less social dependence and hence be less gregarious (and thereby more autistic). This type of result was confirmed for brain opioids by observing the proximity maintenance of pairs of animals in open fields,[38] and in more recent unpublished work we have seen similar antigregariousness effects of administering oxytocin into the brains of both infant and adult rats.[39] However, a corollary of this principle is that such neurochemistries, by promoting social confidence, might at milder levels actually promote social activities, especially in anxiety-provoking situations. This may help make sense of the fact that the same low doses of opiates that reduce gregariousness increase rough-and-tumble play.[40]

Some of these issues may be reconceptualized more simply in relation to "social reward." For some time we have considered the possibility that social reward is a unique process in the brain that can be distinguished from other rewards. Unfortunately, substantive knowledge on the nature of "rewards" in the brain is presently minimal. Certainly, the so-called lateral-hypothalamic self-stimulation "reward" or "reinforcement" system appears to have been misconceptualized, for it appears to mediate the appetitive rather than the consummatory phase of behavior.[41] This leaves the neural nature of all rewards open at the present time. The conceptual issue that needs to be experimentally addressed is whether the various rewards that animals can apparently experience–the pleasures of food, water, warmth, play, sex, and various other forms of social contact–are, in fact, elaborated by distinct and/or shared neural systems in the brain. We currently know very little about such matters, for we have no unambiguous experimental paradigms to study the unconditional nature of such putative processes. Operant approaches are really not ideal for such studies, because all such tasks rely on generalized learning and appetitive mechanisms making it problematic to disentangle distinct reward processes. Certainly, it is well established that animals will learn to exhibit instrumental responses to obtain various social rewards,[42] but to distinguish among different types of reward on a neurophysiological basis, one would have to demonstrate that manipulations that affected one reward would not affect others. That level of functional discrimination remains to be achieved. Indeed, to optimize the search for a distinct type of social reward process in the brain, new methodologies–new social-reward detection systems–need to be developed.

Simply observing the natural social behaviors of animals is not an ideal way to study social reward. Accordingly, we have spent some time devising and evaluating new measures of gregariousness and social reward, so that some of the more subtle underlying psychological and brain issues could eventually be addressed. One of the most promising ethological ways to analyze early affiliative urges is to study social play. A considerable literature is now available on young rats which indicates that the mammalian brain contains specific rough-and-tumble play systems.[43] We would not be surprised if the affect that accompanies ludic activities is in fact the type of social-reward system to which we have alluded. Indeed, young rats readily learn to traverse mazes to obtain access to play partners,[44] but we will not focus on such traditional procedures here. Instead, we are focusing on three new techniques that hold some promise for analyzing social-motivation and reward processes in both older and younger rats that must be studied if we are ever going to fully evaluate the possibility that social reward is a distinct process of the mammalian brain.

The first procedure is a variant of a traditional place-preference paradigm. The second is an apparatus that we recently developed for automatically monitoring gregariousness. Finally, we summarize a new and simple procedure for analyzing maternal reward as a measure of social bonding in infant rats.

CONDITIONED PLACE-PREFERENCE AS A MEASURE OF SOCIAL REWARD

The use of place preference has become routine in the analysis of drug-produced reward in animals,[13,45] and it has been successfully used to evaluate the rewarding qualities of conventional rewards such as food[46] as well as the positive affect derived from juvenile play.[47] In the following work we sought to determine whether the technique could be used to analyze the rewarding effects of social proximity in adult rats.

In the initial experiment, social-interaction induced place preference was measured in 110- to 190-day-old Long-Evans female rats that had had differential social histories. The distribution of subjects for each of four groups was as follows: control animals that received no social reward in the test chambers ($n = 7$); isolated animals that had been weaned at 21 days of age and had no social contact until this experiment ($n = 12$); animals that had been weaned and then allowed to play for six 5-minute play sessions between weaning and 50 days of age ($n = 12$); and animals that had been housed with a like-sexed partner from weaning until the beginning of testing ($n = 12$).

During training, control animals were exposed to both sides of the CPP box in isolation. To optimize conditioning, the right side of each of four test boxes had vertical stripes and a distinctive wire mesh floor. We sponged the walls with a 2% acetic acid solution immediately before animals were placed into that side of the box. That was the social-reward side for all animals except the control group. The other side had horizontal stripes, a grid floor, and no distinct odor. Baseline data were collected on the first day. All rats were given a 20-minute exposure to the boxes with free access to both sides. All rats started that session by being placed into the left side of each two-compartment test chamber.

Conditioning took place on the second and third days. Two 20-minute conditioning sessions were conducted on each day. Half the rats received social-side pairings in the morning and isolate-side pairing in the afternoon; the other half had the reverse order, which was counterbalanced on the next day. During conditioning, a metal barrier was placed between the two sides to block access. The right side of the test chamber (with the vinegar smell) was always paired with social "reward" and the left side with isolation. Social conditioning consisted of placing an experimental rat, along with its partner, in the right side of the box, and in isolate conditioning rats were placed individually in the left side of each test chamber.

Rats were tested three successive times on days 4 through 7. Each testing session consisted of giving individual rats access to both sides of the box for 20 minutes, with time and movement between chambers being automatically recorded by appropriately placed photocells situated 7 cm into each chamber. All animals started the test session on the left. The right side was wiped down with the acetic acid solution before each test session. On the first day of testing, animals received no pretreatment, while on the next 2 test days rats were given 1 mg/kg of naltrexone or vehicle i.p. 20 minutes before testing in a counterbalanced fashion.

The change in preference for the vinegar side by the various groups is summarized in FIGURES 3 and 4. Control animals that had been exposed to both chambers in isolation had a modest increase of about 50 more seconds spent on the vinegar side, whereas the various experimental groups, which did not differ reliably from each other, exhibited four to five times as much time on that socially paired side of the chamber. A comparison of all the experimental groups with the control group yielded a reliable social conditioning effect ($F(1,35) = 6.6$, $p < 0.02$). This pattern of results was sustained on the 2 subsequent test days, with no evident blockade of the effect by preceding opioid blockade with 1 mg/kg of naltrexone. Parenthetically, in follow-

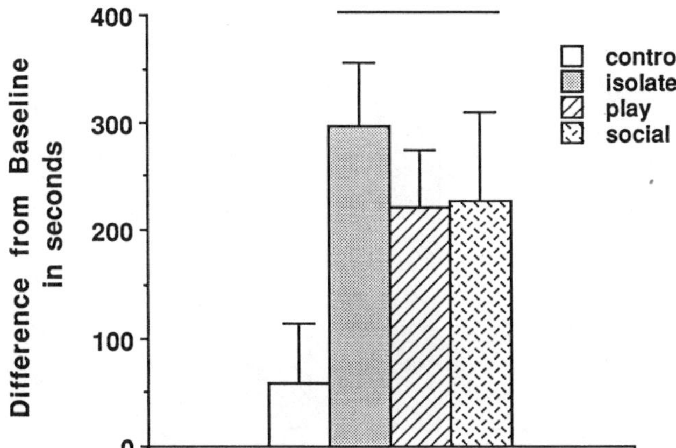

FIGURE 3. Mean (± SEM) changes in time spent in the nonpreferred side of a place-preference chamber in animals with different social histories. All three groups that had received social pairing in the nonpreferred side spent more time on that side during a subsequent 20-minute test session ($*p < 0.05$). The various social histories did not result in differential social reward.

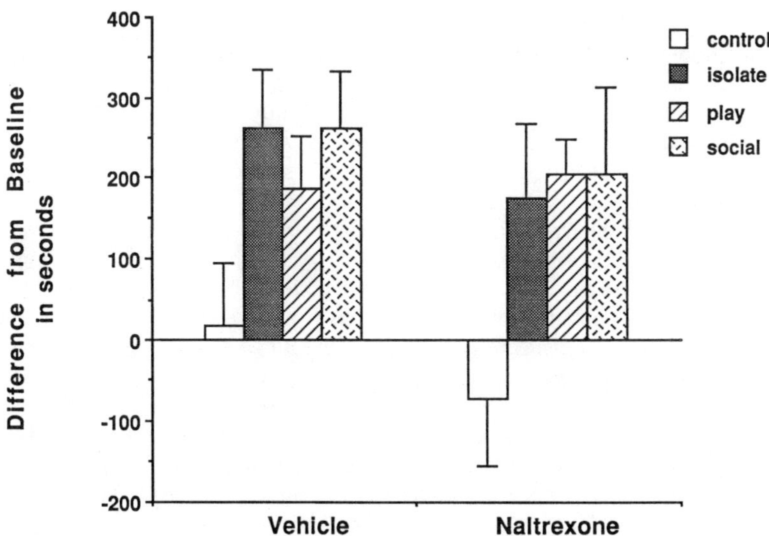

FIGURE 4. Mean (± SEM) place preferences of animals depicted in FIGURE 3 after administration of a vehicle or naltrexone (1 mg/kg) before the test session. Naltrexone did not apparently diminish the socially induced place preference.

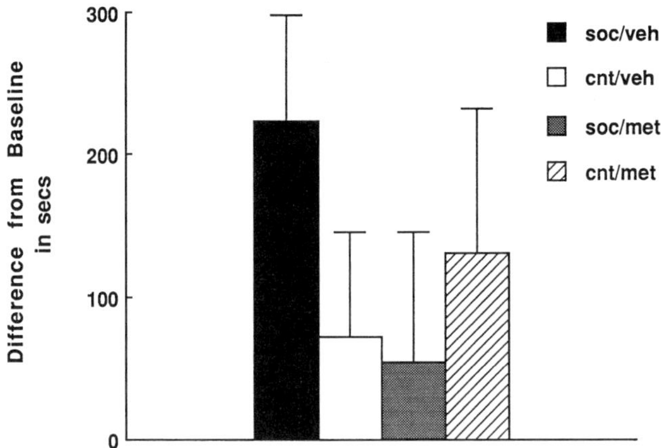

FIGURE 5. Mean (± SEM) summary of a 2 × 2 design evaluating the efficacy of a social-interaction induced place preference in animals that had been treated with 1 mg/kg of methysergide during training. Although the overall social-reward trend was not statistically significant in this study, very little tendency for place preference was seen in animals that had received methysergide during social conditioning.

up experiments we found a clear sex difference in this measure, with female rats generally exhibiting social-reward effects while mature male rats typically did not.

In follow-up work, we have so far failed to demonstrate that the acquisition of this type of social reward is mediated by brain opioids. Animals that received social conditioning while under the influence of naltrexone exhibited essentially the same pattern of choice as did vehicle-treated animals. Thus, even though opioids are very powerful in reducing separation-distress, they apparently are not essential for social reward. This is also indicated by the ability of social stimuli to still significantly reduce DVs in animals given opiate antagonists[48] as well as by their eagerness to seek out social rewards in various other situations.[42,49]

We also provisionally evaluated the role of several other systems, including serotonin and oxytocin. When social conditioning was done under 1 mg/kg of methysergide, the social-reward effect appeared to be completely blocked (FIG. 5). Likewise, we evaluated the possible role of oxytocin in this type of reward phenomenon. First, central intraventricular oxytocin injections (at 1 and 0.1 μg) associated with one side of a CPP chamber yielded no reliable place-preference effect by themselves, suggesting that central oxytocin alone was not perceived to be reinforcing (although the amnesic effects of large doses of oxytocin make the proper evaluation of such a proposition troublesome). However, if oxytocin was administered in conjunction with a social partner, either peripherally (6 ng/kg) or centrally (0.1 μg), we observed a modest elevation (a doubling) of social-reward effects in the conditioned place-preference paradigm. However, because of substantial intersubject variability, that trend has not yet proved statistically reliable in groups of 6–10 animals. Thus, this facilitation effect does not appear to be terribly robust with the techniques used so far. A singular neurochemical system for social-reward system has eluded us, and we might fruitfully consider if certain chemistries need to operate conjointly for social reward to be fully engaged. In any event, we must await further data collection for any definitive conclusions.

AN AUTOMATED APPARATUS FOR MONITORING GREGARIOUSNESS IN RATS

The aim was to devise sensitive instrumentation and a method to quantify social investigation. Here, we summarize a series of validation experiments (i.e., analysis of sex, age, role of sensory systems, and circadian and social deprivation variables) and also provide data indicating that this new procedure is exquisitely sensitive for analyzing the effects of opiates in reducing social motivation.

First, we considered what should be the requisite dimensions of an optimal social-investigation method? An approach with broad applicability should be: (1) fully automated so as to minimize the influence of fallible human perceptual judgments (in terms of both reliability and selecting the behaviors to be coded); (2) sensitive to changes in major social variables (such as social deprivation, gender, and social distance); (3) flexible and easily modified to address a diversity of sociophysiological issues needing clarification; and above all (4) capable of reducing social-investigative tendencies to the simplest analytic terms possible. To fulfill these criteria, we devised a simple investigatory apparatus consisting of two adjacent test chamber boxes (65 cm long × 24 cm wide × 15 cm high), each having two exploration ports, situated on the opposing far walls, with one port designated as the social port (which faced the other box) and the other as the nonsocial one (facing nothing). Each port was designed to allow an adult rat to put its head through but not to escape. The separation of the aligned social holes could be increased systematically to monitor the effects of social distance. To minimize experimenter fatigue, exploration of each hole was monitored automatically via computer-linked photodetectors crossing the center of each hole. In this way, exploration of the nonsocial and social ports (along with coincident frequencies and durations) could be monitored automatically for extended test sessions, simultaneously precluding complex (and analytically troublesome) social interactions that would have emerged had animals been allowed free access to each other.

Preliminary work determined the ideal size for the investigative ports for adult Long-Evans hooded rats. Several colleagues had suggested that such an experiment could never be done because since it was supposed that if a rat could get its head through a hole, the rest of the body could follow. However, from observations of up to 24 hours, this assumption has proven to be incorrect. There are hole diameters that allow easy egress for the head, but that do not allow animals to squeeze through. Of course, the hole size varies depending on the size of the rat. For male and female rats above 200 g, a port diameter of 32 mm allows easy exit of the head, with no animals achieving exit (or getting stuck in failed attempts). At 175 g, over half the animals did escape (or got stuck in the attempt). During prolonged test periods many animals chewed at the edges of the ports, which necessitated reinforcement of the circumference with metal rims. Since then we have encountered no further problems. The 32-mm reinforced hole provides a "golden mean" for the present studies. Male rats above ~375 g have difficulty getting their head through, but they continue to vigorously investigate the ports, especially the social ports, with their nose, pushing their faces forward up to about ear level. A 35-mm diameter hole allows males up to ~600 g (the largest we have tested) head egress, but it allows females up to 250 g to escape with annoying persistence. To use this procedure with younger animals, one will obviously need to use ports of different diameter.

In the preliminary validation work, we pursued the following issues: (1) the evaluation of the distance between investigation ports on the amount of social investigation (the distances between adjacent investigation ports were chosen to be 7 and 12 cm, the shorter distance allowing up to cheek-to-cheek contact and the longer distance little more than nose-to-nose contact; (2) comparison of male-male and female-female responses in this apparatus; and (3) evaluation of 24 hours of social deprivation on proximity maintenance. Because test sessions were 1 hour in length (with six 10 minute recording blocks), we also noted that investigation does decline systematically during a test session. The durations (seconds/10 mins) of port investigations were as follows (frequencies and individual bout durations are not provided, but they paralleled and were statistically more robust than duration results):

1. During a 1-hour test session, isolate-housed animals investigated the social holes (overall average 93.7 s/10 min) more than the nonsocial holes (20.9 s) ($F(1,19) = 114.43$, $p < 0.0001$). This differential effect was sustained, with modest but reliable diminutions across the hour.

2. Isolate-housed females exhibited slightly more overall port investigations (i.e., both social and nonsocial holes combined) than isolate-housed males, the females averaging 70.7 seconds and the males 43.8 seconds ($F(1,19) = 8.47$, $p < 0.01$). However, it is important to note that these elevations were more prominent in females who investigated social holes for 113.4 seconds vs 73.9 seconds for the males, while the respective numbers for nonsocial holes were 28.0 and 13.7 seconds.

3. The two distances yielded highly reliable differences in social investigation, with the closer distance promoting social investigation more ($F = 7.06$ (1,19), $p < 0.02$), with an average of 118.4 seconds at the 7-cm distance and 68.9 seconds at the 12-cm distance and no interaction with sex or the other variables. As expected, investigation of the nonsocial holes was no different as a function of differences in the distance of the social holes (20.7 and 21.0 s/10 min).

4. In comparing social isolation effect, adult female rats that had been pair-housed for 2 weeks before testing were tested either directly from social housing or immediately following 24 hours of prior individual housing. The apparatus was selectively sensitive to social deprivation, yielding a reliable interaction between social-housing condition and social vs nonsocial port investigation. Isolation had no effect on investigation of nonsocial ports (means were 41.9 and 49.6 seconds for isolation and social conditions, respectively), while isolated and social rats explored the social ports for 86.0 and 67.2 s/10 minutes, respectively ($F = 5.29$ (1,27), $p < 0.03$).

5. Finally, we noted that this apparatus could be used as an automated measure of anxiety using the social interaction model developed by File. In bright light (500 lux), animals exhibited reliably less social investigation than they did in complete darkness.

The preliminary results were remarkably clear-cut in demonstrating the sensitivity of this general purpose apparatus for detecting the effects of many variables that should be ideally capable of being detected. This affirms that the apparatus can be used to pursue a systematic analysis of social processes and could be used to routinely monitor the effects of pharmacological treatments on gregariousness. According to our current theoretical view, agents that arouse social-reward processes in the brain would be expected to decrease the amount of social investigation in this apparatus. Indeed, the apparatus is exquisitely sensitive in demonstrating that low doses of opiates (i.e., down to 0.5 mg/kg) can reduce gregariousness, as has been seen with other measures, with no change in the investigation of the nonsocial ports. Likewise, administration of high doses of oxytocin (1 μg) into the region of the third ventricle has reliably reduced social investigation in this apparatus, but because investigation of the nonsocial port was also diminished, we cannot yet conclude that the effect was behaviorally specific. General activity may have been reduced.

To determine if very small doses of oxytocin given peripherally, which were found to facilitate social memories,[50] might have opposite effects, we evaluated the behavior of animals first used in the experiments described in FIGURES 1 and 2 in this apparatus. This experiment was conducted 1 week after the end of the previously described place-preference experiment. Pairs of rats were placed in the social investigation boxes for 4 consecutive days. On days 1 and 2, rats were placed in the boxes, and their previous place-preference partner or a stranger was placed in the adjoining social box. The order of partner and stranger tests was counterbalanced. On days 3 and 4, rats were tested following injections of 6 ng/kg of oxytocin or distilled water vehicle i.p., and their previous partner or a stranger was placed in the adjoining box. Test sessions lasted 10 minutes.

Data (FIG. 6) represent the number of seconds spent investigating the social hole minus the number of seconds in the nonsocial hole for three different variables: (1) whether the rats had had oxytocin or saline solution in the previous CPP test, (2) whether they were tested with the previous CPP partner or a stranger, and (3) whether they were tested after oxytocin or vehicle administration. The only significant effect was evident for the overall oxytocin treatment ($F(1,14) = 12.87$, $p < 0.005$), indicating that all animals tested with the very small peripheral dose of oxytocin spent more time investigating the social port. Although there was a small trend for this effect to be larger in animals tested with their previous partner, none of the subgroup differences was close to significant. The finding that very low peripheral doses of oxytocin can increase gregariousness while high central doses reduce it, highlights the need for a full dose response analysis of both routes of administration, along with oxytocin-receptor antagonists, before any definitive conclusions concerning the natural role of oxytocin in the maintenance of gregariousness can be posited. At present, we might provisionally conclude that mild arousal of the oxytocin system may facilitate gregariousness, while higher doses have opposite effects.

Parenthetically, we noted that the foregoing technology may be effectively deployed to study concepts such as "social readiness." In other words, rather than simply measuring time and duration of social activities during extended test sessions, it could be used to simply monitor the initial urge to indulge in social activities. Also, we used this apparatus to study social cooperation, by linking reward delivery at the nonsocial port to certain amounts of social contact at the social ports. Opiates have diminished the amount of cooperative activity in this variant of the foregoing

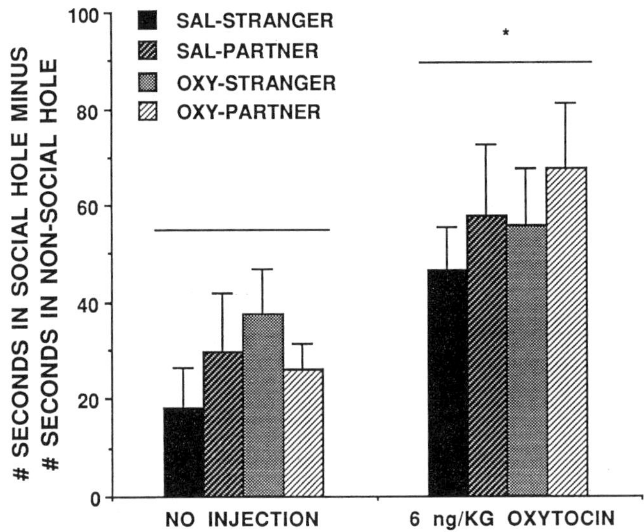

FIGURE 6. Mean (± SEM) increase in the investigation of the social port as compared to the nonsocial port as a function of peripherally administrated oxytocin (6 ng/kg). Animals exhibited more social investigation following oxytocin administration as compared to vehicle treatment.

paradigm. This type of work may eventually help identify neurochemical maneuvers that could help promote social urges in disorders such as autism.

A NEW MODEL SYSTEM FOR ANALYZING SOCIAL BONDING IN INFANT RATS

A critical issue for understanding the neurobiological nature of affiliative behavior is the development of efficient model systems whereby social bonding can be systematically studied in common laboratory mammals. Although the study of imprinting in avian species is well developed,[51] no comparable systems exist for the analysis of attachment processes in mammals. To develop such a model, we capitalized on the acute olfactory sensitivities of the rat and analyzed the tendency of young rats to approach an odor that has been associated with maternal reunion.[52] We found that young rats exhibit an increased tendency to approach an odor that on the previous day was associated with maternal reunion. Indeed, we found that this type of social bonding is partially mediated by opioids[16] as well as oxytocin.[53] The oxytocin effect generally seemed more robust, which is consistent with a great deal of other data implicating oxytocin in social bonding.[12,54]

Considering the apparent importance of vasopressin in sociosexual bonding in adult male voles,[55] we also decided to evaluate the vigor of attachment in young Brattleboro rats who constitutionally lack endogenous vasopressin.[56] The gene for vasopressin is monogenic dominant, so rats that are homozygous recessive (*di/di*) do not produce any endogenous vasopressin and hence exhibit diabetes insipidus. Brattleboro rats which are heterozygous for the vasopressin gene (*di/+*) do produce vasopressin, but at slightly subnormal levels, but they make an excellent control group, because they have a similar breeding history.

Thirty-nine *di/+* pups from four litters and 36 *di/di* pups from four litters were studied for their tendency to exhibit maternal bonding. When pups were 14 days of age, they were removed from their mother and placed along with littermates in a warm environmental chamber. Three times throughout the course of the day the mother was sprayed on the ventral surface with 1 cc of lemon extract, and the pups were returned to her for a 30-minute period. Each conditioning session was proceeded by a 3-hour period of maternal separation. The control animals just received a cottonball odor pairing. At the end of the last session, the ventrum of the mother was washed clean with soap and water, and the pups were returned to the mother overnight.

Approximately 24 hours after the first maternal odor pairing, all pups were isolated from the mother for 3 hours and given five odor approach trials which took place in an 8.5 × 38 cm straight alley. The goal end of this straight alley contained a cottonball freshly soaked in 1 cc of lemon extract. The cottonball was contained in an open-ended jar which faced the start end of the straight alley. Each trial consisted of placing pups at the start end of the straight alley and recording the latency for the pups to reach the goal end. If pups did not reach the goal end in a 60-second period, a no-response was recorded and the trial was terminated. The animals were also tested for place preference for the maternally paired odor.

As can be seen in FIGURE 7, *di/di* pups showed no more rapid approach to the maternally paired odor than the cottonball-paired odor, whereas the *di/+* control animals exhibited a reliably faster approach to the maternally paired odor ($F(1,38) = 5.14$, $p < 0.05$). A similar pattern was observed with the place-preference measure, with *di/di* animals exhibiting a slight aversion for the maternally paired odor side, while the *di/+* animals clearly preferred to spend more time on the maternally paired odor side ($F(1,73) = 5.09$, $p < 0.03$).

These results indicate that vasopressin, like oxytocin and endogenous opioids, may participate in infant-mother bonding. Parenthetically, we would note that the reward value of various aspects of maternal care has also been evaluated in this odor-conditioning paradigm.[52] Active tactile contact is an important aspect of maternal reward in 11-day-old pups (because skin surface anesthetization of the pup with xylocaine or making mothers cataleptic with high doses of opiates eliminates the conditioned attraction). Milk does not appear to be a critical maternal variable (because bromocriptine or covering the nipples does not eliminate the effect). It is especially noteworthy in this context that tactile reward has been indirectly implicated in opioid release.[17,48,57] In short, we believe that touch is a critical variable that mediates this type of social reward/bonding. In this context, it is noteworthy that several other studies have found that opioid blockade can increase the desire for social grooming in primates[17,58] and that tactile and kinesthetic stimulation can increase development in neonates.[59] Although the neural events that lead to this type of infant-mother bonding need to be worked out, the existing pattern of results suggests that various peptide neuromodulators are important in mediating this type of reward.

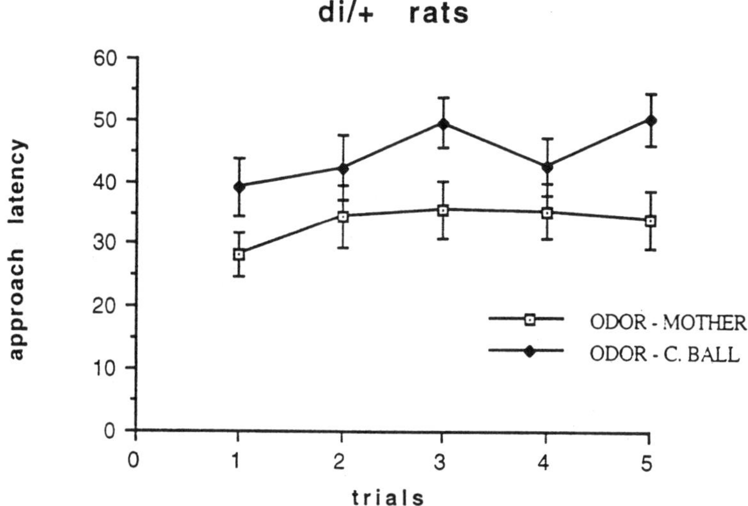

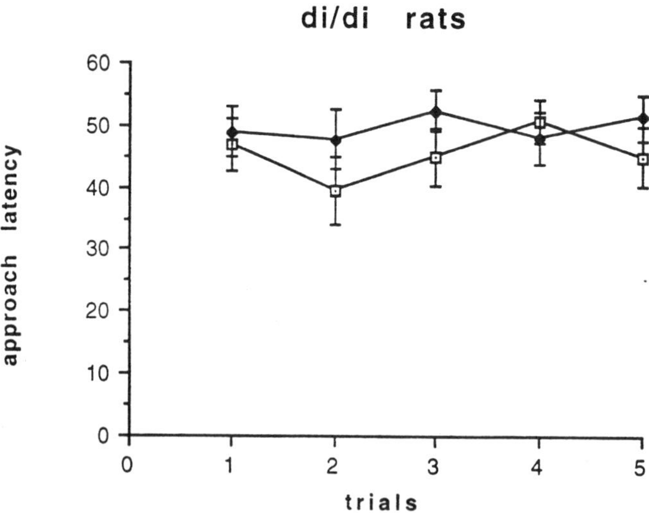

FIGURE 7. Mean (± SEM) latency in seconds to approach an odor that had been paired with the mother (*white squares*) or cottonball (*black diamonds*) three times on the previous day. Vasopressin-producing rats (*di*/+) are depicted in the *top panel* and vasopressin-deficient rat (*di/di*) pups are depicted in the *bottom panel.*

CONCLUSIONS AND IMPLICATIONS

The foregoing studies highlight various new procedures that can be effectively used to analyze affiliative and social-reward tendencies in animals. Unfortunately, the data we collected are preliminary and do not yet conclusively support the supposition that chemistries that suppress distress vocalizations mediate social reward. Thus, social-reward systems, if they exist in the brain, may be at least partially independent of systems that reduce separation distress. For instance, opioid blockade did not clearly diminish social reward in the place-preference paradigm, even though antagonists did block the behavioral indices of infant-mother attachment. In this context, it is noteworthy that male sexual reward, as evaluated with the place-preference procedure, was diminished by opioid blockade induced either peripherally with naloxone or centrally by administration directly into the preoptic area.[60] We have also not yet obtained clear evidence that oxytocin facilitates social-reward effects in adult animals, but it does seem to mediate this process in infants. Oxytocin antagonists clearly diminish the attractive qualities of conditioned maternal cues. Also, vasopressin-deficient animals do not exhibit normal social attachments, suggesting that the same brain chemistries that promote sexual bonding in rodents,[55] may also promote infant-mother bonding. The social-investigation paradigm has indicated that opiates and high central doses of oxytocin reduce investigation, while low peripheral doses of oxytocin increase it. Opiate antagonists do not clearly increase social investigation in that paradigm, and the effect of oxytocin antagonists remains to be evaluated. In sum, although both opioid and oxytocin systems can powerfully modulate various social behaviors, the new techniques that we have developed have not yielded a simple and coherent answer about their role in the mediation of social reward. They seem to be involved in young animals, but comparable effects have not been evident in older ones. Obviously, much more work needs to be done with such models before conclusive statements can be made about the existence and nature of such a brain process. If it does exist as a separate entity from other types of reward, then it is likely to have multiple neurochemical controls, including prolactin, and they may need to operate concurrently to obtain clearer effects in adults.

Hopefully, these lines of reasoning highlight the methodological and conceptual complexities we must address in seeking to understand the substrates of attachment processes in mammals. The view advocated here is that even though there is a key brain system that is the major contributor to normal attachment processes across species, it is constituted of multiple subcomponents that may vary in importance (FIG. 1). At present the part of the system that controls separation distress, along with the chemistries that reduce it is a physiological reality. We cannot yet assert that a form of social reward, independent of the alleviation of separation distress, is also a neurophysiological reality of the mammalian brain. We would like to believe that such a brain process does exist, because it would make it is easier to imagine how social choices within complex social networks might be made, but we are short of having the data to unambiguously affirm that conclusion. If there is a key player in that type of process in the developing brain, it might be closely related to play systems of the brain,[43] for that is where the greatest day-to-day sources of joy seem to arise. Also, the full joy of playfulness can only emerge if the infantile need for the secure base of stable social bond is fulfilled. Postulating the existence of such brain systems might facilitate the understanding of more mature epigenetic forms of bonding such as those that reflect friendships and social coalitions as well as sexual and parental bonds. The psychiatric implications of this type of knowledge should be vast, including important implications for disorders such as early childhood autism,[61] depression,[34] panic, posttraumatic stress, and various personality disorders.[62,63] It may also help us to finally understand the deep neural nature of everyday human love and sadness.

REFERENCES

1. KRAEMER, G. W. 1992. A psychobiological theory of attachment. Behav. Brain Sci. **15:** 493-541.
2. PANKSEPP, J. 1981. Brain opioids: A neurochemical substrate for narcotic and social dependence. *In* Progress in Theory in Psychopharmacology. S. Cooper, Ed.: 149-175, Academic Press. London.
3. HARLOW, C. M., Ed. 1986. Learning to Love: The Selected Papers of H. F. Harlow. Praeger. New York.
4. SCOTT, J. P. 1968. Early Experience and the Organization of Behavior. Brooks/Cole. Monterey, CA.
5. BOWLBY, J. 1980. Attachment and Loss, Vol. 1. Attachment. Basic Books. New York.
6. BOWLBY, J. 1988. A Secure Base: Parent-Child Attachment and Healthy Human Development. Basic Books. New York.
7. MASON, W. A. 1970. Motivational factors in psychosocial development. *In* Nebraska Symposium on Motivation, Vol. **18**. W. J. Arnold & N. M. Page, Eds. University of Nebraska Press. Lincoln.
8. PEDERSEN, C. A., J. D. CALDWELL, G. JIRIKOWSKI & T. R. INSEL. Eds. 1992. Oxytocin in maternal, sexual and social behavior. Ann. N.Y. Acad. Sci. Vol. **652**.
9. PANKSEPP, J. 1982. Toward a general psychobiological theory of emotions. Behav. Brain Sci. **5:** 407-469.
10. PANKSEPP, J. 1991. Affective neuroscience: A conceptual framework for the neurobiological study of emotions. *In* International Reviews of Emotion Research, Vol. **1**. K. Strongman, Ed.: 59-99, Wiley. Chichester.
11. PANKSEPP, J., M. D. NEWMAN & T. R. INSEL. 1992. Critical conceptual issues in the analysis of separation-distress systems of the brain. *In* International Review of Studies on Emotion, Vol. **2** K. T. Strongman, Ed.: 52-72. John Wiley & Sons Ltd. New York.
12. INSEL, T. R. 1992. Oxytocin: A neuropeptide for affiliation-evidence from behavioral, autoradiographic and comparative studies. Psychoneuroendocrinology. **17:** 3-35.
13. SCHECHTER, M. D. & D. J. CALCAGNETTI. 1993. Trends in place preference conditioning with a cross-indexed bibliography; 1957-1991. Neurosci. Biobehav. Rev. **17:** 21-41.
14. BERRIDGE, K. C. 1996. Food reward: Brain substrates of wanting and liking. Neurosci. Biobehav. Rev. **20:** 1-25.
15. PANKSEPP, J., B. H. HERMAN, R. CONNER, P. BISHOP & J. P. SCOTT. 1978. The biology of social attachments: Opiates alleviate separation distress. Biol. Psychiatry **13:** 607-613.
16. PANKSEPP, J., E. NELSON & S. M. SIVIY. 1994. Brain opioids and mother-infant social motivation. Acta Paediatr. Suppl. **397:** 40-46.
17. KEVERNE, E. B., N. MARTENSZ & B. TUITE. 1989. β-endorphin concentrations in CSF of monkeys are influenced by grooming relationships. Psychoneuroendocrinology **14:** 455-161.
18. D'AMATO, F. R. & F. PAVONE. 1993. Endogenous opioids: A proximate reward mechanism for kin selection? Behav. Neural Biol. **60:** 79-83.

19. Kalin, N. H., S. E. Shelton & D. E. Lynn. 1995. Opiate systems in mother and infant primates coordinate intimate contact during reunion. Psychoneuroendocrinology **7:** 735-742.
20. Panksepp, J., P. Lensing, M. Leboyer & M. P. Bouvard. 1991. Naltrexone and other potential new pharmacological treatments of atuism. Brain Dysfunct. **4:** 281-300.
21. Panksepp, J., S. M. Siviy & L. A. Normansell. 1985. Brain opioids and social emotion. *In* The Psychobiology of Attachment and Separation. M. Reite & T. Fields, Eds.: 3-49. Academic Press. New York.
22. Panksepp, J., L. Normansell, B. Herman, P. Bishop & L. Crepeau. 1988. Neural and neurochemical control of the separation distress call. *In* The Physiological Control of Mammalian Vocalizations. J. D. Newman, Ed.: 263-299. Plenum Press, New York.
23. Panksepp, J. 1996. Affective neurocience: A paradigm to study the animate circuits for human emotions. *In* Emotion: Interdisciplinary Perspectives. R. D. Kavanaugh, B. Zimmerberg & S. Fein, Eds.: 29-60. Lawrence Erlbaum Assocs. Mahwah, NJ.
24. Panksepp, J. 1992. Oxytocin effects on emotional processes: Separation distress, social bonding, and relationships to psychiatric disorders. *In* Oxytocin in Maternal, Sexual and Social Behavior. C. A. Pedersen, J. D. Caldwell, G. F. Jirikowski & T. R. Insel. Eds.: Ann. N. Y. Acad. Sci. Vol. **652:** 243-252.
25. Vilberg, T. R., J. Panksepp, A. J. Kastin & D. H. Coy. 1984. The pharmacology of endorphin modulation of chick distress vocalization. Peptides **5:** 823-831.
26. Panksepp, J. 1995. Prolactin reduces separation-distress in young domestic chicks. Soc. Neurosci. Abstr. **20:** 811.
27. Rossi, J., III, T. L. Sahley & J. Panksepp. 1983. The role of brain norepinephrine in clonidine suppression of isolation-induced distress in the domestic chick. Psychopharmacology **79:** 338-342.
28. Normansell, L. 1988. Effects of excitatory amino acids on emotional and sensorimotor behavior in the domestic chick. Unpublished doctoral dissertation, Bowling Green State University, Bowling Green, OH.
29. Turton, M. D., D. O'Shea, I. Gunn, S. A. Beak, C. M. B. Edwards, K. Meeran, S. J. Choi, G. M. Taylor, M. M. Heath, P. D. Lambert, J. P. H. Wilding, D. M. Smith, M. A. Chatel, J. Herbert & S. R. Bloom. 1996. A role for glucagon-like peptide-1 in the central regulation of feeding. Nature. **379:** 69-72.
30. Newman, J. D., Ed. 1988. The Physiological Control of Mammalian Vocalization. Plenum Press. New York.
31. Kalin, N. H., S. E. Shelton & C. M. Barksdale. 1988. Opiate modulation of separation-induced distress in non-human primates. Brain Res. **440:** 285-292.
32. Winslow, J. T. & T. R. Insel. 1991. Endogenous opioids: Do they modulate the rat pup's response to social isolation? Behav. Neurosci. **105:** 253-263.
33. Bouvard, M. P., M. Leboyer, J.-M. Launay, C. Recasens, M.-H. Plumet, D. Waller-Perotte, F. Tabuteau, D. Bondoux, M. Dugas, P. Lensing & J. Panksepp. 1995. Low-dose naltrexone effects on plamsa chemistries and clinical symptoms in autism: A double-blind, placebo-controlled study. Psychiatry Res. **58:** 191-201.
34. Panksepp, J., G. Yates, S. Ikemoto & E. Nelson. 1991. Simple ethological models of depression: Social-isolation induced "despair" in chicks and mice. In Animal Models in Psychopharmacology. B. Olivier, J. Mos & J. L. Slangen, Eds.: 161-181. Birkhauser Verlag. Basel, Switzerland.
35. Kurland, A. A. 1978. Psychiatric Aspects of opiate dependence, CRC Press, Inc. West Palm Beach, FL.
36. Panksepp, J., S. Siviy, L. Normansell, K. White & P. Bishop. 1982. Effects of B-chlornaltexamine on separation distress in chicks. Life Sci. **31:** 2387-2390.
37. Panksepp, J., 1986. The psychobiology of prosocial behaviors: Separation distress, play, and altruism. *In* Altruism and Aggression: Biological and Social Origins. C. Zahn-

Waxler, E. M. Cummings & R. Iannotti, Eds.: 19-57. Cambridge University Press. Cambridge.

38. Panksepp, J., N. Najam & F. Soares. 1980. Morphine reduces social cohesion in rats. Pharmacol. Biochem. Behav. **11:** 131-134.
39. Panksepp, J., E. Nelson & R. Phillips. 1994. Unpublished data.
40. Panksepp, J., J. Jalowiec, F. G. DeEskinazi & P. Bishop. 1985. Opiates and play dominance in juvenile rats. Behav. Neurosci. **99:** 441-453.
41. Panksepp, J. 1981. Hypothalamic integration of behavior. *In* Handbook of the Hypothalamus, Vol. **3**. Part B: Behavioral Studies of the Hypothalamus. P. J. Morgane & J. Panksepp, Eds.: 289-431. Marcel Dekker Inc. New York.
42. Normansell, L. & J. Panksepp. 1990. Effects of morphine and naloxone on play-rewarded spatial discrimination in juvenile rats. Dev. Psychobiol. **23:** 75-83.
43. Panksepp, J. 1993. Rough-and-tumble play: A fundamental brain process. *In* Parent-child play: Descriptions and implications. I. MacDonald, Ed.: 147-184. SUNY Press. Albany, NY.
44. Ikemoto, S. & J. Panksepp. 1992. The effects of early social isolation on the motivation for social play in juvenile rats. Dev. Psychobiol. **25:** 261-274.
45. Carr, G., H. Fibiger & A. Phillips. 1989. Conditioned place preference as a measure of drug reward. *In* The Neuropharmacological Basis of Reward. J. Liebman & S. Cooper, Eds.: 264-319. Clarendon Press, Oxford.
46. Spyraki, C., H. Fibiger & A. Phillips. 1982. Attenuation by haloperidol of place preference conditioning using food reinforcement. Psychopharmacology **77:** 379-382.
47. Calginetti, D. J. & M. D. Schechter. 1992. Place conditioning reveals the rewarding aspect of social interaction in juvenile rats. Physiol. Behav. **51:** 667-672.
48. Panksepp, J., N. J. Bean, P. Bishop, T. Vilberg & T. L. Sahley. 1980. Opioid blockade and social comfort in chicks. Pharmacol. Biochem. Behav. **13:** 673-683.
49. Panksepp, J. & F. G. DeEskinazi. 1980. Opiates and homing. J. Comp. Physiol. Psychol. **94:** 650-663.
50. Popik, P., J. Vetulani & J. M. Van Ree. 1992. Low doses of oxytocin facilitate social recognition in rats. Psychopharmacology **106:** 71-74.
51. Horn, G. 1985. Memory, Imprinting and the Brain: An Inquiry into Mechanisms. Clarendon Press. Oxford. New York.
52. Nelson, E. 1995. Brain substrates of infant-mother attachment in the rat. Unpublished doctoral dissertation, Bowling Green State University, Bowling Green, OH.
53. Nelson, E. & J. Panksepp. 1996. Oxytocin and infant-mother bonding in rats. Behav. Neurosci. **110:** 583-592.
54. Carter, S. C., A. C. DeVries & L. L. Getz. 1995. Physiological substrates of mammalian monogamy: The prairie vole model. Neurosci. Biobehav. Rev. **19:** 303-314.
55. Winslow, J. T., N. Hastings, C. S. Carter, C. R. Harbaugh & T. R. Insel. 1993. A role for central vasopressin in pair bonding in monogamous prairie voles. Nature **365:** 544-548.
56. Sokol, H. W. & H. Valtin, Eds. 1982. The Brattleboro Rat. Ann. N.Y. Acad. Sci. **394:** 1-824.
57. Panksepp, J. & P. Bishop. 1981. An autoradiographic map of (^{3}H) diprenorphine binding in rat brain: Effects of social interaction. Brain Res. Bull. **7:** 405-410.
58. Fabre-Nys, C., R. E. Meller & E. B. Keverne. 1982. Opiate antagonists stimulate affiliative behavior in monkeys. Pharmacol. Biochem. Behav. **16:** 653-659.
59. Schanberg, S. M., G. Evoniuk & C. M. Kuhn. 1984. Tactile and nutritional aspects of maternal care: Specific regulators of neuroendocrine function and cellular development. Proc. Soc. Exp. Biol. Med. **175:** 135-146.
60. Agmo, A. & M. Gomez. 1993. Sexual reinforcement is blocked by infusion of naloxone into the medial preoptic area. Behav. Neurosci. **107**: 812-818.

61. PANKSEPP, J. & T. SAHLEY. 1987. Possible brain opioid involvement in disrupted social intent and language development of autism. *In* Neurobiological Issues in Autism. E. Schopler & G. Mesibov, Eds.: 357-382. Plenum Press. New York.
62. CLYNES, M. & J. PANKSEPP, Eds. 1988. Emotions and Psychopathology. Plenum Press, New York.
63. SCHATZBERG, A. F. & C. B. NEMEROFF, Eds. 1995. American Psychiatric Association Textbook of Psychopharmacology. American Psychiatric Association, Inc. Washington, DC.

16

Physiological and Endocrine Effects of Social Contract

Kerstin Uvnäs-Moberg

ROLE OF INNOCUOUS SENSORY ACTIVATION IN FRIENDLY SOCIAL BEHAVIOR

All kinds of friendly or nonaggressive social contact involve at least three separate phases, an approach or "hunger" phase, an interactive phase during which nonnoxious sensory stimuli are given and received, and a relaxation or "satiety" phase, which actually results from the sensory interaction occurring during the interactive phase. These three aspects of social behavior occur in lactation, sexual behavior, as well as all kinds of less specific interactive behaviors involving touch or other sensory stimuli. Interestingly, they are also part of feeding behavior. In this situation, however, the mucosa of the gastrointestinal tract interacts with "nonliving material" which is to be ingested and incorporated by the living organism. In addition, there are even more unspecific types of interactions in which the "outside" of living beings receives innocuous sensory stimuli such as touch, warm temperature, and pleasant sounds from the environment.

The relaxation or satiety effects induced by activation of sensory neurons during the interactive phase of social behavior have likely evolved from a response pattern originally elicited by benign physical or chemical influences from the environment. The relaxation and sedation of the breastfeeding mother or of pups lying close together could therefore, from a physiological point of view, be related to the satiety and sedation induced by the intake of a meal or simply to the relaxation caused by pleasantly warm surroundings. From a basic physiological perspective, these situations would all favor anabolic metabolism leading to the storage of energy and growth.

The response pattern just described forms an antithesis to the well-defined response pattern characterized by avoidance and activation or fight and flight induced by noxious or dangerous stimuli. In this situation, calories would be used for locomotor activity and other energy-demanding purposes, that is, it is accompanied by a catabolic metabolism (FIG. 1).

PHYSIOLOGICAL AND ENDOCRINE CONSEQUENCES OF NONNOXIOUS VERSUS NOXIOUS STIMULATION (FIG. 2)

Interestingly, nonnoxious and noxius somatosensory information is processed by different nervous pathways. Whereas painful stimuli are transferred in the thin C-fiber or A-delta afferents, stimuli such as touch and pressure mainly activate thicker somatosensory fibers of the A-β type. Furthermore, the central pathways by which

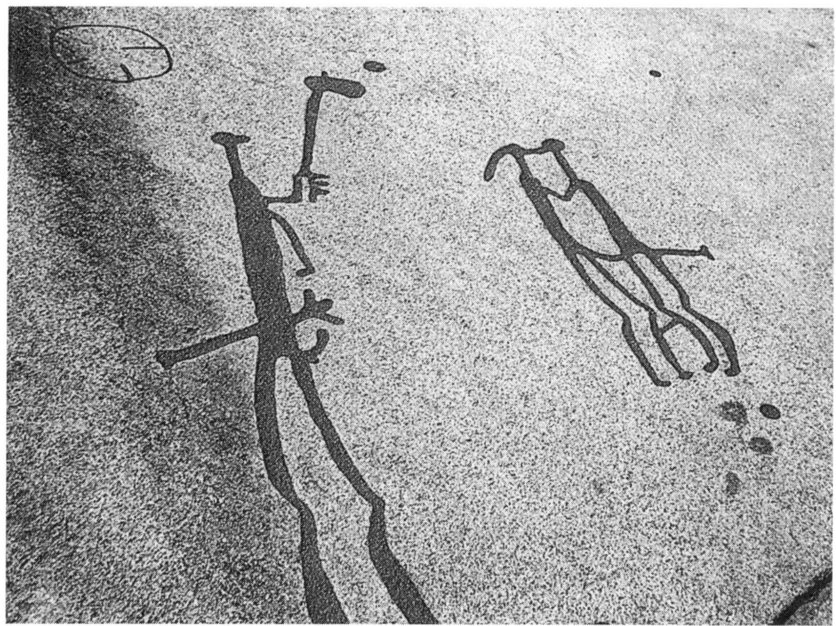

FIGURE 1. Defense or fight-flight reaction and friendly social behavior as illustrated in a bronze age rock-carving from Tanum in Sweden.

these sensory modalities are conveyed are different. Thus, the sensation of pain is transferred in the anterolateral system of the spinal cord, whereas most fibers transmitting innocuous sensory stimulation run in the dorsal column-medial lemniscal system.[1]

Under experimental conditions various subpopulations of somatosensory neurons can be activated separately, and the physiological and endocrine responses to such specific stimuli have been shown to differ. As expected, stimuli leading to activation of C-fiber and A-delta afferents, such as high intensity electrical stimulation of sensory nerves or pinching of a leg in anesthetized rats, cause activation of the cardiovascular system with a rise in pulse rate and blood pressure. The electrical activity in the sympathoadrenal nerve is increased and plasma levels of catecholamines and cortisol rise. On the other hand, vagal nerve activity is inhibited and thereby the function of the gastrointestinal tract.[2-5] By contrast, innocuous or nonnoxious stimulation, such as that induced experimentally by low intensity electrical stimulation or brushing of a leg in anesthetized rats or stroking, lowers blood pressure, decreases electrical activity in the sympathoadrenal nerve as well as levels of catecholamines in the circulation, whereas it increases the activity in the vagal nerve as reflected, for example, by the release of gastrointestinal hormones.[2,3,6-9] Taken together, noxious stimulation increases sympathetic nerve activity and induces a catabolic metabolism, whereas innocuous stimulation tends to promote vagal nerve activity and consequently digestion and anabolic metabolism.

We recently developed a method, first described by Kanetake,[10] to study the effect of nonnoxious somatosensory stimulation in conscious rats. The method involves

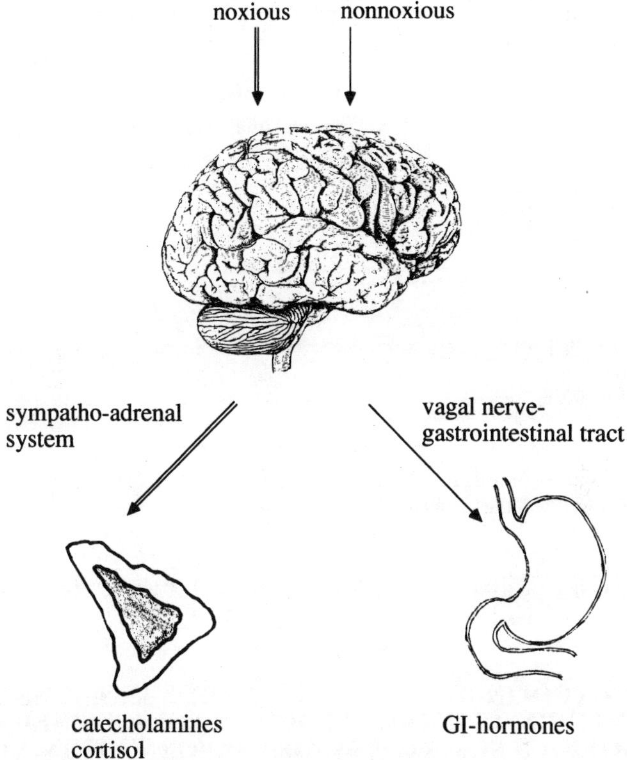

FIGURE 2. Physiological, endocrinological, and behavioral consequences of noxious versus nonnoxious somatosensory stimulation.

stroking the abdomen at a frequency of 40 strokes/m. In response to this treatment, rats express the same physiological and endocrine effect pattern as that induced by nonnoxious stimulation in anesthetized animals, that is, lowering of blood pressure[11] and a release of vagally regulated gastrointestinal hormones (Uvnäs-Moberg *et al.*, to be published), indicating a shift from sympathetic to parasympathetic autonomic dominance. However, in addition, these animals demonstrate some behavioral changes. In an open-field test they are sedated as reflected by reduced locomotor behavior.[12] In addition, their withdrawal latency to heat and mechanical stimuli is prolonged and their tail-skin temperature is reduced[13] (TABLE 1).

Separation of rat pups from their mother is known to induce separation distress calls, which are then followed by a rise in cortisol levels,[14] effects that are abolished after reunion with the mother. However, vagal nerve activity is also activated in this situation. Thus, levels of the vagally controlled hormone cholecystokinin rose even more when dog pups were put together after a period of separation than after suckling.[15]

In further support of an important role for tactile stimuli to promote anabolic metabolism and growth, tactile stimulation may even induce growth in rat pups, an

TABLE 1. Comparison between Effects Induced by Acute Injections of Oxytocin and Abdominal Stroking

	Oxytocin Injection 1 mg/kg sc, 1 mg/kg icv		Abdominal Stroking, 40/minute
	No. 1	No. 5	
Blood pressure	↑↓	↓	↓
Locomotor activity	↓	→	↓
Pain threshold			
Heat stimulation	↑[a]	↑	↑[a]
Mechanical stimulation	↑	nt	↑
Tail-skin temperature	↓	→	↓
Vagal hormone levels	↑	↑	↑
Cortisol levels	↑↓	↓	nt

Abbreviation: nt = not tested.
[a] Reversed by oxytocin antagonist.

effect that has been attributed to a release of growth hormone.[16] The growth rate of premature children has also been shown to increase in response to massage.[17]

CORTICOTROPIN-RELEASING FACTOR, VASOPRESSIN, AND OXYTOCIN AS INTEGRATORS OF NOXIOUS VERSUS NONNOXIOUS SOMATOSENSORY INFORMATION AT THE HYPOTHALAMIC LEVEL

The opposing effects of noxious versus nonnoxious somatosensory stimulation might take place at many anatomic levels, for example, by antagonizing effects of sympathetic and parasympathetic nerve activity at peripheral sites but also at the spinal, brainstem, hypothalamic, or even higher CNS level (FIG. 3).

It is well established that corticotropin-releasing factor (CRF) produced in the paraventricular nucleus of the hypothalamus plays an important integrative role in stress response, such as that induced by noxious somatosensory stimulation, by causing a release of ACTH from the pituitary and thereby cortisol from the adrenal gland.[18] However, it also enhances the activity of the sympathetic nervous system which results in an elevation of pulse rate and blood pressure,[19] and it inhibits digestive function.[20] CRF also exerts behavioral actions when administered intracerebroventricularly (icv). For example, it reduces exploratory behavior[21] and induces defensive withdrawal.[22]

Vasopressin, another peptide produced in the paraventricular nucleus, is also involved in the control of stress responses. It is well established that vasopressin elevates blood pressure by way of circulating actions and by a stimulatory effect on sympathetic function via neurons projecting from the paraventricular nucleus to the brainstem and spinal cord.[23] In addition, however, it enhances the CRF-induced release of ACTH.[24] Vasopressin also promotes aggressive behavior[25] and territorial marking in some species.[26]

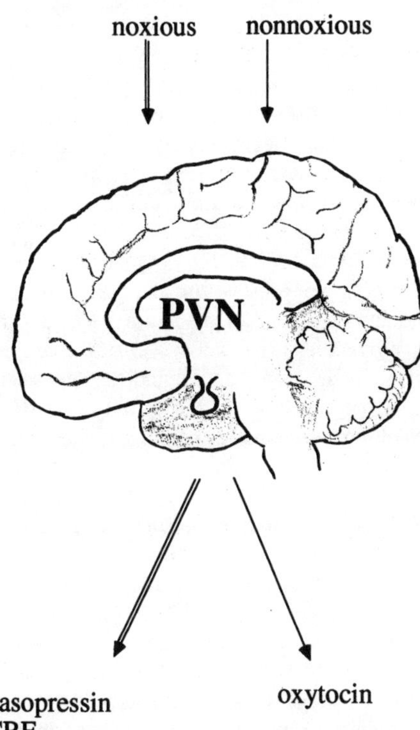

FIGURE 3. Corticotropin-releasing factor (CRF), vasopressin, and oxytocin as hypothalamic integrators of stress and antistress responses.

Oxytocin, another peptide produced in the paraventricular nucleus, has been suggested to contribute to the physiological and endocrine effects of stress.[27] In the following, a potential role for oxytocin as an integrator at the hypothalamic level of physiological, endocrine, and behavioral effects caused by somatosensory stimuli of the nonnoxious type will be proposed, that is, a response pattern characterized by decreased activity in the sympathoadrenal system, enhanced vagal nerve activity, anabolic metabolism and stimulation of growth as well as sedation; in other terms, an antistress pattern. For this purpose the characteristics of the oxytocin neurons will be described and relevant aspects of the effect pattern caused by exogenous administration of oxytocin will be reviewed. Thereafter, experimental data supporting the role of oxytocin as a hypothalamic integrator of the aforedescribed effects will be presented and discussed.

OXYTOCIN

Oxytocin is a nonapeptide produced in the paraventricular nucleus and supraoptic nucleus of the hypothalamus. The structure of oxytocin differs by only two amino acids from that of vasopressin.

Oxytocin produced in magnocellular neurons is transported down to the posterior pituitary from which it is released to the circulation. The magnocellular neurons producing oxytocin exhibit some specific morphological and neurophysiological characteristics. During suckling or in response to other kinds of intense intermittent stimulation, the glia cells normally interposed between the oxytocin neurons retract, and the oxytocin-producing cells come closer to each other.[28,29] The bursting-like electrical activity typical of the magnocellular oxytocin neurons also becomes synchronized, and consequently the cells start to fire together.[30] This synchronized firing pattern is paralleled by a pulsatile release of oxytocin into the circulation.

Oxytocin is also produced in parvocellular neurons within the paraventricular nucleus, and these neurons project to many areas within the brain such as other hypothalamic nuclei, median eminence, amygdala, hippocampus, locus coeruleus, striatum, raphe nuclei, dorsal motor nucleus of the vagus nerve, and nucleus tractus solitarius. In addition, oxytocinergic fibers project down to the spinal cord, where they terminate on the presynaptic neurons of the sympathetic chain in the intermediolateral cell column and also in the dorsal horn in the area in which pain modulation takes place.[31]

Until now only one oxytocin receptor has been identified and characterized.[32] However, data are emerging showing that subpopulations of oxytocin receptors exist. Steroids, estrogen in particular, stimulate the synthesis of oxytocin and the affinity to its receptors in certain regions.[33]

Taken together, these morphological characteristics of the oxytocinergic system indicate that activation of oxytocin release may in fact cause an integrative effect pattern. Furthermore, different effect profiles may be induced depending on the prevailing steroid levels. Oxytocin may or may not be released in parallel into the circulation and the brain. In addition, subpopulations of oxytocinergic fibers may be activated separately.

PHYSIOLOGICAL AND ENDOCRINOLOGICAL EFFECTS OF OXYTOCIN

The physiological and endocrinological effect pattern caused by the administration of oxytocin is complex. Many different and often opposing effects have been described. The complexity may be related to the fact that oxytocin induces opposite effects on one and the same physiological or endocrinological function at different anatomical sites innervated by oxytocinergic nerves. Therefore, depending on species, route of administration, dose given, time of observation, and other experimental factors, different effects in response to oxytocin may be observed.

As regards cardiovascular effects, oxytocin both increases and decreases blood pressure and pulse rate. It may increase blood pressure and pulse rate by activating the presynaptic sympathetic neurons in the spinal cord or by influencing centra in the brainstem.[34] Furthermore, it may cause bradycardia by activation of a cholinergic mechanism in the dorsal motor nucleus of the vagus nerve,[35] and electrical stimulation of the paraventricular nucleus invariably leads to a lowering of blood pressure.[36] In primates or humans, administration of oxytocin always seems to be associated with decreased blood pressure. Circulating oxytocin may also under special circumstances induce vasodilatation.[37]

Oxytocin also stimulates acid secretion[38] and a release of various gastrointestinal hormones such as insulin, cholecystokinin, somatostatin, and gastrin by activation of vagal fibers in the dorsal motor nucleus of the vagus nerve. These effects are blocked by atropine, suggesting that they are mediated by cholinergic fibers.[39,40] From a functional point of view, this leads to stimulation of the digestive process and an anabolic metabolism.

Oxytocin may also influence glucose metabolism by peripheral effects. Insulin and, in particular, glucagon can be released by the actions of oxytocin in the pancreas, and peripheral administration of oxytocin results in an elevation of glucose levels.[41] Obviously, oxytocin has two opposite effects in the handling of nutrients. By way of a central vagal cholinergic mechanism, insulin is released which leads to storing of energy or anabolic metabolism.[39] By contrast, circulating oxytocin mobilizes energy by stimulating glucagon release and thereby glucose levels.[41]

Locomotor behavior is also influenced by oxytocin. Depending on the dose, oxytocin may induce an anxiolytic-like effect or a sedative effect. When administered to rats, low amounts of oxytocin (ng icv or μg sc) induce an anxiolytic-like effect, whereas higher amounts of oxytocin (μg icv or mg sc) cause a sedative effect.[42] In addition, oxytocin causes delayed withdrawal latency to heat stimuli and to mechanical stimuli.[43]

Because oxytocinergic neurons project to the median eminence, oxytocin may be released into the hypothalamic pituitary portal system to influence the hormones produced in the anterior pituitary. Oxytocin, for example, was shown to be one of the mechanisms by which prolactin release is stimulated.[44] In addition, it was shown to either stimulate or inhibit the secretion of growth hormone.[45] A short-term release of ACTH and cortisol was demonstrated in rats but not in primates and humans in which the effect is inhibitory.[46,47]

Repeated administration of oxytocin causes an effect profile that in part differs from that induced by single injections (Table 1). The effects cannot be attributed to direct effects of oxytocin, because of the short half-life of this substance (minutes). The mechanisms involved are only partly known but are presently being explored. In the following, the effects of 1 mg/kg sc or 1 μg/kg icv for 5 days will be described.

Blood pressure, both systolic and diastolic, is lowered by 15–20 mm Hg without affecting pulse rate in female and male rats. There is a sex difference in that 10 days after the last oxytocin treatment blood pressure has normalized in the male rats, but not in the females, that is, the difference between saline-treated controls and oxytocin-treated animals persists.[48] Female rats have a slow spontaneous weight gain without an increase in food intake, suggesting a change in metabolism in a direction favoring energy storage.[49]

The withdrawal latency to heat stimuli as measured in the tail-flick test is increased. The effect is maximal 5 days after the last injection and gradually subsides to reach pretreatment values within 10 days. The acute increase in withdrawal latency caused by oxytocin can be antagonized by an oxytocin antagonist. By contrast, the sustained effect induced by repeated administration of oxytocin cannot be antagonized by the oxytocin antagonist. Instead, naloxone temporarily inhibits the enhanced delay in withdrawal latency, suggesting that endogenous opiates mediate this effect.[50] Five days after the last injection, cortisol levels are significantly lower and CCK levels significantly higher than those in saline-treated controls.

In summary, repeated oxytocin injections cause sustained physiological and endocrine and behavioral changes consistent with inhibited activity in the sympathoadrenal system and enhanced vagal nerve tone and therefore decreased catabolic and enhanced anabolic metabolism.

DO PHYSIOLOGICAL, ENDOCRINOLOGICAL, AND BEHAVIORAL EFFECTS CAUSED BY NONNOXIOUS SENSORY STIMULATION INVOLVE OXYTOCINERGIC MECHANISMS?

As just mentioned, activation of somatosensory afferents by nonnoxious stimulation in anesthetized animals leads to an effect pattern characterized by inhibited activity in the sympathoadrenal system (lowering of pulse rate and blood pressure, reduced firing activity in the adrenal nerve, and lowered plasma levels of catecholamines) and enhanced activity of the vagus, causing, for example, a release of gastrointestinal hormones. In addition, the withdrawal latency to noxious stimuli is prolonged, and behavioral sedation may be induced following stroking in conscious animals. A similar shift in autonomic nervous tone from sympathetic to parasympathetic dominance in addition to the behavioral changes described may also be induced by the administration of exogenous oxytocin, in particular when studied in a long-term perspective and after repeated administration of oxytocin.[48–50]

It has been assumed that oxytocin is released into the circulation and brain only in response to very specific types of somatosensory stimulation, such as suckling of the nipple and vaginocervical stimulation during birth or sexual behavior.[51–53] However, it has long been known that it is indeed possible to trigger oxytocin release by afferent vagal nerve stimulation. Such stimulation causes a rise in oxytocin levels and even milk ejection in lactating animals.[54] Also, feeding or intraperitoneal injections of CCK cause a release of oxytocin as well as increased levels of oxytocin mRNA in the paraventricular nucleus.[55–57] These effects are abolished by vagotomy and are consequently mediated via the vagal nerves.[57,58]

However, oxytocin can also be released by nonnoxious activation of somatosensory neurons in general. Several types of innocuous stimuli such as touch, warm temperature, vibration, and electroacupuncture increase oxytocin levels in plasma and particularly in cerebrospinal fluid.[59,60] In conscious rats the massage-like stroking of the abdomen just described is also followed by increased oxytocin levels.[13]

Obviously, oxytocin may not only cause effects that are similar to those induced by various types of innocuous somatosensory stimulation. It is also released in these situations, suggesting that oxytocin may indeed take part in the control of effects triggered by such stimuli.

One more direct way to show that oxytocin is involved in mediation of physiological and endocrine effects caused by nonnoxious somatosensory stimulation would be to show that such effects are blocked by specific oxytocin antagonists. Warm temperature, vibration, and electroacupuncture, stimuli that all cause a release of oxytocin in anesthetized rats, increase the withdrawal latency to heat as determined in the tail-flick test. When treated with the oxytocin antagonist 1-deamino-2-D-Tyr-(Oet)-4-Thr-8-Orn-oxytocin (Ferring AB, Malmö, Sweden), the effect on withdrawal latency in response to these stimuli is blocked.[60] Moreover, the increased withdrawal latency following massage in conscious animals as studied in the hot-plate test is also reversed by the oxytocin antagonist. By contrast, elevation of the pain threshold to mechanical stimuli is not reversed by the oxytocin antagonist and neither are some other effects such as reduced locomotor behavior, decreased tail-skin temperature, and decreased blood pressure caused by massage-like stroking.[13] Interestingly, the oxytocin antagonist also fails to inhibit these effects when induced by administration of exogenous oxytocin[13,42] (TABLE 1). It is therefore possible that some of the central oxytocinergic effects are mediated via an as yet unidentified oxytocin receptor. Indeed, evidence in favor of different subpopulations of oxytocin receptors has started to emerge.[61]

LACTATION AS A MODEL FOR SOCIAL CONTACT

Lactation is a specialized form of social contact during which not only sensory stimulation is exchanged between mother and young in the suckling situation, but milk, that is, nourishment, is also transferred from mother to young (FIG. 3). Naturally, milk production which is extremely energy demanding requires specific metabolic and physiological adjustments. Nutrients have to be mobilized from maternal stores and transported to the mammary gland, and milk production must be stimulated. On the other hand, it is important that maternal energy is handled in an economical way to make production of milk possible.[62–64] However, even if the purely nutritional aspects of suckling/breastfeeding are disregarded, the sensory stimulation (e.g., touch and warmth) is mutually given and received.

Oxytocin is released by the suckling stimulus to cause milk ejection. Milk ejection, however, is also accompanied by an oxytocin-mediated increased blood flow to the skin overlying the mammary gland.[37] Interestingly, breastfeeding women have also shown elevated chest-skin temperature.[65] The increase in cutaneous blood flow may serve special purposes. A warm nipple may encourage to attachment by the offspring. However, more importantly it indicates that warmth may also be transmitted to the offspring to induce physiological effects of a calming and nurturing nature. (Perhaps transmission of warmth represents a more original form of giving in friendly social relationships.)

Suckling or breastfeeding, however, is also associated with the aforedescribed changes that occur in response to nonnoxious somatosensory stimulation. In women, each suckling episode is followed by a fall in blood pressure and cortisol levels.[66,67] As a sign of more chronic depression of the sympathoadrenal system during lactation, cortisol levels induced by physical stress are lower in breastfeeding women than in bottle-feeding control women.[68] Furthermore, in rats blood pressure is lowered during the entire lactation period (Uvnäs-Moberg *et al.,* to be published). Suckling is also associated with a release of gastrointestinal hormones which ascertains a optimal digestion and stimulates anabolic metabolism.[62–64] In rat experiments, these effects are abolished following vagotomy or administration of oxytocin antagonists, suggesting that they involve oxytocinergic activation of vagal neurons in the dorsal motor nucleus of the vagus nerve.[69,70] Taken together, these physiological and endocrinological changes are similar to the aforedescribed effect pattern that occurs in response to nonnoxious stimulation of somatosensory nerves in general and to repeated injections of oxytocin.[69,70]

Obviously, oxytocin serves two different functions during lactation. The mother gives calories to the offspring as milk and warmth. In addition, she saves energy by increasing vagal nerve tone and decreasing activity in the sympathoadrenal axis.

Interestingly, milk ejection and cutaneous vasodilatation allowing transmission of warmth (and even mobilization of glucose from maternal stores to provide substrate for milk production), that is, all the "giving" effects of oxytocin, are induced by peripheral circulating effects of oxytocin.[37,63,64] By contrast, the energy-conserving effects of oxytocin similar to those induced by any kind of nonnoxious somatosensory stimulation are exerted by the central actions of oxytocin.[63,64]

LACTATION AND BEHAVIOR

Lactation is also accompanied by behavioral changes which may be linked to central actions of oxytocin. Their interactive maternal behavior and attachment to the young are facilitated by oxytocin.[63] In addition, lactating rats exhibit more unspecific behavioral changes; they express slow-wave sleep when ejecting milk[71] and react less to stressful stimuli such as noise or light.[72] The fact that oxytocin may induce sedation and also delays withdrawal latency to heat and mechanical stimuli indicate that oxytocin may be responsible for these effects; however, direct experimental proof is still lacking.

Oxytocin may also be involved in behavioral adaptations in breastfeeding women. Women feel relaxed and sedated while nursing, but there are also signs of deep temporary changes in the personality profile of women postpartum. In the first days after delivery, women taking the personality inventory, the Karolinska Scales of Personality, report themselves to be calmer and more socially interactive than similar aged nonpregnant and nonbreastfeeding women.[73,74] When the scores obtained in the various personality traits were related to the breastfeeding-induced oxytocin pattern in each woman, basal oxytocin levels correlated with the level of calm. By contrast, oxytocin pulsatility (a release pattern typical of the magnocellular neurons) was related to the level of social desirability, that is, to the wish to please, give, and interact. Assuming that circulating oxytocin levels indirectly reflect central oxytocinergic activity, these findings indicate that a causal relationship may exist between endogenous oxytocin and "personality" in the postpartum woman and also that calm and social skills could possibly reflect different aspects of central oxytocinergic activity, calm being related to basal levels of oxytocin and social skills with the pulsatility of the oxytocin pattern. In further support of a role for oxytocin in these personality changes, women having had an acute cesarean section not only fail to develop a pulsatile breastfeeding-induced oxytocin pattern, but also lack the change in their personality profile to the calm and increased socialization seen in women having vaginal delivery.[67,73,74]

Interestingly, oxytocin pulsatility was correlated not only to the personality item social desirability, but also to the amount of milk given to the child during the breastfeed, and the amount of milk was in turn also related to the level of social desirability.[74] These data suggest that a relationship may exist between physiological and psychological expressions of generosity and that an oxytocinergic mechanism, reflected by oxytocin pulsatility in the circulation, may underly both effects.

energy saving (CNS)
- sedation
- decreased reactivity
- increased digestion and anabolic metabolism
- decreased blood pressure (and cortisol secretion in humans)

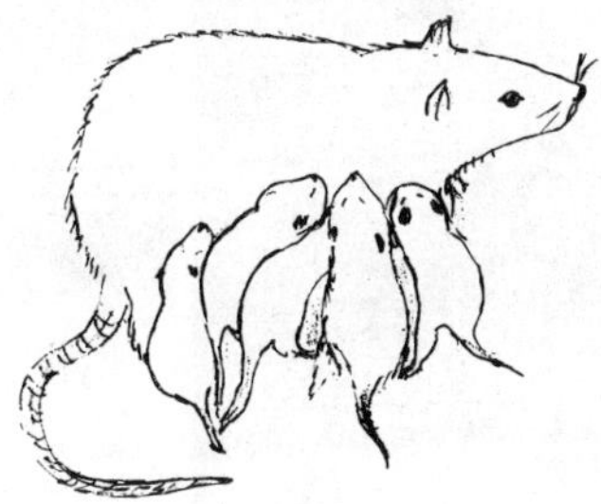

energy transfer (periphery)
- milk ejection
- cutaneous vasodilation (transmission of warmth)
- elevation of plasma levels of glucose and glucagon

FIGURE 4. Oxytocin-induced effects in a lactating rat.

In the suckling-breastfeeding situation the offspring or the baby obviously receives not only milk from the mother, but also warmth and touch, stimuli that influence the baby. Bolus-fed premature infants grow better if given to a pacifier or massage,[17,75] in part because of activation of the vagal nerve and consequent release of gastrointestinal hormones.[15,76] They also become calmer and more tolerant to pain.[77,78] A newborn baby put on its mother's chest does not cry, whereas it does if placed beside the mother in a cot.[79] Whether the effects of the sensory stimuli just described in the baby involve central oxytocinergic mechanisms remains to be established.[64]

OTHER TYPES OF SOCIAL CONTACT IN WHICH EFFECTS OF OXYTOCIN MAY BE INVOLVED

As discussed in the beginning of this article, all friendly social behaviors include an approach, an interactive, and a relaxation phase. This article has focused on oxytocin as a possible hypothalamic integrator of sensory information obtained during the interactive phase of social interaction to cause the effects of the relaxation phase. Lactation has been used as a model in which oxytocin was experimentally shown to cause these effects. It is very likely, however, that oxytocin plays a similar role in other kinds of social interaction. Oxytocin, for example, is released in response to sexual behavior in both rats and humans and is likely linked to many effects that form part of sexual behavior in both females and males, as recently reviewed by

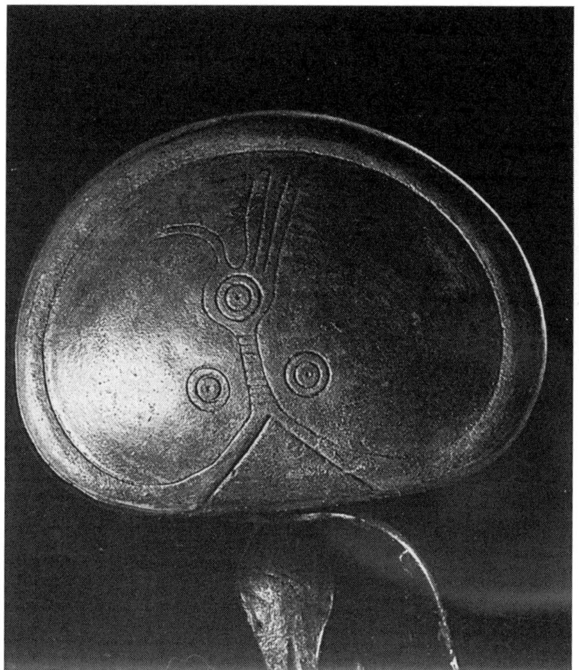
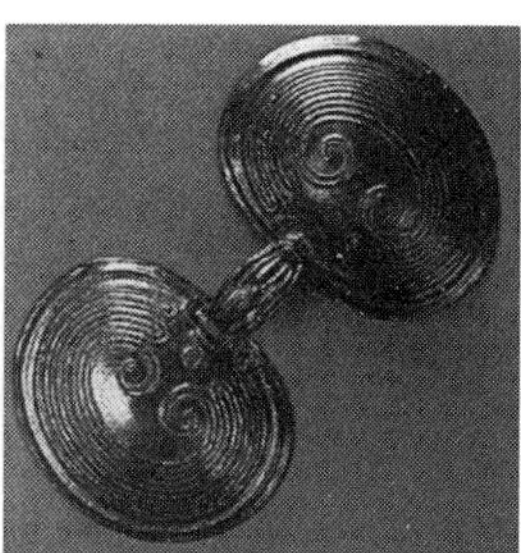

FIGURE 5. A symbol of protection, a hand on the back of a bronze age brooch from Sweden.

Carter.[80] Feeding behavior is also associated with oxytocin release in, for example, pigs, dogs, and cows[81] and has been suggested to take part in the satiety effect, such as that caused by CCK released from the duodenum in response to feeding in rats.[58] However, also under special circumstances it may increase food intake.[82] Grooming and other kinds of less specific types of social interaction are also likely to be accompanied by a rise in oxytocin[59,60] and oxytocin-induced effects, and administration of oxytocin may also cause grooming[83] and increase social contact.[84]

OXYTOCIN-INDUCED ATTACHMENT FOR DEVELOPMENT OF HEALTH-PROMOTING OR ANTISTRESS EFFECTS BY SOCIAL INTERACTION

In various animal experimental models, oxytocin was shown to facilitate bonding or attachment or simply to increase the amount of social contact between individuals.[84,85] A specific bond between two individuals or an increased wish or need for contact (in opposite terms, a lowered level of suspicion or aggression) also has interesting physiological consequences in that it allows for repetitive exposure to friendly interaction involving tactile or other kinds of sensory activation and therefore to the physiological consequences of this kind of stimuli. Assuming that oxytocin is repeatedly released by the sensory stimulation exchanged in social interaction, a situation similar to the experiments in which oxytocin was administered repeatedly should follow. If so, decreased sympathoadrenal activity and enhanced vagal nerve activity leading to anabolic metabolism and possibly to growth as well as sedation ought to be induced (see above). The literature showing that good relationships have a positive effect on health is indeed extensive. A good marriage and access to a confident or supportive family or social network has been shown in many studies to have health-promoting effects. In particular, the risk of cardiovascular disease seems to be decreased as reflected by lower blood pressure values and also by a decreased incidence of cardiac infarction and stroke.[86]

In humans, warm and friendly interaction does not necessarily involve tactile interaction but rather psychological interaction of this character (FIG. 5). That oxytocin is released in response to such friendly, warm interaction remains to be shown, but it is highly possible. In support of the role of oxytocin in human interactive behaviors are correlational studies performed on healthy nonpregnant or breastfeeding individuals, in which oxytocin was shown to correlate with personality traits such as attachment and calm and social dependency.[87,88]

It is also likely that certain kinds of physical therapies such as massage activate nonnoxious somatosensory afferents and thereby just like social relationships cause antistress effects of the type described herein. Indeed, massage has been shown to reduce anxiety and to lower cortisol levels in humans.[89,90]

In conclusion, in the language of physiology it is very likely that the beneficial effects of good relationships may be a consequence of repetitive nonnoxious sensory stimulation, leading to a release of oxytocin. The effect spectrum caused by oxytocin, that is, a lowered sympathoadrenal tone, elevated vagal nerve tone, anabolic metabolism, relaxation, and behavioral calm, actually runs counter to that of the stress axis and therefore constitutes an antithesis to the fight-flight response (FIG. 1).

SUMMARY

Nonnoxious sensory stimulation associated with friendly social interaction induces a psychophysiological response pattern involving sedation, relaxation, decreased sympathoadrenal activity, and increased vagal nerve tone and thereby an endocrine and metabolic pattern favoring the storage of nutrients and growth. It is suggested that oxytocin released from parvocellular neurons in the paraventricular nucleus (PVN) in response to nonnoxious stimulation integrates this response pattern at the hypothalamic level. The response pattern just described characterized by calm, relaxation, and anabolic metabolism could be regarded as an antithesis to the well known fight-flight response in which mental activation, locomotor activity, and catabolic metabolism are expressed. Furthermore, the health-promoting aspect of friendly and supportive relationships might be a consequence of repetitive exposure to nonnoxious sensory stimulation causing the physiological endocrine and behavioral changes just described.

REFERENCES

1. GUYTON, A. C. & J. E. HALL. 1996. The nervous system. A. General principles and sensory physiology. *In* Textbook of Medical Physiology, 9th Ed., chapt. **45:** 565-582. W. B. Saunders. Philadelphia, PA.

2. Sato, A., Y. Sato & R. F. Schmidt. 1981. Heart rate changes reflecting modifications of efferent cardiac sympathetic outflow by cutaneous and muscle afferent volleys. J. Auton. Nerv. Syst. **4:** 231-247.
3. Araki, T., K. Ito, M. Kurosawa & A. Sato. 1984. Responses of adrenal sympathetic nerve activity and catecholamine secretion to cutaneous stimulation in anesthetized rats. Neuroscience **12:** 289-299.
4. Tsuchiya, T., Y. Nakayama & A. Sato. 1991. Somatic afferent regulation of plasma corticosterone in anesthetized rats. Jpn. J. Physiol. **41:** 169-176.
5. Uvnäs-Wallensten, K. & J. Järhult. 1982. Reflex activation of the sympatho-adrenal system inhibits the gastrin release caused by electrical vagal stimulation in cats. Acta Physiol. Scand. **114:** 297-302.
6. Kurosawa, M., A. Suzuki, K. Utsugi & T. Araki. 1982. Response of adrenal efferent nerve activity to non-noxious mechanical stimulation of the skin in rats. Neurosci. Lett. **34:** 295-300.
7. Kurosawa, M., H. Saito, A. Sato & T. Tsuchiya. 1985. Reflex changes in sympatho-adrenal medullary functions in response to various thermal cutaneous stimulations in anesthetized rats. Neurosci. Lett. **56:** 149-154.
8. Uvnäs-Moberg, K., B. Posloncec & L. Åhlberg. 1986. Influence on plasma levels of somatostatin, gastrin, glucagon, insulin and VIP-like immunoreactivity in peripheral venous blood of anaesthetized cats induced by low intensity afferent stimulation of the sciatic nerve. Acta Physiol. Scand. **126:** 225-230.
9. Uvnäs-Moberg, K., T. Lundeberg, G. Bruzelius & P. Alster. 1992. Vagally mediated release of gastrin and cholecystokinin following sensory stimulation. Acta Physiol. Scand. **146:** 349-356.
10. Kanetake, C. 1982. A method for continuous drawing of blood from the jugular vein and drug injection in mice and rats. Jpn. J. Bacteriol. **37:** 943-947. (In Japanese.)
11. Kurosawa, M., T. Lundeberg, G. Ågren, I. Lund & K. Uvnäs-Moberg. 1995. Massage-like stroking of the abdomen lowers blood pressure in anesthetized rats: Influence of oxytocin. J. Auton. Nerv. Syst. **56:** 26-30.
12. Uvnäs-Moberg, K., P. Alster, I. Lund, T. Lundeberg, M. Kurosawa & S. Ahlenius. 1996. Stroking of the abdomen causes decreased locomotor activity in conscious male rats. Physiol. Behav. **6:** in press.
13. Ågren, G., T. Lundeberg, K. Uvnäs-Moberg & A. Sato. 1995. The oxytocin antagonist 1-deamino-2-D-Tyr-(Oet)-4-Thr-8-Orn-oxytocin reverses the increase in the withdrawal response latency to thermal, but not mechanical nociceptive stimuli following oxytocin administration or massage-like stoking in rats. Neurosci. Lett. **187:** 49-52.
14. Kuhn, C. M., J. Pauk & S. M. Schanberg. 1990. Endocrine responses to mother-infant separation in developing rats. Dev. Psychobiol. **23:** 395-410.
15. Uvnäs-Moberg, K., A. M. Widström, G. Marchini & J. Winberg. 1987. Release of GI hormones in mother and infant by sensory stimulation. Acta Paediatr. Scand. **76:** 851-860.
16. Pauk, J., C. M. Kuhn, T. M. Field & S. M. Schanberg. 1986. Positive effects of tactile versus kinesthetic or vestibular stimulation on neuroendocrine and ODC activity in maternally-deprived rat pups. Life Sci. **39:** 2081-2087.
17. Scafidi, F. A., T. Field & S. M. Schanberg. 1993. Factors that predict which preterm infants benefit most from massage therapy. J. Dev. Behav. Pediatr. **14:** 176-180.
18. Grossman, A., L. Perry, A. V. Schally, L. H. Rees, A. C. N. Kruseman, S. Tomlin, D. H. Coy, A. M. C. Schally & G. M. Besser. 1982. New hypothalamic hormone, corticotropin-releasing factor, specifically stimulates the release of adrenocorticotropic hormone and cortisol in man. Lancet **24:** 921-922.
19. Kurosawa, M., A. Sato, R. S. Swenson & Y. Takahashi. 1986. Sympatho-adrenal medullary functions in response to intracerebroventricularly injected corticotropin-releasing factor in anesthetized rats. Brain Res. **367:** 250-257.

20. SMEDH, U. & K. UVNÄS-MOBERG. 1994. Intracerebroventricularly administered corticotropin-releasing factor releases somatostatin through a vagal pathway in freely fed, but not in food-deprived, rats. Acta Physiol. Scand. **151:** 241-248.
21. SPADARO, F., C. W. BERRIDGE, H. A. BALDWIN & A. J. DUNN. 1990. Corticotropin-releasing factor acts via a third ventricle site to reduce exploratory behavior in rats. Pharmacol. Biochem. Behav. **36:** 305-309.
22. YANG, X. M. & A. J. DUNN. 1990. Central β_1-adrenergic receptors are involved in CRF-induced defensive withdrawal. Pharmacol. Biochem. Behav. **36:** 847-851.
23. PITTMAN, Q. J., W. L. VEALE & K. LEDERIS. 1982. Central neurohypophyseal pathways: Interactions with endocrine and other autonomic functions. Peptides **5:** 515-520.
24. GILLIES, G. E., E. A. LINTON & P. J. LOWRY. 1982. Corticotropin releasing activity of the new CRF is potentiated several times by vasopressin. Nature (Lond.) **299:** 355-357.
25. FERRIS, C. F. & Y. DELVILLE. 1994. Vasopressin and serotonin interactions in the control of agonistic behavior. Psychoneuroendocrinology **19:** 593-601.
26. FERRIS, C. F., H. E. ALBERS, S. M. WESOLOWSKI, B. D. GOLDMAN & S. E. LEEMAN. 1984. Vasopressin injected into the hypothalamus triggers a stereotypic behavior in golden hamsters. Science **224:** 510-523.
27. GIBBS, D. M. 1984. Dissociation of oxytocin, vasopressin and corticotropin secretion during different types of stress. Life Sci. **35:** 487-491.
28. THEODOSIS, D. T., D. B. CHAPMAN, C. MONTAGNESES, D. A. POULAIN & J. F. MORRIS. Structural plasticity in the hypothalamic supraoptic nucleus at lactation affects oxytocin. Neuroscience **17:** 661-678.
29. HATTON, G. I. & C. D. TWEEDLE. 1982. Magnocellular neuropeptidergic neurons in hypothalamus: Increases in membrane apposition and number of specialized synapses from pregnancy to lactation. Brain Res. Bull. **8:** 197-204.
30. POULAIN, D. A. & J. B. WAKERLEY. 1982. Electrophysiology of hypothalamic magnocellular neurons secreting oxytocin and vasopressin. Neuroscience **7:** 773-808.
31. SOFRONIEW, M. W. 1983. Vasopressin and oxytocin in the mammalian brain and spinal cord. Trends Neurosci. **6:** 467-472.
32. JARD, S. 1983. Vasopressin isoreceptors in mammals: Relation to cyclic-AMP dependent and cyclic-AMP independent transduction. Curr. Top. Membr. Transp. **18:** 255-285.
33. SCHUMACHER, M., H. COIRINI, D. W. PFAFF & B. S. MCEWEN. 1990. Behavioral effects of progesterone associated with rapid modulation of oxytocin receptors. Science **250:** 691-694.
34. RIPHAGEN, C. & Q. J. PITTMAN. 1986. Oxytocin and (1-deamino,8-D-arginine)-vasopressin (dDAVP): Intrathecal effects on blood pressure, heart rate and urine output. Brain Res. **374:** 371-374.
35. DREIFUSS, J., M. RAGGENBASS, S. CHARPAK, M. DUBOIS-DAUPHIN & E. TRIBOLLET. 1988. A role of central oxytocin in autonomic functions: Its action in the motor nucleus of the vagus nerve. Brain Res. Bull. **20:** 765-770.
36. YAMASHITA, H., H. KANNAN, M. KASAI & T. OSAKA. 1987. Decrease in blood pressure by stimulation of the rat hypothalamic paraventricular nucleus with l-glutamate or weak current. J. Auton. Nerv. Syst. **19:** 229-234.
37. ERIKSSON, M., T. LUNDEBERG & K. UVNÄS-MOBERG. 1996. Studies on cutaneous blood flow in the mammary gland of lactating rats. Acta Physiol. Scand. In press.
38. ROGERS, R. C. & G. E. HERMAN. 1985. Dorsal medullary oxytocin, vasopressin, oxytocin antagonist, and TRH effects on gastric acid secretion and heart rate. Peptides **6:** 1143-1148.
39. BJÖRKSTRAND, E., M. ERIKSSON & K. UVNÄS-MOBERG. 1996. Evidence of a peripheral and a central effect of oxytocin on pancreatic hormone release in rats. Neuroendocrinology **63:** 377-383.
40. BJÖRKSTRAND, E., S. AHLENIUS, U. SMEDH & K. UVNÄS-MOBERG. 1996. The oxytocin receptor antagonist 1-deamino-2-D-Tyr-(OEt)-4-Thr-8-Orn-oxytocin inhibits effects of

the 5-HT_{1A} receptor agonist 8-OH-DPAT on plasma levels of insulin, cholecystokinin and somatostatin. Regul. Pept. **63:** 47-52.

41. Stock, S., J. Fastbom, E. Björkstrand, U. Ungerstedt & K. Uvnäs-Moberg. 1990. Effects of oxytocin on in vivo release of insulin and glucagon studied by microdialysis in the rat pancreas and autoradiographic evidence for [^{3}H]oxytocin binding sites within the islets of Langerhans. Regul. Pept. **30:** 1-13.
42. Uvnäs-Moberg, K., S. Ahlenius, V. Hillegaart & P. Alster. 1994. High doses of oxytocin cause sedation and low doses cause an anxiolytic-like effect in male rats. Pharmacol. Biochem. Behav. **49:** 101-106.
43. Lundeberg, T., K. Uvnäs-Moberg, G. Ågren & G. Bruzelius. 1994. Anti-nociceptive effects of oxytocin in rats and mice. Neurosci. Lett. **170:** 153-157.
44. Mori, M., S. Vigh, A. Miayata, T. Yoshihara, S. Oka & A. Arimura. 1990. Oxytocin is the major prolactin releasing factor in the posterior pituitary. Endocrinology **125:** 1009-1013.
45. Björkstrand, E., A. L. Hulting & K. Uvnäs-Moberg. 1996. Evidence for a dual function of oxytocin in the control of growth hormone secretion in rats. NeuroReport. In press.
46. Gibbs, D. M., M. W. Vale, J. Rivier & S. S. C. Yen. 1984. Oxytocin potentiates the ACTH-releasing activity of CRF (41) but not vasopressin. Life Sci. **34:** 2245-2249.
47. Page, S. R., V. T. Y. Ang, R. Jackson, A. White, S. S. Nussey & J. S. Jenkins. 1990. The effect of oxytocin infusion on adenohypophyseal function in man. Clin. Endocrinol. **32:** 307-313.
48. Petersson, M., P. Alster, T. Lundeberg & K. Uvnäs-Moberg. 1996. Oxytocin causes a long-term decrease of blood pressure in female and male rats. Physiol. Behav. In press.
49. Uvnäs-Moberg, K., P. Alster & M. Petersson. 1996. Dissociation of oxytocin effects on body weight in two variants of female Sprague-Dawley rats. Integr. Physiol. Behav. Sci. **31:** 44-55.
50. Petersson, M., P. Alster, T. Lundeberg & K. Uvnäs-Moberg. 1996. Oxytocin increases nociceptive threshold in a long-term perspective in female and male rats. Neurosci. Lett. **212:** 87-90.
51. Kendrick, K. M., E. B. Keverne, C. Chapman & B. A. Baldwin. 1988. Intracranial dialysis measurement of oxytocin monoamine and uric release from the olfactory bulb and substantia nigra of sheep during parturition, suckling, separation from lambs and eating. Brain Res. **439:** 1-10.
52. Kendrick, K. M., E. B. Keverne, C. Chapman & B. A. Baldwin. 1988. Microdialysis measurement of oxytocin, aspartate, gamma-aminobutyric acid and glutamate release from olfactory bulb of the sheep during vaginocervical stimulation. Brain Res. **422:** 171-174.
53. Neumann, I., J. A. Russel & R. Landgraf. 1993. Oxytocin and vasopressin release within the supraoptic and paraventricular nuclei of pregnant, parturient and lactating rats: A microdialysis study. Neurosciences **53:** 65-75.
54. Moos, F & P. Richard. 1975. Importance de la libération d'oxytocine induite par la dilatation vaginale (réflexe de Furguson) et la stimulation vagale (réflexe vagopituitaire) chez la ratte. J. Physiol. **70:** 307-314.
55. Svennersten, K., L. Nelson & K. Uvnäs-Moberg. 1990. Feeding induced oxytocin release in dairy cows. Acta Physiol. Scand. **140:** 295-296.
56. Lindén, A., K. Uvnäs-Moberg, P. Eneroth & P. Södersten. 1989. Stimulation of maternal behavior in rats with cholecystokinin octapeptide. J. Neuroendocrinol. **1:** 389-392.
57. Verbalis, J. G. & J. Dohanics. 1991. Vasopressin and oxytocin secretion in chronically hyposmolar rats. Am. J. Physiol. **30:** R1028-R1038.
58. Uvnäs-Moberg, K. 1994. Role of efferent and afferent vagal nerve activity during reproduction: Integrating function of oxytocin on metabolism and behaviour. Psychoneuroendocrinology **19:** 687-695.

59. STOCK, S. & K. UVNÄS-MOBERG. 1988. Increased plasma levels of oxytocin in response to afferent electrical stimulation of the sciatic and vagal nerves and in response to touch and pinch in anesthetized rats. Acta Physiol. Scand. **132:** 29-34.
60. UVNÄS-MOBERG, K., G. BRUZELIUS, P. ALSTER & T. LUNDEBERG. 1993. The antinociceptive effect of non-noxious sensory stimulation is partly mediated through oxytocinergic mechanisms. Acta Physiol. Scand. **149:** 199-204.
61. CHAN, W. Y., D. L. CHEN & M. MANNING. 1993. Oxytocin receptor subtypes in the pregnant rat myometrium and decidua: Pharmacological differentiations. Endocrinology **132:** 1381-1386.
62. UVNÄS-MOBERG, K. 1989. The gastrointestinal tract in growth and reproduction. Sci. Am. **261:** 78-83.
63. UVNÄS-MOBERG, K. & M. ERIKSSON. 1996. Breastfeeding: Physiological, endocrine and behavioural adaptations caused by oxytocin and local neurogenic activity in the nipple and the mammary gland. Acta Paediatr. **85:** 525-530.
64. UVNÄS-MOBERG, K. 1996. Neuroendocrinology of the mother-child interaction. Trends Endocrinol. Metab. **7:** 126-131.
65. LIND, J., V. VUORENKOSKI & O. WASZ-HÖCKERT. 1971. The effect of cry stimulus on the temperature of the lactating breast of primipara. A thermographic study. Psychosom. Med. Obstet. Gynecol. Third International Congress, London, pp.: 293-295.
66. AMICO, J., J. M. JOHNSTON & A. H. VAGNUCCI. 1944. Suckling induced attenuation of plasma cortisol concentration in postpartum lactating women. Endocrinol. Res. **20:** 79-87.
67. NISSEN, E., K. UVNÄS-MOBERG, K. SVENSSON, S. STOCK, A. M. WIDSTRÖM & J. WINBERG. 1996. Different patterns of oxytocin, prolactin but not cortisol release during breastfeeding in women delivered by caesarean section or by the vaginal route. Early Hum. Dev. **45:** 103-118.
68. ALTEMUS, M., P. A. DEUSTER, E. GALLIVEN, C. S. CARTER & P. W. GOLD. 1995. Suppression of hypothalamic-pituitary-adrenal axis responses to stress in lactating women. J. Clin. Endocrinol. Metab. **80:** 2954-2959.
69. LINDÉN, A., M. ERIKSSON, S. HANSEN & K. UVNÄS-MOBERG. 1990. Suckling-induced release of cholecystokinin into plasma in the lactating rat: Effects of abdominal vagotomy and lesions of central pathways concerning with milk ejection. J. Endocrinol. **127:** 257-263.
70. ERIKSSON, M. 1994. Neuroendocrine Mechanisms in the Control of Milk Ejection. Thesis, Stockholm.
71. VOLOCHIN, L. M. & J. H. TRAMEZANNI. 1979. Milk ejection reflex linked to slow wave sleep in nursing rats. Endocrinology **105:** 1202-1207.
72. HANSEN, S. & A. FERREIRA. 1986. Food intake, aggression, and fear behavior in the mother rat: Control by neural systems concerned with milk ejection and maternal behavior. Behav. Neurosci. **100:** 64-70.
73. UVNÄS-MOBERG, K., A. M. WIDSTRÖM, E. NISSEN & H. BJÖRVELL. 1990. Personality traits in women 4 days post partum and their correlation with plasma levels of oxytocin and prolactin. J. Psychosom. Obstet. Gynaecol. **11:** 261-273.
74. NISSEN, E. & K. UVNÄS-MOBERG. 1996. Oxytocin, prolactin and cortisol levels in response to nursing in women after Sectio Caesarea and vaginal delivery: Relationship with changes in personality patterns post partum. Psychoneuroendocrinology. Submitted.
75. BERNBAUM, J. C., G. PEREIRA, J. WATKINS & G. PECKHAM. 1983. Nonnutritive sucking during gavage feeding enhances growth and maturation in premature infants. Pediatrics **71:** 41-45.
76. UVNÄS-MOBERG, K., G. MARCHINI & J. WINBERG. 1993. Plasma cholecystokinin concentrations after breast feeding in healthy 4 day old infants. Arch. Dis. Childhood **68:** 46-48.
77. FIELD, T. & E. GOLDSON. 1984. Pacifying effects of nonnutritive sucking on term and preterm neonates during heelstick procedures. Pediatrics **74:** 1012-1015.

78. Field, T. M., S. M. Schanberg, F. Scafadi *et al.* 1986. Tactile/kinesthetic stimulation effects on preterm neonates. Pediatrics **77:** 654.
79. Christensson, K., T. Cabrera, E. Christensson, K. Uvnäs-Moberg & J. Winberg. 1995. Separation distress call in the human neonate in the absence of maternal body contact. Acta Paediatr. **84:** 468-473.
80. Carter, C. S. 1992. Oxytocin and sexual behavior. Neurosci. Biobehav. Rev. **16:** 131-144.
81. Uvnäs-Moberg, K. 1989. Neuroendocrine regulation of hunger and satiety. *In* Obesity in Europe. P. Björntorp & S. Rössner, Eds. Vol. **1:** 1-13. John Libbey & Company Ltd. London.
82. Björkstrand, E. & K. Uvnäs-Moberg. 1996. Central oxytocin increases food intake and daily weight gain in rats. Physiol. Behav. **59:** 947-952.
83. Argiolas, A. & G. L. Gessa. 1991. Central functions of oxytocin. Neurosci. Biobehav. Rev. **15:** 217-231.
84. Witt, D. M., J. T. Winslow & T. R. Insel. 1992. Enhanced social interactions in rats following chronic, centrally infused oxytocin. Pharmacol. Biochem. Behav. **43:** 855-886.
85. Carter, C. S., A. C. DeVries & L. L. Getz. 1995. Physiological substrates of mammalian monogamy: The prairie vole model. Neurosci. Biobehav. Rev. **19**.
86. Shumaker, S. A. & S. M. Czajkowski. 1994. Social Support and Cardiovascular Disease. Plenum Press. New York, NY.
87. Uvnäs-Moberg, K., I. Arn, T. Theorell & C. O. Jonsson. 1991. Personality traits in a group of individuals with functional disorders of the gastrointestinal tract and their correlation with gastrin, somatostatin and oxytocin levels. J. Psychosom. Res. **35:** 515-523.
88. Uvnäs-Moberg, K., I. Arn, C. O. Jonsson, S. Ek & Å. Nilsonne. 1993. The relationships between personality traits and plasma gastrin, cholecystokinin, somatostatin, insulin, and oxytocin levels in healthy women. J. Psychosom. Res. **37:** 581-588.
89. Field, T., C. Morrow, C. Valdeon, S. Larson, C. Kuhn & S. Schanberg. 1992. Massage reduces anxiety in child and adolescent psychiatric patients. J. Am. Acad. Child Adolesc. **31:** 125-131.
90. Gonzalez, J., T. Field, R. Yando, K. Gonzalez, D. Lasko & D. Bendell. 1994. Adolescent's perceptions of their risk-taking behavior. Adolescence **29:** 701-709.

17
Early Learning and the Social Bond

Eric B. Keverne, Claire M. Nevison, and Frances L. Martel

There are many groups of mammals that display complex social behavior, but all have in common two important features that are interrelated. These features are, first, the increased size of the executive neocortex compared with the rest of the forebrain, and second, the importance of the matriline in maintaining social cohesion and group stability. These generalizations apply to wolves, elephants, hyenas, dolphins, and lions, as representatives of their order. However, the mammalian order that provides the greatest number of examples is that of the primates. Indeed, many primate societies are referred to as being female bonded,[1] while it has been suggested that the push for a larger neocortex in primates stems from social living.[2] Social relationships in primates require the deployment of complex and intelligent behavioral strategies.

Among primates the term female bonding signifies the importance of the matriline for group continuity and social cohesion. High ranking females tend to produce high ranking daughters and high ranking lineages grow faster. This is because infants in high ranking lineages have lower mortality rates and begin reproducing earlier than do females of lower ranking lineages.[3] Male rank does not ultimately depend on that of mothers, and there is less social stability and more mobility among males. They frequently become peripheral to the group at puberty and may leave to form male subgroups or become part of new groups.

A question of some importance concerns the neural mechanisms subserving social behavior and how these might have evolved. In principle, evolution is conservative on mechanisms. It therefore, would not make good biological sense for natural selection to produce new mechanisms underpinning social behavior if existing mechanisms, such as those that subserve maternal bonding and infant attachment, could be deployed equally well. In order for such established mechanisms to work, the brain has had to develop a means whereby other social relationships, and the complexity of behaviors that represent them, gain access to those neural processes that subserve the mother-infant social relationship.

In most mammals the neural and hormonal mechanisms of importance to maternal care are called into action from the moment of conception.[4] These endocrine mechanisms not only sustain pregnancy, but also suspend sexual activity and increase feeding, while priming other central neural mechanisms that ensure the mother's undivided attention to her offspring at parturition. Those neural events that are primed during pregnancy and triggered by the onset of parturition have much in common across mammals.[5] They are fundamental to maternal homeostasis, not only synchronizing the onset of maternal behavior with parturition and maternal effect, but also ensuring that its maintenance is accompanied by lactation and reproductive quiescence. Once established, maternal behavior can be called upon by a wide variety of sensory cues which may differ across species and may change within a species over the developmental period of the neonate.

The growth of the neocortex, a social lifestyle, and the emancipation of behavior from endocrine determinants have played a large part in the evolution of primate behavior, including parental behavior.[6] The importance of hormonal priming in pregnancy, which is critical for a rapid onset of maternal behavior in most mammals, is not required for the spontaneity of primate parental care, but experiental and cognitive factors are crucial.[7]

Thus, among monkeys and apes the findings that primiparous mothers give less adequate maternal care than do multiparous mothers have invariably been conducted on captive reared animals. Caged gorillas have been known to kill their first infant, and captive chimpanzee mothers are often afraid of their firstborn, refusing to touch them or allow them to suckle. In the wild, the case for incompetent care of infants rests on observations of nulliparous juveniles, because primiparous mothers normally give adequate care.[8] The only significant difference between multiparous and primiparous monkeys is the high anxiety and possessiveness of primiparae which contrasts with the firmness in rejection that is accomplished among multiparous mothers. Hence, the impaired maternal care of primiparous captive primates is likely to be a consequence of their lack of prior experience with infants, which in feral primates is rare even for primiparous females. In social primates, most females will have had some contact with infants prior to motherhood. Maternal behavior is a highly skilled performance, and because few infants are born to any one female, the loss of an infant through inexperience would be very costly. It is therefore significant that nulliparous females are frequently seen participating in the care of younger siblings.

Experimentally depriving monkeys of maternal or social contact for the first 8 months of their life has profound effects on their ability to be competent mothers. Their maternal care is at best indifferent or at worst abusive, requiring intervention for the infants to survive. Permitting social contact with peers does procure improvements in subsequent maternal care, but even this is less satisfactory than is that of feral mothers.[9] Although a socially deprived monkey may show inadequate maternal behavior to her first offspring, improvements have been found with subsequent offspring.[10] Once adequate care has been displayed to an infant, it is then likely to be shown to subsequent offspring, whereas if a mother is abusive, she is also likely to have been abusive to previous infants.

MOTHER-INFANT BONDING AND MANIPULATIONS OF THE MOTHER'S OPIOID SYSTEM

In recent years, interest has focused on the endogenous opioid system in learning, maternal behavior, and social reward.[11] Endogenous opioids are generally thought to mediate "the positive affect created by a rewarding situation."[12,13] Opioids are implicated in maternal behavior, as demonstrated by the effects of naloxone in preventing its induction in sheep,[14] and the potentiating effects of morphine on maternal acceptance in nonparturient ewes.[15] Suckling promotes the release of opioids in the medial preoptic area of sheep, while plasma levels of endorphins double in lactating women when

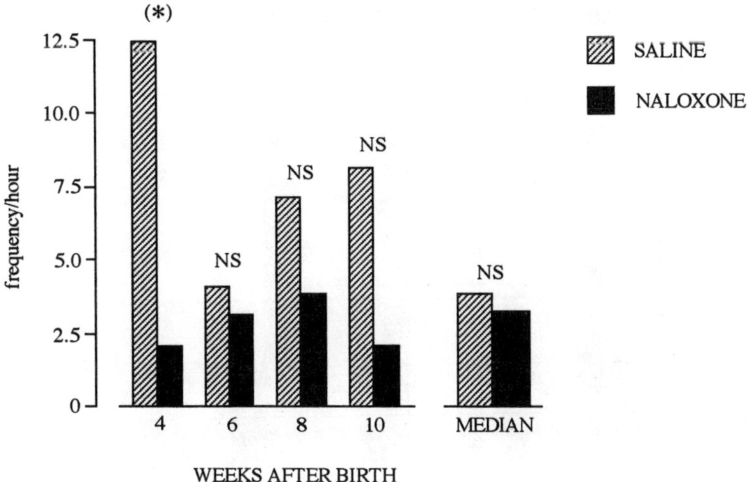

FIGURE 1. Median frequency (restrains/hour) of mother restraining infant. $^{*}p < 0.01$, Mann-Whitney U test.

their infants are suckling.[16] It has been suggested that activation of the endogenous opioid system in late pregnancy and suckling promote the "positive affect arising from maternal behaviour," and the mechanisms subserving this bonding might provide the neural basis from which other socially rewarding systems have evolved.[17] Our studies on naloxone treatment of rhesus monkey mothers have addressed the importance of opioids in primate maternal behavior. Naloxone reduced mother's grooming with other group members, and more significantly, they were less care-giving and protective towards their infants.[18] In the first weeks of life, when infant retrieval is normally very high, naloxone-treated mothers neglect their infants and show less retrieval when the infant moves away (FIG. 1). As infants approach 8 weeks of age, when a strong grooming relationship normally develops between mother and infant, mothers treated with naloxone failed to develop such a grooming relationship (FIG. 2). Moreover, they permitted other females to groom their infants (FIG. 2), while saline-treated control mothers were very possessive and protective of their infants.

In the postpartum period, a mother's social interactions are predominantly with her infant, and as just outlined, opiate receptor blockade has marked effects on this relationship. The infant is seldom rejected from suckling, but the mother's possessive preoccupation with the infant declines, she is not the normal attentive caregiver, and mother-infant interactions are invariably infant initiated. It is clear, therefore, that primates are not unlike other mammals in this respect; however, the consequences of opioid blockade in nonprimate mammals are much greater for the biological aspects of maternal behavior. In rodents and sheep, interference with the endogenous opioid system severely impairs maternal behavior including suckling, whereas monkeys neglect their caregiving but still permit suckling. Such differences may reflect the degree of emancipation from neuroendocrine influences that maternal behavior has

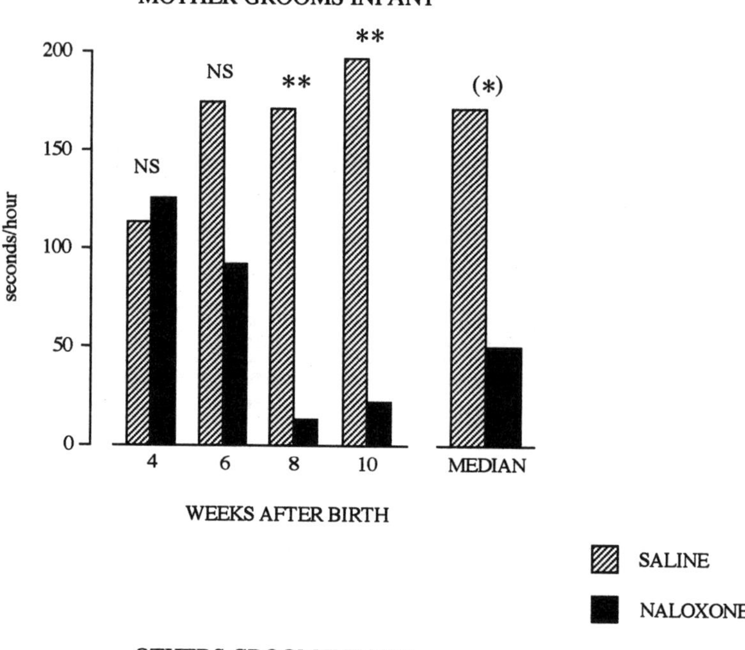

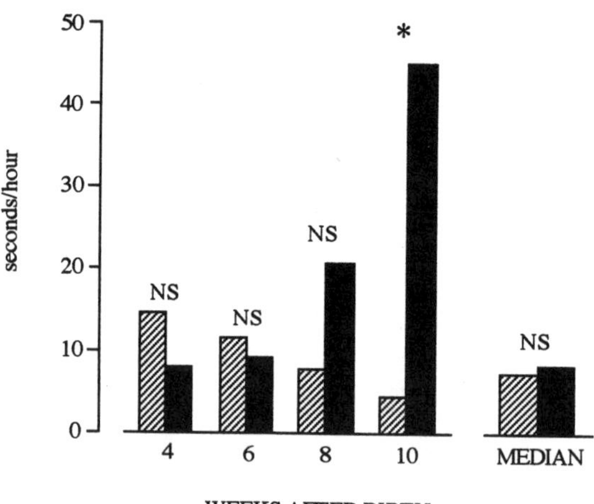

FIGURE 2. (**Top**) Median duration (seconds/hour) for grooming received by infants from their own mothers. $^{**}p < 0.01$; $^{*}p < 0.1$, Mann-Whitney U test. There was a tendency for the grooming by naloxone-treated mothers to decrease as the experiment progressed ($p < 0.1$, Friedman chi-squared = 13.4, $df = 3$). (**Bottom**) Median duration (seconds/hour) for grooming received by infants from monkeys other than their own mothers. $^{*}p < 0.05$, Mann-Whitney U test.

undergone in primates, while the affective components remain strongly linked with these hormonal limbic influences.

INFANT DEVELOPMENT AND INVOLVEMENT OF THE OPIOID SYSTEM IN ATTACHMENT

The early development of monkey social behavior occurs exclusively in the context of interactions with the mother. These early social interactions are almost totally under the mother's control in terms of both the amount and the kinds of interaction permitted. By 40 weeks of age, infants are considerably more independent from their mother, and much of their behavior is oriented towards peers. Nevertheless, mothers continue to monitor their infants and quickly intervene in response to risks arising during play.[19] The mother serves as a secure base from which the infant can obtain contact and grooming while developing and strengthening its social bonds with peers or other kin.

Administration of opioids has reduced the distress shown by diverse species of infants when separated from their mothers. For example, the opiate agonist morphine reduces distress vocalization rates in chicks,[20] guinea pigs,[21] puppies,[22] and rhesus monkeys.[23] Processes involving opioid reward may therefore play a role in infant attachment and in the development of social behavior as well as in maternal bonding. We investigated this in a study of young rhesus monkeys given acute treatment with naloxone and observed in their natal group.[24] Naloxone increased the duration of affiliative infant-mother contact and the time the infant spent on the nipple (FIG. 3). This occurred even at 1 year of age when the mothers were no longer lactating. Indeed, feeding was unaffected by naloxone treatment of infants, but play activity decreased and distress vocalizations increased (FIG. 4). These results may be interpreted in terms of opiate receptor blockade reducing the positive affect arising from new and developing social relationships with peers, as a result of which the young infant returns to mother as a secure base.

In the first 2 years of life, no difference was found between male and female infants with respect to the effects of naloxone on increasing their contact with mother. However, at puberty, the picture changes. Males spend equal portions of their time in the group with mother, with others, and alone. Treatment with naloxone results in significant increases in time with mother and decreases in time spent with others and alone (FIG. 5). Females, on the other hand, spend more than half their time alone, usually foraging and eating, and the remaining time is shared equally with mother and with others. Treatment with naloxone significantly increases the time spent with others, but not with mother, and decreases the time alone (FIG. 5). This suggests that at puberty females have developed other socially meaningful relationships to which they respond when challenged with naloxone, while males still rely on mother. Of course, pubertal males running to mother could invite aggression from the dominant males in the group, and the lack of other social affiliations would be a significant driving force to peripheralize such males and result in the well recognized male mobility from the natal social group.

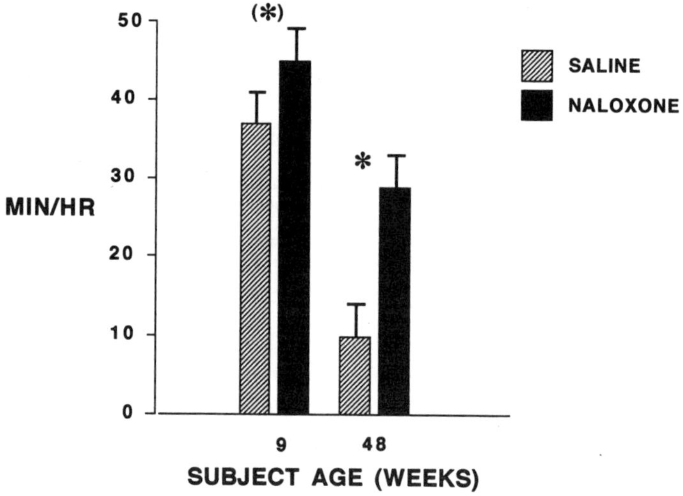

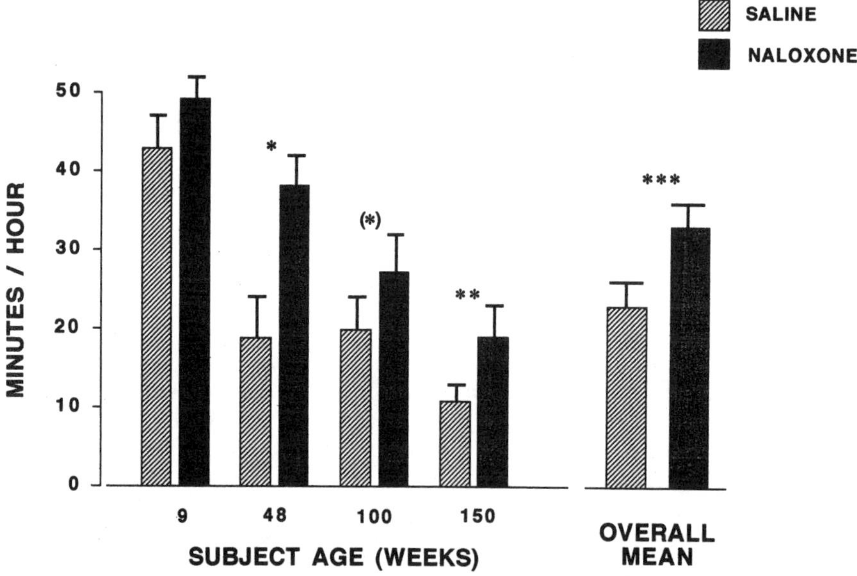

FIGURE 3. (**Top**) Duration of nipple contact. The 9- and 48-week old infants spent longer on the nipple after naloxone treatment, even though mothers attempted to get their infants off the nipple. (**Bottom**) Duration of infant mother contact. Apart from the earliest stages of the study when contact with mother was at a ceiling, infants spent longer in contact with their mothers when treated with naloxone. $^*p < 0.05$, $^{**}p < 0.01$, $^{***}p < 0.001$.

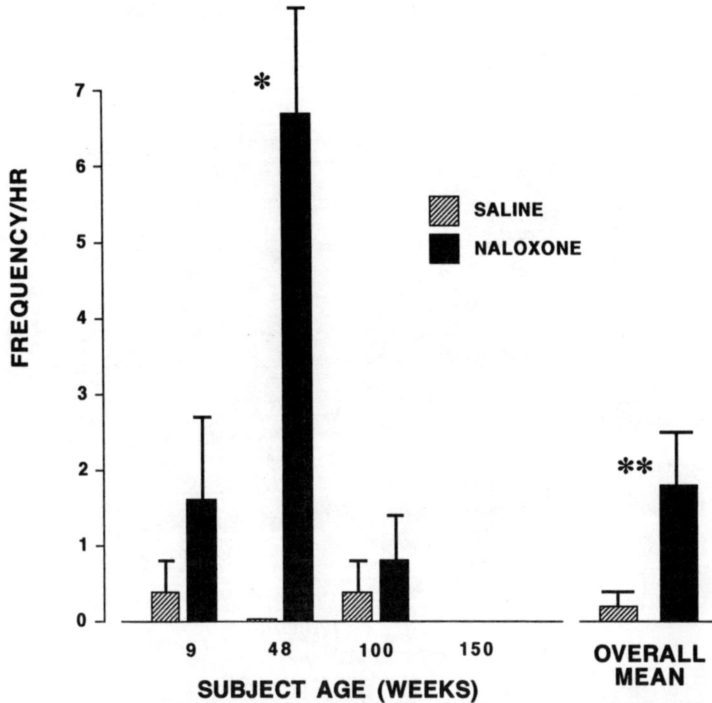

FIGURE 4. Young subjects increased contact "whoo" calls when treated with naloxone. Anova, $p < 0.01$. "Whoo" calls were seldom made when subjects were in contact with the mother.

OPIOIDS AND ADULT SOCIAL BEHAVIOR

This effect of opioid antagonism on the developing socialization of monkeys and its differential effects in males and females are maintained in the adult. Here, the way the endogenous opioid system is deployed differs in males and females according to differences in intrasexual behavioral strategies. Behavioral interactions in the monkey social group cluster into four main categories: investigation, aggression, affiliation, and sexual interaction. Investigation is high among and between males and females and invariably leads to another behavioral category. Among these, grooming is an important affiliative behavior that is influenced by naloxone and produces acute increases in CSF β-endorphin,[25] whereas the receipt of aggression leads to chronic increases in CSF β-endorphin.[26] As sexual behavior also has a substantial affiliative grooming component, it is likely that sexual behavior will also be accompanied by increased β-endorphin; but this has not been measured directly in the sexual context. However, naloxone treatment in both rhesus and talapoin monkeys blocks sexual activity.[27,28]

The way social behaviors are deployed is very different between males and females, and within sex it is very different according to rank.[17] Intrasexual aggression

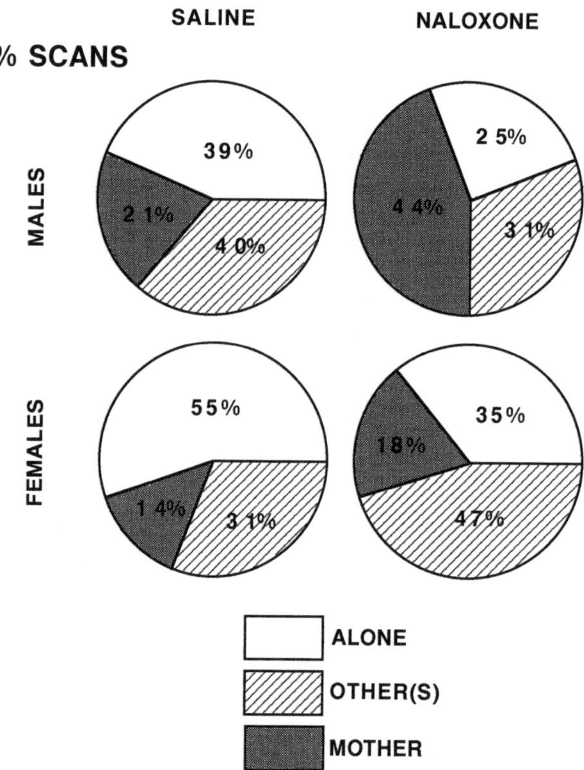

FIGURE 5. Both males and females spent increasingly more time alone as they increased in age. At 3 years of age a clear sex difference was seen in the effects of naloxone on the time infants spent with mother. Males increased contact time with mother, but females increased contact time with others when treated with naloxone.

is low among females and high among males, while the reverse is true for affiliative behavior, being high among females. No differences exist in chronic levels of β-endorphin in females, but among males, those of lowest rank have significantly higher levels of CSF β-endorphin than do others in the group.[17] Moreover, the opioid receptor seems to be downregulated in low ranking males, because challenges with naloxone fail to produce increases in levels of luteinizing hormone or testosterone, which are normally held low by opioid inhibition.[26] Hence, low ranking males that receive little affiliation and high levels of aggression paradoxically have a nonfunctional opioid system because of sustained activity in the system downregulating the receptor. If the endogenous opioids serve as the ''glue'' for social cohesion, then the attraction of the group for subordinate males is lost and may further explain why it is mainly males of low rank that are more likely to leave their natal group in the wild.

These experimental studies with naloxone in primates reveal an important role for the opioid system in a wide variety of social interactions including mother-infant,

infant-peer, and the affiliative, sexual, and aggressive interactions of adults. Release of central opioids is achieved by somatosensory stimulation, but the type of sensory stimulus and the context for its release are very different, ranging from parturition, suckling, and grooming to aggression. Moreover, the way that these life events and behaviors occur varies according to rank and is also very different in males and females. The outcome of these behavioral strategies for social cohesion is therefore very different in males and females. Females engage in the sort of behavior that is likely to acutely activate the opioid system at intervals contingent on affiliative social interactions. Males are more likely to activate the opioid system in the context of aggressive behavior, which in the case of subordinates is continuously a threatening presence. This chronic activation of the opioid system effectively deprives them of any social reward. Subordinate males are therefore more likely to leave their natal group, or if they stay, it is essential that they learn the social rules in order to reduce the aggression they receive from others. These rules entail a very low priority in the pecking order for females, for food, and for the receipt of affiliative behavior.

CONCLUSIONS

These studies illustrate the continuing significance of the brain's opioid system for the affective component of relationships throughout early social development and into the adult life of primate mammals. In evolutionary terms the mechanisms that underlie affect in these contexts have much in common with the mother-infant affect in other mammals. This is not to imply that the endorphins are the "affectional" peptide, because they have been shown to influence the release of other peptide transmitters in the limbic brain (oxytocin, vasopressin) as well as the classical neurotransmitters (noradrenaline, acetylcholine). Oxytocin and vasopressin are closely tied to "pair-bonding" in other mammals.[29,30]

What are the evolutionary developments that have enabled expansion of the affectional system deployed in mother-infant bonding to incorporate other contexts of social/affiliative relationships? In considering primates, strong interrelationships are beginning to emerge between the two important features noted earlier, neocortical expansion and matrilineal inheritance. These are common to all mammals that exhibit complex social organizations. The development of a larger neocortex has enabled behavior to occur at will, such that maternal affiliation may take place without pregnancy and parturition. This unique development in primate evolution has matched parturient females with nonparturient females in sustaining the behavioral potential for infant caregiving. Such an emancipation has only been evolutionarily possible with the development of a bigger brain, because any decision-taking processes in the context of maternal behavior need to be the right decision. Progression away from the synchronization of maternal behavior with the hormones of pregnancy and replacement with a system of cognitive control require exceptional cognitive abilities. These abilities are not inherited, but a larger brain enables social factors to take over from hormonal factors in predicting reproductive success. Hence, the requirement for maternal experience for adequate maternal care, experience that can be acquired during early social development outside the context of pregnancy and parturition.

From the available fossil records it appears that many mammalian lineages have evolved increased cranial capacity, but because it is claimed that the push for an exceptionally larger neocortex in primates has developed from complex social living, then differences in maternal and paternal lifestyles may have subjected brain evolution to differential selection pressures. Females provide social stability and group cohesion, are more affiliative than males, and maintain the continuity of the group over successive generations. Females are the primary caregivers with social rank of daughter, but not sons, being related to the matriline. This kind of inheritance is compatible with genomic imprinting which not only results in the development of a larger forebrain from maternally expressed alleles,[31] but the advantages of genomically imprinted inheritance are transmitted to both sons and daughters. Hence, the differential selection pressures operating through the matriline result in a larger neocortex which enables greater cognitive control over behavior.[32] For such control over behavior to be successful, the process of early social learning is essential for the development of normal affiliative relationships.

REFERENCES

1. WRANGHAM, R. W. 1987. Evolution of social structure. *In* Primate Societies. B. B. Smuts, D. L. Cheney, R. M. Seyfarth, R. W. Wrangham & T. T. Struhsaker, Eds.: 282-296. University of Chicago Press. Chicago, IL.
2. DUNBAR, R. I. M. 1992. Neocortex size as a constraint on group size in primates. J. Human Evol. **20:** 469-493.
3. BERMAN, C. 1983. Differentiation of relationships among rhesus monkey infants. *In* Primate Social Relationships: An Integrated Approach. Blackwell. Oxford.
4. ROSENBLATT, J. S. & H. I. SIEGEL. 1981. Factors governing the onset and maintenance of maternal behavior among nonprimate mammals: The role of hormonal and nonhormonal factors. *In* Parental Care in Mammals. D. J. Gubernick & P. H. Klopfer, Eds.: 13-76. Plenum Press. New York.
5. KEVERNE, E. B. 1988. Central mechanisms underlying the neural and neuroendocrine determinants of maternal behaviour. Psychoneuroendocrinology **14:** 155-161.
6. KEVERNE, E. B. 1995. Neurochemical changes accompanying the reproductive process: Their significance for maternal care in primates and other mammals. *In* Motherhood in Human and Nonhuman Primates. C. R. Pryce, R. D. Martin & D. Skuse, Eds.: 69-77. Karger. Basel.
7. HOLMAN, S. D. & R. W. GOY. 1995. Experimental and hormonal correlates of care-giving in rhesus macaques. *In* Motherhood in Human and Nonhuman Primates. C. R. Pryce, R. D. Martin & D. Skuse, Eds.: 87-93. Karger. Basel.
8. BLAFFER-HRDY, S. 1976. Care and exploitation of primate infants. Adv. Study Behav. **6:** 101-158.
9. RUPPENTHAL, G. C., M. K. HARLOW, C. D. EISELE, H. F. HARLOW & S. F. SUOMI. 1974. Development of peer interactions of monkeys reared in a nuclear family environment. Child Dev. **45:** 670-682.
10. RUPPENTHAL, G. C., G. L. ARLING, H. F. HARLOW, G. P. SACKETT & S. J. SUOMI. 1976. A 10-year perspective of motherless mother monkey behaviour. J. Abnorm. Psychol. **85:** 341-349.
11. OLSON, G. A., R. D. OLSON & A. J. KASTIN. 1990. Endogenous opiates. Peptides **11:** 1277-1304.
12. DUM, J. & A. HERZ. 1987. Opioids and motivation. Interdisciplinary Sci. Rev. **12:** 180-190.
13. PANKSEPP, J. 1981. Brain opioids—A neurochemical stubstrate for narcotic and social dependence. *In* Theory in Psychopharmacology. S. J. Cooper, Ed.: 149-175. Academic Press. London.
14. KENDRICK, K. M. & E. B. KEVERNE. 1989. Effects of intracerebroventricular infusions of naltrexone and phentolamine on central and peripheral oxytocin release and on

maternal behaviour induced by vaginocervical stimulation in the ewe. Brain Res. **505:** 329-332.

15. KEVERNE, E. B. & K. M. KENDRICK. 1991. Morphine and corticotrophin-releasing factor potentiate maternal acceptance in multiparous ewes after vaginocervical stimulation. Brain Res. **540:** 55-62.
16. FRANCESCHINI, R., P. L. VENTURINI, A. CATALDI, T. BARRECS, N. RAGNI & E. ROLANDI. 1989. Plasma beta-endorphin concentration during suckling in lactating women. Br. J. Obst. Gynaecol. **96:** 711-713.
17. KEVERNE, E. B. 1992. Primate social relationships: Their determinants and consequences. Adv. Study Behav. **21:** 1-37.
18. MARTEL, F. L., C. M. NEVISON, F. D. RAYMENT, M. J. A. SIMPSON & E. B. KEVERNE. 1993. Opioid receptor blockade reduces maternal affect and social grooming in rhesus monkeys. Psychoneuroendocrinology **18:** 307-321.
19. SIMPSON, M. J. A., M. A. GORE, M. JANUS & F. D. G. RAYMENT. 1989. Prior experience of risk and individual differences in enterprise shown by rhesus monkey infants in the second half of their first year. Primates **30:** 493-509.
20. PANKSEPP, J., T. VILBERG, N. J. BEAN, D. H. COY & A. J. GASKIN. 1978. Reduction of distress vocalization in chicks by opiate-like peptide. Brain Res. Bull. **3:** 663-667.
21. HERMAN, B. H. & J. PANKSEPP. 1978. Effects of morphine and naloxone on separation distress and approach attachment: Evidence of opiate mediation of social effect. Pharmacol. Biochem. and Behav. **9:** 213-220.
22. PANKSEPP, J., B. HERMAN, R. CONNER, P. BISHOP & J. O. P. SCOTT. 1978. The biology of social attachment: Opiates alleviate separation distress. Biol. Psychiatry **13:** 607-618.
23. KALIN, N. H., S. E. SHELTON & C. M. BARKSDALE. 1988. Opiate modulation of separation-induced distress in nonhuman primates. Brain Res. **440:** 285-292.
24. MARTEL, F. L., C. M. NEVISON, M. J. A. SIMPSON & E. B. KEVERNE. 1995. Effects of opioid receptor blockade on the social behavior of rhesus monkeys living in large family groups. Dev. Psychobiol. **28:** 71-84.
25. KEVERNE, E. B., N. D. MARTENEZ & B. TUITE. 1989. Beta-endorphin concentrations in cerebrospinal fluid of monkeys are influenced by grooming relationships. Psychoneuroendocrinology **14:** 155-161.
26. MARTENSZ, N. D., S. V. VELLUCCI, E. B. KEVERNE & J. HERBERT. 1986. β-endorphin levels in the cerebrospinal fluid of male talapoin monkeys in social groups related to dominance status and the luteinizing hormone response to naloxone. Neuroscience **3:** 651-658.
27. MELLER, R. E., E. B. KEVERNE & J. HERBERT. 1980. Behavioural and endocrine effects of naltrexone in male talapoin monkeys. Pharmacol. Biochem. Behav. **13:** 663-672.
28. FABRE-NYS, C., R. E. MELLER & E. B. KEVERNE. 1982. Opiate antagonists stimulate affiliative behavior in monkeys. Pharmacol. Biochem. and Behav. **16:** 653-659.
29. CARTER, C. S., J. R. WILLIAMS, D. WITT & T. R. INSEL. 1992. Oxytocin and social bonding. Ann. N.Y. Acad. Sci. **652:** 204-211.
30. WINSLOW, J. T., N. HASTINGS, C. S. CARTER, C. R. HARBAUGH & T. R. INSEL. 1993. A role for central vasopressin in pair bonding in monogamous voles. Nature **365:** 545-548.
31. ALLEN, N., K. LOGAN, G. LALLY, D. J. DRAGE, M. NORRIS & E. B. KEVERNE. 1995. Distribution of parthenogenetic cells in the mouse brain and their influence on brain development and behaviour. Proc. Natl. Acad. Sci. USA **92:** 10733-10717.
32. KEVERNE, E. B., F. L. MARTEL & C. M. NEVISON. 1996. Primate brain evolution: Genetic and functional considerations. Proc. Roy. Soc. Biol. Sci. **262:** 689-696.

18

Neuroanatomical Circuitry for Mammalian Maternal Behavior

Michael Numan and Teige P. Sheehan

This paper presents an overview of the neural circuitry underlying maternal behavior in mammals. Because most of this work has been done on the rat, our review concentrates on that species. The hormonal events of late pregnancy, in particular, rising estrogen and prolactin levels and declining progesterone levels, are necessary for stimulating the onset of maternal behavior at parturition in primiparous females of many mammalian species.[1] An important process to understand is the neural mechanisms influenced by "maternal hormones." Several recent reviews argue that maternal behavior is facilitated when the tendency to approach infant stimuli and engage in maternal behavior is greater than the tendency to avoid or withdraw from such stimuli.[2–4] This kind of analysis suggests that the hormonal events of late pregnancy act on brain mechanisms to either decrease fear/aversion of infant stimuli or increase attraction/approach towards infant stimuli, or both. These possibilities are illustrated in FIGURE 1.

Several pieces of evidence support this scheme: (1) Nulliparous females of many mammalian species avoid or attack neonates.[1] Indeed, nulliparous female rats move out of the preferred part of their home cage if pups are placed there.[5] (2) Although nonpregnant rats and sheep either show no preference for or actively avoid olfactory stimuli associated with neonates, animals that have been exposed to the hormonal events of late pregnancy show a strong attraction to such stimuli.[6,7] (3) Although the nulliparous female rat will not show immediate maternal responsiveness towards its young, if she is cohabited with them, she will come to show maternal behavior after about 5-7 days.[1] This latency to respond can be shortened by a hormone regimen that mimics the endocrine changes of late pregnancy.[1] Importantly, this latency can also be reduced in nonhormone-primed nulliparous females by making them anosmic.[8] Such females show maternal behavior after about only 24 hours of pup exposure. These findings have been interpreted to mean that nulliparous females find olfactory stimuli from young aversive and that maternal behavior will occur only after the aversive nature of such stimuli has been reduced by either habituation, hormonal effects, or experimentally induced anosmia.[2,4] The effects of anosmia on maternal behavior in nulliparous rats support the model shown in FIGURE 1A: approach and attraction to nonolfactory stimuli may be relatively high in the absence of hormone treatment, and the hormonal events of late pregnancy downregulate the aversion-producing influence of pup odors.[3] However, the fact that anosmic virgins do not

This work was supported by National Science Foundation grant IBN 9319315 (to M.N.).

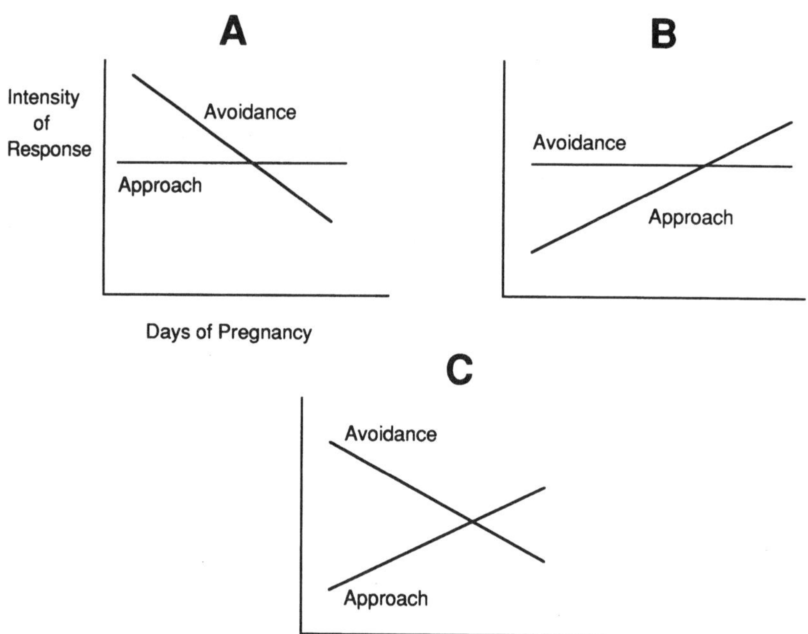

FIGURE 1. Three alternative approach-avoidance models of the onset of maternal behavior at parturiton. Maternal behavior occurs when central neural approach systems are more active than central neural avoidance systems with respect to infant-related stimuli. In **A** the physiological events of pregnancy primarily decrease avoidance, in **B** these physiological factors promote approach responses, and in **C** avoidance systems are depressed and approach systems are activated towards the end of pregnancy.

show immediate maternal behavior suggests that hormones probably act to both decrease the aversive qualities and increase the attractive qualities of young in parturient females.

The present chapter provides a partial and preliminary neural substrate for approach-avoidance models of maternal responsiveness. First, we discuss elements of an excitatory neural system for maternal behavior in the rat that may regulate approach and attraction to pup-related stimuli as well as the performance of particular maternal behaviors. Then we discuss evidence for a neural system that may regulate avoidance and aversion of pup-related stimuli.

THE APPROACH/PERFORMANCE SYSTEM

FIGURE 2A shows a cross-section through the rostral hypothalamus at the level of the medial preoptic area (MPOA) and ventral part of the bed nucleus of the stria terminalis (VBST). These two regions play a pivotal role in the regulation of maternal behavior in rats:[1] Application of estradiol or prolactin to the MPOA/VBST stimulates

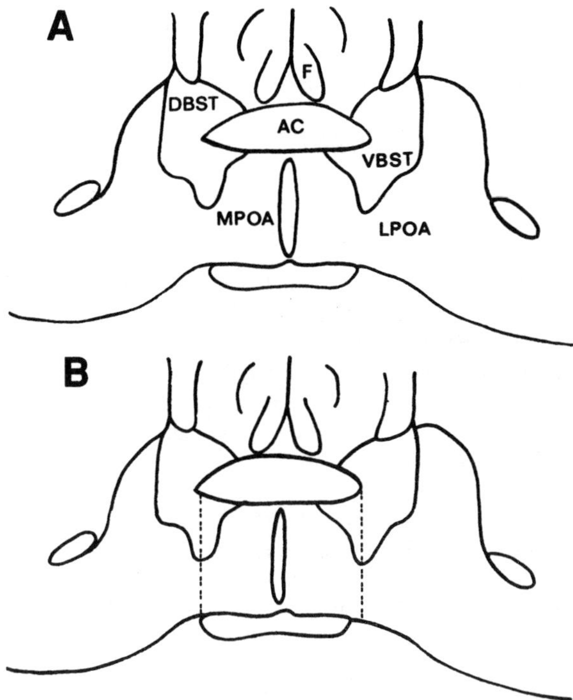

FIGURE 2. Frontal sections through the level of the preoptic area. (**A**) Location of critical cell nuclei. (**B**) A diagrammatic representation of knife cuts (shown in *dashed lines*) that sever the lateral connections of the medial preoptic area and part of the ventral bed nucleus of the stria terminalis. Such cuts disrupt maternal behavior. AC = anterior commissure; DBST = dorsal bed nucleus of the stria terminalis; F = Fornix; LPOA = lateral preoptic area; MPOA = medial preoptic area; VBST = ventral bed nucleus of the stria terminalis.

maternal behavior,[9,10] and destruction of MPOA/VBST cell bodies with an excitotoxic amino acid disrupts established maternal behavior.[11,12] Finally, knife cuts that sever the lateral connections of MPOA/VBST neurons (Fig. 2B) also disrupt maternal behavior.[13]

Species-typical behaviors have been divided into appetitive (motivational) and consummatory (performance) components.[14,15] The appetitive component consists of those behaviors that bring the organism in contact with an attractive or desired stimulus object, whereas the consummatory component is made up of behaviors that are performed once contact has been made with the stimulus object. Because the appropriate behavioral tests have not been performed, it is currently not clear if MPOA/VBST lesions interfere with the appetitive or the motivational aspects of maternal behavior; however, they clearly interfere with the consummatory component. In some cases MPOA/VBST damage completely eliminates maternal behavior. After a brief investigatory period, the pups are basically ignored, and retrieving, nest building, and nursing do not occur. Such behavior is certainly consistent with an interference with motivational mechanisms. In other cases, however, although preoptic damage produces complete elimination of retrieval behavior (hoarding behavior still occurs, which shows that the lesions do not produce a general oral motor deficit), some nursing and nest building still occur.[1] Clearly, in these cases preoptic damage does not globally interfere with all aspects of maternal motivation. Future work is needed to determine if these differential lesion effects are due to differences in lesion size and/or location. Also, we need to examine preoptic-lesioned females on tests that can dissociate motivational disturbances from interference with the neural mechanisms regulating consummatory responses.[14]

To understand the function of the MPOA/VBST in maternal behavior, we have taken a neuroanatomical approach. By uncovering the structures to which preoptic efferents project to influence maternal responsiveness, we might understand the neural mechanism of action. Our ongoing research indicates that MPOA/VBST efferents project to a variety of regions to influence maternal behavior and that this circuitry appears to interact with structures that may promote both the appetitive and the consummatory aspects of maternal behavior and, in addition, may depress avoidance responses to pup-related stimuli.

An initial hypothesis was that MPOA projections to the ventral tegmental area (VTA) in the midbrain influenced maternal responsiveness.[16] The ventral tegmental area contributes neurons to the mesotelencephalic dopamine system, with major termination sites in ventral striatal structures, which include the nucleus accumbens.[17] The mesotelencephalic dopamine system is involved in the appetitive or motivational aspects of a variety of behaviors, and the system acts to potentiate the ability of biologically significant stimuli to activate appropriate responses.[14,17] Our initial findings supported this hypothesis. When a unilateral knife cut that severed the lateral connections of the MPOA/VBST region was paired with a contralateral electrical lesion of the ventral tegmental area, the maternal behavior of postpartum females, particularly retrieving behavior, was disrupted.

Other evidence also supports the importance of ventral tegmental area dopaminergic systems in maternal behavior. Hansen's group[18,19] has shown that the application of 6-hydroxydopamine (6OHDA), a dopamine neurotoxin, to either the ventral tegmental area or the nucleus accumbens specifically disrupts retrieval behavior in postpartum rats. This disruption of maternal retrieving does not occur under all conditions, however. If females with 6OHDA lesions of the nucleus accumbens are separated from their pups for 3 hours, when the pups are returned, they are quickly retrieved.[19] This finding, in particular, suggests that the mesotelencephalic dopamine system may regulate the motivation to retrieve pups rather than the ability to perform the retrieval response.

Although damage to the mesotelencephalic dopamine system does not interfere with retrieval behavior under all conditions, damage to MPOA/VBST efferents does appear to permanently abolish retrieval behavior.[20] This latter finding suggests that MPOA/VBST efferents may project to other regions in addition to ventral tegmental area dopamine neurons to influence maternal behavior. This view fits with the findings of Numan and Numan[21] which indicate that preoptic efferents not only may synapse in the ventral tegmental area to influence maternal behavior, but also may pass through the ventral tegmental area to terminate in more caudal brainstem structures. They found that when a unilateral knife cut that severed the lateral connections of the MPOA/VBST region was paired with a contralateral coronal knife cut caudal to the ventral tegmental area, all aspects of maternal behavior were disrupted in postpartum rats. FIGURE 3 diagrams the effective brain damage. Note that the brainstem knife cut passes through the retrorubral field. Importantly, the retrorubral field contains the A8 dopamine neurons which also contribute to the mesotelencephalic dopamine system.[22] Perhaps it is this dopamine system, rather than that arising from the ventral tegmental area, which is important in certain aspects of maternal behavior.

The evidence just presented indicates that preoptic projections to the brainstem are important in maternal behavior, but the exact site of termination has not been clearly defined. If the preoptic area is an important integrative region for maternal behavior, it is certainly possible that the preoptic area projects to more than just one region to influence maternal behavior. Indeed, an extreme "maternal behavior center" hypothesis would argue that the hormonally primed preoptic area projects to some regions to facilitate the appetitive aspects of maternal behavior, projects to other regions to potentiate consummatory components, and projects to still other neuronal groups to depress aversive reactions to pup stimuli. If the particular neurons within the MPOA/VBST region that are involved in maternal behavior were known, then we could trace their connections to get a more complete understanding of the neural circuitry of maternal behavior. To reach this objective, we turned to the use of Fos immunocytochemistry. Fos is a nuclear protein, the product of the immediate early gene c-*fos,* and it serves as a transcriptional factor that can alter the expression of other genes.[23] Importantly, Fos detection has been used as a marker for neuronal activation,[23] and our initial approach was to compare the expression of Fos in MPOA/VBST of postpartum females under two different conditions.[24] Primiparous lactating females were separated from their pups on day 5 postpartum. On day 8 postpartum, females were exposed to pups or candy for 2 hours. All females exposed to pups showed full maternal behavior. Following the 2-hour test the females were sacrificed, and their brains were immunocytochemically processed for the detection of Fos. FIGURE 4 shows that maternal females had many more Fos-labeled cells in the MPOA/VBST than did females that were not exposed to pups. We observed a similar difference when we compared the preoptic Fos pattern of nulliparous females that had shown maternal behavior after cohabitation with pups with that of nulliparous females that had not yet shown maternal behavior towards pups. The finding that parental animals show a greater Fos response in the preoptic area than do nonparental animals has been confirmed in several laboratories.[25–27] In a second study,[28] we showed that the increased expression of Fos in MPOA/VBST neurons of maternal females occurred even if such females had their olfactory bulbs and nipples removed (such females show normal maternal behavior). This result suggested that the induction of Fos in the MPOA/VBST was not simply the result of olfactory and suckling stimulation; rather, it was closely tied to the performance of maternal behavior. This finding lent credence to the view that Fos was marking those neurons that were regulating maternal responsiveness and that if we could uncover the regions to which these neurons projected, we would begin to outline some of the circuits of maternal behavior.

To this end we first performed a neural tract-tracing study using the sensitive anterograde tracer *Phaseolus vulgaris* leucoagglutinin (PHAL).[12] In postpartum rats, PHAL was iontophoretically injected into the VBST and adjoining MPOA. After a 1-week survival period the brains were immunocytochemically processed for the

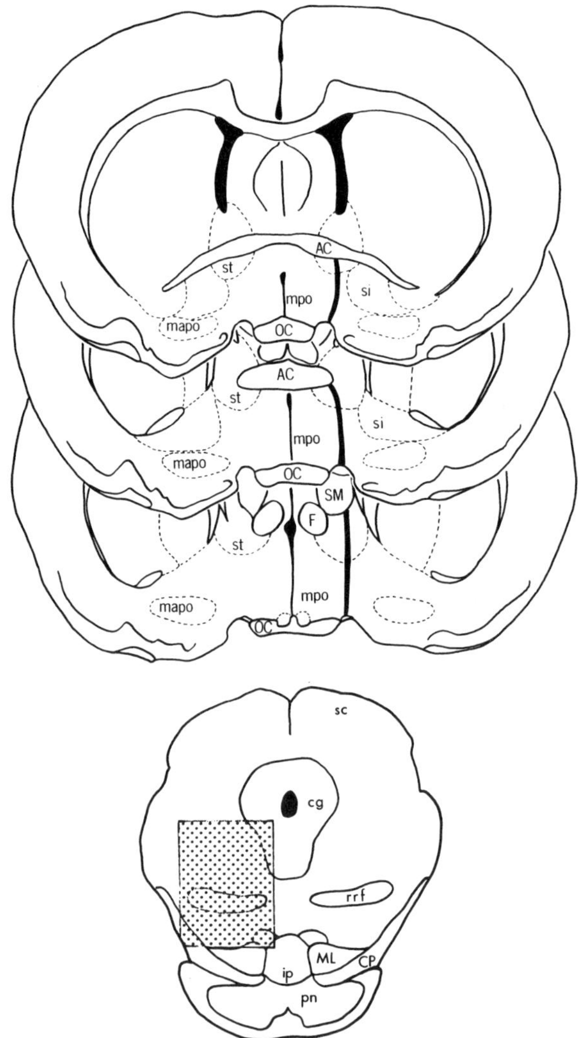

FIGURE 3. Diagram of a unilateral knife cut that severs the lateral connections of the medial preoptic area paired with a contralateral knife cut caudal to the ventral tegmental area. The *top three sections* show the extent of the preoptic knife cut (*heavy black line*). The *last section* illustrates the knife cut located caudal to the ventral tegmental area (*stippled area*). AC = anterior commissure; cg = central gray (same as periaqueductal gray); CP = cerebral peduncle; F = fornix; ip = interpeduncular nucleus; mapo = magnocellular preoptic nucleus; ML = medial lemniscus; mpo = medial preoptic area; OC = optic chiasm; pn = pontine nuclei; rrf = retrorubral field; sc = superior colliculus; si = substantia innominata; SM = stria medullaris; st = bed nucleus of stria terminalis. Reproduced with permission from Numan and Numan.[21]

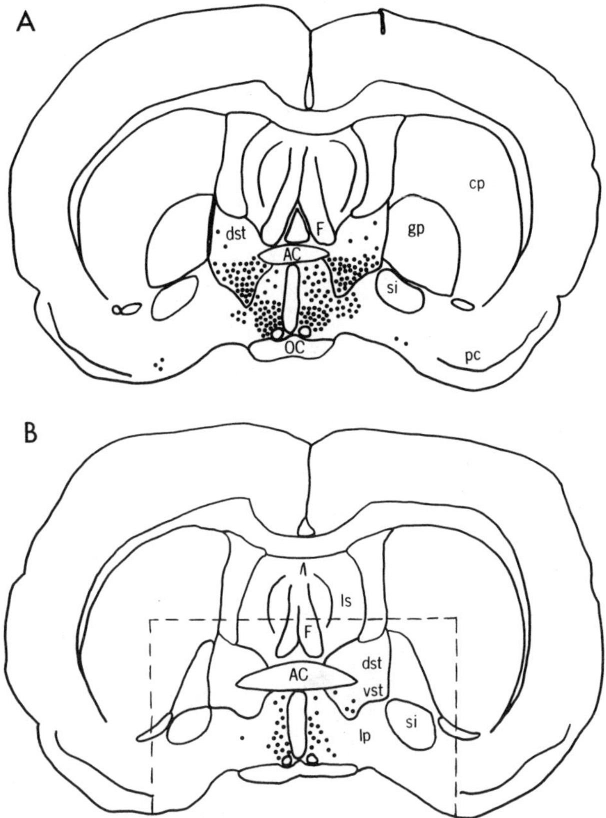

FIGURE 4. Distribution of cells labeled with Fos-like immunoreactivity on a single frontal section through the preoptic area of a postpartum female rat that was exposed to pups and showed maternal behavior (**A**) and from a postpartum female that was exposed to candy and therefore did not show maternal behavior (**B**). Each dot represents five labeled cells. The area analyzed in both sections is represented in the lower section by *dashed lines.* cp = caudate-putamen; dst = dorsal bed nucleus of stria terminalis; F = fornix; gp = globus pallidus; lp = lateral preoptic area; ls = lateral septum; OC = optic chiasm; pc = piriform cortex; si = substantia innominata; vst = ventral bed nucleus of stria terminalis. Modified from Numan and Numan.[24]

localization of PHAL-labeled neural pathways. Some of the results are shown in FIGURE 5. Ascending projections from the MPOA/VBST had a major termination site in the lateral septum, while descending efferents provided significant input to the ventromedial nucleus of the hypothalamus, ventral tegmental area, retrorubral field, and periaqueductal gray. This study provided candidate sites to which MPOA/VBST neurons might project in their influence over maternal behavior. Because the PHAL procedure traced the efferents of a heterogeneous population of neurons, many of these neurons may not have been involved in maternal behavior. What we really needed to determine was the sites of termination of MPOA/VBST neurons that

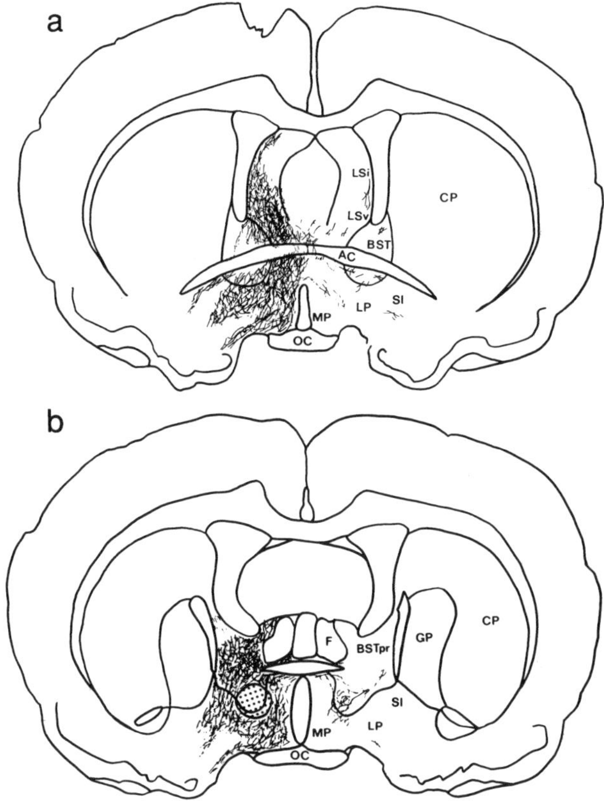

FIGURE 5. *Legend is on facing page.*

express Fos during a maternal episode. To do this we recently completed a double-labeling immunocytochemical study[29] which detected the presence of both Fos and a sensitive retrograde tracer, wheat germ agglutinin. Using the PHAL findings as a guide, wheat germ agglutinin was injected into different sites in different postpartum rats and the degree to which MPOA and VBST Fos neurons projected to each of these regions was determined.

Fully maternal primiparous rats were separated from their litters on the afternoon of day 4 postpartum. On day 5 postpartum a 1% wheat germ agglutinin solution was iontophoretically injected unilaterally into one of the following regions: lateral septum, ventromedial nucleus of the hypothalamus, ventral tegmental area, retrorubral field, and periaqueductal gray. We also injected wheat germ agglutinin into a sixth site, the lateral habenula. (See FIGURE 5 for the locations of these regions.) Although the lateral habenula receives only weak inputs from MPOA/VBST,[12] there is evidence for its involvement in maternal behavior.[30] On day 7 postpartum, pups were returned to females for a 2-hour test, and only those females showing full maternal behavior

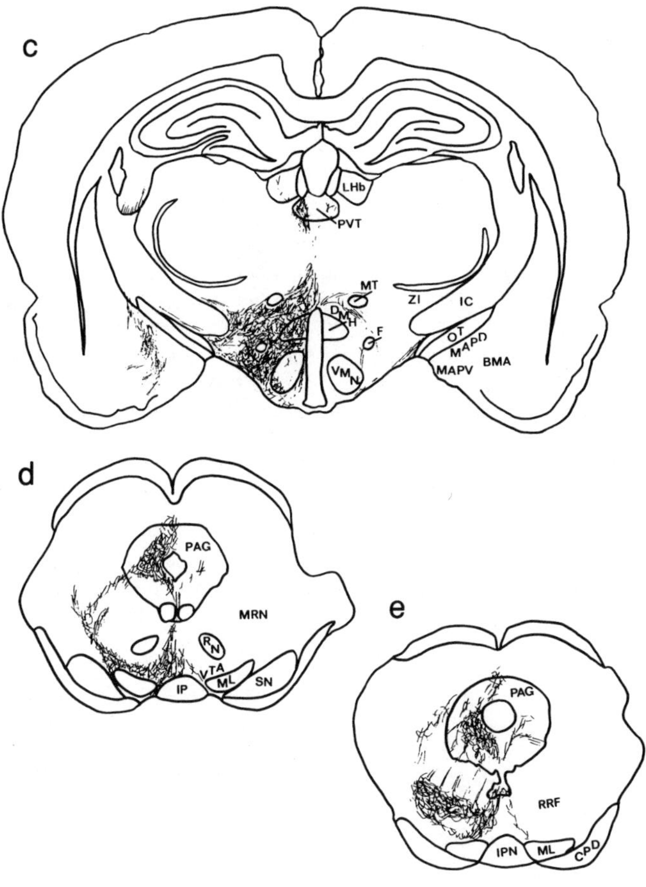

FIGURE 5. A series of frontal sections from rostral to caudal (**a** through **e**) showing the distribution of PHAL fibers after an injection of PHAL into the ventral bed nucleus of the stria terminalis and adjoining medial preoptic area. The injection site is indicated by *stippling* in section **b.** AC = anterior commissure; BMA = basomedial nucleus of amygdala; BST = bed nucleus of stria terminalis; BSTpr = principal subnucleus of bed nucleus of stria terminalis; CP = caudate-putamen; CPD = cerebral peduncle; DMH = dorsomedial hypothalamus; F = fornix; GP = globus pallidus; IC = internal capsule; IP or IPN = interpeduncular nucleus; LHb = lateral habenula; LP = lateral preoptic area; LSi = lateral septum, intermediate part; LSv = lateral septum, ventral part; MAPD = posterodorsal medial amygaloid nucleus; MAPV = posteroventral medial amygdaloid nucleus; ML = medial lemniscus; MP = medial preoptic area; MRN = midbrain reticular nucleus; MT = mammillothalamic tract; OC = optic chiasm; OT = optic tract; PAG = periaqueductal gray; PVT = paraventricular thalamus. RN = red nucleus; RRF = retrorubral field; SI = substantia innominata; SN = substantia nigra; VTA = ventral tegmental area; ZI = zona incerta. Modified from Numan and Numan.[12]

TABLE 1. Mean (± SEM) Number of Fos-Expressing Neurons in the MPOA and VBST of Females Tested with or without Pups

Group	n	MPOA	VBST
VTA	10	798.40 ± 69.75	459.60 ± 39.23
PAG	8	861.13 ± 97.07	415.25 ± 17.35
LHb	8	907.50 ± 55.23	376.63 ± 28.86
RRF	5	774.60 ± 65.95	423.40 ± 28.86
LS	3	908.67 ± 175.06	381.33 ± 47.74
VMN	7	738.86 ± 49.55	406.29 ± 29.04
No pup	17	261.65 ± 27.30[a]	94.42 ± 11.32[a]

Abbreviations: LHb = lateral habenula; LS = lateral septum; MPOA = medial preoptic area; PAG = periaqueductal gray; RRF = retrorubral field; VBST = ventral part of the bed nucleus of the stria terminalis; VMN = ventromedial nucleus of the hypothalamus; VTA = ventral tegmental area.

[a] Significantly different from remaining groups, $p < 0.05$.

TABLE 2. Mean (± SEM) Number of WGA-Labeled Neurons in the MPOA and VBST of Maternal Females with WGA Injections into Different Sites

Group	n	MPOA	VBST
VTA	10	430.50 ± 63.46[a]	522.10 ± 66.55[b]
PAG	8	181.25 ± 31.14	219.00 ± 39.19[c]
LHb	8	79.13 ± 21.61	59.00 ± 15.31
RRF	5	252.00 ± 35.15	523.80 ± 38.53[b]
LS	3	1278.67 ± 245.98[d]	187.00 ± 31.57
VMN	7	1820.57 ± 114.22[e]	558.71 ± 49.46[b]

Abbreviations: LHb = lateral habenula; LS = lateral septum; MPOA = medial preoptic area; PAG = periaqueductal gray; RRF = retrorubral field; VBST = ventral part of the bed nucleus of the stria terminalis; VMN = ventromedial nucleus of the hypothalamus; VTA = ventral tegmental area; WGA = wheat germ agglutinin.

[a] Significantly greater than PAG and LHb, $p < 0.05$.

[b] Significantly greater than PAG, LHb, and LS, $p < 0.05$.

[c] Significantly greater than LHb, $p < 0.05$.

[d] Signficantly greater than VTA, PAG, LHb, and RRF, $p < 0.05$.

[e] Significantly greater than remaining groups, $p < 0.05$.

upon reexposure to pups remained in the study. Following the 2-hour test the females were perfused and their brains were immunocytochemically processed for the localization of wheat germ agglutinin and Fos. Neurons labeled with wheat germ agglutinin contained blue cytoplasm, neurons labeled with Fos contained a brown nucleus, and double-labeled cells had both a brown nucleus and blue cytoplasm. Brain sections were microscopically examined, and the number and location of each type of labeled neuron were determined for three consecutive frontal hemisections (ipsilateral to the

TABLE 3. Mean (± SEM) Number of Double-Labeled Neurons in MPOA and VBST of Maternal Females with WGA Injections into Different Sites

Group	*n*	MPOA	VBST
VTA	10	26.10 ± 5.20	46.30 ± 5.67[a]
PAG	8	27.50 ± 5.32	31.38 ± 5.44[a]
LHb	8	3.88 ± 0.99	4.13 ± 1.43
RRF	5	12.80 ± 3.86	53.40 ± 6.98[b]
LS	3	98.33 ± 23.56[c]	12.00 ± 2.08
VMN	7	170.00 ± 19.17[d]	44.71 ± 6.16[a]

Abbreviations: LHb = lateral habenula; LS = lateral septum; MPOA = medial preoptic area; PAG = periaqueductal gray; RRF = retrorubral field; VBST = ventral part of the bed nucleus of the stria terminalis; VMN = ventromedial nucleus of the hypothalamus; VTA = ventral tegmental area; WGA = wheat germ agglutinin.

[a] Significantly greater than LHb and LS, $p < 0.05$.

[b] Significantly greater than LHb, LS, and PAG, $p < 0.05$.

[c] Significantly greater than VTA, PAG, LHb, and RRF, $p < 0.05$.

[d] Significantly greater than remaining groups, $p < 0.05$.

site of wheat germ agglutinin injection) through the MPOA and VBST. A separate series of postpartum females was treated exactly like the maternal females just described except that they were exposed to candy instead of pups for their 2-hour test on day 7. These females will be referred to as the no-pup (NP) females.

TABLE 1 shows the mean number of Fos-labeled neurons in the MPOA and VBST for each group. Each group that interacted with pups, irrespective of the site of wheat germ agglutinin injection, had more neurons that expressed Fos-like immunoreactivity than did females that were not exposed to pups. TABLE 2 shows the mean number of wheat germ agglutinin-labeled cells in the MPOA and VBST of maternal females with wheat germ agglutinin injections into different sites. The results indicate that the MPOA projects most strongly to the lateral septum, ventromedial nucleus of the hypothalamus, and ventral tegmental area, while the VBST projects most strongly to the ventral tegmental area, retrorubral field, and ventromedial nucleus of the hypothalamus. The important question, however, is the degree to which these various projections are comprised of Fos-containing neurons that are activated during maternal behavior. TABLE 3 shows the number of double-labeled cells in the MPOA and VBST for each of the maternal groups, and FIGURE 6 depicts the percentage of Fos-expressing neurons in the MPOA and VBST that projected to each wheat germ agglutinin injection site. Fos-expressing neurons in the MPOA of maternal females project most strongly to the ventromedial nucleus of the hypothalamus and lateral septum. Fos-expressing neurons in the VBST project most strongly to the retrorubral field, ventral tegmental area, and ventromedial nucleus of the hypothalamus.

FIGURE 7 depicts the degree to which a particular circuit contains Fos-labeled neurons for maternal females in each of the wheat germ agglutinin injection groups, and the data, expressed as the percentage of wheat germ agglutinin-labeled cells that also contain Fos, emphasize the importance of MPOA and VBST projections to

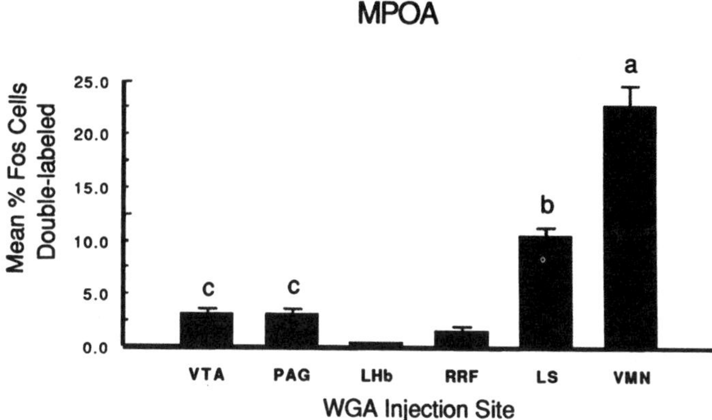

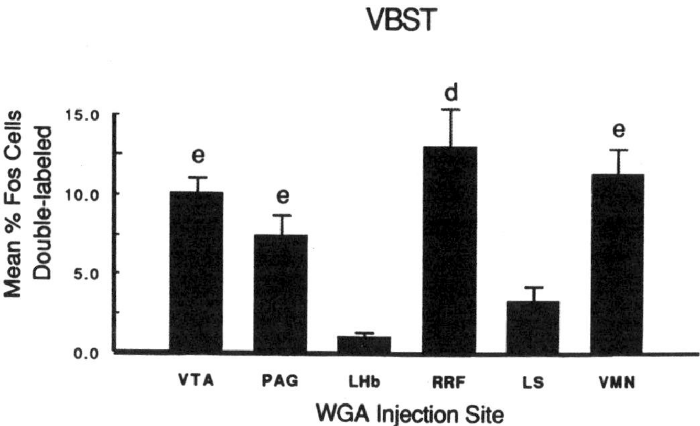

FIGURE 6. Mean (+ SEM) percentage of Fos-containing cells in the medial preoptic area (MPOA) and ventral bed nucleus of stria terminalis (VBST) that are also labeled with wheat germ agglutinin (WGA) after WGA injections into one of the following sites: ventral tegmental area (VTA); periaqueductal gray (PAG); lateral habenula (LHb); retrorubral field (RRF); lateral septum (LS); or ventromedial hypothalamus (VMN). [a]Significantly greater than remaining groups; [b]significantly greater than VTA, PAG, LHb, RRF; [c]significantly greater than LHb; [d]significantly greater than LHb, PAG, LS; [e]significantly greater than LHb, LS. p's < 0.05.

periaqueductal gray. In comparing FIGURE 7 with FIGURE 6, we can conclude that although a relatively small percentage of Fos-expressing neurons in the MPOA and VBST projects to periaqueductal gray, those neurons make up a relatively large percentage of the VBST-to-periaqueductal gray and MPOA-to-periaqueductal gray projection.

Comparisons of the data for maternal females with the data for no-pup females indicated that the number of double-labeled cells was much greater in the maternal

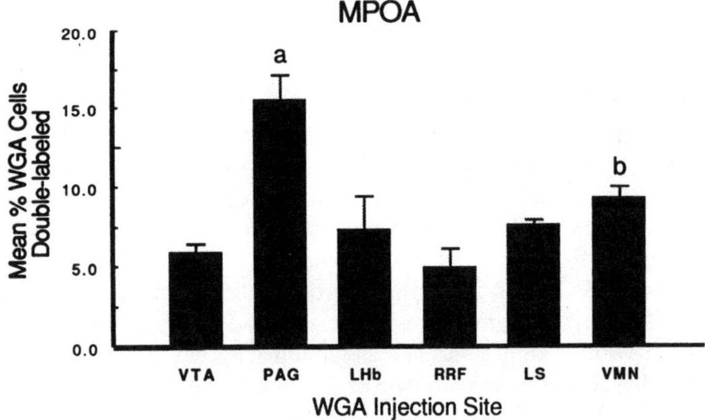

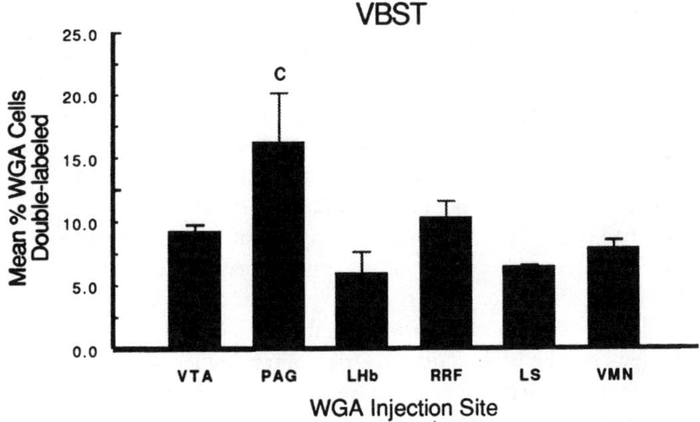

FIGURE 7. Mean (+ SEM) percentage of wheat germ agglutinin (WGA) containing cells in the medial preoptic area (MPOA) and ventral bed nucleus of stria terminalis (VBST) that are also labeled with Fos after WGA injections into one of the following sites: ventral tegmental area (VTA); periaqueductal gray (PAG); lateral habenula (LHb); retrorubral field (RRF); lateral septum (LS); or ventromedial hypothalamus (VMN). [a]Significantly greater than remaining groups; [b]significantly greater than RRF; [c]significantly greater than VTA, LHb, LS, and VMN. p's < 0.05.

females. This data suggests that our anatomical findings are relevant to neuronal circuits that are activated during maternal behavior.

In examining FIGURE 6, if we assume that each Fos-expressing neuron projected to only one of the sites into which we injected wheat germ agglutinin, then we can conclude that we have accounted for the termination sites of approximately 40% of the neurons in the MPOA and VBST that express Fos during maternal behavior. Although this number is impressive, it still leaves 60% of the critical neurons unaccounted for. Many of these neurons may be local interneurons, and the remainder would have to project to regions outside the sites of our wheat germ agglutinin injections.

To summarize, these results emphasize the importance of MPOA projections to the lateral septum, ventromedial nucleus of the hypothalamus, and periaqueductal gray and VBST projections to the retrorubral field, periaqueductal gray, and ventral tegmental area for maternal behavior control. Other projections may also be important, but a picture is now emerging which suggests that the MPOA/VBST may project to a variety of regions to influence maternal behavior.

Projections of MPOA Fos-expressing neurons to the lateral septum and ventromedial nucleus of the hypothalamus fit with work on the involvement of these regions in parental behavior.[31,32] Since the lateral septum may be involved in suppressing aggressive tendencies,[33] perhaps preoptic projections to the lateral septum play a role in decreasing the likelihood of pup-attacking behavior. In the next section we discuss the ventromedial nucleus of the hypothalamus in more detail in the context of a central aversion system. For the time being, note that MPOA projections to this region may suppress aversive reactions toward pup-related stimuli.

The strong projection of VBST neurons to the retrorubral field in maternal females fits well with previous work from our laboratory. We argued that MPOA/VBST neurons involved in maternal behavior project through the ventral tegmental area to terminate in more caudal brainstem regions,[21] and the retrorubral field lies caudal to the ventral tegmental area. Since the retrorubral field contributes to the ascending mesotelencephalic dopamine system,[22] it may be the source of dopaminergic influences over maternal behavior. Therefore, VBST projections to the retrorubral field may play a role in the appetitive aspects of maternal behavior, enhancing the attraction value of pup-related stimuli and the rewarding effects of behaving maternally.[34] The retrorubral field may also be concerned with the consummatory aspects of maternal behavior, particularly the regulation of retrieving and other oral maternal activities. Descending efferents from the retrorubral field project to the pontomedullary reticular formation which contains neurons that project to trigeminal sensory and motor nuclei.[35]

Our double-labeling Fos-wheat germ agglutinin study also emphasizes the importance of MPOA and VBST projections to the periaqueductal gray. This is important because coronal knife cuts caudal to the ventral tegmental area which disrupt maternal behavior[21] would sever projections of the MPOA/VBST to parts of the periaqueductal gray. Inasmuch as recent anatomical work has revealed that the caudal periaqueductal gray projects strongly to the trigeminal sensory complex, including the principal sensory nucleus,[36] it seems likely that MPOA/VBST projections to periaqueductal gray are involved in regulating trigeminal sensorimotor integration related to retrieval behavior.[37] Another role for preoptic to periaqueductal gray projections may be related to findings which indicate the involvement of the periaqueductal gray in fear and defensive behavior.[38] Perhaps preoptic projections to the periaqueductal gray depress aversive or avoidance responses toward pup-related stimuli.

Our results indicate that very few Fos-expressing neurons in the MPOA and VBST project to the lateral habenula. However, the role of the lateral habenula in maternal behavior control may be exerted in other ways, for example, through its direct projections to midbrain dopamine neurons.[30]

The Fos-wheat germ agglutinin double-labeling results implicate several circuits in maternal behavior control. These results are correlational in nature, however, and therefore some of the circuits may not be involved in directly influencing maternal behavior. For example, some of the projections may be involved in regulating neuroendocrine processes associated with lactation. Stronger and more complete evidence for the involvement of each pathway would be forthcoming if we could determine the neurotransmitter contained in each circuit. Then, through application of the relevant agonists and antagonists to the appropriate termination site, we could determine the nature of the involvement of the particular projection in maternal behavior control. One neurotransmitter that may be contained in MPOA/VBST efferents regulating aspects of maternal behavior is neurotensin. Neurotensin-containing neurons are located in both the VBST and the MPOA,[39,40] and estrogen increases neurotensin mRNA expression in some of these neurons.[39] Also important are findings that neurotensin mRNA expression may involve transcription activation by Fos.[41] Finally, neurotensin axon terminals and receptors are located in the ventral tegmental area, retrorubral field, and periaqueductal gray,[42–44] and neurotensin microinjection into the ventral mesencephalon activates dopamine neurons and produces a rewarding effect.[45]

Another peptide within the MPOA/VBST region relevant to maternal behavior is oxytocin. Central oxytocin systems potentiate maternal behavior in rodents and sheep,[1] and the hormones of pregnancy and lactation increase the expression of oxytocin mRNA within MPOA and VBST neurons.[46,47] Most recently, Pedersen *et al.*[48] detected an increase in oxytocin binding sites in the ventral mesencephalon of parturient rats, and they also showed that microinjection of an oxytocin antagonist into this region disrupts the onset of maternal behavior. Perhaps a VBST-to-ventral tegmental area/retrorubral field oxytocinergic system is involved in promoting maternal responsiveness. It should also be pointed out that the ventromedial nucleus of the hypothalamus contains a high density of oxytocin receptors[49] which suggests involvement of an MPOA/VBST-to-ventromedial nucleus of the hypothalamus oxytocinergic circuit in maternal behavior control.

THE AVERSION/AVOIDANCE SYSTEM

Recall that nulliparous female rats not exposed to the endocrine events of late pregnancy do not engage in maternal behavior and tend to avoid pup-related stimuli; but if such females are made anosmic, they will show maternal behavior. These findings have given rise to the view that the nulliparous female rat finds the smell of pups aversive and that this aversion must be counteracted at parturition for maternal behavior to occur. This hypothesis fits well with the finding that while nulliparous females do not find olfactory stimuli from pups attractive, parturient females do. Although the physiological events associated with the end of pregnancy change the valence of pup-related olfactory inputs from negative to positive, the important aspect of this olfactory modification is that it removes the aversive nature of such inputs. That is, being attracted to pup-related odors is not necessary for maternal behavior to occur in rats, because anosmic females show such behavior.

The neural mechanism by which pup-related olfactory cues inhibit maternal behavior in virgins is only partly understood. For example, do such stimuli cause

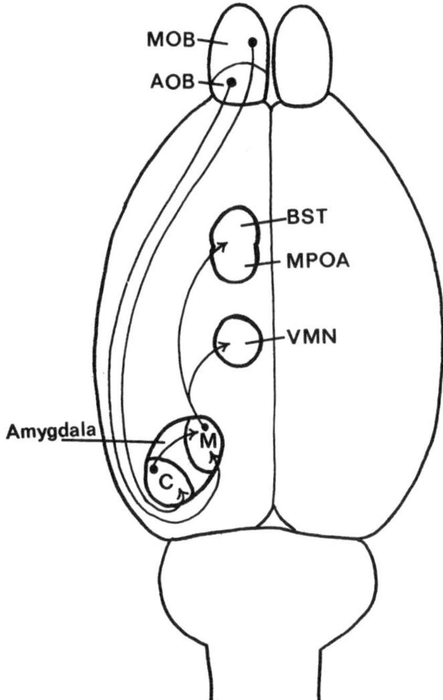

FIGURE 8. Diagrammatic representation of olfactory bulb connections to the corticomedial amygdala, and amygdaloid projections to the hypothalamus and bed nucleus of the stria terminalis (BST). Projections are shown on only one side of the brain. Not all known projections are shown. The main olfactory bulb has projections to the anterior cortical amygdaloid nucleus (C) and the accessory olfactory bulb projects to the medial amygdaloid nucleus (M). C projects to M. The medial amygdala projects to the BST, medial preoptic area (MPOA), and ventromedial nucleus of the hypothalamus (VMN).

direct inhibition of the neural nuclei that promote maternal behavior or do they stimulate a neural aversion system, causing withdrawal from pups and inhibiting maternal behavior indirectly? Although both answers may be correct, the fact that virgins do not simply fail to show maternal behavior but actually withdraw from pups suggests involvement of the second of these possibilities.

Two major chemosensory (olfactory) receptor systems are present in the nasal cavity of female rats: vomeronasal system and primary olfactory system. Research suggests that both systems are involved in inhibiting maternal behavior in the nulliparous female.[8] An important anatomical finding is that chemosensory inputs from both of these systems can be integrated within the medial amygdala.[1] This finding, coupled with the long-standing knowledge of the role of the amygdala in emotion, fear, and anxiety,[50] has given rise to the hypothesis that novel olfactory stimuli from pups inhibit maternal behavior in nulliparous females, because such input activates fear-inducing mechanisms in the amygdala.[51] In support of such a view, it was shown that electrical or excitotoxic amino acid lesions of the medial amygdala facilitate the maternal responsiveness of nulliparous female rats.[51,52] Such females no longer actively avoid the pups with which they are cohabited, and they begin to show maternal behavior after only 2-3 days of pup exposure in comparison with the 7-8 days required of control females.

If the output of the medial amygdala inhibits maternal behavior, where might this output act? FIGURE 8 diagrams some olfactory-amygdala-hypothalamic pathways.

A major efferent pathway from the medial amygdala is the stria terminalis, and Fleming *et al.*[51] reported that stria terminalis lesions are just as effective as medial amygdala lesions in facilitating maternal behavior. Medial amygdala efferents via the stria terminalis reach several regions, including the MPOA and ventromedial nucleus of the hypothalamus.[53,54] One hypothesis is that when novel pup odors activate the medial amygdala in nulliparae, medial amygdala efferents in turn inhibit the MPOA, in this way preventing the occurrence of maternal behavior.

Alternatively, medial amygdala efferents may activate an inhibitory region outside the MPOA. One such area may be the ventromedial nucleus of the hypothalamus. Recent work by Bridges and Mann[31] suggests that the ventromedial nucleus of the hypothalamus may inhibit maternal behavior in that damage to this area appeared facilitatory, and they suggested that the ventromedial nucleus of the hypothalamus may be part of an amygdala-to-hypothalamic inhibitory circuit for maternal behavior. There is abundant evidence that the ventromedial nucleus of the hypothalamus and nearby regions of the medial hypothalamus participate in an amygdalo-hypothalamic-brainstem circuit mediating anxiety, fear, aversion, and defensive behavior: (a) Electrical stimulation in the vicinity of the ventromedial nucleus of the hypothalamus is aversive, and animals will perform an operant response to terminate such stimulation;[55] (b) electrical and chemical stimulation of the ventromedial nucleus of the hypothalamus produces defensive aggression and escape/flight behavior in a variety of mammalian species, including rats;[56,57] (c) the ventromedial nucleus of the hypothalamus has strong projections to the periaqueductal gray,[58] a region that is critically involved in regulating diverse reactions related to fear, anxiety, escape responses, and defensive aggression.[38,56,57] Therefore, medial amygdala input to the ventromedial nucleus of the hypothalamus may inhibit maternal behavior by activating a fear or aversion system.

To better understand the nature of medial amygdala inhibition over maternal behavior, we have attempted to identify a neurotransmitter present in the medial amygdala-to-hypothalamus pathway that may be involved in this inhibition. Our attention has been focused on the tachykinins, a prominent family of neuropeptides in such a pathway. FIGURE 9 provides a general overview of the biosynthesis of several tachykinins.[59] As a result of alternative splicing of the precursor RNA transcript of the preprotachykinin (PPT)-I gene, one of three types of PPT mRNA can be produced, each of which can be translated to produce a precursor PPT peptide. Posttranslational processing of the precursor peptides can yield the following tachykinins: substance P (SP), neurokinin A (NKA), neuropeptide K (NPK), and neuropeptide γ (NPγ). Importantly, tachykinin immunoreactive (TKir) cell bodies are located in the medial amygdala, TKir axon terminals are located in MPOA and ventromedial nucleus of the hypothalamus,[54,60,61] and some TKir neurons in the medial amygdala project to the hypothalamus.[54,62]

In addition to their prominence in the amygdalo-to-hypothalamic pathway, other evidence drew our attention to the tachykinins. Systemic treatment of rodents and primates with tachykinin receptor antagonists has shown anxiolytic effects.[63] Furthermore, Shaikh *et al.*[62] found that the defensive aggression elicited in the cat by electrical stimulation of the ventromedial nucleus of the hypothalamus is potentiated by concurrent electrical stimulation of the medial amygdala and that this potentiating effect of

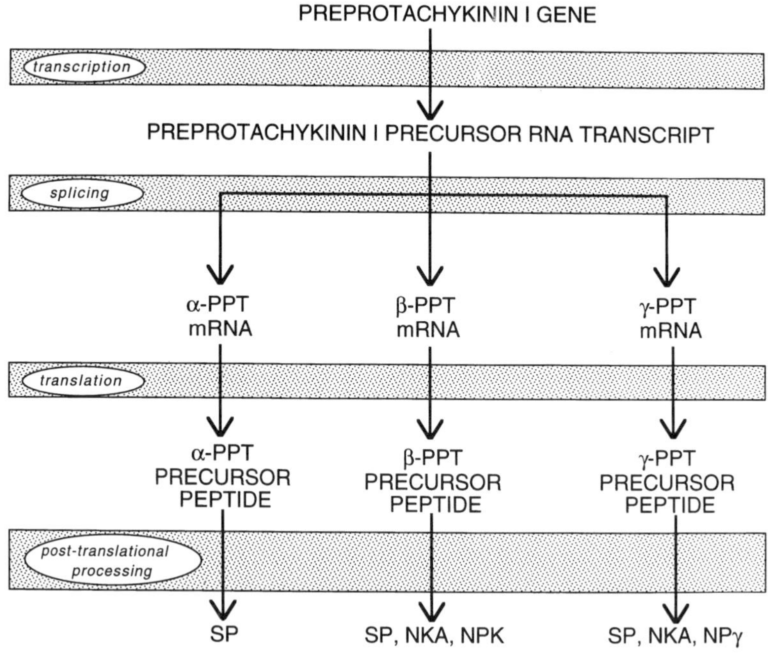

FIGURE 9. Diagrammatic representation of the biosynthesis of the various tachykinin peptides from the preprotachykinin (PPT) I gene. SP = substance P; NKA = neurokinin A; NPK = neuropeptide K; NPγ = neuropeptide γ.

medial amygdala stimulation is blocked when a tachykinin receptor antagonist is applied to the ventromedial nucleus of the hypothalamus.

Using the foregoing analysis, Sheehan and Numan[64] began a research program that is based on the hypothesis that in the nulliparous female, novel olfactory stimuli from pups activate the medial amygdala which, in turn, releases a tachykinin peptide into the ventromedial nucleus of the hypothalamus that antagonizes maternal responsiveness. Furthermore, we hypothesized that the hormonal events of late pregnancy must in some way downregulate this inhibitory tachykinin effect. If this were the case, then application of the appropriate tachykinin to the hypothalamus of *hormonally primed* females should antagonize maternal responsiveness.

In designing experiments to test these hypotheses we used the model developed by Siegel and Rosenblatt.[65] When primigravid female rats were hysterectomized and ovariectomized on day 16 of pregnancy and treated with estradiol, they showed near immediate maternal responsiveness towards pups that were presented to them 48 hours later. We wanted to test whether central administration of a tachykinin could inhibit this hormonally induced maternal behavior. In our initial experiments we examined whether applying NPK to the ventromedial nucleus of the hypothalamus could inhibit maternal behavior. We chose to examine NPK because previous work had shown that the central administration of NPK had potent inhibitory effects on male sexual behavior in rats.[66]

Nulliparous female rats were mated (day 1 of pregnancy), and on day 2 of pregnancy bilateral cannulas were stereotaxically aimed at the ventromedial nucleus of the hypothalamus. On day 16 of pregnancy all females were subjected to hysterectomy and ovariectomy and were injected with 20 μg/kg of estradiol benzoate subcutaneously. Forty-eight hours later, on day 0 of testing, females received microinjections of various doses of NPK or physiological saline solution into the ventromedial nucleus of the hypothalamus region. This injection procedure was repeated on the morning of day 1 of testing. Behavioral testing began on the morning of day 0 and continued through day 5. On each day each female was presented with three test pups (provided by donor mothers), with one pup being placed in each quadrant of the test female's cage outside her sleeping or nesting area. On days 0 and 1, pups were presented approximately 45 minutes after the intracranial injection. Females were observed for 1 hour following pup presentation and again for 15 minutes at 4 PM, the end of the test day. A female was classified as showing full maternal behavior if she retrieved all of her pups to a single location and adopted a nursing crouch over them.

In the first experiment we compared the effects of injecting 1,110 ng NPK into the ventromedial nucleus of the hypothalamus with the effects of injecting physiological saline solution.[64] FIGURE 10 shows the cumulative percentage of females in each group showing maternal behavior by the end of each daily 1-hour test and by the end of each test day. NPK disrupted maternal behavior throughout day 0 and for the first hour of the day 1 test. Whereas 75% of the saline-injected females were showing full maternal behavior by the end of day 0 of testing, this was true for only 15% of the NPK females.

In a second experiment the effectiveness of various doses of NPK was tested.[64] Females received either 0 ng (physiological saline solution), 740 ng, 463 ng, or 264 ng of NPK into the ventromedial nucleus of the hypothalamus on days 0 and 1. Subjects that received 740 ng and those that received 463 ng were combined into a single group. The results are shown in FIGURE 11. All doses of NPK inhibited the onset of maternal behavior. This was particularly apparent for the 1-hour test on day 1 of testing, when nearly 90% of the 0 ng group was showing maternal behavior while less than 25% of the females in the NPK injected groups were doing so.

Although NPK microinjections into the ventromedial nucleus of the hypothalamus disrupted the onset of maternal behavior, they did not disrupt the general arousability of the females. On days 0 and 1, the days of NPK administration, the latency for each female to approach and sniff the pups following their placement in her cage was recorded, and these results are shown in TABLE 4. The NPK-injected females responded as quickly as did the saline-injected females.

An experiment we currently have in progress shows some anatomical specificity to the inhibitory effects of NPK. Although 264-ng microinjections of NPK into the ventromedial nucleus of the hypothalamus disrupt maternal behavior, similar injections into the thalamic region dorsal to the ventromedial nucleus of the hypothalamus are without effect.

These results show that NPK has potent inhibitory effects on maternal behavior. Much remains to be done however to validate the hypothesis on which these initial experiments were based. It will be important to compare the effects of NPK with those of the other tachykinins and to determine if the MPOA is a site where tachykinins might also act to inhibit maternal behavior. Another important question is whether

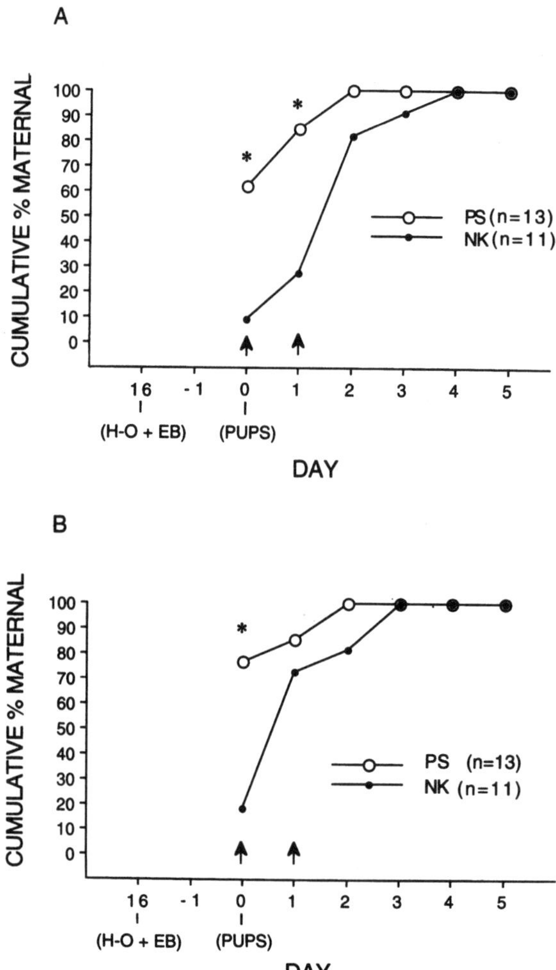

FIGURE 10. Cumulative percentage of females showing full maternal behavior either within the first hour of behavioral testing on each test day (shown in **A**) or by the end of each test day (4 pm, shown in **B**). Females received microinjections of either physiological saline (PS) or 1,110 ng of neuropeptide K (NK) into the ventromedial hypothalamus. *Arrows* indicate days on which intracranial injections took place. Females were subjected to hysterectomy (H) and ovariectomy (O) and treated with 20 μg/kg of estradiol benzoate (EB) on day 16 of pregnancy. Pups were presented for maternal behavior tests beginning 48 hours after H-O + EB. *Significantly greater than NK group, $p < 0.05$.

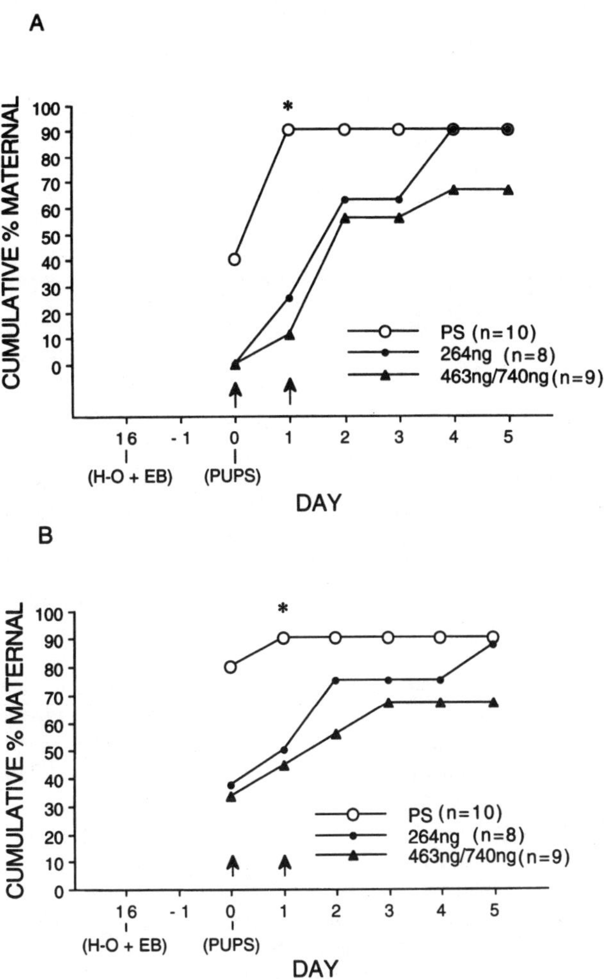

FIGURE 11. Cumulative percentage of females showing full maternal behavior either within the first hour of behavioral testing on each test day (shown in **A**) or by the end of each test day (4 pm, shown in **B**). Females received microinjections of either physiological saline (PS), 264 ng, 463 ng, or 740 ng of neuropeptide K into the ventromedial hypothalamus. Females receiving 463 and 740 ng of neuropeptide K were combined into a single group. *Arrows* indicate days on which intracranial injections took place. Females were subjected to hysterectomy (H), ovariectomy (O), and treated with 20 μg/kg of estradiol benzoate (EB) on day 16 of pregnancy. Pups were presented for maternal behavior tests beginning 48 hours after H-O + EB. For graph **A,** * significantly greater than remaining groups, $p < 0.05$. For graph **B,** * significantly greater than 463/740 ng group, $p < 0.05$.

TABLE 4. Mean (± SEM) Latencies to Approach and Sniff Pups after Intracranial Injections of Either Physiological Saline Solution or Various Doses of Neuropeptide K

		Mean (± SEM) Sniff Latencies (s)	
Group	*n*	Day 0	Day 1
PS	10	18.20 ± 4.56	6.40 ± 1.78
264 ng	8	11.50 ± 4.28	4.63 ± 0.75
463/740 ng	9	7.56 ± 3.35	9.56 ± 1.91

Abbreviation: PS = physiological saline solution.

the inhibitory effect of NPK on maternal behavior is the result of directly activating inhibitory neurobehavioral mechanisms or if NPK is having neuroendocrine effects that disrupt maternal behavior. The latter possibility must be considered, because central administration of NPK and other tachykinins does have hormonal effects.[67] It will also be important to determine if tachykinin receptor antagonists can facilitate maternal behavior under conditions of suboptimal hormonal stimulation. Finally, it will be necessary to determine if the medial amygdala is the source of inhibitory tachykinin input to the hypothalamus and if novel olfactory stimuli from pups activate this system in nonhormone-primed nulliparae.

If the homonal events of late pregnancy counteract our hypothetical inhibitory amygdala-to-hypothalamus tachykininergic circuit, what might be the mechanism of action? One possibility is that the critical hormones decrease the synthesis and/or release of NPK. Tachykinin immunoreactive neurons in the medial amygdala and medial hypothalamus bind estradiol, and estradiol treatment can influence the number of neurons in these regions that contain tachykinin immunoreactivity, in most cases causing an increase.[60] Using an RNA probe that was complementary to all three PPT-I mRNA species (α, β, and γ), Simerly *et al.*[54] reported that estrogen does not affect the level of PPT-I mRNA in the medial amygdala. Perhaps steroids can influence splicing mechanisms and regulate the particular mRNA variants that are produced, an effect that may not have been detectable with the nonspecific RNA probe used by Simerly *et al.*[54] The available evidence, however, does not support this idea.[68]

Even if steroids do not influence transcription or splicing mechanisms, they could influence tachykinin levels and maternal behavior by altering posttranslational mechanisms.[68] For example, estrogen may cause an increase in the synthesis of NKA over that of NPK from the β-PPT mRNA transcript (FIG. 9), thereby decreasing inhibition of maternal behavior. Finally, endocrine events might alter release mechanisms in tachykininergic medial amygdala neurons. More complete answers to the issues raised here will be obtained once we begin to explore the effects of pregnancy and its particular hormonal milieu on transcriptional, splicing, posttranslational, and release mechanisms in tachykinin neurons.

Although we have stressed the importance of NPK in the inhibitory circuit from the medial amygdala to the hypothalamus, it should be noted that other peptides might also be involved. In particular, corticotropin releasing hormone (CRH) is present in the neural pathway from the medial amygdala to the ventromedial nucleus of the hypothalamus,[69] and intracerebroventricular administration of CRH has disruptive effects on maternal behavior in rats.[70] Interestingly, there is some evidence that the central administration of NPK may cause the central release of CRH.[67]

CONCLUSIONS

In this review we suggest that efferent circuits from MPOA/VBST neurons regulate the consummatory and possibly the appetitive aspects of maternal behavior and that such circuits are stimulated by the endocrine events of late pregnancy. In contrast, an amygdala-to-hypothalamus circuit probably depresses maternal behavior by activating a central aversion system, and it is suggested that the endocrine events of late pregnancy act to downregulate activity in this system. Although we created a hypothetical scheme from a limited amount of data, we hope that our outline focuses future research. Some examples of how our model has helped us think about the neural mechanisms of parental behavior follow.

If a preoptic output circuit regulates excitatory influences over maternal behavior, while an amygdala-to-ventromedial nucleus of the hypothalamus circuit regulates inhibitory influences, an interesting question is the degree to which the two systems need to interact. Although potential points of neural interaction exist between the two systems (for example, the ventromedial nucleus of the hypothalamus projects to the MPOA[58] and both the MPOA/VBST and ventromedial nucleus of the hypothalamus project to the periaqueductal gray[12,58]), it is also possible that these systems act in parallel. The parallel view would argue that as long as activation of the aversion system is greater than activation of the approach system, females will not be exposed to those stimuli that foster maternal behavior because they will avoid neonates.

In our model we presented evidence that medial amygdala output systems inhibit maternal responsiveness in rats. These data need to be reconciled with data from other species which show that the medial amygdala exerts a positive influence on parental responsiveness.[71] It will be important to compare the particular nuclei involved in these disparate influences, the connections of the relevant nuclei, and their neurochemical makeup.

An important aspect of the regulation of maternal responsiveness in a variety of mammalian species is the role played by experiential factors.[1,3] In particular, although hormones are essential for the immediate onset of maternal behavior at parturition in naive primiparous female rats, the need for hormonal facilitation is reduced in females with previous breeding experience (for a review, see ref. 1). These findings suggest that previous maternal experience may decrease the aversive nature of pup-related olfactory stimuli. Perhaps maternal experience activates learning mechanisms in the olfactory bulb or the amygdala so that pup-related olfactory stimuli no longer gain access to our hypothesized central aversion system.[1]

REFERENCES

1. Numan, M. 1994. *In* The Physiology of Reproduction. E. Knobil & J. D. Neill, Eds. Vol. **2:** 221-302. Raven Press. New York, NY.

2. Fleming, A. & G. Orpen. 1986. *In* Origins of Nurturance. A. Fogel & G. F. Melson, Eds.: 141-207. Lawrence Erlbaum Associates. Hillside, NJ.
3. Pryce, C. R. 1992. Anim. Behav. **43:** 417-441.
4. Rosenblatt, J. S. & A. D. Mayer. 1995. *In* Behavioral Development. K. E. Hood, G. Greenberg & E. Tobach, Eds.: 177-230. Garland Press, NY.
5. Fleming, A. S. & C. Luebke. 1981. Physiol. Behav. **27:** 863-868.
6. Fleming, A. S., U. Cheung, N. Myhal & Z. Kessler. 1989. Physiol. Behav. **46:** 449-453.
7. Levy, F., P. Poindron & P. Le Neindre. 1983. Physiol. Behav. **31:** 687-692.
8. Fleming, A. S., F. Vaccarino, L. Tambosso & P. Chee. 1979. Science **203:** 372-374.
9. Bridges, R. S., M. Numan, P. M. Ronsheim, P. E. Mann & C. E. Lupini. 1990. Proc. Natl. Acad. Sci. USA **87:** 8003-8007.
10. Numan, M., J. S. Rosenblatt & B. R. Komisaruk. 1977. J. Comp. Physiol. Psychol. **91:** 146-164.
11. Numan, M., K. P. Corodimas, M. J. Numan, E. M. Factor & W. D. Piers. 1988. Behav. Neurosci. **102:** 381-396.
12. Numan, M. & M. J. Numan. 1996. Dev. Psychobiol. **29:** 23-51.
13. Numan, M., J. McSparren & M. J. Numan. 1990. Behav. Neurosci. **104:** 964-979.
14. Everitt, B. J. 1990. Neurosci. Biobehav. Rev. **14:** 217-232.
15. Pryce, C. R., M. Dobeli & R. D. Martin. 1993. J. Comp. Psychol. **107:** 99-115.
16. Numan, M. & H. G. Smith. 1984. Behav. Neurosci. **98:** 712-727.
17. Blackburn, J. R., J. G. Pfaus & A. G. Phillips. 1992. Prog. Neurobiol. **39:** 247-279.
18. Hansen, S., C. Harthon, E. Wallin, L. Lofberg & K. Svennson. 1991. Behav. Neurosci. **105:** 588-598.
19. Hansen, S. 1994. Physiol. Behav. **55:** 615-620.
20. Numan, M. 1990. Behav. Neural Biol. **53:** 284-290.
21. Numan, M. & M. J. Numan. 1991. Behav. Neurosci. **105:** 1013-1029.
22. Deutch, A. Y., M. Goldstein & R. H. Roth. 1988. Ann. N.Y. Acad. Sci. **537:** 27-50.
23. Morgan, J. I. & T. Curran. 1991. Annu. Rev. Neurosci. **14:** 421-451.
24. Numan, M. & M. J. Numan. 1994. Behav. Neurosci. **108:** 379-394.
25. Calamandrei, G. & E. B. Keverne. 1994. Behav. Neurosci. **108:** 113-120.
26. Fleming, A. S., E. J. Suh, M. Korsmit & B. Rusak. 1994. Behav. Neurosci. **108:** 724-734.
27. Kirkpatrick, B., J. W. Kim & T. R. Insel. 1994. Brain Res. **658:** 112-118.
28. Numan, M. & M. J. Numan. 1995. Behav. Neurosci. **109:** 135-149.
29. Numan, M. & M. J. Numan. 1995. Soc. Neurosci. Abstr. **21:** 465.
30. Corodimas, K. P., J. S. Rosenblatt, M. E. Canfield & J. I. Morrell. 1993. Behav. Neurosci. **107:** 827-843.
31. Bridges, R. S. & P. E. Mann. 1994. Psychoneuroendocrinology **19:** 611-622.
32. Wang, Z., C. F. Ferris & G. J. De Vries. 1994. Proc. Natl. Acad. Sci. USA **91:** 400-404.
33. Albert, D. J. & G. L. Chew. 1980. Behav. Neural Biol. **30:** 357-388.
34. Fleming, A. S., M. Korsmit & M. Deller. 1994. Psychobiology **22:** 44-53.
35. Von Krosigk, M. & A. D. Smith. 1991. Eur. J. Neurosci. **3:** 260-273.
36. Li, Y. Q., M. Takada, Y. Shinonaga & N. Mizuno. 1993. Neuroscience **54:** 431-443.
37. Stern, J. M. & J. M. Kolunie. 1991. Behav. Neurosci. **105:** 984-997.
38. Behbehani, M. M. 1995. Prog. Neurobiol. **46:** 575-605.
39. Alexander, M. J. & S. E. Leeman. 1994. J. Comp. Neurol. **345:** 496-509.
40. Ju, G., L. W. Swanson & R. B. Simerly. 1989. J. Comp. Neurol. **280:** 603-621.
41. Merchant, K. M. 1994. Molec. Cell. Neurosci. **5:** 336-344.
42. Nicot, A., W. Rostene & A. Berod. 1995. J. Neurosci. Res. **40:** 667-674.
43. Shipley, M. T., J. H. McLean & M. Behbehani. 1987. J. Neurosci. **7:** 2025-2034.
44. Woulfe, J & A. Beaudet. 1992. J. Comp. Neurol. **321:** 163-176.
45. Rompre, P. & A. Gratton. 1993. Brain Res. **616:** 154-162.
46. Broad, K. D., K. M. Kendrick, D. J. S. Sirinathsinghji & E. B. Keverene. 1993. J. Neuroendocrinol. **5:** 435-444.
47. Brooks, P. J., P. Lund, W. Stumpf & C. Pedersen. 1990. J. Neuroendocrinol. **2:** 621-626.

48. PEDERSEN, C. A., J. D. CALDWELL, C. WALKER, G. AYERS & G. A. MASON. 1994. Behav. Neurosci. **108:** 1163-1171.
49. KREMARIK, P., M. J. FREUND-MERCIER & M. E. STOECKEL. 1995. Brain Res. Bull. **36:** 195-203.
50. DAVIS, M. 1992. Annu. Rev. Neurosci. **15:** 353-375.
51. FLEMING, A. S., F. VACCARINO & C. LUEBKE. 1980. Physiol. Behav. **25:** 731-743.
52. NUMAN, M., M. J. NUMAN, & J. B. ENGLISH. 1993. Horm. Behav. **27:** 56-81.
53. CANTERAS, N. S., R. B. SIMERLY & L. W. SWANSON. 1995. J. Comp. Neurol. **360:** 213-245.
54. SIMERLY, R. B., B. J. YOUNG, M. A. CAPOZZA & L. W. SWANSON. 1989. Proc. Natl. Acad. Sci. USA **86:** 4766-4770.
55. HOEBEL, B. G. 1988. *In* Steven's Handbook of Experimental Psychology, 2nd Ed. R. C. Atkinson, R. J. Hernstein, G. Lindzey & R. Duncan Lace, Eds. Vol. 1: 547-625. John Wiley & Sons. New York, NY.
56. BANDLER, R. 1988. Prog. Psychobiol. Physiol. Psych. **13:** 67-153.
57. ROELING, T. A. P., J. G. VEENING, M. R. KRUK, J. P. W. PETERS, M. E. J. VERMELIS & R. NIEUWENHUYS. 1994. Neuroscience **59:** 1001-1024.
58. CANTERAS, N. S., R. B. SIMERLY & L. W. SWANSON. 1994. J. Comp. Neurol. **348:** 41-79.
59. KRAUSE, J. E., A. D. HERSHEY, P. E. DYKEMA & Y. TAKEDA. 1990. Ann. N.Y. Acad. Sci. **579:** 254-272.
60. AKESSON, T. R. & P. E. MICEVYCH. 1995. *In* Neurobiological Effects of Sex Steroid Hormones. P. E. Micevych & R. P. Hammer, Eds.: 207-233. Cambridge University Press. Cambridge, England.
61. VALENTINO, K. L., K. TATEMOTO, J. HUNTER & J. D. BARCHAS. 1986. Peptides **7:** 1043-1049.
62. SHAIKH, M. B., A. STEINBERG & A. SIEGEL. 1993. Brain Res. **625:** 283-294.
63. WALSH, D. M., S. C. STRATTON, F. J. HARVEY, I. J. M. BERESFORD & R. M. HAGAN. 1995. Psychopharmacology **121:** 186-191.
64. SHEEHAN, T. P. & M. NUMAN. 1995. Paper presented at the 27th Annual Conference on Reproductive Behavior, Boston, MA. June 1995.
65. SIEGEL, H. I. & J. S. ROSENBLATT. 1975. Horm. Behav. **6:** 211-222.
66. DORNAN, W. A., K. L. VINK, P. MALEN, K. SHORT, W. STRUTHERS & C. BARRETT. 1993. Physiol. Behav. **54:** 249-258.
67. KALRA, P. S. & S. P. KALRA. 1993. Brain Res. **610:** 330-333.
68. BROWN, E., R. E. HARLAN & J. E. KRAUSE. 1990. Endocrinology **126:** 330-340.
69. SAKANAKA, M., T. SHIBASAKI & K. LEDERIS. 1986. Brain Res. **382:** 213-238.
70. PEDERSEN, C. A., J. D. CALDWELL, M. MCGUIRE & D. EVANS. 1991. Life Sci. **48:** 1537-1546.
71. KIRKPATRICK, B., C. S. CARTER, S. W. NEWMAN & T. R. INSEL. 1994. Behav. Neurosci. **108:** 501-513.

19

Oxytocin Control of Maternal Behavior: Regulation by Sex Steroids and Offspring Stimuli

Cort A. Pedersen

The evolution of maternal behavior (MB) revolutionized reproduction. Sustained maternal protection and nurturing of offspring until they were able to fend for themselves allowed a much higher rate of survival. Mothering also permitted a much longer period of brain development and was therefore an essential prerequisite for the evolution of higher intelligence. Species that mother their offspring have dominated every ecological niche in which they dwell. The ever increasingly complex social behavior that has been a major feature of mammalian evolution has probably been built on brain systems that originally evolved to generate MB.

The remarkable success of MB as a reproductive behavioral strategy has depended on evolution of mechanisms to assure that maternal responses towards offspring (1) are exhibited only by females that are lactating (i.e., can feed offspring), (2) are not exhibited by females that are not lactating, and (3) are sustained for the prolonged period necessary for offspring to mature despite rapid postpartum dissipation of the hormonal conditions that were necessary for the initial activation of MB. This chapter focuses on the now overwhelming evidence that the neuropeptide oxytocin (OT) is centrally involved in activating MB at the appropriate time as well as on new evidence that OT may play a less essential but significant role in sustaining MB during lactation.

ROLE OF OXYTOCIN IN HORMONAL ACTIVATION OF MATERNAL BEHAVIOR

Nature has arranged for MB to emerge in subprimate mammalian species at precisely the right time, that is, when offspring are being born. The precision between birth and the activation of parental interest in newborns comes about because many of the same hormonal events that exert effects on the uterus and mammary glands that lead to parturition and lactation also exert effects in the brain that activate

This study was conducted with funds provided by National Institute of Child Health and Human Development grant HD25255 as well as grants MH33127 and HD18968.

Tel: 919 966-1480; fax: 919 966-7659; e-mail: cpedersen@css. unc. edu mothering. Of first importance are the changes in the serum concentrations of the ovarian steroids estrogen and progesterone during pregnancy.[1–3] A prolonged period of elevated progesterone levels and a rise in estrogen levels during pregnancy appear to be necessary for the rapid postpartum onset of MB in all subprimate mammalian species that have been studied. In some species, including the rat, a decline in progesterone levels over the last few days of pregnancy is also necessary for both the onset of parturition and the activation of MB. Treatment with estrogen and progesterone doses that replicate changes in the concentrations of these hormones over the last half of pregnancy significantly accelerates the onset of MB in virgin rats.

Clearly, ovarian steroids activate MB by exerting effects on OT systems in the brain. This theme emerged in early studies in which intracerebroventricular (icv) administration of OT was observed to rapidly stimulate MB in virgin rats.[4,5] Ovariectomy abolished and estrogen priming reinstated sensitivity to this effect of OT. Later studies consistently found that interference with central OT activity by icv administration of OT antiserum or OT receptor antagonists potently blocked the onset of MB in ovarian steroid-treated or parturient rats.[6–8] The same icv treatments that so successfully inhibited the onset of MB had no effect on rat mothers that had been allowed several or more days of mothering experience.[7,8] Lesions of the paraventricular nucleus of the hypothalamus, the source of most extrahypothalamic OT projections within the brain,[9,10] markedly disrupted the postpartum onset of MB[11] but had no discernible effect on MB when performed in lactating rats that had 5 days of postpartum mothering experience.[12] These findings suggested that central OT was critical for the initial activation of MB but played no role in sustaining established MB. This was also consistent with the conclusion that OT was exclusively a mediator of ovarian steroid effects on MB. Although the postpartum onset of MB had clearly been shown to depend upon ovarian steroids, it had been as irrefutably demonstrated that once initiated, the continuing expression of MB rapidly became independent of ovarian steroid conditions.[1–3] Therefore, OT appeared to be necessary for the expression of MB when ovarian steroids were also necessary (i.e., during the initiation of MB), whereas while OT was not necessary for the expression of MB when ovarian steroids no longer played a role (i.e., during the maintenance of established MB).

Oxytocin has been implicated in the activation of MB in mice and sheep. Peripheral or central administration of OT to wild house mice markedly suppressed the high spontaneous rate of infanticide usually displayed by these animals and increased somewhat maternal nurturing behavior towards pups.[13,14] Much more work has been done in sheep. Intracerebroventricular administration of OT rapidly stimulated species' typical maternal responses towards young lambs in multiparous, nonpregnant ewes that were estradiol-primed.[15] Cerebrospinal fluid (CSF) concentrations of OT increased in sheep during parturition as well as during vaginocervical stimulation which also activated MB in ewes.[16,17] Peridural anesthesia of primiparous ewes blocked both the onset of MB and the rise in CSF concentrations of OT; icv administration of OT reversed the inhibitory effect of peridural anesthesia on the onset of MB.[18] Intracerebroventricular injection of OT in estradiol-primed, nonpregnant nulliparous ewes did not stimulate active nurturing behavior, but it did suppress rejection behavior towards lambs.[19] These findings suggest that OT may be important in the activation of MB in many, if not all, mammalian species.

Progress has been made in identifying sites in the brain where OT activates MB. When radiolabeled analogs of OT with very high affinity for the OT receptor became available in the 1980s, many investigators began to use autoradiographic methods to locate and quantifiy OT binding in the brain.[20–23] As their findings emerged, a discrepancy became apparent between brain sites identified by autoradiography to contain OT receptors and brain sites implicated by lesion studies in the control of MB. Numan and his colleagues[2] conducted a series of careful lesion studies which established that a dorsolateral projection from the medial preoptic area (MPOA) that connects with the ventral tegmental area (VTA) and more caudal midbrain sites is critical for the expression of MB in the rat. The ventral bed nucleus of the stria terminalis (vBNST) appeared to be an important junction in this projection. These connections were conceptualized as the vital motivational link between the region in which ovarian steroids exerted their influence and critical sensory inputs from pups were processed (the MPOA) and the midbrain monoaminergic systems that focused the mother's attention and interest on pups and guided the motoric components of MB.[2] However, autoradiographic studies employing tritiated OT or the iodinated OT analog, $[d(CH_2)_5[Tyr(Me)^2, Thr^4, Tyr\text{-}NH_2^9]$ornithine-vasotocin (OTA[24]), did not find appreciable OT binding in these brain sites.[20–23]

Other lines of evidence suggested that OT might exert some of its MB-facilitating effects in the MPOA and/or the VTA. Some immunohistochemical studies had described OT projections that either terminated or passed through these brain sites.[9,25] Fahrbach *et al.*[26] had also reported on a preliminary study in which OT infusion into the VTA significantly stimulated MB in estrogen-primed nulliparous rats; infusion of OT into the MPOA, however, had no significant effect. With these findings in mind, we decided to employ a different method to measure OT binding in these sites. Saturation radioligand assays were conducted on the MPOA and the ventral midbrain (containing the VTA and the substantia nigra [SN]) as well as the amygdala after they were dissected out of whole brains.[27] We used the same iodinated OT analog used in most of the autoradiography studies (^{125}I-OTA[24]). With this method, we compared OT binding between rats sacrificed in midparturition (when MB began), on days 15-17 of pregnancy (P15-17, when MB had not yet emerged), on days 5-7 of lactation (L5-7, when MB was well established and no longer dependent upon ovarian steroids), or, in nulliparous rats, 2 weeks or more after ovariectomy. We found a considerable amount of OT binding in the MPOA and a smaller amount in the ventral midbrain. The B_{max} and K_D values for each brain area obtained in each of the four separate groups are presented in TABLE 1. B_{max} values were significantly different among these groups in the VTA/SN and MPOA ($F = 4.79$, $p = 0.03$; $F = 5.61$, $p = 0.02$, respectively) but not in the amygdala ($F = 0.63$, $p = 0.62$). Posthoc pairwise comparisons of B_{max} values using the Bonferroni test were nearly significant ($p = 0.06$) between P15-17 and midparturition in the VTA/SN and in the MPOA and significant between midparturition and L5-7 in the MPOA ($p = 0.04$). K_D values were significantly different among groups in the amygdala and MPOA ($F = 4.72$, $p = 0.04$; $F = 4.03$, $p = 0.05$, respectively), but not in the VTA/SN ($F = 0.96$, $p = 0.46$). However, posthoc analysis of K_D values revealed that the only pairwise comparisons that approached significance were between ovariectomized and P15-17 rats in the amygdala ($p = 0.08$) and between ovariectomized and L5-7 rats in the amygdala ($p = 0.09$) and the MPOA ($p = 0.08$). These results suggested that the

TABLE 1. B_{max} (fmol/mg protein, mean ± SEM) and K_D (nM, mean ± SEM) from Three Scatchard Plots of ^{125}I-OTA Binding in Brain Tissue[a]

Measure	Pregnancy Days 15-17	Mid-parturition	Lactation Days 5-7	Ovariectomy
B_{max}				
VTA/SN	4.4 ± 0.32	6.2 ± 0.59	4.7 ± 0.20	4.6 ± 0.23
MPOA	23.7 ± 1.5	34.0 ± 1.6	22.6 ± 2.6	26.2 ± 2.7
Amygdala	19.3 ± 0.8	22.9 ± 1.4	21.8 ± 2.8	21.6 ± 2.0
K_D				
VTA/SN	0.072 ± 0.004	0.098 ± 0.009	0.073 ± 0.008	0.088 ± 0.022
MPOA	0.092 ± 0.010	.1105 ± 0.009	0.086 ± 0.003	0.142 ± 0.021
Amygdala	0.082 ± 0.003	0.085 ± 0.005	0.084 ± 0.008	0.141 ± 0.024

Abbreviation: MPOA = medial preoptic area; VTA/SN = ventral tegmental area/substantia nigra.

[a] Reprinted from Pedersen *et al.*,[27] 1994, with the publisher's permission.

parturition-associated onset of MB may be (1) stimulated by activation of OT receptors in the MPOA and the VTA, and (2) dependent upon an increase in OT binding in both of these sites, possibly driven by the hormonal changes of late pregnancy.

Testing the first implication of our binding results simply involved infusion of OT antagonists or control substances into the MPOA or VTA of parturient rats.[27] Repeated (× 4) bilateral infusions of 1 μg/side of the selective OT antagonist [Pen[1], Phe[2], Thr[4], delta[3,4] Pro[7], Orn[8]]OT (PPT[28]) into the VTA beginning with the delivery of the first pup significantly diminished pup retrieval and crouching over pups in a nursing posture compared to infusions of 1 μg/side of a selective V_{1a} antagonist, [d$(CH_2)_5$[1], O-Me-Tyr[2], Arg[6]]-vasopressin[29] or a normal saline vehicle alone. Bilateral infusions of the more potent OT antagonist, OTA, into the MPOA (0.25 μg/side × 4) also significantly inhibited the display of these components of rat MB when compared to normal saline infusions. In this site, infusion of the selective V_{1a} antagonist was almost as potent as OTA in blocking the postpartum onset of MB. FIGURE 1 summarizes the effects of treatments in the VTA or MPOA on latency to retrieve pups. Thus, OT receptors in both the MPOA and VTA and V_{1a} receptors in the MPOA were shown to be critical for the postpartum onset of MB. In our early studies, we observed that icv administration of arginine vasopressin (AVP) stimulated the onset of MB in estrogen-primed virgin rats.[30] We seem to have identified one brain site (MPOA) at which AVP exerted this effect.

Now that we have demonstrated that the MPOA and VTA are sites at which OT plays a necessary role in the initial postpartum activation of MB, we are beginning to investigate the location of the OT perikarya that give rise to the OT projections to these brain sites. By combining injection of a retrograde tract tracer into the VTA of intact animals with OT immunohistochemistry of brain sections, we (in collaboration with Dr. Michael Numan) have preliminarily found that OT neurons that project to the VTA are located in the vBNST-lateral preoptic region as well as the paraventricular nucleus. These are very exciting results because they are consistent

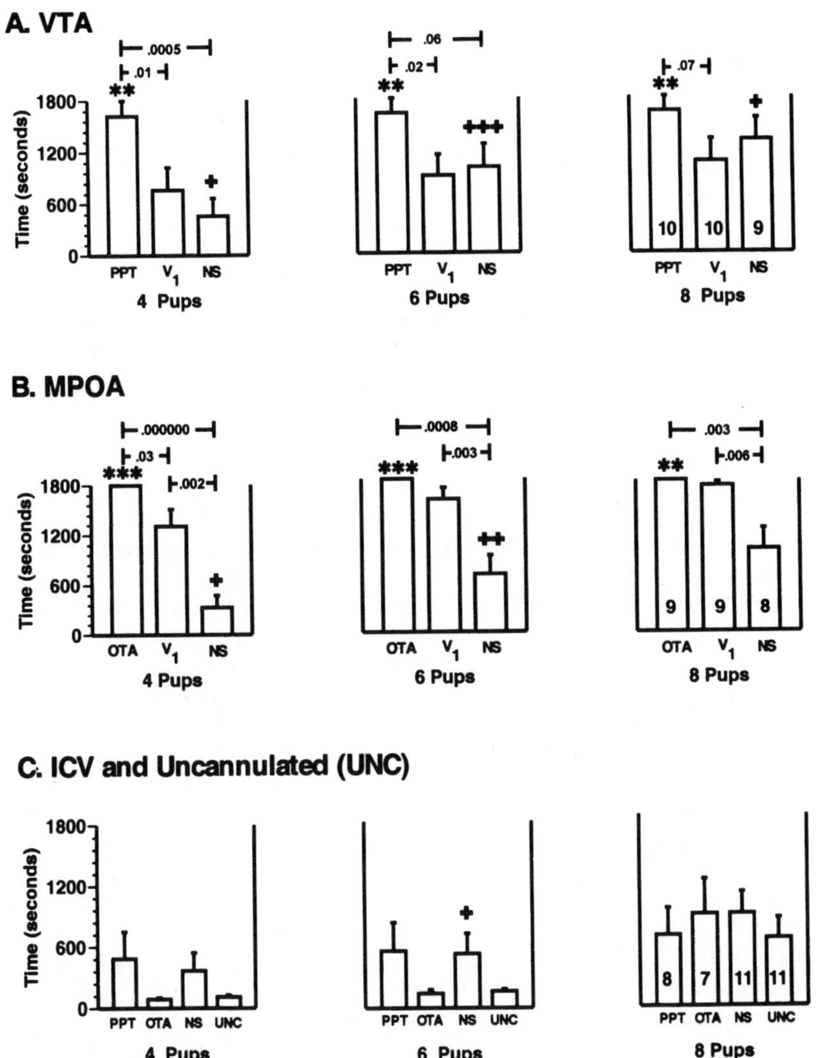

FIGURE 1. Mean (± SEM) latencies to retrieve 4, 6, or 8 pups exhibited by intracerebrally cannulated parturient rats given four infusions of the specific oxytocin (OT) antagonist PPT (1 μg/side), a specific V_1 antagonist (1 μg/side), or normal saline (NS) vehicle (0.25 μl/side) alone bilaterally into or rostral to the ventral tegmental area (VTA); specific OT antagonist OTA (0.25 μg/side), V_1 antagonist (1 μg/side), or NS vehicle bilaterally into the medial preoptic area (MPOA); or PPT (2 μg), OTA (0.5 μg), or NS vehicle (2 μl) into the lateral cerebral ventricle (LCV); and by uncannulated (UNC) parturient rats that received no treatments. *p* values are for pairwise ANOVA comparisons between treatments within each brain site. Reprinted from Pedersen *et al.*,[27] 1994, with the publisher's permission. $**p < 0.01$; $***p < 0.001$ (site vs ICV); $\dagger p < 0.10$; $\dagger\dagger p < 0.05$; $\dagger\dagger\dagger p < 0.01$ (NS vs UNC).

with previous studies that found that lesions in these sites disrupted the onset of MB.[2,11]

The VTA is the origin of the ascending mesolimbic dopamine projections which play a key role in stimulating specific motor sequences and mediating the rewarding aspects of pleasurable activities.[31] Evidence has accumulated that this dopamine system plays an important role in MB. Neurotoxic lesions of dopamine cells in the VTA disrupted MB.[32] Hansen *et al.*[33] measured increased dopamine release in the nucleus accumbens during maternal interactions with pups. It is tempting to speculate that direct or indirect OT stimulation of dopaminergic neurons in the VTA that give rise to the mesolimbic projections may both activate the specific movements necessary to gather and nurture newborns and trigger the pleasurable emotions that strongly reinforce the execution of those maternal behaviors.

We next examined the relationships during late pregnancy between changes in OT binding in the MPOA and the VTA and changes in concentrations of ovarian steroids. This was done to determine if the rise in OT binding in these brain sites coincided with the onset of MB and to provide clues as to which of the hormonal features of pregnancy may stimulate the increased OT binding we had found in parturient rats. Three components of the ovarian steroid environment of pregnancy were shown to be necessary for the rapid postpartum onset of MB: (1) the sustained elevation of progesterone levels during most of pregnancy, (2) the rise in estrogen levels during the last half of pregnancy, and (3) the precipitous fall in progesterone over the last few days of pregnancy.[1-3] Our initial hypothesis was that the increase in OT binding in the MPOA and the VTA in parturient rats was similar in time course and ovarian steroid correlates as the rise in OT binding previously described in the uterus. Soloff[34] found that elevated estrogen levels and rapidly declining progesterone levels at the end of pregnancy in the rat stimulated a dramatic increase in OT binding in the uterus that immediately preceded and contributed to the onset of labor.

Our hypothesis was wrong. FIGURE 2 demonstrates that most of the increase in OT binding in the MPOA and VTA region originally observed in parturient rats occurred between days 15 and 18 of pregnancy, a time frame corresponding with the late gestational rise in estradiol levels. To our surprise, the increase in OT binding in both of these brain sites occurred well before the prepartum drop in progesterone levels, suggesting that the latter exerted no effect on the former. This impression was confirmed when we, using a saturating concentration of ^{125}I-OTA (1.3 μM) in the radioligand assay, found that OT binding (fmol/mg protein $\pm$ SEM) in the VTA region and the MPOA was not significantly different between rats treated with progesterone from day 18 to day 23 of pregnancy (the usual day of parturition) at a daily dose (4 mg) sufficient to keep concentrations at peak gestational levels and rats treated with sesame oil alone (VTA, 2.3 $\pm$ 0.1 vs 1.9 $\pm$ 0.2; MPOA, 9.4 $\pm$ 0.4 vs 8.7 $\pm$ 0.5). We conclude that the elevation of OT binding in these brain sites is probably driven by some but not all of the ovarian steroid components of pregnancy that contribute to the postpartum onset of MB. The rise in estrogen levels during late pregnancy seems very likely to be involved. It will be important to test this directly and to determine if the lengthy period of elevated progesterone levels that precedes and coincides with the rise in estrogen also contributes to the increase in OT binding in the MPOA and the VTA.

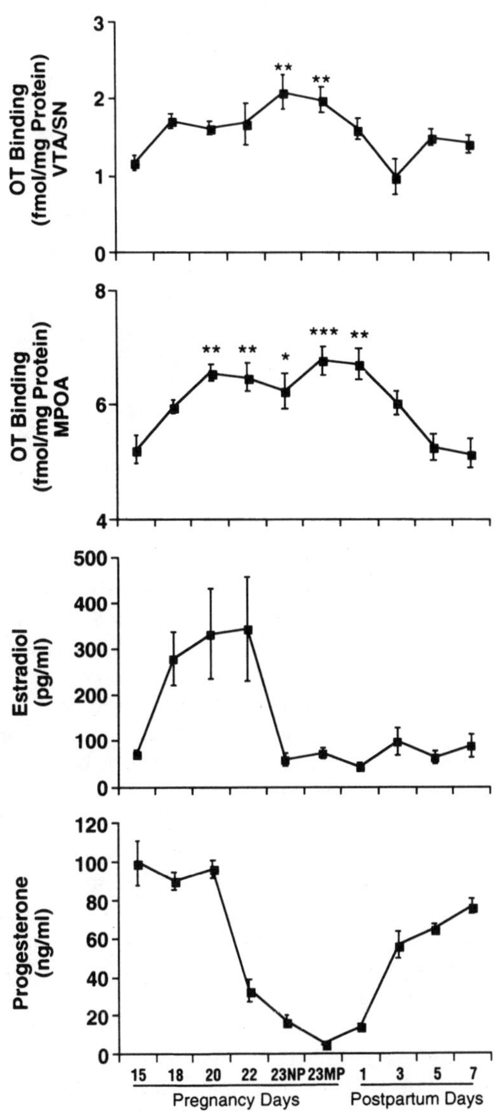

FIGURE 2. Mean (± SEM) OT binding in the ventral tegmental area/substantia nigra (VTA/SN) and medial preoptic area (MPOA), serum 17 β-estradiol and progesterone levels on pregnancy days 15, 18, 20, 22, 23NP (no parturition), 23 MP (midparturition), and postpartum days 1, 3, 5, and 7. *$p < 0.05$, **$p < 0.01$, ***$p < 0.001$ (in the VTA/SN, compared to pregnancy day 15 and/or postpartum day 3; in the MPOA, compared to pregnancy day 15 and/or postpartum day 7; Tukey HSD).

An impressive body of evidence indicates that ovarian steroids have powerful effects on OT binding in the brain. Several days of estrogen treatment increased OT binding in the ventromedial nucleus of the hypothalamus and in the lateral BNST.[20–22] This appears to be a genomic effect, because two days of estrogen treatment markedly increased OT receptor mRNA in the ventromedial nucleus.[35] Ovarian steroids can also exert brief effects on OT binding that are probably not genomically mediated. For example, 4-6 hours after progesterone treatment in estrogen-primed rats, a significant lateral extension of OT binding in the ventromedial nucleus had occurred.[36] In some brain sites, changes in OT binding at parturition appear to be very similar to those produced by brief estrogen treatment. For instance, total OT binding capacity increases in the ventromedial nucleus under both of these conditions.[20–22,37] However, in the MPOA, which is critically involved in MB, OT binding changes are qualitatively different during late pregnancy and after estrogen treatment. Oxytocin binding affinity but not binding capacity increased significantly in the MPOA after estrogen treatment,[38] whereas late pregnancy produced the inverse, a rise in OT binding capacity with no change in affinity.

The ovarian steroid changes of pregnancy may also stimulate the rapid postpartum onset of MB by increasing OT synthesis, transport, and release within the brain. Some groups have measured an increase in OT mRNA in the hypothalamus or magnocellular nuclei towards the end of pregnancy.[39,40] We[41] found that OT immunoreactive content in the magnocellular nuclei of the hypothalamus was significantly higher in late pregnant rats than in ovariectomized rats and that OT content rose significantly in sites that receive OT projections such as the lateral septum and the lower brainstem between the day before and the day after parturition. These observations suggest that the ovarian steroid conditions of late pregnancy promote OT synthesis and transport to or release within extrahypothalamic brain sites in some of which OT may stimulate the onset of MB. Ovarian steroid changes during late pregnancy may also indirectly stimulate central OT release by increasing OT binding in the uterus and subsequently vaginocervical dilation during labor. Landgraf *et al.*[42] measured an increase in OT release in the dorsal hippocampus during parturition in rats, while Kendrick *et al.*[43,44] found that mechanical vaginocervical stimulation in sheep increased CSF concentrations of OT and parturition increased OT release in the MPOA and the BNST. Estrogen and progesterone may also promote OT release by direct membrane effects on OT neurons. Caldwell *et al.*[45] found that 30 minutes of incubation with estadiol conjugated to BSA released OT from synaptosome-containing homogenates prepared from MPOA tissue; progesterone blocked this effect.

Oxytocin very likely exerts effects in other brain sites that contribute to the activation of MB. Olfactory stimuli from pups play a major role in suppressing MB in nulliparous rats. Experimental manipulations that temporarily or permanently eliminate olfaction (intranasal zinc sulfate treatment, olfactory bulbectomy, severing vomernasal nerves, and lesions of the lateral olfactory tracts) markedly decrease the latency of onset of MB in virgin rats that are cohoused with young pups.[2] Oxytocin projections to the olfactory bulbs may promote the onset of MB by suppressing or altering olfactory perception of newborns. Kendrick *et al.*[43] measured a rise in OT concentrations in the olfactory bulbs of sheep during vaginocervical stimulation which induces MB in this species. Other brain sites that have been implicated by lesion studies in the regulation of MB, including the amygdala,[46] hippocampus,[47,48] and the septum,[49] all contain OT projections and/or receptors.[9,10,20–22]

PUP STIMULI AND REGULATION OF OXYTOCIN CONTROL OF MATERNAL BEHAVIOR

Recent findings in our laboratory have forced a reevaluation of our assumptions, cited above herein, as to why OT no longer plays a necessary role in the expression of MB once parturient rats have acquired some mothering experience. Our new data indicate that effects of pup stimuli, rather than the postpartum decline in ovarian steroids, diminish the importance of OT in the maintenance of established MB.[50] This insight emerged from studies originally intended to examine the importance of somatosensory stimuli from pups in the changes in OT immunostaining pattern within the preoptic-anterior hypothalamic region of the brain that we had previously observed in postpartum, lactating rats.[25] In our initial approach to this question, we subjected rat dams that had 5 days of postpartum mothering experience to one of the following three conditions:

Proximal Separation. Pups were removed from each mother's home cage, the mother was placed in a clean cage with fresh bedding, and then 8 pups were placed inside a washbasket that was placed in the mother's new cage.

Total Separation. Pups were removed from each mother's home cage, and the mother was placed in a clean cage with fresh bedding in a room that contained no pups.

No Separation. Pups were taken from each mother's cage, the mother was moved to a clean cage with fresh bedding, and then 8 of the pups were returned to the mother.

Proximally separated dams were unable to push their snouts through the gaps in the walls of the washbaskets. However, dams could touch pups that were near the inside wall of the washbaskets either by extending their tongues, whiskers, or paws through the gaps. Pups were unable to push their heads or torsos through the gaps but did sometimes extend their legs or tails through the gaps. When this occurred, dams could directly touch those portions of the pups with their perioral area. Thus, under the proximal separation condition, rat mothers could readily hear, smell, and see pups but could only occasionally touch the pups with their paws, tongues, and perioral area and could never touch pups with their ventral trunks or nipples. Freshly nourished pups replaced used pups every 8 - 16 hours in the proximal and no separation conditions.

Animals were sacrificed after 6 days in these conditions. Analysis of OT-immunostained sections through the preoptic-anterior hypothalamic region of their brains revealed that there were significantly fewer discernible OT immunostaining perikarya in a number of brain sites within this region in the proximally separated compared to the totally or nonseparated rat dams (TABLE 2). We also noted that proximally separated dams continued to attempt to make contact with the isolated pups throughout the entire 6-day period. We hypothesized that proximal separation may maintain a higher level of maternal responsivity to pups than would be exhibited by rat dams totally separated from pups for the same interval of time. We tested this in other groups of rat dams that were subjected to each of these three separation conditions

TABLE 2. Mean (± SEM) Number of Oxytocin Immunostaining Perikarya Found on 50 μm Coronal Brain Sections through the Periventricular Nuclei, Anterior Hypothalamic Area, the Lateral Hypothalamus; the Medial Preoptic Area, and Lateral Preoptic Area from Rat Dams Subjected to 6 Days of Proximal, Total, or No Separation from Pups Beginning on Postpartum Day 5[a]

Brain Area	Proximal	Total	None
Perivent	10.7 ± 3.5	65.7 ± 3.5***	32.0 ± 8.1*
AHA	9.7 ± 9.7	26.3 ± 4.3	26.0 ± 3.0
LH	10.7 ± 6.1	61.0 ± 20.5*	37.3 ± 5.0**
MPOA	3.7 ± 1.8	19.7 ± 7.4*	13.3 ± 7.8
LPOA	0.7 ± 0.7	5.0 ± 3.6	8.0 ± 3.1*

Abbreviations: AHA = anterior hypothalamic area; LH = lateral hypothalamus; LPOA-lateral preoptic area; MPOA = medial preoptic area; perivent = periventricular nuclei.

[a] Reprinted from Pedersen *et al.*,[50] 1995, with the publisher's permission.

* $p < 0.10$; ** $p < 0.05$; *** $p < 0.01$ (compared to proximal separation, ANOVA).

for 4-6 days. Indeed, proximally separated dams began to exhibit MB significantly more quickly than did totally separated dams when they were again given unimpeded access to pups.[50] In fact, in our behavioral tests, proximally separated dams began mothering pups as rapidly as did nonseparated rat dams.

We hypothesized that the much greater depletion of OT immunostaining in the brains of proximally separated dams may have resulted from a release of central OT that could then have contributed to the more rapid reemergence of MB observed in this group of animals. To test this theory, we bilaterally infused the OT antagonist OTA (1 μg/side) into the VTA of dams that had been proximally separated or not separated from pups for 4-6 days beginning 5 days postpartum; some proximally separated dams were infused into the VTA with saline vehicle alone. In support of our hypothesis, OTA infusion into the VTA significantly inhibited the reemergence of pup retrieval and crouching in a nursing posture compared to saline infusion in proximally separated dams; OTA infusion was ineffective in blocking MB in nonseparated dams. (See FIG. 3 for a summary of the pup retrieval results.) Subsequently, we found that OTA infusion into the VTA significantly inhibited the reemergence of retrieval and crouching after 3 days of proximal separation, but not as potently as after 4 or more days of proximal separation. Oxytocin infusion into the VTA was ineffective in blocking the reemergence of MB after only 2 days of proximal separation. (See FIG. 4 for a summary of the pup retrieval results.)

Our finding that denying experienced rat mothers normal somatosensory stimuli from pups for 3 or more days reestablished sensitivity to OTA inhibition of MB suggests that pup stimuli alter the mechanisms that sustain MB such that OT is no longer essential for the expression of this behavior. Prior studies have repeatedly confirmed that somatosensory stimulation of the dam's ventral trunk or perioral area by pups regulates pup retrieval and crouching over pups, central components of rat MB.[51–57]

The simplest explanation for sensitization of experienced rat mothers to OTA inhibition of MB during proximal separation involves changes in central OT binding.

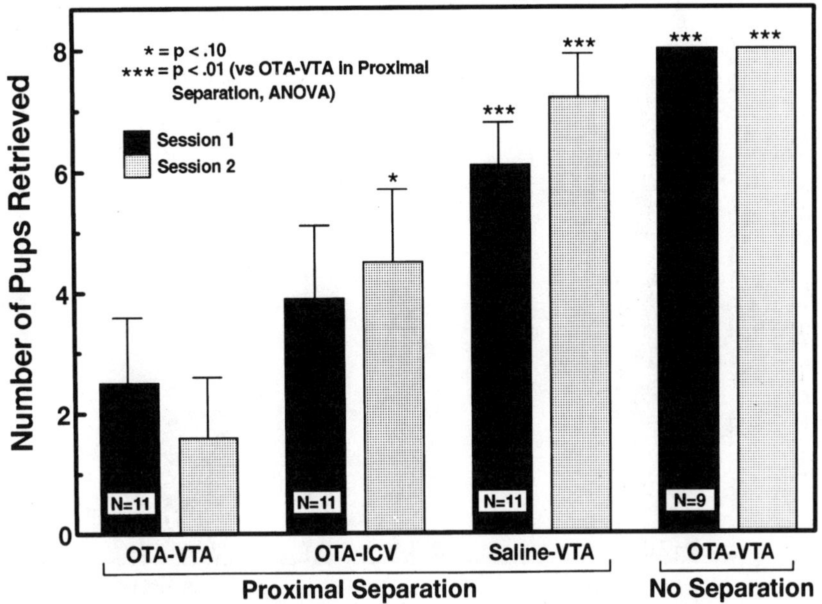

FIGURE 3. Mean (± SEM) number of pups retrieved during observation sessions 1 and 2 which began 1 hour after infusion of the oxytocin (OT) antagonist OTA or normal saline into the ventral tegmental area (VTA) and immediately after reintroduction of pups (8) to rat dams subjected to 4-6 days of proximal separation or no separation from pups beginning on day 5 postpartum. (Reprinted from Pedersen *et al.*,[50] 1995, with the publisher's permission.)

If increased release of central OT occurs in dams during interactions with pups and especially during suckling stimulation, there may be downregulation of central OT receptors. If so, one would expect during proximal separation, when nipple and other somatosensory stimulation from pups is absent or diminished, that central OT release would fall and OT receptors would upregulate. This could possibly resensitize the brain to the MB-stimulating effects of OT control of MB and reestablish OT control of MB. To test this hypothesis, we compared OT binding in the ventral midbrain (containing the VTA) and the MPOA between rat dams that had been proximally separated or had not been separated from pups for 5 days using a saturating concentration of ^{125}I-OTA (1.3 μM) in the radioligand assay. Binding (fmol/pg of protein ± SEM) was not significantly different between proximally separated and nonseparated dams in the ventral midbrain (1.7 ± 0.1 vs 1.7 ± 0.1; F = 0.003, [1,14], p = 0.96) or the MPOA (6.0 ± 0.2 vs 5.5 ± 0.5; F = 0.973, [1,14], p = 0.34). Therefore, alterations in OT binding could not account for proximal separation reinstatement of OT control of MB. Also, the depletion of OT immunostaining within the preoptic-anterior hypothalamic region that we found in proximally separated dams is not consistent with decreased central release of OT in these animals.

Two other quite different mechanisms of pup stimulus regulation of the role of OT in the control of MB can be invoked to account both for our recent finding that

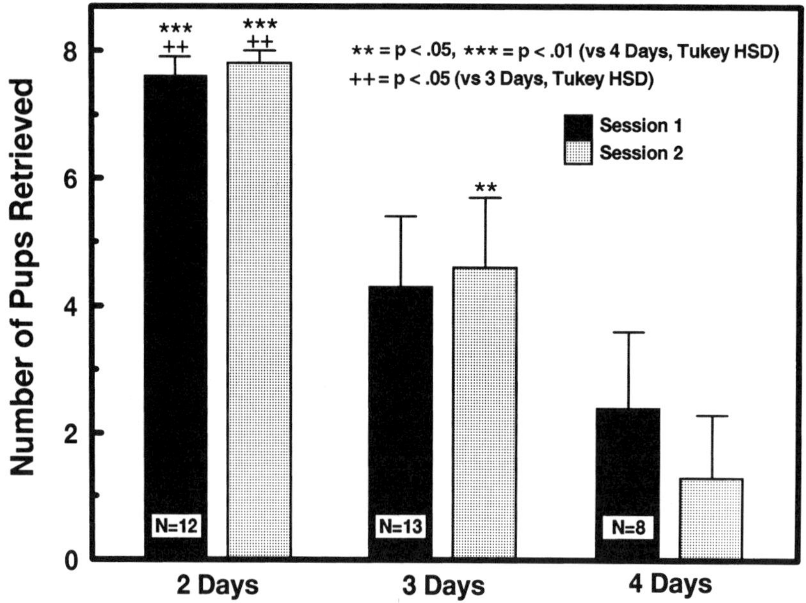

FIGURE 4. Mean (± SEM) number of pups retrieved during observation sessions 1 and 2 which began 1 hour after infusion of the oxytocin (OT) antagonist OTA into the ventral tegmental area and immediately after reintroduction of pups (8) to rat dams subjected to 2, 3, or 4 days of proximal separation from pups beginning on day 5 postpartum. (Reprinted from Pedersen *et al.*,[50] 1995, with the publisher's permission.)

proximal separation for 3 or more days establishes sensitivity to inhibition of MB by a single dose of OTA and prior findings, summarized herein, that brief central treatment with OT antiserum or antagonists blocks the onset of MB but not the maintenance of established MB. In the first hypothetical mechanism (see Model 1 in FIG. 5), somatosensory stimulation from pups during the early puerperium activates a system, other than the OT system, that sustains maternal responses to pups during the maintenance phase of MB. The OT system of MB stimulation may or may not remain active in parallel with the non-OT system (see below). Administration of an OT antagonist during the maintenance phase would block the OT system but not MB, because the non-OT system would sustain mothering behavior. During proximal separation, the absence of normal somatosensory stimulation from pups, over a 3-4 day period, would deactivate the non-OT system. Administration of OT antagonist after this period of proximal separation would block MB because OT would be the only MB-activating system remaining.

In the second hypothetical mechanism (see Model 2 in FIG. 5), somatosensory stimulation from pups causes a shift during the early puerperium from a short duration OT-activating effect on MB that we and others have shown to be necessary for the onset of MB and that can be blocked by brief treatment with an OT antagonist[8,27] to a much longer duration MB-sustaining effect during the maintenance phase of MB.

While the OT activation of the onset of MB is short-lived, once the behavior-mediating neural circuitry has been fully activated and has developed "momentum," the OT activation effect would persist for considerably longer periods. We have found that the inhibitory effect on the onset of MB of a brief period of OT antagonist administration lasts at least 1 day but no more than 2 days in most rat mothers. If, during the maintenance phase of MB, the OT facilitating effect persists longer than 2 days, the brief periods of OT antiserum or OT antagonist treatment that have been effective in blocking the onset of MB[6–8,27] would not exert their effects long enough to inhibit established MB. Three or more days of proximal separation may be necessary to establish sensitivity to single-dose OTA inhibition of MB, because this period exceeds the hypothesized long duration MB-activating effect of OT that depends upon normal somatosensory stimulation from pups during the maintenance phase of MB. The "momentum" in the neural apparatus that sustains established MB may be lost during a 3 or more day proximal separation period, returning the OT-activating effect to the short duration seen during the onset of MB.

An obvious initial experiment that would help distinguish which of these two hypothetical mechanisms best characterizes the effect of pup somatosensory stimuli on OT systems that stimulate MB would be to determine if maintaining OT receptor blockade with repeated daily infusions of an antagonist would eventually inhibit established MB in experienced, lactating rat mothers.

Our observation that 6 days of proximal separation from pups, but not 6 days of total separation from pups, markedly depleted OT immunostaining in many brain sites (see Preliminary Studies) suggests that proximal separation affects CNS OT much differently than does total separation. Some of the unique aspects of proximal separation (e.g., exposure to olfactory and auditory stimuli from the pups) rather than loss of normal somatosensory stimulation from pups, which is common to both proximal and total separation, probably exert this differential effect. Sensitization to OTA inhibition of MB in experienced rat mothers may also depend upon sustained exposure to olfactory and/or auditory stimuli from pups, which are unique to proximal separation, as well as a lack of normal somatosensory stimulation from pups. This concept is illustrated as Model 3 in FIGURE 5. Prior studies have established that olfactory and auditory stimuli from pups are very attractive to maternally responsive dams,[58,59] although neither of these sensory inputs is necessary for the onset or maintenance of MB.[2]

The importance of nonsomatosensory stimuli from pups for the proximal sensitization reinstatement of OT control of MB can be relatively easily determined by testing whether central administration of an OT antagonist will block the resurgence of MB in experienced rat mothers after a period of total separation from pups of 3 or more days. If the antagonist has no effect on the resurgence of MB after total separation, it would strongly suggest that nonsomatosensory stimuli from pups, as well as interference with normal somatosensory stimuli from pups, are necessary to reestablish OT control of MB in experienced rat mothers.

It is also possible that endocrine changes that occur during proximal separation may play a role in reinstating OT control of MB. Proximal separation is very likely stressful to maternal dams. The adrenal axis is markedly unresponsive to stress during lactation,[60] and total separation from pups does not increase dams' corticosterone levels.[61] Nonetheless, proximal separation may stimulate the release of corticosterone, especially if it is sustained long enough for the adrenal axis-inhibiting effect of lactation to wane. There are reasons for speculating that a rise in corticosterone during proximal separation may play a role in establishing sensitivity to OTA inhibition of MB. Oxytocin is known to be released and to facilitate ACTH and corticosterone release in rats under some stressful conditions.[82] Glucocorticoid receptors have been found in some OT neurons.[83] The depletion of OT immunostaining that we have seen during proximal separation may reflect mobilization of this neuropeptide to sustain corticosterone release. It will be interesting to determine if corticosterone levels increase during proximal separation and if adrenalectomy alters proximal separation reinstatement of OT control of MB.

It is also possible that estrous cycling may resume during 3 or more days of proximal separation. The rapid induction of MB by central administration of OT is estrogen dependent.[4] If estrogen levels rise during proximal separation because of a resumption of estrous cycling, the brain may be sensitized to the MB-stimulating effects of OT. This may contribute to the reinstatement of OT control of MB that occurs during proximal separation. If so, ovariectomy should block this effect of proximal separation.

Pup somatosensory stimulation of the dam's ventral trunk, nipples, and perioral region are each known to regulate the display of certain components of MB.[51–57] For two reasons, we hypothesize that pup contact with the dam's ventral trunk, and especially the nipples, is the component of somatosensory stimulation from pups that prevents OT (or the short duration activating effect of OT) from controlling MB in experienced rat mothers. First, pup contact with the dam's ventral trunk and nipples is the one component of somatosensory stimulation that is completely eliminated during proximal separation. Although difficult, dams do manage some paw, tongue, and perioral contact with pups through the openings in the mesh of the washbaskets used to isolate pups during proximal separation.

Second, pup stimulation of the dam's ventral trunk, especially the nipples, is well known to stimulate magnocellular OT neurons that project to the posterior pituitary and is thought to promote glial retraction and other morphological changes that increase electrotonic coupling of OT neurons in the paraventricular and supraoptic nuclei.[64,65] Although they enhance peripheral release of OT, it is possible that morphological changes induced by somatosensory stimulation of the dam's ventral surface may possibly inhibit OT neurons that project centrally to MB-mediating sites such as the VTA and the MPOA. This concept is supported by the observation that it requires several days, after lactating dams have been separated from pups, for plastic changes affecting OT neurons to revert to their prelactational state.[65] This is very similar to the minumum period of proximal separation (3-4 days) required to sensitize experienced rat mothers to single-dose OTA inhibition of MB. Perhaps the reversal of the morphological changes that enhance peripheral release of OT during separation from normal somatosensory stimulation from pups disinhibits central OT projections and allows resumption of their control of MB.

Our findings on the effects of proximal separation on OT control of MB have psychopathophysiological implications. Proximal separation of rat dams from pups, more so than total separation, may be a useful model of relationship loss. In people, many aspects of attachments persist after they are severed. These include memories of the person who is no longer available, frequent encounters with objects, situations,

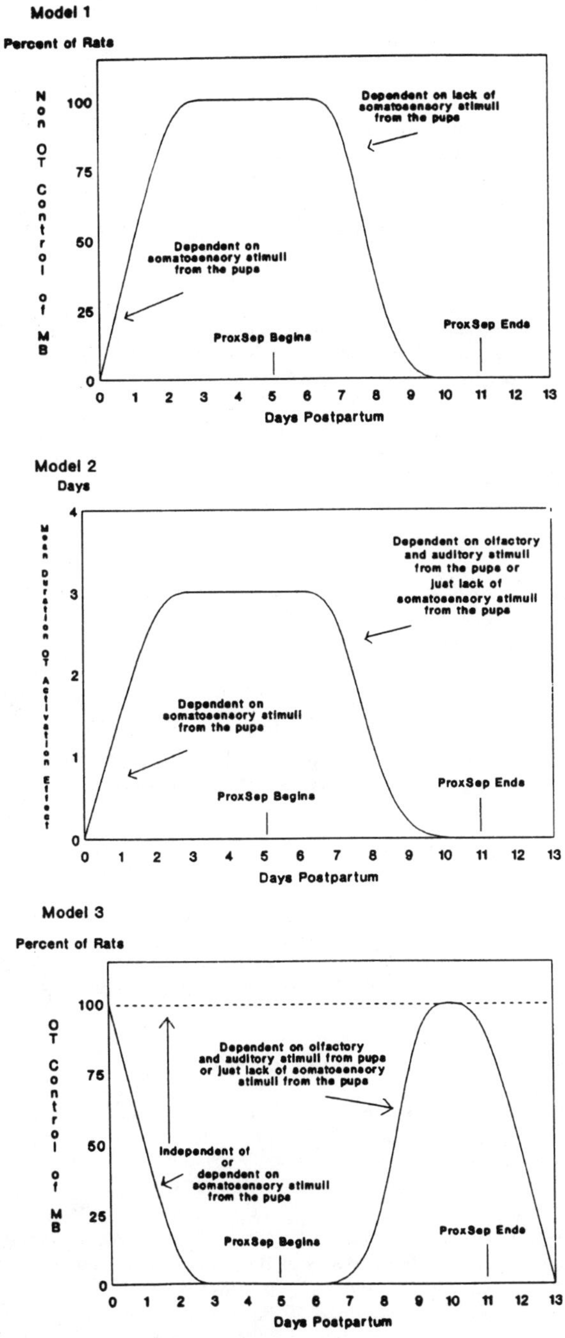

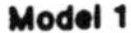

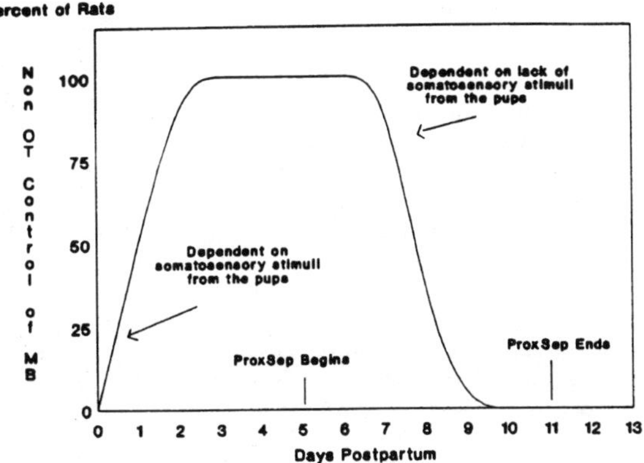

Model 1
Percent of Rats
Non OT Control of MB
100
75
50
25
0
Dependent on lack of somatosensory stimuli from the pups
Dependent on somatosensory stimuli from the pups
ProxSep Begins
ProxSep Ends
0 1 2 3 4 5 6 7 8 9 10 11 12 13
Days Postpartum
Model 2
Days
4
3
2
1
0
Dependent on olfactory and auditory stimuli from the pups or just lack of somatosensory stimuli from the pups
Dependent on somatosensory stimuli from the pups
ProxSep Begins
ProxSep Ends
0 1 2 3 4 5 6 7 8 9 10 11 12 13
Days Postpartum
Model 3
Percent of Rats
OT Control of MB
100
75
50
25
0
Dependent on olfactory and auditory stimuli from pups or just lack of somatosensory stimuli from the pups
Independent of or dependent on somatosensory stimuli from the pups
ProxSep Begins
ProxSep Ends
0 1 2 3 4 5 6 7 8 9 10 11 12 13
Days Postpartum

FIGURE 5. *Legend is on next page.*

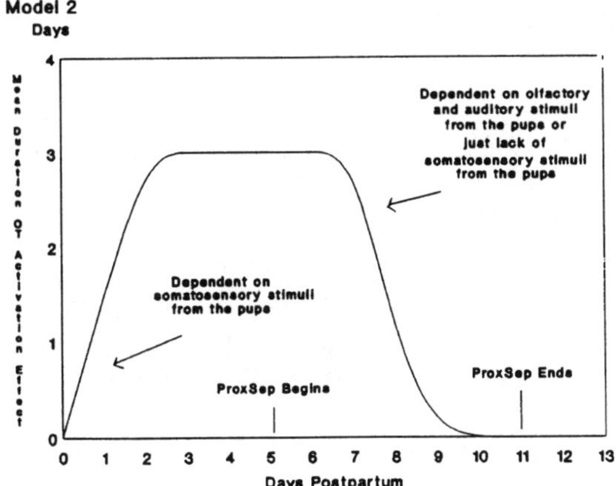

FIGURE 5. Three hypothetical models illustrating mechanisms that may account for the observations in rats that brief central treatment with an oxytocin (OT) antagonist (1) blocks the postpartum onset of maternal behavior (MB), (2) has no effect on established MB in dams with several days of postpartum mothering experience, but (3) blocks the resurgence of MB in lactating rat dams with 5 days of postpartum mothering experience that have been proximally separated from pups for 3 or more days. Model 1 illustrates the hypothetical time courses over which activation of MB by a non-OT mechanism may increase postpartum under the influence of somatosensory stimuli from pups and then decrease in the absence of normal somatosensory stimuli from pups during proximal separation. Model 2 illustrates the hypothetical time courses over which the duration of OT activation of neural systems that mediate MB may increase postpartum under the influence of somatosensory stimuli from pups and then decrease in the absence of normal somatosensory stimuli and, possibly, the presence of nonsomatosensory stimuli (e.g., olfactory and auditory) from pups during proximal separation. Model 3 illustrates the time courses over which OT activation of MB may decrease postpartum under the influence of somatosensory stimuli from pups and then increase in the absence of normal somatosensory stimuli and, possibly, the presence of nonsomatosensory stimuli from pups during proximal separation. Model 3 also illustrates that, alternatively, OT activation of MB may not be influenced at all by pup stimuli.

locations, and other people that were experienced together. After some losses, the partner in the former relationship may continue to be encountered on a regular basis. Our findings suggest that under these conditions, neural systems that contributed to the initial formation of the attachment (e.g., central OT) may be reactivated by stimuli from and about the former partner who is no longer available. This may contribute to the resurgence of longing and other strong emotions that typically occur after a close relationship is lost. Thus, investigation of the mechanisms underlying proximal separation reinstatement of OT control of MB may provide clinically useful insights into the psychobiology of grief, loss, and their potential psychopathological consequences, such as depression.

ACKNOWLEDGMENT

We wish to recognize the excellent secretarial help from Betsy Shambley.

REFERENCES

1. Bridges, R. S. 1990. Endocrine regulation of parental behavior in rodents. *In* Mammalian Parenting. N. A. Krasnegor & R. S. Bridges, Eds.: 93-117. Oxford University Press. Oxford, England.
2. Numan, M. 1994. Maternal behavior. *In* The Physiology of Reproduction, 2nd Ed. E. Knobil & J. D. Neill, Eds: 221-302. Raven Press. New York.
3. Rosenblatt, J. S., A. D. Mayer & H. I. Siegel. 1985. Maternal behavior among the nonprimate mammals. *In* Handbook of Behavioral Neurobiology. N. Adler, D. Pfaff & R. W. Goy, Eds: 229-298. Plenum Press. New York.
4. Pedersen, C. A. & A. J. Prange, Jr. 1979. Induction of maternal behavior in virgin rats after intracerebroventricular administration of oxytocin. Proc. Natl. Acad. Sci. USA **76:** 6661-6665.

5. Fahrbach, S. E., J. I. Morrell & D. W. Pfaff. 1984. Oxytocin induction of short-latency maternal behavior in nulliparous, estrogen-primed female rats. Horm. Behav. **18:** 267-286.
6. Pedersen, C. A., J. D. Caldwell, M. F. Johnson, S. A. Fort & A. J. Prange, Jr. 1985. Oxytocin antiserum delays onset of ovarian steroid-induced maternal behavior. Neuropeptides **6:** 175-182.
7. Fahrbach, S. E., J. I. Morrell & D. W. Pfaff. 1985. Possible role of endogenous oxytocin in estrogen-facilitated maternal behavior in rats. Neuroendocrinology **40:** 526-532.
8. Van Leengoed, E., E. Kerker & H. H. Swanson. 1987. Inhibition of postpartum maternal behavior in the rat by injecting an oxytocin antagonist into the cerebral ventricles. J. Endocrinol. **112:** 275-282.
9. Kozlowski, G. P. & G. Nilaver. 1986. Localization of neurohypophyseal hormones in the mammalian brain. *In* Neuropeptides and Behavior: The Neurohypophyseal Hormones. D. de Wied, W. H. Gispen & Tj B. van Wimersma Greidanus, Eds.: **2:** 23-38. Pergamon Press. Oxford.
10. Nieuwenhuys, R. 1985. Neurohypophyseal peptides. *In* Chemoarchitecture of the Brain.: 84-87. Springer-Verlag. Berlin.
11. Insel, T. R. & C. R. Harbaugh. 1989. Lesions of the hypothalamic paraventricular nucleus disrupt the initiation of maternal behavior. Physiol. Behav. **45:** 1033-1041.
12. Numan, M. & K. P. Corodimas. 1985. The effects of paraventricular hypothalamic lesions on maternal behavior in rats. Physiol. Behav. **35:** 417-425.
13. McCarthy, M. M., J. E. Bare & F. S. Vom Saal. 1986. Infanticide and parental behavior in wild female house mice: Effects of ovariectomy, adrenalectomy, and administration of oxytocin and prostaglandin F_2 alpha. Physiol. Behav. **36:** 17-23.
14. McCarthy, M. M. 1990. Oxytocin inhibits infanticide in wild female house mice (*Mus domesticus*). Horm. Behav. **24:** 365-375.
15. Kendrick, K. M., E. B. Keverne & B. A. Baldwin. 1987. Intracerebroventricular oxytocin stimulates maternal behaviour in the sheep. Neuroendocrinology **46:** 56-61.
16. Kendrick, K. M., E. B. Keverne, B. A. Baldwin & D. F. Sharman. 1986. Cerebrospinal fluid levels of acetylcholinesterase, monoamines and oxytocin during labour, parturition, vaginocervical stimulation, lamb separation and suckling in sheep. Neuroendocrinology **44:** 149-156.
17. Kendrick, K. M., E. B. Keverne, M. R. Hinton & J. A. Goode. 1991. Cerebrospinal fluid and plasma concentrations of oxytocin and vasopressin during parturition and vaginocervical stimulation in sheep. Brain Res. Bull. **26:** 803-807.
18. Levy, F., E. B. Keverne, K. M. Kendrick, V. Piketty & P. Poindron. 1992. Intracerebral oxytocin is important for the onset of maternal behavior in inexperienced ewes delivered under peridural anesthesia. Behav. Neurosci. **106:** 427-432.
19. Keverne, E. B. & K. M. Kendrick. 1991. Morphine and corticotropin-releasing factor potentiate maternal acceptance in multiparous ewes after vaginocervical stimulation. Brain Res. **540:** 55-62.
20. De Kloet, E. R., T. A. M. Voorhuis & J. Elands. 1986. Estradiol induces oxytocin binding sites in rat hypothalamic ventromedial nucleus. Eur. J. Pharmacol. **118:** 185-186.
21. Insel, T. R. 1986. Postpartum increases in brain oxytocin binding. Neuroendocrinology **44:** 515-518.
22. Insel, T. R. 1990. Regional changes in brain oxytocin receptors post-partum: Time-course and relationship to maternal behaviour. J. Neuroendocrinol. **2:** 539-545.
23. Tribolet, E., C. Barberis, S. Jard, M. Dubois-Dauphin & J. J. Dreifuss. 1988. Localization and pharmacological characterization of high affinity binding sites for vasopressin and oxytocin in the rat brain by light microscopic autoradiography. Brain Res. **442:** 105-118.

24. Elands, J., C. Barberis, S. Jard, E. Tribollet, J.-J. Dreifuss, K. Bankowski, M. Manning & W. Sawyer. 1987. ^{125}I-Labelled $d(CH_2)_5[Tyr(Me)^2, Thr^4, Tyr\text{-}NH_2^9]$OVT: A selective oxytocin receptor ligand. Eur. J. Pharmacol. **147:** 197-207.
25. Jirikowski, G. F., J. D. Caldwell, C. Pilgrim, W. E. Stumpf & C. A. Pedersen. 1989. Changes in immunostaining for oxytocin in the forebrain of the female rat during late pregnancy, parturition and early lactation. Cell Tissue Res. **256:** 411-417.
26. Fahrbach, S. E., J. I. Morrell & D. W. Pfaff. 1985. Role of oxytocin in the onset of estrogen-faciliated maternal behavior. *In* Oxytocin: Clinical and Laboratory Studies. J. A. Amico & A. G. Robinson, Eds. **666:** 372-388. Elsevier Science Publishers. Amsterdam.
27. Pedersen, C. A., J. D. Caldwell, C. Walker, G. Ayer & G. A. Mason. 1994. Oxytocin activates the postpartum onset of rat maternal behavior in the ventral tegmental and medial preoptic areas. Behav. Neurosci. **108:** 1163-1171.
28. Hruby, V. J. 1986. Structure-activity of the neurohypophyseal hormones and analogues and implications for hormone receptor interactions. *In* Biochemical Actions of Hormones. G. Litwack, Ed.: 191-241. Academic Press. New York.
29. Kruszynski, M., B. Lamarc, M. Manning, J. Seto, J. Haldar & W. H. Sawyer. 1980. [1-(β-mercapto-β,β-cyclopentamethylenepropionic acid),2-(0-methyl)tyrosine]arginine vasopressin, two highly potent antagonists of the vasopressor response to arginine-vasopressin. J. Med. Chem. **23:** 364-368.
30. Pedersen, C. A., J. A. Ascher, Y. L. Monroe & A. J. Prange, Jr. 1982. Oxytocin induces maternal behavior in virgin female rats. Science **216:** 648-649.
31. Le Moal, M. 1995. Mesocorticolimbic dopaminergic neurons functional and regulatory roles. *In* Psychopharmacology: The Fourth Generation of Progress. F. E. Bloom & D. J. Kupfer, Eds.: 283-294. Raven Press. New York.
32. Hansen, S., C. Harthon, E. Wallin, L. Lofberg & K. Svensson. 1991. Mesotelencephalic dopamine system and reproductive behavior in the female rat: Effects of ventral tegmental 6-hydroxydopamine lesions on maternal and sexual responsiveness. Behav. Neurosci. **105:** 588-598.
33. Hansen, S., A. H. Bergvall & S. Nyiredi. 1993. Interaction with pups enhances dopamine release in the ventral striatum of maternal rats: A microdialysis study. Pharmacol. Biochem. Behav. **45:** 673-676.
34. Soloff, M. S. 1985. Oxytocin receptors and mechanisms of oxytocin action. *In* Oxytocin: Clinical and Laboratory Studies. J. A. Amico & A. G. Robinson, Eds.: 259-276, Elsevier Science Publishers. Amsterdam.
35. Bale, T. L. & D. M. Dorsa. 1995. Sex differences in and effects of estrogen on oxytocin receptor messenger ribonucleic acid expression in the ventromedial hypothalamus. Endocrinology **136:** 27-32.
36. Schumacher, M., H. Coirini, M. Frankfurt & B. S. McEwen. 1989. Localized actions of progesterone in hypothalamus involve oxytocin. Proc. Natl. Acad. Sci. USA **86:** 6798-6801.
37. Bale, T. L., C. A. Pedersen & D. M. Dorsa. 1995. CNS oxytocin receptor mRNA expression and regulation by gonadal steroids. *In* Oxytocin: Cellular and Molecular Approaches in Medicine and Research. R. Ivell & J. Russell, Eds. Plenum Press. New York. In Press.
38. Caldwell, J. D., C. H. Walker, C. A. Pedersen, A. S. Barakat & G. A. Mason. 1994. Estrogen increases affinity of oxytocin receptors in the medial preoptic area—anterior hypothalamus. Peptides **15:** 1079-1084.
39. Van Tol, H. H. M., E. L. M. Bolwerk, B. Liu & J. P. H. Burbach. 1988. Oxytocin and vasopressin gene expression in the hypothalamo-neurohypophyseal system of the rat during the estrous cycle, pregnancy, and lactation. Endocrinology **122:** 945-951.
40. Zingg, H. H. & D. Lefebvre. 1988. Oxytocin and vasopressin gene expression during gestation and lactation. Mol. Brain Res. **4:** 1-6.

41. CALDWELL, J. D., E. R. GREER, M. F. JOHNSON, A. J. PRANGE, JR. & C. A. PEDERSEN. 1987. Oxytocin and vasopressin immunoreactivity in hypothalamic and extrahypothalamic sites in late pregnancy and post-partum rats. Neuroendocrinology **46:** 39-47.
42. NEUMANN, I., J. A. RUSSELL, B. WOLFF & R. LANDGRAF. 1991. Naloxone increases the release of oxytocin, but not vasopressin, within limbic brain areas of conscious parturient rats: A push-pull perfusion study. Neuroendocrinology **54:** 545-551.
43. KENDRICK, K. M., E. B. KEVERNE, C. CHAPMAN & B. A. BALDWIN. 1988. Microdialysis measurement of oxytocin, aspartate, γ-aminobutyric acid and glutamate release from the olfactory bulb of the sheep during vaginocervical stimulation. Brain Res. **442:** 171-174.
44. KENDRICK, K. M., E. B. KEVERNE, M. R. HINTON & J. A. GOODE. 1992. Oxytocin, amino acid and monoamine release in the region of the medial preoptic area and bed nucleus of the stria terminalis of the sheep during parturition and suckling. Brain Res. **569:** 199-209.
45. CALDWELL, J. D., M. A. MORRIS, C. H. WALKER, R. B. CARR, B. M. FAGGIN & G. A. MASON. 1996. Estradiol conjugated to BSA releases oxytocin from synaptosome-containing homogenates from the medial preoptic area-hypothalamus. Horm. Metab. Res. **28:** 119-121.
46. FLEMING, A. S., F. VACCARINO & C. LUEBKE. 1980. Amygdaloid inhibition of maternal behavior in the nulliparous female rat. Physiol. Behav. **25:** 731-743.
47. KIMBLE, D. P., L. ROGERS & C. W. HENDRICKSON. 1967. Hippocampal lesions disrupt maternal, not sexual, behavior in the albino rat. J. Comp. Physiol. Psychol. **63:** 401-407.
48. TERLECKI, L. J. & R. S. SAINSBURY. 1978. Effects of fimbria lesions on maternal behavior in the rat. Physiol. Behav. **21:** 89-97.
49. FLEISCHER, S. & B. M. SLOTNICK. 1978. Disruption of maternal behavior in rats with lesions of the septal area. Physiol. Behav. **21:** 189-200.
50. PEDERSEN, C. A., J. M. JOHNS, I. MUSIOL, M. PEREZ-DELGADO, G. AYERS, B. M. FAGGIN & J. D. CALDWELL. 1995. Interfering with somatosensory stimulation from pups sensitizes experienced, postpartum rat mothers to oxytocin antagonist inhibition of maternal behavior. Behav. Neurosci. **109:** 980-990.
51. KENYON, P., P. CRONIN & S. KEEBLE. 1981. Disruption of maternal retrieving by perioral anesthesia. Physiol. Behav. **27:** 313-321.
52. KENYON, P., P. CRONIN & S. KEEBLE. 1983. Role of the infraorbital nerve in retrieving behavior in lactating rats. Behav. Neurosci. **97:** 255-269.
53. MORGAN, H. D., A. S. FLEMING & J. M. STERN. 1992. Somatosensory control of the onset and retention of maternal responsiveness in primiparous Sprague-Dawley rats. Physiol. Behav. **51:** 549-555.
54. STERN, J. M. & S. K. JOHNSON. 1990. Ventral somatosensory determinants of nursing behavior in Norway rats. I. Effects of variations in the quality and quantity of pup stimuli. Physiol. Behav. **47:** 993-1011.
55. STERN, J. M. & J. M. KOLUNIE. 1989. Perioral anesthesia disrupts maternal behavior during early lactation in Long-Evans rats. Behav. Neural Biol. **52:** 20-38.
56. STERN, J. M. & J. M. KOLUNIE. 1991. Trigeminal lesions and maternal behavior in Norway rats. I. Effects of cutaneous rostral snout denervation on maintenance of nurturance and maternal aggression. Behav. Neurosci. **105:** 984-987.
57. STERN, J. M., L. DIX, C. BELLOMO & C. THRAMANN. 1992. Ventral trunk somatosensory determinants of nursing behavior in Norway rats. 2. Role of nipple and surrounding sensation. Psychobiology **20:** 71-80.
58. ALLIN, J. T. & E. M. BANKS. 1972. Functional aspects of ultrasound production by infant albino rats *(Rattus norvegicus).* Anim. Behav. **20:** 175-185.
59. SMOTHERMAN, W. P., R. W. BELL, J. STARZEC, J. ELIAS & T. A. ZACHMAN. 1974. Maternal responses to infant vocalizations and olfactory cues in rats and mice. Behav. Biol. **12:** 55-66.

60. Stern, J. M., L. Goldman & S. Levine, S. 1973. Pituitary-adrenal responsiveness during lactation in rats. Neuroendocrinology **12:** 179-191.
61. Smotherman, W. P., S. G. Wiener, S. P. Mendoza & S. Levine. 1977. Maternal pituitary-adrenal responsiveness as a function of differential treatment of rat pups. Dev. Psychobiol. **10:** 113-122.
62. Gibbs, D. M. 1986. Vasopressin and oxytocin: Hypothalamic modulators of the stress response. A review. Psychoneuroendocrinology **22:** 131-140.
63. Jirikowski, G. F., W. C. McGimsey, J. D. Caldwell & M. Sar. 1993. Distribution of oxytocinergic glucocorticoid target neurons in the rat hypothalamus. Horm. Metab. Res. **25:** 543-544.
64. Hatton, G. I., B. K. Modney & A. K. Salm. 1992. Increases in dendritic bundling and dye coupling of supraoptic neurons after the induction of maternal behavior. *In* Oxytocin in Maternal, Sexual, and Social Behaviors. C. A. Pedersen, J. D. Caldwell, G. F. Jirikowski & T. R. Insel, Eds. Ann. N. Y. Acad. Sci. **652:** 142-155.
65. Theodosis, D. T. & D. A. Poulain. 1992. Neuronal-glial and synaptic plasticity of the adult oxytocinergic system. *In* Oxytocin in Maternal, Sexual, and Social Behaviors. C. A. Pedersen, J. D. Caldwell, G. F. Jirikowski & T. R. Insel, Eds. Ann. N. Y. Acad. Sci. **652:** 303-325.

20
Mating-Induced c-fos Expression Patterns Complement and Supplement Observations after Lesions in the Male Syrian Hamster Brain

Sarah Winans Newman, David B. Parfitt, and Sara Kollack-Walker

Experimental efforts to define the functional neuroanatomical circuitry underlying male sexual behavior in rodents have relied in the past on the observation of behavioral deficits in males with selectively placed brain lesions. More recently, experiments in our laboratory and several other laboratories have attempted to selectively stimulate or eliminate Fos protein production associated with mating by controlling either the past sexual experience of the animal or the stimuli and behavioral events immediately preceding perfusion-fixation of the brain,[1–5] by altering the hormonal status of the behaving animal,[6] or by observing Fos-ir patterns ipsilateral to unilateral lesions in key nuclei of the mating behavior pathway.[4] In this chapter we summarize the results of several studies in the male Syrian hamster in light of previously reported behavioral effects of lesions in the same areas.

MATING BEHAVIOR CIRCUITS REVEALED BY LESION STUDIES

In 1970 Murphy and Schneider[7] reported that olfactory bulbectomy, which destroys both olfactory and vomeronasal inputs to the CNS, completely eliminated male sexual behavior and greatly diminished intermale aggression in golden hamsters and that these effects were not secondary to reduced testosterone stimulation of the brain. Subsequent studies indicated that the peripheral sensory afferents and the centrally projecting efferents of both the main (olfactory) and accessory (vomeronasal) bulbs

This research was supported by the National Institutes of Health (NINCD-NS 20629 and the Morphology Core Facility of NICHD-P-30, HD 18258).

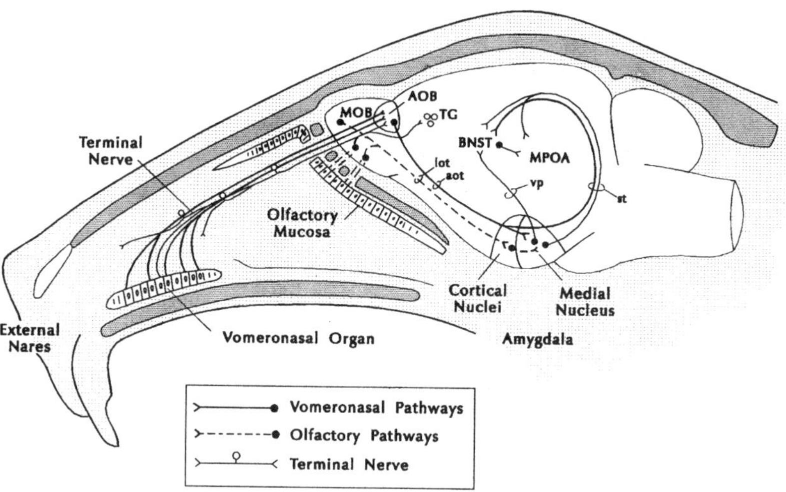

FIGURE 1. Sagittal view of a hamster head illustrating the chemosensory pathways critical to male hamster sexual behavior. Abbreviations: AOB = accessory olfactory bulb; aot = accessory olfactory tract; BNST = bed nucleus of the stria terminalis; lot = lateral olfactory tract; MPOA = medial preoptic area; st = stria terminalis; TG = terminal ganglion; vp = ventral pathway.

were contributing to the maintenance of mating behavior[8–11] and that the essential chemosensory pathways included the lateral olfactory tract projections to the corticomedial amygdala.[12]

Further analysis of behavior after amygdaloid lesions focused attention on the anterior part of the medial nucleus of the amygdala (MeA), where damage mimicked the effect of olfactory bulbectomy and completely abolished both phases of sexual behavior, the chemoinvestigatory phase (sniffing and licking the female's head, flanks and, anogenital area) and the copulatory phase (mounts, intromissions and ejaculations). In contrast, males with lesions of the posterior part of this nucleus, MeP, exhibited partial reduction in chemoinvestigation, with no deficits in copulatory behavior; however, they did show changes in the temporal pattern of copulation.[13] Neither lesions in the basolateral amygdala nor those in other nuclei of the corticomedial amygdala produced these effects.[14,15]

From the medial nucleus the behaviorally relevant efferents follow both the stria terminalis and the ventral amygdaloid pathway[16–18] to the bed nucleus of the stria terminalis BNST and the medial preoptic area (MPOA). These pathways are illustrated in FIGURE 1. However, unlike the effects of damage to the medial amygdaloid nucleus, lesions in the BNST and MPOA revealed a dissociation of effects on the two major components of the male hamster's mating activities. Whereas some animals with lesions of either the BNST or the MPOA showed severe deficits in both phases of mating, many animals with BNST damage showed a deficit in chemoinvestigation without any alteration in copulation, and the reverse effect was observed after lesions of the MPOA.[19] The differential effects of these lesions in the chemosensory pathways are summarized in FIGURE 2.

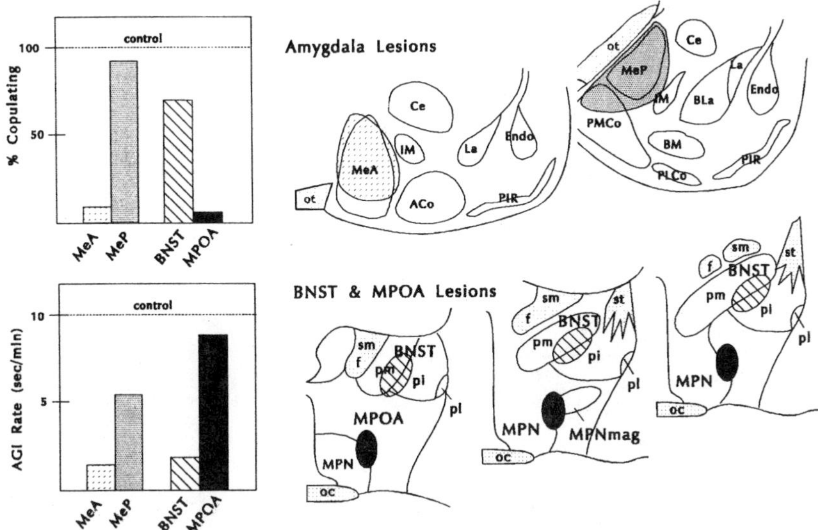

FIGURE 2. Effects of lesions placed within the anterior or posterior subdivisions of the medial amygdaloid nucleus (MeA or MeP), bed nucleus of the stria terminalis (BNST), or medial preoptic area (MPOA) on the percentage of males copulating with receptive females and on the rate of investigation of the female's anogenital region (AGI). Each *shaded* or *patterned area* represents the area that was damaged in common in a group of males. See TABLE 1 for additional abbreviations.

MATING-INDUCED EXPRESSION OF FOS PROTEIN

Fos-Immunoreactivity Reveals Activation of Neurons Not Only in Areas Where Lesions Eliminate the Behavior, But Also in Areas Where Lesions Have Subtle Effects

The observations of Robertson *et al.*,[5] that immunohistochemistry for Fos protein could be used to visualize neuronal activation after male sexual behavior in the rat, presented an opportunity to localize and study directly the neurons activated as a result of mating in the Syrian hamster. In the first experiment in this species, in which each sexually naive male mated for 55 minutes with three females,[1] Fos immunoreactivity (Fos-ir) was elevated above control levels in numerous nuclei within the corticomedial amygdala, BNST, and MPOA (FIGS. 3 and 4). Furthermore, quantitative analysis revealed a broad range of differences across nuclei, from 35% more Fos-ir cells in the posterolateral cortical nucleus of the amygdala to a 20-fold difference, or a 2000% increase, in the posteromedial BNST.

It was immediately clear, however, that no correlation existed between the magnitude of the increase in Fos-ir cells in a given area and the significance of that area, as determined by lesions, for initiation of sexual behavior. In the MeA, where bilateral lesions completely eliminate both phases of the behavior,[15] the number of Fos-ir cells

A

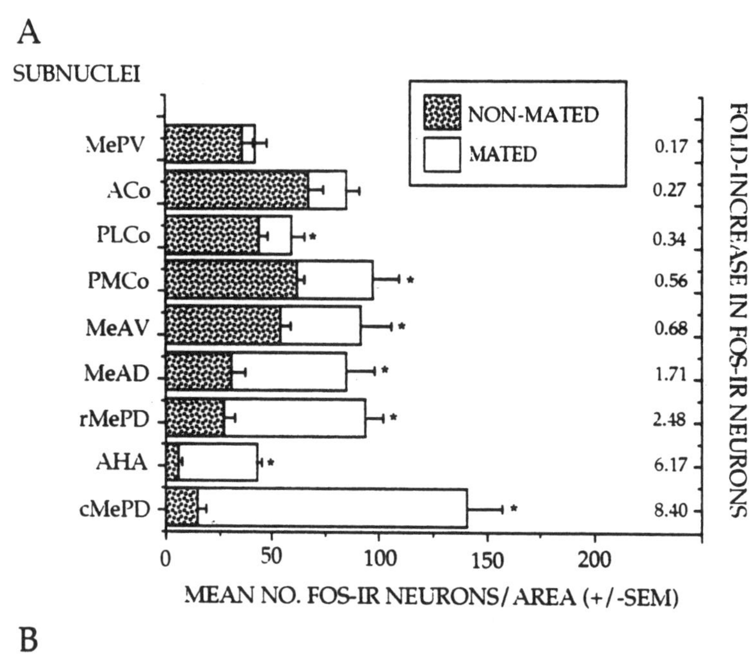

B

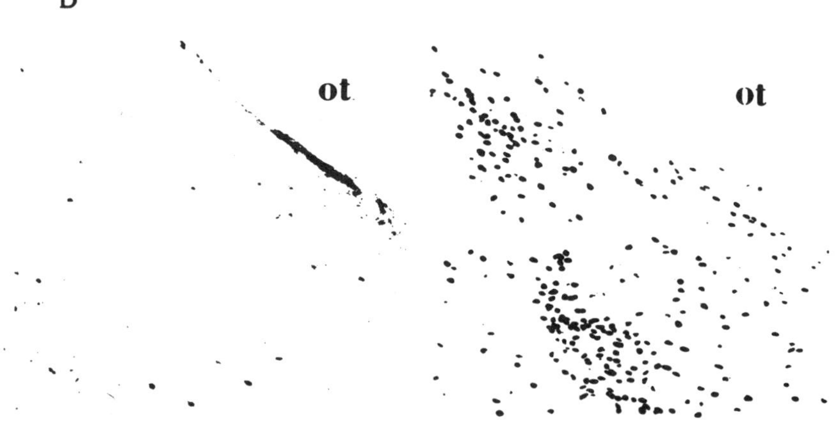

FIGURE 3. (**A**) Mean number of Fos-ir neurons per 0.21 mm^2 in subnuclei of the amygdala in nonmated (n = 5) and mated (n = 6) groups of male hamsters. The fold-increase in Fos-ir neurons indicates the mating-induced increase above control levels. * = area that contained significantly more Fos-ir neurons following mating. For abbreviations see TABLE 1. (**B**) Photomicrographs of Fos-ir neurons in the caudal posterodorsal division of the medial nucleus of the amygdala (cMePD) of nonmated (*left*) and mated (*right*) hamsters. ot = optic tract.

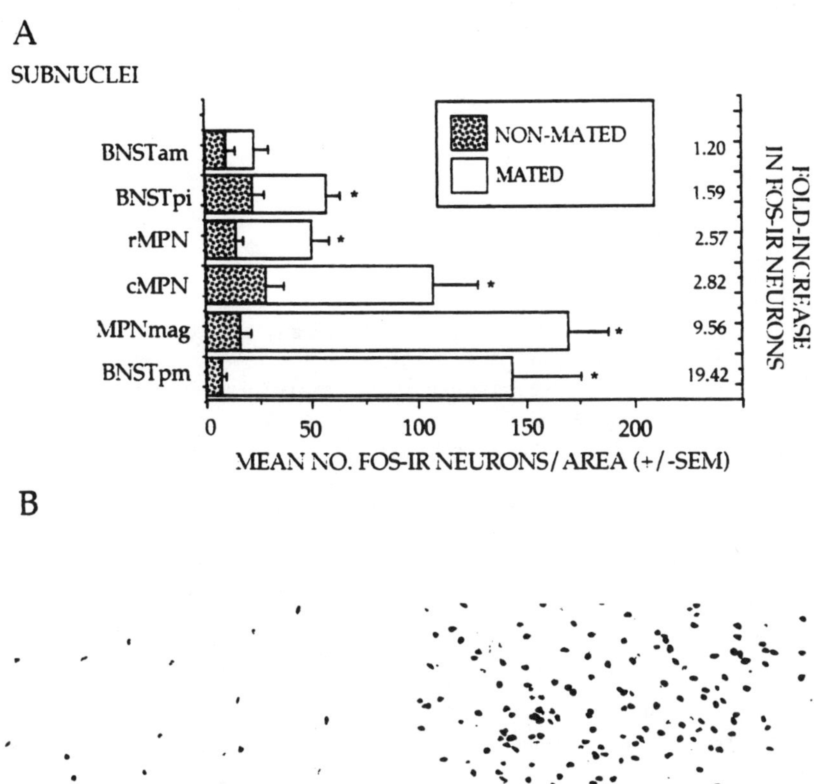

B

FIGURE 4. (**A**) Mean number of Fos-ir neurons per 0.21 mm^2 in subnuclei of the bed nucleus of the stria terminalis and medial preoptic area in nonmated (n = 5) and mated (n = 6) groups of male hamsters. The fold-increase in Fos-ir neurons indicates the mating-induced increase above control levels. * = area that contained significantly more Fos-ir neurons following mating. For abbreviations see TABLE 1. (**B**) Photomicrographs of Fos-ir neurons in the magnocellular medial preoptic nucleus (MPNmag) of nonmated (*left*) and mated (*right*) hamsters.

was elevated only 100% above control levels in the mated males (FIG. 3), while in the same animals an 800% increase was observed in the MeP, where lesions alter only the temporal pattern of copulation.[13] Similarly, in the caudal MPOA, where lesions abolish the copulatory phase of the behavior,[19] we observed a 1000% difference (FIG. 4), whereas in the posteromedial BNST (BNSTpm), where lesions interfere with the chemoinvestigatory phase of the behavior,[19] mated males had almost 2000% more Fos-ir cells than did controls. Finally, a 200% increase in Fos-ir was observed in a specific area of the paraventricular nucleus of the hypothalamus, a nucleus with no known involvement in sexual behavior. Although these results indicated that Fos-ir could be detected in brain regions shown previously to be important in male sexual behavior, it was unclear whether this pattern reflected activity associated selectively with male copulation or associated with social behaviors in general.

Comparison of Fos-ir after Mating and Agonistic Behavior Reveals Activation in a "Mating-Specific" Circuit and in a "Nonspecific" Circuit Activated Equally by Mating and Aggression

Identification of the "Mating-Specific" Circuit

To narrow the investigation to neurons specifically activated by mating in the male, we compared the Fos-ir pattern in three groups of sexually naive males that had lived in isolation for 1 week and on the day of the experiment either (1) engaged in sexual behavior with a receptive female or (2) agonistic behavior with a male or (3) were left alone after handling by the experimenter (Experiment 2). All of these males remained in their own cages during behavioral testing.[2] The rationale for this experiment was based on the observation that both mating and aggression are diminished by removal of the olfactory bulbs[7,20] and by bilateral lesions of the amygdala[21] and on the assumption that both behaviors require emotional arousal, autonomic activation, and strenuous motor activity on the part of the males, whereas the specific chemosensory stimuli and motor patterns are different. We therefore hypothesized that we could identify mating-specific areas of the limbic system by subtraction of the areas activated equally by the two behaviors, recognizing that in doing so we might be eliminating from further consideration areas in which equal but different populations of cells in one region are active during the two different social behaviors.

Analysis of 26 limbic areas in these male hamsters showed significant increases in Fos-ir above control levels in 20, but in only 4 of these 20 areas was Fos-ir increased in the copulating males and not at all in the agonistic males. All four of these nuclei were in the preoptic region, including medial preoptic nucleus (MPN), the magnocellular medial preoptic nucleus (MPNmag, a small nucleus in the lateral part of the medial preoptic area of the hamster[22]), the dorsolateral medial preoptic area (MPOA), and the preoptic portion of the BNST (the posteroventral portion of the posteromedial BNST or BNSTpm[pv]). These results are summarized in FIGURE 5.

In addition to these selectively activated nuclei in the preoptic region, two nuclei were activated by both mating and agonistic behavior, but to a greater degree by mating. Both the lateral part of the caudal posterodorsal division of the medial amygdaloid nucleus (cMePD) and the rostral part of the posteromedial BNST (BNSTpm[ad]) contained 2-3 times as many Fos-ir cells in the copulating males as in the fighting males, although the Fos-ir cell populations were intermingled and indistinguishable by location in both areas. However, in addition, an easily distinguishable group of cells, close to the optic tract in cMePD, was always labeled in the brains of mated but not aggressing males (FIGS. 5 and 6). The behavioral significance of this activation pattern in BNSTpm(ad) and cMePD was revealed by work in other laboratories and confirmed in our recent studies, and we will return to this topic.

Of the six areas that were significantly activated by mating (MPN, MPNmag, MPOA, BNSTpm[ad], BNSTpm[pv], and cMePD), four belong to a neuroanatomical

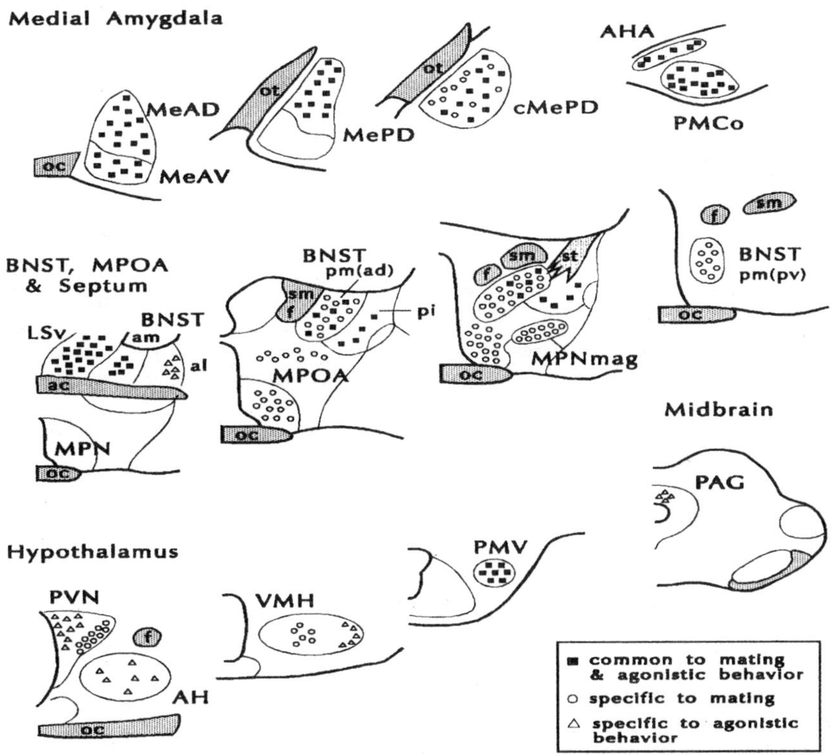

FIGURE 5. Summary of the net effect of copulation and agonistic behavior on the pattern of Fos-immunostaining within limbic regions of the male Syrian hamster brain. The intermingling of "common" and "mating-specific" activation symbols in BNSTpm and in cMePD reflects activation of neurons above control after both behaviors, but with mating producing significantly greater numbers of Fos-ir neurons than agonistic encounters. For abbreviations see TABLE 1.

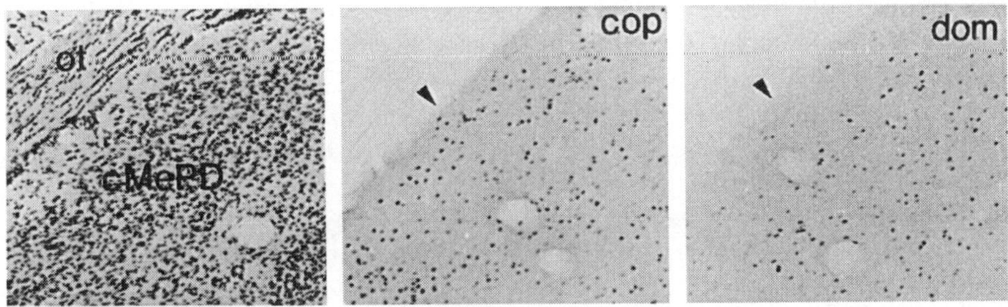

FIGURE 6. Photomicrographs of the caudal posterodorsal subdivision of the medial amygdaloid nucleus (cMePD), illustrating the cytoarchitecture of this subnucleus in a cresylviolet-stained section and the distribution of Fos-ir neurons within this area in a representative animal from copulator (cop) and dominant (dom) groups. Arrowhead identifies the boundary between the molecular layer of cMePD and the optic tract (ot).

circuit that can be defined in the hamster[23] and rat[24] by the projections of the posterior division of the medial amygdaloid nucleus (MePD). Iontophoresis of PHA-L into MePD of the hamster reveals projections to the BNSTpm (including BNSTpm[ad] and BNSTpm[pv]) and the medial region of the MPOA, including the MPN. Furthermore, these are the subdivisions of Me, BNST, and MPOA that are most densely populated with androgen- and estrogen-receptor producing neurons,[25–29] where delivery of gonadal steroids can reinstate sexual behavior in castrated males that have stopped mating.[30]

Specific Antecedents for Fos Production within the "Mating-Specific" Circuit

With evidence that structures in a neuroanatomically definable circuit of sex steroid-sensitive areas were selectively activated by sexual behavior, we were anxious to try to determine the specific components of mating that induced Fos production in each of these areas. In our next experiment (Experiment 3), six groups of six male hamsters were given prior mating experience in a testing arena. On the day of the experiment all males were placed in the mating arena. Males in the handled-control group with experience (HC-Exp) were left alone. A second group received female hamster vaginal secretion (FHVS) presented on a cotton swab. The remaining groups were given free access to a receptive female, but their mating behavior was interrupted after either five intromissions (5-INTRO), one ejaculation (1-EJAC), five ejaculations (5-EJAC), or the first long intromission (Long-INTRO). (In the male hamster, the long intromission at the termination of mating is an extended period of intromissions with repeated pelvic thrusting, but without ejaculation.[31,32]) A seventh group of six males, that had no prior mating experience but had been placed in the clean testing arena alone on pretest days (HC-Naive), were again placed in the arena on the day of the experiment.

The results from this third experiment provided both new data and data confirming the results from other laboratories.[3,4,33,39,40] Quantification of the number of Fos-ir neurons per nuclear area was analyzed using a one-way ANOVA and post hoc comparisons with the Tukey test for significant differences. This analysis identified discrete patterns of activation in association with specific aspects of male mating behavior, including sexual conditioning, pheromonal stimulation, chemosensory investigation of the female, copulation, and sexual satiety.

Sexual Conditioning. Significant differences in Fos-ir cell numbers were found in cMePD, MPN, and MPNmag of sexually experienced and naive control males (Figs. 7 and 8, Exp 3). On the day of the experiment these males were treated identically; both were placed in the empty testing arena for an hour. The only difference was that the experienced controls had mated on three previous occasions in an identical arena, whereas the naive males had simply been placed in the empty arena on those occasions. This sexual experience-associated neuronal activation presumably reflects a conditioned response to environmental cues and may be the basis of previously documented changes in mating behavior following experience.[34,35] Alternatively or in addition, it may indicate brain areas that regulate neuroendocrine reflexes that are known to be enhanced after sexual encounters.[36–38]

Pheromonal Stimulation and Chemosensory Investigation of the Female. The second distinctive activation pattern within this circuit is associated with pheromonal

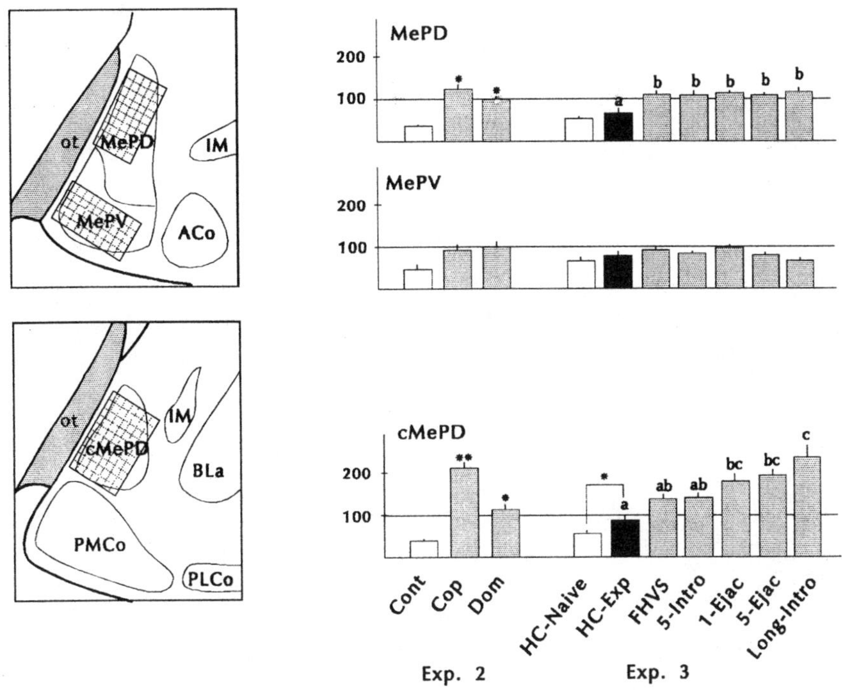

FIGURE 7. Location of cell counts within the posterior subdivisions of the medial nucleus of the amygdala and the resultant mean number of Fos-ir neurons (± SEM) per subdivision for control (Cont), copulator (Cop), and dominant (Dom) groups in Experiment 2 and for Handled Control-Naive (HC-Naive), Handled Control-Experienced (HC-Exp), female hamster vaginal secretion (FHVS), 5-Intromissions (5-Intro), 1-Ejaculation (1-Ejac), 5-Ejaculations (5-Ejac), and Long-Intromission (Long-Intro) groups of males in Experiment 3. A significant increase in the number of Fos-ir neurons (above Cont in Exp 2; HC-Exp above HC-Naive in Exp 3) is indicated with an *asterisk* ($p < 0.05$). In Experiment 3 a significant difference ($p < 0.05$) between groups (excluding HC-Naive) is identified by different lowercase letters.

stimulation. In 1993 Fiber *et al.*[39] reported that female hamster vaginal secretion (FHVS) induced Fos production in the areas we designated MePD, BNSTpm(ad), and MPNmag but not in the MPN. Fernandez-Fewell and Meredith[3] also observed activation after FHVS alone in the MePD and BNSTpm(ad) (their "mBNSTpc"). They did not report on MPNmag, but, like Fiber *et al.*,[39] they found that MPN was not activated. Our study replicated these findings in MePD (FIG. 7), MPNmag (FIG. 8), and BNSTpm(ad) (FIG. 9). In addition, our histological material presented a distinctive qualitative difference in the location of Fos-ir neurons in cMePD between control animals and all other groups, including both FHVS-stimulated and mated males. Illustrations in Fiber *et al.*[39] and Fernandez-Fewell and Meredith[3] also show this distinctive pattern of immunolabeling. In these two reports and in all three of our studies, a strip of cells close to the optic tract in cMePD of the medial amygdaloid nucleus is activated in all animals that have been exposed to FHVS (FIG. 6).

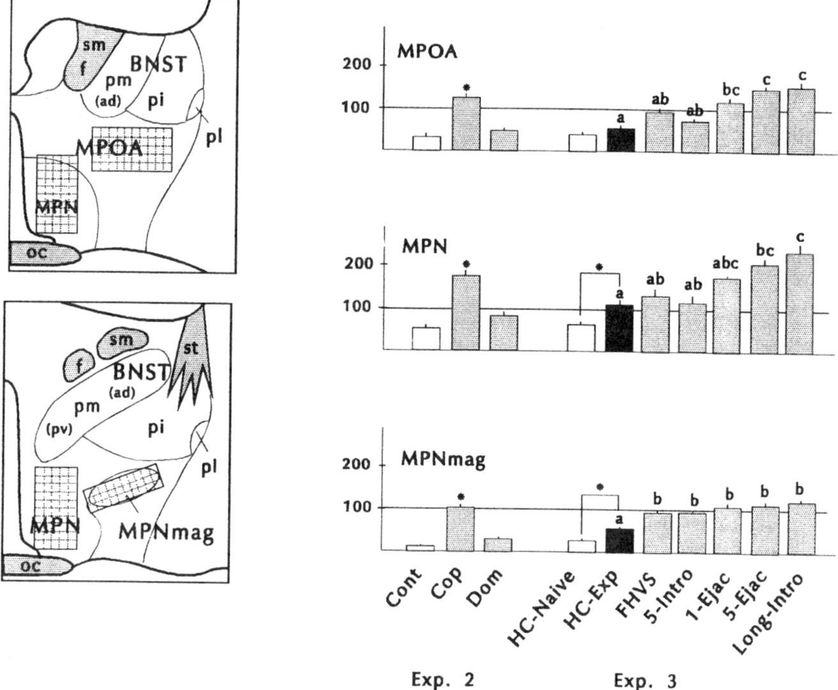

FIGURE 8. Location cell counts and mean number of Fos-ir neurons counted within the medial preoptic area. For explanation see legend for FIGURE 7.

Although each of these three areas is activated by the presentation of FHVS alone, the functional significance of this pheromonal stimulation may be different. Whereas lesions of MePD reduce anogenital investigation of the female (AGI) and affect only the temporal pattern of copulation, small lesions of BNSTpm(ad) can virtually eliminate AGI without altering copulation, and lesions that include the MPNmag can abolish copulatory behavior without affecting AGI. Thus, it would appear that projections from MePD to BNSTpm may process FHVS-associated information to drive the chemoinvestigatory behavior. Additional evidence to support this hypothesis comes from Fernandez-Fewell and Meredith[3] who report that male hamsters in which the vomeronasal organ has been removed prepubertally (at 17 days of age) show no Fos-ir induction in BNSTpm(ad) (their mBNSTpc) when exposed to FHVS, but do show statistically significant increases in Fos-ir if they engage in chemoinvestigatory behavior with a receptive female, regardless of whether they show any copulatory responses.

In the MPNmag, in contrast, FHVS stimulation may be required for the pheromonal elicitation of mounts, intromissions, and ejaculations. Although this empirically derived explanation is clear and consistent with the hamster's dependence on chemosensory inputs for mating, the specific pathways that might be responsible for mediating these pheromonal effects in MPNmag have not been identified.

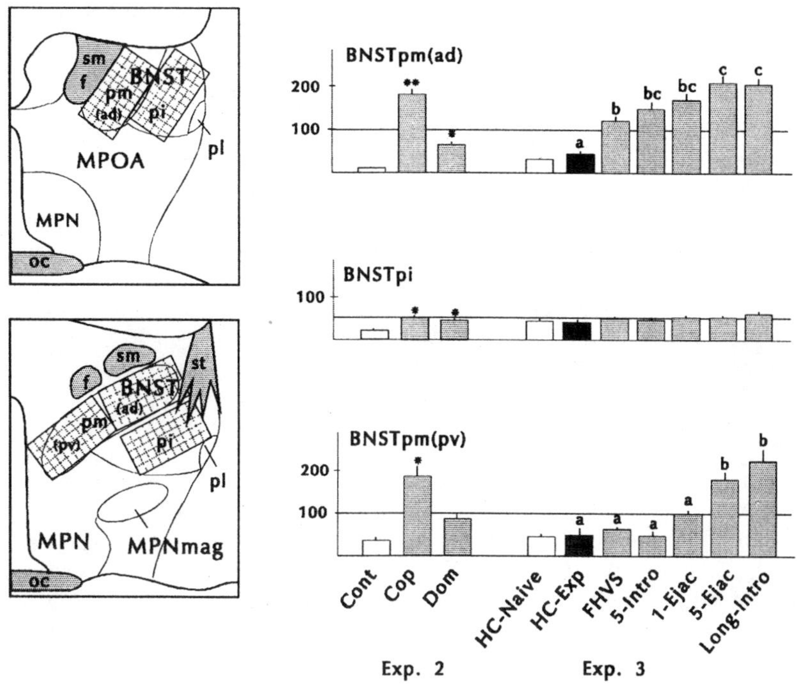

FIGURE 9. Location cell counts and mean number of Fos-ir neurons counted within the bed nucleus of the stria terminalis. For explanation see legend for FIGURE 7.

Copulation. Mating to intromissions did not selectively increase Fos production in any of the areas we analyzed. However, in males that were allowed to mate to ejaculation, several areas along this pathway, including cMePD, BNSTpm(ad), BNSTpm(pv), MPOA, and MPN, and the central tegmental field of the midbrain (CTF), appeared to reach a new level of activation. In our sexually experienced animals this represented a further significant increase in the number of Fos-ir cells, adding to the populations in cMePD and MPN that had already been stimulated to express Fos on exposure to the testing arena. However, in both of these areas, and in BNSTpm(ad), what was actually observed was a gradual and continual increase in the levels of activation, rather than an abrupt increase associated with ejaculations (FIGS. 7, 8, and 9). Only in BNSTpm(pv) (FIG. 9) and the CTF did it appear that the population was stimulated for the first time in the behavioral sequence by the occurrence of ejaculations. This is in agreement with the observations of Coolen[40] in the male rat, but in contrast to the findings of Baum and Everitt,[4] who reported the induction of Fos protein in the CTF after five intromissions.

Sexual Satiety. Finally, investigations of Fos-ir in the male hamster after copulation have produced evidence for selective activation of cell "clusters," small groups of cells (approximately 150-250 cells in an area no more than 250 μm in diameter), that have not, to date, been observed as discrete populations with any other markers or histological methods (FIG. 3). These cells were reported in cMePD by Kollack and Newman[1] and by Fernandez-Fewell and Meredith[3] in cMePD and rostral BNST (corresponding to rostral BNSTpm[ad] in this paper; called mBNSTpr by Fernandez-Fewell and Meredith). In both of these studies each male mated for at least 45 minutes with three females. In Experiments 2 and 3 described above,[2,42] we determined that these Fos-ir clusters of cells are readily distinguishable in 40 μm sections of cMePD and BNSTpm(ad) only in males that had mated to multiple ejaculations. They were never present in males that had been stopped after one ejaculation but were found in one half to two thirds of males that had achieved five ejaculations, and in all males that had mated to long intromissions.

These findings led one of us (D.B.P.) to hypothesize that the appearance of the Fos-ir cell clusters was associated with the culmination of a mating behavior sequence and not with multiple ejaculations per se. In the first of two experiments he compared the brains of males that were mated for 4 consecutive days to long intromissions or rested and then mated only on the fourth day to long intromissions. The rationale for this paradigm was based on observations by Huck and Lisk,[41] who showed that rested male hamsters (i.e., animals that have not mated for at least 2 weeks) will ejaculate an average of 13 times before reaching long intromissions, whereas males mated on succeeding days will reliably ejaculate only four times, on average, before stopping. Thus, this study was designed to determine if the number of ejaculations preceding long intromissions influences the appearance of clusters in cMePD.

In six rested male hamsters mated to long intromissions, after an average of 10 ejaculations, all 6 brains had clusters in cMePD. A second group of males were mated to long intromissions for 4 consecutive days and averaged only four ejaculations on the fourth day, but five of six males in this group also had Fos-ir clusters in the cMePD. In a third group, male hamsters mated to long intromissions for 3 consecutive days were placed in an empty clean cage on the fourth day to serve as controls, and none of these males showed the cell clusters. These results were consistent with the hypothesis that activation of cMePD cell clusters is correlated with the onset of sexual satiety rather than the number of ejaculations per se. However, because all animals that exhibited clusters had ejaculated more than once, we could not exclude the possibility that cluster activation was dependent on multiple ejaculations.

As already noted, we had never seen this activation pattern in rested male hamsters stopped after one ejaculation. Therefore, in a second experiment one of us (DBP) compared the Fos-ir pattern in a group of rested animals that had been interrupted after one ejaculation with the pattern in a second group of males that were mated to long intromissions for 3 consecutive days and then interrupted after one ejaculation on the fourth day. Although none of the rested animals had Fos-ir cell clusters, five of six males in the second group did (FIG. 10). Therefore, we conclude that the appearance of cell clusters in cMePD does not depend on multiple ejaculations, but is associated with the onset of sexual satiety.

In contrast to the neuronal activation observed along the optic tract in the medial part of cMePD, which appears following exposure to FHVS (FIG. 6), activation of the cell clusters in the lateral part of this same region may be independent of chemosensory stimulation. Fernandez-Fewell and Meredith[3] report that these lateral Fos-ir cell clusters were present in the brain of one male that mated following removal of the vomeronasal organ (7 of 9 animals in this group did not mate). Instead, based

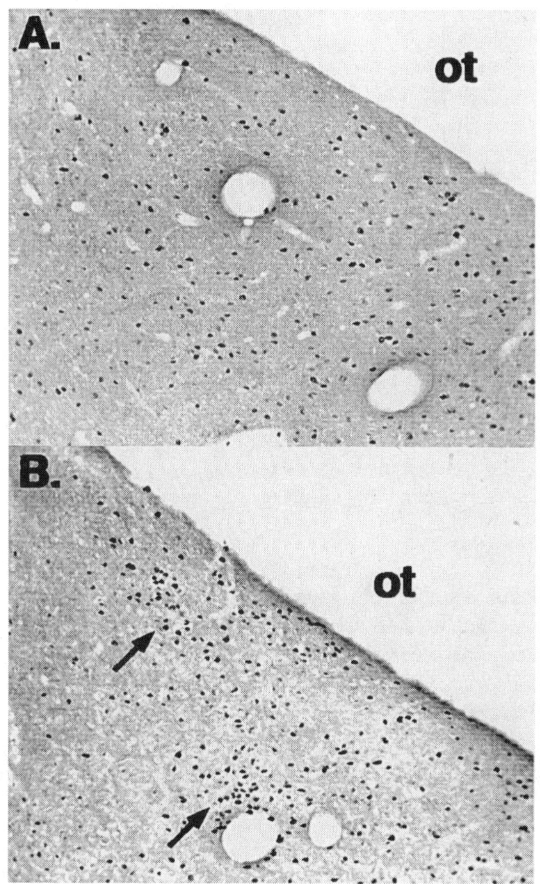

FIGURE 10. Photomicrographs of Fos-ir neurons within the cMePD of a rested male hamster stopped after one ejaculation (**A**) and a male hamster mated to one ejaculation on the fourth of 4 consecutive days of mating to long intromissions (**B**). *Arrows* indicate the location of Fos-ir cell clusters.

largely on data from the male rat, it appears more likely that these cell clusters are activated by somatosensory stimuli and/or visceral stimuli processed through ascending spinal cord pathways reaching the amygdala via the midbrain, where a field of cells in the ventral tegmentum show Fos-ir after copulation in both the rat[4,40] and the hamster.[42]

Given the observations that within the cMePD there may be separate cells groups activated specifically by FHVS, sexual conditioning, copulation to ejaculation, and sexual satiety, it is surprising that lesions destroying this area do not eliminate any of the behavioral components of male sexual behavior. These lesions cause decreases in chemoinvestigatory behavior and an increase in latency to the first ejaculation in

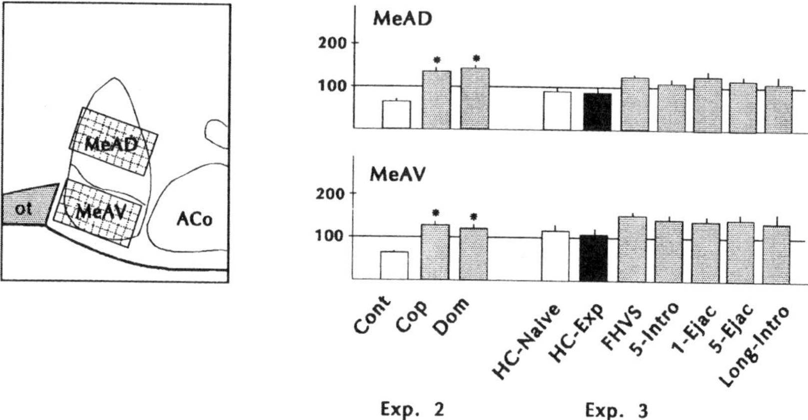

FIGURE 11. Location of cell counts and mean number of Fos-ir neurons counted within the anterior subdivisions of the medial amygdaloid nucleus. For explanation see legend for FIGURE 7.

a series,[13] but over 4–8 weeks following the lesions the only behavioral changes that have been documented to date are changes in the temporal pattern of mating by experienced males. These deficits appear insignificant when compared to the total loss of mating following lesions of the MeA. However, work by Lanier *et al.*[43] and Huck and Lisk[44] suggests that the timing of the copulatory bout, which in the Syrian hamster is controlled largely by the male, and particularly the occurrence of long intromissions, are of great importance for successful conception, the ultimate goal of mating.

A Separate "Nonspecific" Circuit May be an Essential "Arousal Circuit" for Social Behaviors

In contrast to the projections of MePD, axons of the cells in MeA preferentially terminate in the posterointermediate BNST (BNSTpi) and the lateral part of the MPOA including MPNmag.[23] It was the integrity of this circuit which the results of lesion studies had indicated was absolutely essential for mating to occur in the hamster.[15,19] What did the results of Fos expression after mating or agonistic behavior tell us about this circuit? Quantitative analysis of the data indicated that cells in MeA and BNSTpi were equally activated after these two behaviors (FIGS. 9 and 11, Exp 2), and histological analysis indicated that the activated cells were equally distributed. Acknowledging that future research might reveal separate but equal, intermingled populations of activated cells in these two circumstances, we tentatively concluded that the Fos-ir cells in MeA and BNSTpi belong to an arousal circuit, providing essential background activation for discrete stimuli to elicit appropriate social responses.

This conclusion would lead to the prediction that any animal engaging in mating would show increased Fos-ir in these areas, but quantitative analysis of Fos-ir neurons in MeA (MeAD and MeAV) and BNSTpi in the seven groups of males in Experiment 3 revealed no significant increase in any of the stimulated groups of animals relative to controls (FIGS. 9 and 11, Exp 3), even though comparison of the data from Experiments 2 and 3 revealed that the number of Fos-ir cells in the mated males were equivalent. This comparison indicated that an increase in the number and variance of immunolabeled cells in the control groups (HC-Exp and HC-Naive) in Experiment 3 was, in fact, responsible for the failure to replicate the results of Experiment 2. FIGURE 12 presents data from individual animals in these two experiments, showing comparable levels of activation in the copulators from Experiment 2 and the males mated to five ejaculations in Experiment 3, but a striking difference between the number of Fos-ir neurons in the control groups in these two experiments.

Although the basis for the apparent changes in Fos production in the control animals remains to be investigated, the explanation may be attributable to differences in the amount of prior handling and in the location where the experiments were conducted. In the first study in this series and in Experiment 2, males were handled by the experimenter only briefly[2] or not at all[1] before being anesthetized for perfusion fixation of the brain. In these experiments the control, mated, and dominant animals all remained in their home cages. In the third study all males were handled on three testing days before the day of the experiment and again on the day of the experiment, when in each case all males were placed in a testing arena. Although it might be argued that repeated handling and experience in the arena should have acclimated the animals to this procedure, the fact remains that all of these animals spent the hour before anesthetization in a testing arena, whereas all of the animals in the first two experiments were in their home cages during this period. We hypothesize that being placed in the arena aroused both control and stimulated animals in the third experiment sufficiently to eliminate differences between these groups in a circuit that is active during arousal.

CONCLUSIONS

Exposure of male Syrian hamsters to female pheromones, or copulation with the female, increases immunohistochemically detectable Fos protein and Fos-related antigens in a number of discrete populations of limbic system neurons where lesions eliminate male sexual behavior. Although in the initial stages of this work it was tempting to conclude that Fos-immunoreactive cell populations in the lesion-sensitive areas are essential for the initiation of mating, it is now evident that Fos immunoreactivity is also elevated in regions where lesions have less impact on the occurrence of the behavior. Furthermore, no correlation appears to exist between the magnitude of the increase of Fos-ir in a given area and the significance of that area, as determined by lesions, for initiation of mating. Perhaps areas essential for triggering the behavior are activated by appropriate stimuli only briefly, at the onset of the behavior and, depending on the previous experience of the individual animal, are responsible for activating other circuits that pace and maintain the events of copulation. We must also keep in mind, however, that the Fos-defined neuroanatomical substrate does not necessarily represent the entire circuitry underlying mating, because many, but by no means all, neurons employ *c-fos* as a transcription factor following excitation.

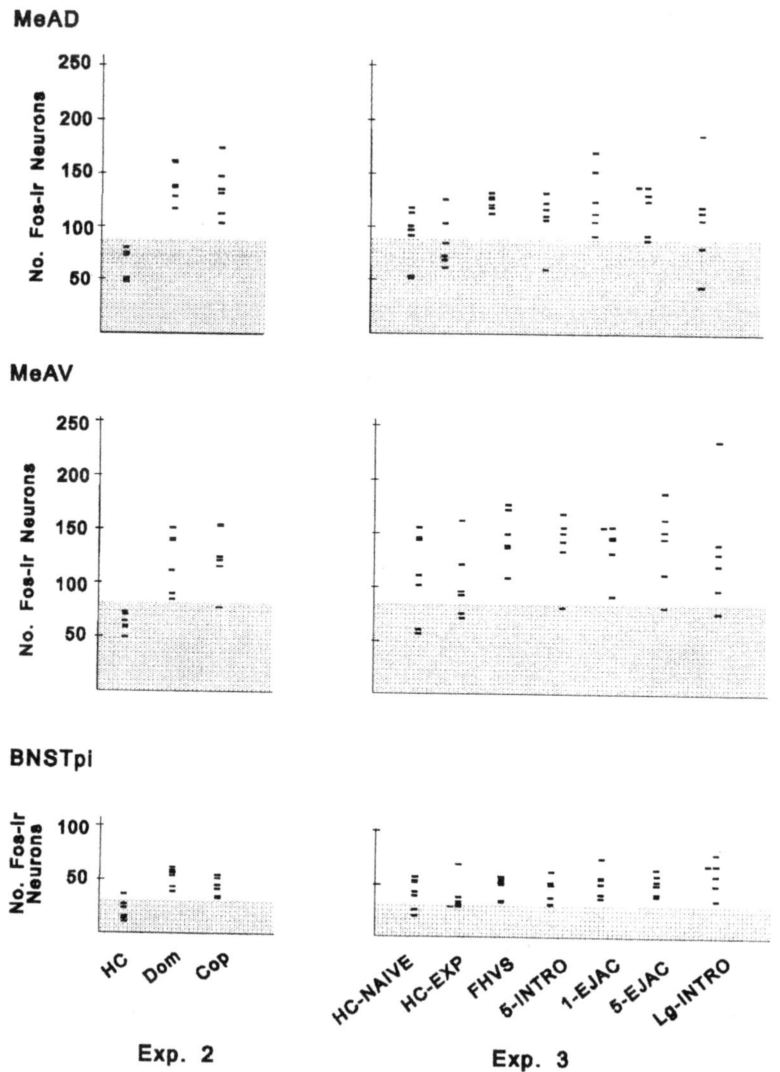

FIGURE 12. Distribution of cell counts (number of Fos-ir neurons) in the anterodorsal medial amygdaloid nucleus (MeAD), the anteroventral medial nucleus (MeAV) and the postero-intermediate division of the bed nucleus of the stria terminalis (BNSTpi) taken from individual male hamsters in control and experimental groups in Experiments 2 and 3, showing the increase in number and variance in the control groups in Experiment 3 (HC-NAIVE and HC-EXP) compared to the control group in Experiment 2 (HC).

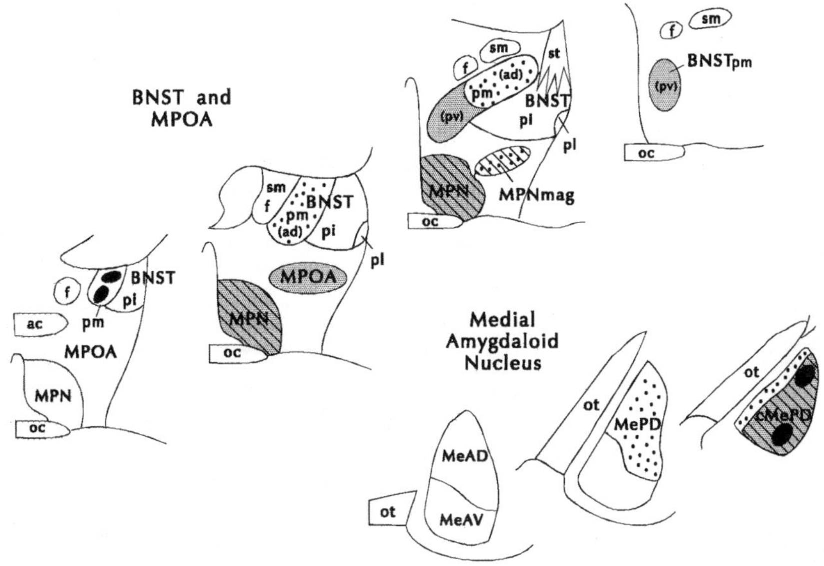

FIGURE 13. Interpretation of the results of Experiment 3, suggesting that specific subdivisions of the amygdala, bed nucleus of the stria terminalis, and medial preoptic area are selectively activated by sexual conditioning (*diagonal cross-hatching*), exposure to female hamster vaginal secretion FHVS (*stippling*), ejaculations (*gray*), and sexual satiety (*black*). See TABLE 1 for abbreviations.

Clearly, Fos-ir resulting from male sexual activity does not define function for the Fos-containing neurons; rather it identifies a neuroanatomical substrate with which to work, a substrate within which many challenges remain to determine experimentally the specific antecedents and results of neuronal activation.

With these caveats in mind, FIGURE 13 presents our interpretation of the results of studies just presented in which prior sexual experience, pheromonal stimulation, or the sequence of mating was associated with activation of individual cell groups within subdivisions of the medial amygdaloid nucleus, bed nucleus of the stria terminalis, and medial preoptic area. With the exception of the dorsolateral MPOA and the MPNmag, the areas illustrated in FIGURE 13 belong to a neuroanatomically definable network[23] characterized by dense populations of sex steroid-concentrating cells that supply essential hormonal signals for mating in this species.[30]

Some of the cell groups in this network show gradual increases in Fos-immunoreactivity as mating proceeds, suggesting either continual recruitment of neurons in a functionally homogeneous population or sequential activation of separate functional populations. Other areas, however, appear to be specialized in function within the context of mating, such as the cell clusters in cMePD and the BNSTpm[ad] that are activated at the onset of sexual satiety. Although lesion studies did not reveal these areas to be critical for the initiation of mating, Fos-ir evidence for their role in the sequencing and termination of a copulatory bout suggests that they may be essential for the success of mating, conception.

TABLE 1. Neuroanatomical Abbreviations

ac	anterior commissure
Aco	anterior cortical nucleus of the amygdala
AH	anterior hypothalamic nucleus
AHA	amygdalohippocampal area
BLa	basolateral nucleus of the amygdala, anterior
BM	basomedial nucleus of the amygdala
BNST	bed nucleus of the stria terminalis
BNSTam	BNST, anteromedial
BNSTal	BNST, anterolateral
BNSTpi	BNST, posterointermediate
BNSTpl	BNST, posterolateral
BNSTpm	BNST, posteromedial
BNSTpm (ad)	BNSTpm, anterodorsal
BNSTpm (pv)	BNSTpm, posteroventral
ce	central nucleus of the amygdala
cMePD	MePD, caudal extension
Endo	endopiriform nucleus
f	fornix
IM	intercalated mass
La	lateral nucleus of the amygdala
LSv	ventral lateral septum
MeAD	Me, anterodorsal
MeAV	Me, anteroventral
MePD	Me, posterodorsal
MePV	Me, posteroventral
MPOA	medial preoptic area
MPN	medial preoptic nucleus
cMPN	medial preoptic nucleus, caudal region
rMPN	medial preoptic nucleus, rostral region
MPNmag	medial preoptic nucleus, magnocellular
oc	optic chiasm
ot	optic tract
PAG	periaqueductal gray
PIR	piriform cortex
PLCo	posterolateral nucleus of the amygdala
PMCo	posteromedial nucleus of the amygdala
PMV	ventral premammillary nucleus
PVN	paraventricular nucleus of the hypothalamus
rMePD	MePD, rostral
sm	stria medullaris
st	stria terminalis
VMH	ventromedial nucleus of the hypothalamus

REFERENCES

1. KOLLACK, S. S. & S. W. NEWMAN. 1992. Mating behavior induces selective expression of Fos protein within the chemosensory pathways of the male Syrian hamster brain. Neurosci. Lett. **143:** 223-228.
2. KOLLACK-WALKER, S. S. & S. W. NEWMAN. 1995. Mating and agonistic behavior produce different patterns of Fos immunolabeling in the male Syrian hamster. Neuroscience **66:** 721-736.
3. FERNANDEZ-FEWELL, G. D. & M. MEREDITH. 1994. c-Fos expression in vomeronasal pathways of mated or pheromone-stimulated male golden hamsters: contributions from vomeronasal sensory input and expression related to mating performance. J. Neurosci. **14:** 3643-3654.
4. BAUM, M. J. & B. J. EVERITT. 1992. Increased expression of c-fos in the medial preoptic area after mating in male rats: Role of afferent inputs from the medial amygdala and midbrain central tegmental field. Neuroscience **50:** 627-646.
5. ROBERTSON, G. S., J. G. PFAUS, L. J. ATKINSON, H. MATSUMURA, A. G. PHILIPS & H. C. FIBIGER. 1991. Sexual behavior increases c-fos expression in the forebrain of the male rat. Brain Res. **564:** 352-357.
6. BAUM, M. J. & S. R. WERSINGER. 1993. Equivalent levels of mating-induced neural c-fos immunoreactivity in castrated male rats given androgen, estrogen, or no steroid replacement. Biol. Reprod. **48:** 1341-1347.
7. MURPHY, M. R. & G. E. SCHNEIDER. 1970. Olfactory bulb removal eliminates mating behavior in the male golden hamster. Science **167:** 302-304.
8. POWERS, J. B. & S. S. WINANS. 1975. Vomeronasal organ: Critical role in mediating sexual behavior of the male hamster. Science **187:** 961-963.
9. WINANS, S. S. & J. B. POWERS. 1977. Olfactory and vomeronasal deafferentation of male hamsters: Histological and behavioral analyses. Brain Res. **126:** 325-344.
10. DEVOR, M. & M. R. MURPHY. 1973. The effect of peripheral olfactory blockade on the social behavior of the male golden hamster. Behav. Biol. **9:** 31-42.
11. MEREDITH, M. 1986. Vomeronasal organ removal before sexual experience impairs male hamster mating behavior. Physiol. Behav. **36:** 737-743.
12. DEVOR, M. 1973. Components of mating dissociated by lateral olfactory tract transection in male hamsters. Brain Res. **64:** 437-441.
13. LEHMAN, M. N., J. B. POWERS & S. S. WINANS. 1983. Stria terminalis lesions alter the temporal pattern of copulatory behavior in the male golden hamster. Behav. Brain Res. **8:** 109-128.
14. LEHMAN, M. N., S. S. WINANS & J. B. POWERS. 1980. Medial nucleus of the amygdala mediates chemosensory control of male hamster sexual behavior. Science **210:** 557-560.
15. LEHMAN, M. N. & S. S. WINANS. 1982. Vomeronasal and olfactory pathways to the amygdala controlling male hamster sexual behavior: Autoradiographic and behavioral analyses. Brain Res. **240:** 27-41.
16. KEVETTER, G. A. & S. S. WINANS. 1981. Efferents of the corticomedial amygdala in the golden hamster. I. Efferents of the 'vomeronasal amygdala.' J. Comp. Neurol. **197:** 81-98.
17. LEHMAN, M. N. & S. S. WINANS. 1983. Evidence for a ventral non-strial pathway from the amygdala to the bed nucleus of the stria terminalis in the male golden hamster. Brain Res. **268:** 139-146.
18. LEHMAN, M. N. 1982. Neural pathways of the vomeronasal and olfactory systems controlling sexual behavior in the male golden hamster. Unpublished Ph.D. dissertation, University of Michigan.
19. POWERS, J. B., S. W. NEWMAN & M. L. BERGONDY. 1987. MPOA and BNST lesions in male Syrian hamsters: Differential effects on copulation and chemoinvestigatory behaviors. Behav. Brain Res. **23:** 181-195.
20. MURPHY, M. R. 1976. Olfactory stimulation and olfactory bulb removal: Effects on territorial aggression in male Syrian golden hamsters. Brain Res. **113:** 95-110.

21. Bunnell, B. N., F. J. Sodetz, Jr. & D. I. Shalloway. 1970. Amygdaloid lesions and social behavior in the golden hamster. Physiol. Behav. **5:** 153-161.
22. Maragos, W. F., S. W. Newman, M. N. Lehman & J. B. Powers. 1989. Neurons of origin and fiber trajectory of amygdalofugal projections to the medial preoptic area in Syrian hamsters. J. Comp. Neurol. **280:** 59-71.
23. Gomez, D. M. & S. W. Newman. 1992. Differential projections of the anterior and posterior regions of the medial amygdaloid nucleus in the Syrian hamster. J. Comp. Neurol. **317:** 195-218.
24. Canteras, N. S., R. B. Simerly & L. W. Swanson. 1995. Organization of projections from the medial nucleus of the amygdala: A PHAL study in the rat. J. Comp. Neurol. **360:** 213-245.
25. Wood, R. I., R. K. Brabec, J. M. Swann & S. W. Newman. 1992. Androgen and estrogen receptor-containing neurons in the chemosensory pathways of the male Syrian hamster brain. Brain Res. **596:** 89-98.
26. Wood, R. I. & S. W. Newman. 1993. Mating activates androgen-receptor containing neurons in chemosensory pathways of the male Syrian hamster brain. Brain Res. **614:** 65-77.
27. Wood, R. I. & S. W. Newman. 1995. Androgen and estrogen receptors coexist within individual neurons in the brain of the Syrian hamster. Neuroendocrinology **62:** 487-497.
28. Doherty, P. L. & P. J. Sheridan. 1981. Uptake and retention of androgen in neurons in the brain of the golden hamster. Brain Res. **219:** 327-334.
29. Krieger, M. S., J. I. Morrell & D. W. Pfaff. 1976. Autoradiographic localization of estradiol-concentrating cells in the female hamster brain. Neuroendocrinology **22:** 193-205.
30. Wood, R. I. & S. W. Newman. 1995. The medial amygdaloid nucleus and medial preoptic area mediate steroidal control of sexual behavior in the male Syrian hamster. Horm. Behav. **29:** 338-353.
31. Beach, F. A. & R. G. Rabedeau. 1959. Sexual exhaustion and recovery in the male hamster. J. Comp. Physiol. Psychol. **52:** 56-61.
32. Bunnell, B. N., B. D. Boland & D. A. Dewsbury. 1977. Copulatory behavior of golden hamsters (*Mesocricetus auratus*). Behaviour **61:** 180-206.
33. Heeb, M. M. & P. Yahr. 1996. c-Fos immunoreactivity in the sexually dimorphic area of the hypothalamus and related brain regions of male gerbils after exposure to sex-related stimuli or performance of specific sexual behaviors. Neuroscience **72:** 1049-1071.
34. Macrides, F., P. A. Johnson & S. P. Schneider. 1977. Responses of the male golden hamster to vaginal secretion and dimethyl sulfide: Attraction versus sexual behavior. Behav. Biol. **20:** 377-386.
35. Murphy, M. R. 1973. Effects of female hamster vaginal discharge on the behavior of male hamsters. Behav. Biol. **9:** 367-375.
36. Kamel, F. & A. I. Frankel. 1978. Hormone release during mating in the male rat: Time course, relation to sexual behavior, and interaction with handling procedures. Endocrinology **103:** 2172-2179.
37. Graham, J. M. & C. Desjardins. 1980. Classical conditioning: Induction of luteinizing hormone and testosterone secretion in anticipation of sexual activity. Science **210:** 1039-1041.
38. Pfeiffer, C. A. & R. E. Johnston. 1994. Hormonal and behavioral responses of male hamsters to females and female odors: Roles of olfaction, the vomeronasal system, and sexual experience. Physiol. Behav. **55:** 129-138.
39. Fiber, J. M., P. Adames & J. M. Swann. 1993. Pheromones induce c-*fos* in limbic areas regulating male hamster mating behavior. Neuroreport **4:** 871-874.
40. Coolen, L. M. 1995. The neural organization of sexual behavior in the male rat: A functional neuroanatomical Fos-study. Unpublished Ph.D. dissertation. University of Nijmegen.

41. HUCK, U. W. & R. D. LISK. 1985. Determinants of mating success in the golden hamster (*Mesocricetus auratus*): I. male capacity. J. Comp. Psychol. **99:** 98-107.
42. KOLLACK-WALKER, S. S. & S. W. NEWMAN. 1996. Mating-induced expression of c-fos in the male Syrian hamster brain: Role of experience, pheromones and ejaculations. J. Neurobiol., in press.
43. LANIER, D. L., D. Q. ESTEP & D. A. DEWSBURY. 1975. Copulatory behavior of golden hamsters: Effects on pregnancy. Physiol. Behav. **15:** 209-212.
44. HUCK, U. W. & R. D. LISK. 1985. Determinants of mating success in the golden hamster (*Mesocricetus auratus*): II. pregnancy initiation. J. Comp. Psychol. **99:** 231-239.

21
Regulatory Mechanisms of Oxytocin-Mediated Sociosexual Behavior

Diane M. Witt

A combination of behavioral, neuroanatomical, and pharmacological evidence underscores a critical and interactive role for oxytocin (OT) and gonadal steroids in mammalian sociosexual behavior. Underlying mechanisms of OT's action include variations in the gonadal steroid milieu *in vivo,* species-specific differences in steroidal regulation of the densities of OT receptors in discrete brain regions, behavioral control of central OT release, and other mechanisms such as the activation of neurotransmitter networks that affect OT gene expression and secretion, or homologous modulation of OT neurosecretion. The precise signal transduction mechanisms and second messenger systems in the hypothalamus that regulate stimulus-coupled OT gene expression and behavioral responses, however, have been difficult to study *in vivo* because of the inherent complexities of the neuroanatomic pathways involved. We have developed an *ex vivo* system to study neurotransmitter regulation of hypothalamic gene expression. This system, slice explants of acutely dissected brain regions, preserves neuroanatomic detail and specific interneuronal circuitry to allow for the systematic examination of rapid cellular regulation of gene expression that occurs within minutes or hours after neuronal activation by a variety of techniques.

This review summarizes studies that elucidate the concomitant roles of OT and gonadal steroids on species-specific sociosexual interactions and provides a short overview of our on-going *ex vivo* investigations of the role of neuronal activation in hypothalamic gene expression.

OXYTOCIN REGULATION OF SOCIOSEXUAL BEHAVIOR

Perhaps one of the most elucidating animal models for the study of the interactive effects of gonadal steroids and OT on sociosexual behavior is the prairie vole. Unlike other laboratory rodents, prairie voles do not exhibit spontaneous estrous cycles or cyclic fluctuations in ovarian steroid secretion. Instead, prairie voles require social stimuli to activate reproductive processes. Heterosexual encounters involve reciprocal olfactory investigations of anogenital regions followed by stereotypic autogrooming

Address for correspondence: Diane M. Witt, PhD, Department of Psychology, Binghamton University, Science 4, Rm 255, Binghamton, NY 13902-6000.

which directly delivers a male urinary chemosignal to the female's olfactory epithelium.[1] This pheromonal stimulation, acting via the vomeronasal organ, induces a series of neuroendocrine responses in the female, including increased norepinephrine and luteininzing hormone-releasing hormone levels in the olfactory bulb, elevated serum luteinizing hormone and estrogen, and increased densities of estrogen and progesterone receptors in the hypothalamus (see review in ref. 2). Mating commences 24-48 hours after pheromonal stimulation, and the associated vaginocervical stimulation induces ovulation. However, plasma progesterone levels do not increase until 24-72 hours after the onset of mating.[3] This first estrus period (male-induced) consists of prolonged sexual receptivity (>30 hours), frequent mating bouts, and extended periods of social contact.[1] Coincident with parturition, the female enters postpartum estrus, which is not induced by pheromones, but rather is a consequence of neuroendocrine processes associated with birth. In contrast to male-induced estrus, postpartum estrus is characterized by markedly shorter periods of mating (<9 hours) involving only occasional bouts of sexual activity; however, frequent social interactions persist despite the cessation of copulatory activity.[4]

The specific neuroendocrine mechanisms regulating the abbreviated mating response during postpartum estrus were unknown. Postpartum females simultaneously mate, give birth, and nurse pups, all of which are potent stimuli for OT release.[5] We examined the hypothesis that OT release in the central nervous system during sexual interactions, parturition, and lactation truncates postpartum sexual activity. To test this, pups were removed immediately upon birth (interrupting lactational OT release) and females were exposed to a variety of sexually experienced males.[4] Partner familiarity was not a factor in mating duration, but the absence of pups significantly increased the duration and frequency of postpartum mating, independent of other social activity, suggesting OT mediation of mating behavior.

Initial OT experiments used estrogen-primed voles in confirmed, behavioral estrus. Intracerebroventricular (icv), but not intraperitoneal (ip) OT administration produced a dose-dependent decrease in the number of estrous females that continued to be sexually receptive.[6] Unexpectedly, OT markedly increased the duration of social contact and decreased male-directed agonistic encounters. This study, simulating the endogenous postcopulatory release of OT, showed not only that OT plays a major role in the sexual behavior of this species, but also that OT is implicated in numerous other nonsexual behaviors. These data support the hypothesis that in prairie voles the cumulative release of OT may function as a sexual satiety signal, facilitating other social encounters even in the absence of mating behavior.[6–9] Thus, OT, acting centrally, affects sociosexual behavior in prairie voles through neuronal pathways that are modulated by estrogen priming.

In contrast to the inhibitory effect of OT observed in prairie voles, studies conducted on female rats suggest a markedly different role for OT in the expression of feminine sexual behavior. Exogenous OT (icv), in concert with estrogen and progesterone, enhances sexual receptivity in females optimally primed with these ovarian steroids.[10–13] Estrogen and progesterone are essential for expression of the lordosis reflex.[14] In estrogen-primed rats, the addition of progesterone markedly enhances behaviors such as proceptive hopping and darting, ear wiggling, and whisker twitching, all solicitous copulatory behaviors.[15] The effects of central OT on social behavior in rats were examined by administering OT (100-1,000 ng, icv) to hormonally primed females. Lordosis quotients were potentiated (by 20-30%), proceptive behaviors increased significantly, and rejection behaviors (kicking) decreased dramatically.[16] These OT behavioral responses were blocked by concurrent icv administration of the selective OT receptor antagonist $d(CH_2)_5[Tyr(Me)^2,Thr^4,Tyr\text{-}NH_2^9]$ornithine vasotocin (OTA). This pharmacological blockade provides additional evidence that central OT modulates both social and sexual behavior in female rats that have received optimal estrogen and progesterone priming. OTA blockade of endogenous OT receptors likewise produces a dose-dependent decrease in lordosis quotients and proceptive behaviors and a concomitant increase in rejection behaviors in ovariectomized females receiving gonadal steroid priming.[17] However, a single icv injection of OTA is only effective if administered at the same time with a subcutaneous progesterone injection, 4 hours *prior* to the onset of sexual receptivity.[17,18] Blockade of endogenous OT receptors provides evidence of a physiological role for OT in the expression of female sexual interactions and for the first time implicates OT in the mediation of solicitation behaviors. These observations stimulated investigations into the CNS nuclei where interactions between OT, estrogen, and progesterone might likely occur.

The medial preoptic area and the ventromedial nucleus of the hypothalamus, areas where estrogen and progesterone receptors are localized, have been implicated in the regulation of lordosis. Central infusion of OT into the medial preoptic area produces a marked increase in lordosis quotients in females primed with either estrogen alone or estrogen together with progesterone.[19,20] However, infusions of OT into the ventromedial nucleus require both estrogen and progesterone priming for OT to enhance lordosis.[21] In more detailed studies, microinjections of OTA into discrete brain regions implicate the medial preoptic area and the ventromedial nucleus in OT-mediated lordosis, whereas the ventral tegmental area appeared to regulate OT-mediated social behavior.[18,20]

Only a few studies exist on OT-mediated behavioral responses in male prairie voles (see other chapters in this volume). Administration of OT (300 ng, icv) immediately inhibits mating behavior in otherwise sexually active male prairie voles. This inhibition is similar to that observed in female prairie voles; however, comparable OT doses are without effect on nonsexual, social interactions in males.[22]

In contrast to male prairie voles, but similar to female rats, administration of low acute doses of OT (1 ng, icv) in male rats can facilitate male copulatory performance.[11] Higher acute doses (62.5-500 ng), however, attenuate male sexual responses, such as lengthening the postejaculatory interval.[23] Chronic OT (icv) infusion in male rats has no lasting effects on sexual behavior, such as mounting, intromission, ejaculation, or the postejaculatory interval; however, a dramatic increase occurs in the length of time during which OT-infused males position themselves in direct physical contact with the female rat (even in the absence of copulatory interactions).[24] In males, OT infusion also increases upper body autogrooming and anogenital sniffing of the female, important features of the male's social repertoire. This OT infusion study was the first to link OT with the expression of social behavior in male rats independent of mating activity. The enhanced social contact is not the result of thermoregulatory, anxiolytic, or anxiogenic reactions to central OT infusion, because basal body temperature, nociception, or exploratory behavior in an open field are unaffected. Thus, chronic infusion of OT in male rats is associated with social, nonsexual interactions possibly acting via olfactory or somatosensory processing pathways in the brain.

GONADAL STEROID REGULATION OF OXYTOCIN RECEPTORS IN THE CNS

The behavioral antagonism studies just described indicate that certain aspects of social and sexual behaviors are regulated by distinct subpopulations of oxytocin receptors (OTRs) localized in telencephalic nuclei. Limbic structures that contain OTRs appear to be conserved across mammalian phylogeny. Therefore, multi-species comparisons of the distribution of OTRs and gonadal steroid regulation of OTRs may elucidate the specific cellular mechanisms that differentially modulate OT-mediated behaviors.

The specific radiolabeled OTR antagonist [^{125}I]-OTA is typically used to map the distribution of binding sites for the OTR in the CNS.[25,26] [^{125}I]-OTA exhibits an affinity for OTRs (k_i = 0.031 nM) that differs dramatically from its affinity for AVP receptors (k_i = 13.6 nM for the V_1 subtype, 10.2 nM for the V_2 subtype). The CNS distribution of OTRs in prairie voles resembles that found in most other rodent species,[27] suggesting an evolutionary conservation in neuroanatomic expression.[28,29] The densities of hypothalamic OTRs in prairie voles do not show the typical regional changes following increases in either endogenous or exogenous estrogen stimulation that are observed in other species.[30] For example, in prairie voles, only the anterior olfactory nucleus shows a marked increase in the density of OTR (2 fold above nonhormonally primed animals) with either endogenous or exogenous estrogen stimulation.[27] Thus, olfactory pathways may be involved in OT-mediated behaviors in the vole, a species whose neuroendocrinology is pheromonally regulated. Olfactory processes that might be modulated by OT include estrus induction, reflex ovulation, mate discrimination, and pair bond formation (see other chapters in this volume) in this species.[7–9,27,31] Reported differences between prairie voles and montane voles, a closely related species, in the density of OTRs in montane voles have led to the speculation that OTR densities may reflect evolutionary variations in social organization as well[32] (see other chapters in this volume).

Autoradiographic analyses have demonstrated site-specific localization of OTRs in the forebrain, and the density of OTRs can be selectively modulated by gonadal steroids in neuronal subpopulations known to regulate reproductive behavior. For example, rat gonadal steroids selectively increase the density of OTRs in the olfactory tubercle, nucleus accumbens, central amygdaloid nucleus, ventromedial nucleus, and bed nucleus of the stria terminalis.[29,33–43] The ventromedial nucleus contains neurons that regulate the lordosis reflex in many rodent species and may be involved in the orchestration of OT-mediated social behavior. Johnson *et al.*[40] showed that the time course for estrogen-dependent increases in OTRs in the ventromedial nucleus closely parallels the cyclic fluctuations of ovarian steroids in female rats. In support of these findings is the demonstration that exogenous[44] as well as endogenous steroid levels across the estrous cycle account for the incremental increase of OTR mRNA expressed in the ventrolateral ventromedial nucleus at the time of sexual receptivity; OTR mRNA levels are lowest during diestrus, when ovarian steroid levels are low and sexual behavior is nonexistent.[45] In addition, the density of OTRs in the ventromedial nucleus dramatically increases after estrogen stimulation,[36,37,40] and progesterone further expands the neuroanatomic field where OTRs are expressed to include more lateral regions of the ventromedial nucleus.[42] Estrogen requires 1-2 days for its effect in the ventromedial nucleus, whereas progesterone's effects are apparent within 30 minutes. Schumacher and associates theorize that progesterone may act either directly on the OTR, on the neuronal membrane, or perhaps through recruitment of preexisting receptor pools, because this receptor phenomenon was observed both *in vivo* and *in vitro* after progesterone stimulation.[36,37,40–42] These data provide strong evidence linking gonadal steroid regulation of OTRs, specifically in the ventromedial nucleus, with the expression of female sexual receptivity. Questions about the neuroplasticity of OTRs, however, had not addressed the possibility of sexual dimorphism in the distribution of steroid-regulated OTRs that might account for male behavioral responses to OT secretion.

Initial studies indicated that no inherent sex differences in the distribution of OTRs were found when gonadally intact male and female rats were compared.[43] However, more quantitative experiments to date show that male rats actually express higher basal levels of OTR mRNA in the medial hypothalamus than do gonadally intact females. Females exhibit more variability in the levels of OTR mRNA, possibly due to cyclic fluctuations in gonadal steroid levels.[44,45] In both sexes, gonadectomy significantly decreases the binding of [^{125}I]-OTA to OTRs in the islands of calleja and the ventrolateral portion of the ventromedial nucleus, the bed nucleus of the stria terminales, and posterior portion of the central amygdaloid nucleus,[43] and exogenous steroids reverse the effects of gonadectomy on OTR density. For example, in gonadectomized females, exogenous estradiol significantly increases the density of OTRs in the islands of calleja, the ventromedial nucleus, and the central amygdaloid nucleus. Also, testosterone given to gonadectomized males or females restores OTR levels in steroid-responsive regions to those observed in gonadally intact animals.[39,43] In males, aromatase inhibitors reduce OTR density in the islands of calleja to levels observed in castrated males, suggesting that the effects of testosterone on OTR may depend on its conversion to estradiol.[43] These data support the hypothesis that distinct OTR fields are responsive to gonadal steroids in both male and female rats and that estrogen and possibly progesterone may selectively regulate subpopulations of OTRs.

Homologous regulation of OT receptors has also been reported. Autoradiographic analyses of brain sections obtained from the male rats *chronically* infused with OT (100 ng/h) demonstrate that prolonged OT exposure causes a 50% decrease in OTR density in both steroid-responsive and steroid-nonresponsive fields throughout the brain.[46] Thus, both heterologous (gonadal steroid) and homologous (OT autoregulation) modulation of OTRs within distinct brain nuclei provides the requisite neuroplasticity for OT to influence multiple aspects of sociosexual interactions.

MECHANISMS REGULATING OT RELEASE

The ability of OT to influence behavior depends not only on the availability and functionality of OTRs, but also on transsynaptic activity in neurons within the hypothalamus. Thus, mechanisms controlling neuropetide gene expression, processing, and secretion would play a critical role in OT-mediated behavior. Peripheral actions of OT, such as uterine contractions during parturition and milk ejection during lactation, are the result of synchronous release of OT from neurons in the magnocellular regions of the supraoptic nucleus and the paraventricular nucleus, most of which project to the posterior pituitary.[47] In addition, neurons in the parvocellular regions of the paraventricular nucleus project to both limbic structures and autonomic regions in the brainstem,[48] areas which may coordinate OT-mediated behavioral responses. Numerous OT neurons distribute terminals rostrally towards the olfactory bulbs, septum, medial preoptic area, and the amygdaloid nucleus in the brain, and caudally to the substantia nigra, tractus solitarious, locus coeruleus, and parasympathetic outflow of the spinal cord.[49,50] Terminal projection sites where gonadal steroid stimulation or behavioral activation of the oxytocinergic system results in OT release may be important neuronal subpopulations that regulate homeostasis and coordinate sociosexual behaviors, thus facilitating species survival.

Previous studies showed that fluctuations in levels of endogenous gonadal steroids affect electrical activity in magnocellular neurons[51] and may lead to some of the ultrastructural changes observed in magnocellular nuclei when OT pathways are activated.[52] Oxytocin mRNA levels are significantly elevated at times when gonadal steroid levels are increasing, as during puberty and estrous periods in the rat. During proestrus in the female rat, OT surges at times when estrogen and progesterone are typically elevated. As previously mentioned, these gonadal steroids, essential for the display of sexual behavior in rats, are known to regulate endogenous OT secretion, which in turn affects proceptivity, receptivity, and the lordosis posture itself.[10] Estrogen enhances both OT immunoreactivity and mRNA levels in the medial preoptic area,[53,54] and progesterone has similar effects on OT immunoreactivity in estrogen-primed females. Exogenous estrogen priming, followed by injections of progesterone, selectively increases OT mRNA in paraventricular nucleus, but not supraoptic nucleus neurons.[55] Thus, gonadal steroids affect OT secretion in addition to regulating OTRs.

Based on the numerous species examined, OT neurons are equally represented in males and females, and sexual dimorphism in OT neuronal organization is not apparent in the paraventricular nucleus and supraoptic nucleus.[56] Oxytocin is released during vaginocervical stimulation in females,[57–59] and in both genital[60,61] and nongenital contact in males.[62] Mating stimuli significantly affects OT varicosities in the anterior hypothalamus and ventromedial nucleus when females are primed with both estrogen and progesterone.[10,19] Thus OT synthesis and release are directed not only by the gonadal steroid milieu, but also by reproductive and somatosensory interactions. Sociosexual behavior itself may be viewed as a mechanism that regulates neuronal responses and subsequent gene expression.

FACTORS REGULATING GENE EXPRESSION IN THE PARAVENTRICULAR NUCLEUS

Both parvocellular and magnocellular OT neurons are known to be transsynaptically stimulated by multiple neuronal circuits during parturition and lactation in the female.[63,64] Yet, little is known about how external stimuli, such as mating or social behavior, directly affect gene expression in OT neurons of the paraventricular nucleus. Studies of stimulus-coupled activation of gene expression have been made possible by recent research that has defined the role of transacting factors termed immediate early genes (IEGs).[65] IEGs, such as c-*fos*, are involved in both transient transcriptional regulation of gene expression and more prolonged functional changes in neurons that respond to a multitude of environmental stimuli (reviewed in refs. 66 and 67). Fos, the gene product of c-*fos*, is a transcription factor that regulates gene expression by binding to AP-1 sites, resulting in the activation of secondary genetic programs. A possible target for Fos transcription might be the rat OT gene which has a potential AP-1 binding site (TGAC*C*CA, located 144 bases upstream from the 5′ coding region) that differs by only one base pair from AP-1 binding sites (TGAC*T*CA) found on other genes. Thus, the OT gene may contain possible elements for transcriptional regulation by heterodimers of Fos or other IEG products. Other important targets for Fos regulation may include dynorphin and cholecystokinin,[68] galanin,[69] and corticotropin-releasing factor,[70] all of which are neuropeptides known to modulate masculine reproductive behavior and are coexpressed in OT neurons in the paraventricular nucleus.

Supportive evidence comes from early immunocytochemical studies in which changes in Fos identified specific nuclei subserving masculine sexual behavior.[71–73] Subsequent dual-label immunocytochemical analyses revealed that increasing masculine copulatory interactions incrementally increases Fos, primarily in parvocellular OT neurons in the caudal/lateral regions of the male paraventricular nucleus.[74] Specific OT neurons in this subpopulation of the paraventricular nucleus project to the brain stem and lumbar levels of the spinal cord where sensorimotor neurons regulate penile erection.[75] These data implicate Fos and OT gene expression in male copulatory interactions and suggest a possible neurochemical circuit for controlling penile erection.

MECHANISMS REGULATING IMMEDIATE EARLY GENE EXPRESSION IN THE PARAVENTRICULAR NUCLEUS

Neuronal depolariztion, calcium influx, or second messenger activation of IEGs is typically studied in primary, dissociated neurons or cultures of transformed cell lines. In neuronal cultures, the fundamental neuroanatomic specificity and innate synaptic organization are absent, and many of the regulatory mechanisms operating within interneuronal circuits *in vivo* may not be represented. In response to this problem we developed an *ex vivo* preparation for studying neurotransmitter regulation of hypothalamic gene expression. Slice explants are generated from brains recently dissected from postnatal day 5 rat pups (FIG. 1). Neuroanatomic detail and interneuronal circuitry is preserved within a 400-μm thick slice. This preparation permits systematic examination of acute cellular responses that occur within minutes or hours after neuronal depolarization; thus, we have termed the slice explants "acute" slice explants. Within 2 hours slice explants exhibit electrical excitability such as spontaneous action potentials and conductance responses to GABA and glutamate.

In initial experiments, the effect of neuronal depolarization on Fos expression was examined in the paraventricular nucleus. Potassium chloride increases Fos expression nonspecifically throughout the PVN and surrounding striatal areas. To specifically examine Fos expression in neurons, we used veratridine, an activator of voltage-dependent sodium channels. Veratridine-induced Fos expression requires the presence of extracellular Ca^{2+}. Furthermore, pretreatment with blockers of voltage-gated Ca^{2+} channels, such as nifedipine (L-type) or ω-conotoxin (N-type), revealed that specific

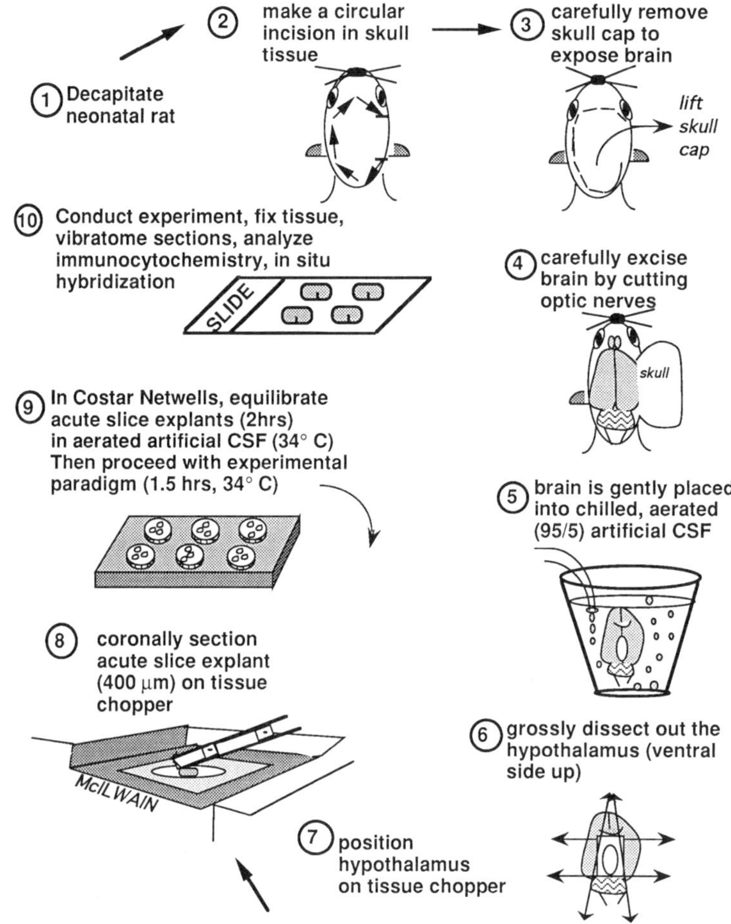

FIGURE 1. Schematic drawing of the methodology used to generate acute slice explants of the hypothalamus (based on ref. 80) and experimental procedures for *ex vivo* gene expression.

Ca^{2+} channels are involved in Fos gene expression in distinct neuronal subpopulations of the paraventricular nucleus. Specifically, both L- and N-type channels are involved in veratridine-induced Fos expression in parvocellular, but not in magnocellular areas. In contrast, only L-type channels regulate veratridine-induced Fos expression in periventricular regions. These data demonstrate that distinct topographical patterns in depolarization-induced Fos expression exist in subpopulations of the PVN, rich in OT neurons, suggesting that regional specificity of cellular responses to external stimuli may occur in the hypothalamus. With the acute slice explant system, regulatory mechanisms associated with receptor activation, transcription, neuropeptide processing, and secretion can be analyzed by a variety of techniques that identify distinct neuronal phenotypes, maintained and manipulated in a controlled environment. This *ex vivo* approach will make possible the neuroanatomic study of neurotransmitter and both classical steroid and neurosteroid effects on gene expression and neuropeptide secretion.

DISCUSSION

Overwhelming evidence supports the hypothesis that OT plays a major role in controlling behavioral interactions in both females and males of various mammalian species. The differential behavioral responses and sensitivity to OT may be directly linked to species differences in neural mechanisms that are modulated by gonadal steroids. We now may be able to examine the specific neurocircuitry and exact cellular mechanisms underlying some of these OT-mediated behaviors.

Oxytocin and Sexual Behavior. Although sexual behavior may include aspects of social interactions, sexual behavior is operationally defined as those behaviors that are directly associated with copulation, such as lordosis, mounting, intromission, and ejaculation. Oxytocin inhibits lordosis in estrogen-primed prairie voles, whereas in rats OT enhances lordosis in females primed with both estrogen and progesterone. In female prairie voles, physical interactions and chemosensory stimulation lead to estrogen secretion which is required for lordosis. In female rats, lordosis directly correlates with cyclic fluctuations in both plasma estrogen and progesterone levels. Species variations in gonadal steroid priming may account for these differential responses in females. The role of OT in masculine sexual behavior is more ambiguous, and the biological significance of OT in male prairie voles remains to be determined. However, in the male rat, low OT levels facilitate and high levels inhibit masculine sexual behavior, suggesting that OT may function as a sexual satiety signal.

Oxytocin and Social Behavior. Social behaviors can be classified as selective affiliative interactions, such as prolonged physical contact, olfactory investigation, and frequent directed approaches. In both species and sexes, OT markedly facilitates social contact, suggesting that certain affiliative behaviors persist in the absence of copulatory interactions. Both female and male prairie voles are innately social, and OT further enhances social contact. Likewise, female rats seek tactile stimulation after exposure to OT. In less social male rats, chronic OT infusion also results in a dramatic increase in nonsexual, social interactions. These phenomena may be due to OT's effects on somatosensory thresholds or olfactory processes, thus activating mechanisms that encourage affiliation through direct physical contact. As with sexual behaviors, species-specific differences in the gonadal steroid milieu may impart differences in sensitivity to OT and thus regulate OT-mediated social responses.

Oxytocin Receptors and Gonadal Steroids. Differences in gonadal steroid regulation of OTRs may be an additional, critical factor in determining the timing of OT-mediated behavioral responses. Estrogen increases OTRs in both species, but with regional distinctions. In prairie voles, estrogen increases OTRs in the anterior olfactory nucleus, most likely with biological significance in a species whose neuroendocrinology is pheromonally regulated. In the female rat, estrogen elevates OTRs in the ventromedial nucleus, one of the nuclei involved in the expression of lordosis. With the addition of progesterone the density of OTRs further increases in the ventromedial nucleus. These data support the hypothesis that OTRs display regional differences in regulation by estrogen, progesterone, and testosterone. Thus, gonadal steroid regulation of OTRs may impart differential sensitization to OT in select brain regions and provides another mechanism regulating species-specific expression of sociosexual behaviors.

Oxytocin and Gonadal Steroids. Estrogen is viewed as a ''permissive'' steroid with respect to OT-mediated behaviors, that is, progesterone is largely without effect in the absence of elevated estrogen levels. Thus, progesterone may play a central role in modulating neuronal responses involved in OT-directed behaviors. The critical timing of progesterone's involvement in the sexual receptivity of female rats is a key factor in facilitating OT's effects on sexual and social behavior. Genomic mechanisms via estrogen-induced progesterone receptors in the medial preoptic area and ventromedial nucleus may account for progesterone's effect. However, recent data indicate that progesterone, acting as a neurosteroid, may also exert its effects through nongenomic mechanisms such as modulation of ion channel receptors in select brain areas.[76] These findings have prompted a reexamination of the physiological role of progesterone in females and have initiated studies designed to dissociate which neural substrates rely on nongenomic versus genomic actions.

More recently, studies in male rats have shown that at physiological levels, progesterone facilitates masculine sexual behavior in the absence of androgen stimulation.[77] Interactions between OT and progesterone have not been studied in the male. Progesterone acts directly by altering OT gene expression and neuropeptide release or indirectly by affecting other neurotransmitter networks involved in sexual/social behavior. Such neurochemical interactions remain to be studied with new methodologies such as the acute slice explants described earlier.

Oxytocin Neurocircuitry and Gene Expression. *In vivo* studies show changes in Fos immunoreactivity in OT neurons during sexual activity in males. These OT neurons, confined to parvocellular regions of the paraventricular nucleus, project to sensorimotor nuclei regulating penile erection. Studies have demonstrated that OT receptors in the paraventricular nucleus mediate penile reflexes, as microinjections of OT into the PVN induce erections that are blocked by selective OTR antagonists (reviewed in ref. 78). Furthermore, OTR activation in the paraventricular nucleus involves Ca^{2+} influx, because microinjections of the N-type Ca^{2+} channel blocker ω-conotoxin antagonize OT-induced penile erections *in vivo.* The acute slice explant system should allow us to colocalize specifically activated Ca^{2+} channels in OT neurons in subpopulations in the paraventricular nucleus. These *ex vivo* studies will support and expand the information derived from the *in vivo* experiments just described. We have shown that depolarization-induced Fos expression in parvocellular nuclei (regions projecting to the spinal cord and brain areas under autonomic control) involves both L-type and N-type Ca^{2+} channels. In contrast, depolarization-induced Fos expression in periventricular subdivisions of the paraventricular nucleus involves N-type Ca^{2+} channels, suggesting neuroanatomic specificity in IEG signal transduction mechanisms.[79] We plan to assess transcriptionally active neural factors involved in gene expression by using antisense approaches to determine if Fos is directly involved in OT gene expression in the paraventricular nucleus. We are also interested in studying the effects of neurosteroids on OT gene expression to better understand the neurocircuitry and cellular mechanisms involved in the expression of OT-mediated behaviors.

ACKNOWLEDGMENT

Many thanks to Dr. Larry Mahan for his insightful comments and editorial review of this paper.

REFERENCES

1. Witt, D. M., C. S. Carter, K. Carlstead & L. D. Read. 1988. Sexual and social interactions preceding and during male-induced oestrus in prairie voles, *Microtus ochrogaster*. Anim. Behav. **36:** 1465-1471.
2. Witt, D. M. 1995. Oxytocin and rodent sociosexual responses: From behavior to gene expression. Neurosci. Biobehav. Rev. **19:** 315-324.
3. Carter, C. S., D. M. Witt, S. R. Manock, K. A. Adams, J. M. Bahr & K. Carlstead. 1989. Hormonal correlates of sexual behavior and ovulation in male-induced and postpartum estrus in female prairie voles. Physiol. Behav. **46:** 941-948.
4. Witt, D. M., C. S. Carter, R. Chayer & K. Adams. 1990. Patterns of behaviour during postpartum oestrus in prairie voles (*Microtus ochrogaster*). Anim. Behav. **39:** 528-534.
5. Tindal, J. S. 1974. Stimuli that cause the release of oxytocin. *In* Handbook of Physiology. S. R. Geiger, E. Knobil, W. H. Sawyer, R. O. Greef & E. B. Astwoods. 257-267. American Physiological Society, Washington, DC.
6. Witt, D. M., C. S. Carter & D. M. Walton. 1990. Central and peripheral effects of oxytocin administration in prairie voles (*Microtus ochrogaster*). Pharmacol. Biochem. Behav. **37:** 63-69.
7. Carter, C. S., J. R. Williams & D. M. Witt. 1990. The biology of social bonding in a monogamous mammal. *In* Hormones, Brain and Behavior in Vertebrates. 2. Behavioral Activation in Males and Females-Social Interactions and Reproductive Endocrinology. Eds Balthazart, J., S. Karger & Basel, A G.
8. Carter, C. S., J. Williams, D. M. Witt & T. R. Insel. 1992. Oxytocin and social bonding. *In* Oxytocin in Maternal Sexual, and Social Behaviors. C. Pedersen, G. Jirikowski, J. Caldwell & T. Insel, Eds. Ann. N.Y. Acad. of Sci. **652:** 204-211.
9. Williams, J. R., T. R. Insel, C. R. Harbaugh & C. S. Carter. 1994. Oxytocin administered centrally facilitates formation of a partner preference in female prairie voles (*Microtus ochrogaster*). J. Neuroendocrinol. **6:** 247-250.
10. Caldwell, J. D., G. F. Jirikowski, E. R. Greer, W. E. Stumpf & C. A. Pedersen. 1988. Ovarian steroids and sexual interaction alter oxytocinergic content and distribution in the basal forebrain. Br. Res. **446:** 236-244.
11. Arletti, R. & A. Bertolini. 1985. Oxytocin stimulates lordosis behavior in female rats. Neuropeptides **6:** 247-253.
12. Caldwell, J. D., A. J. Prange, Jr. & C. A. Pedersen. 1986. Oxytocin facilitates the sexual receptivity of estrogen-treated female rats. Neuropeptides **7:** 175-189.
13. Gorzalka, B. B. & G. L. L. Lester. 1987. Oxytocin-induced facilitation of lordosis behaviour in rats is progesterone-dependent. Neuropeptides **10:** 55-65.
14. Pfaff, D. W. & S. Schwartz-Giblin. 1988. Cellular mechanisms of female reproductive behaviors. *In* Physiology of Reproduction. E. Knobil & J. Neill, Eds: 1487-1568. Raven Press, Ltd. New York, NY.
15. Fadem, B. H., R. J. Barfield & R. E. Whalen. 1979. Dose-response and time-response relationships between progesterone and the display of patterns of receptive and proceptive behavior in the female rat. Horm. Behav. **13:** 40-48.

16. WITT, D. M. & T. R. INSEL. 1992. Central oxytocin antagonism decreases female reproductive behavior. *In* Oxytocin in Maternal, Sexual and Social Behaviors. C. Pedersen, J. Caldwell, G. Jirikowski & T. Insel, Eds.: 445-447. Ann. of the N.Y. Acad. of Sci. **652:** 445-447
17. WITT, D. M. & T. R. INSEL. 1991. A selective oxytocin antagonist attenuates gonadal steroid facilitation of female sexual behavior. Endocrinology **128:** 3269-3276.
18. CALDWELL, J. D., J. M. JOHNS, B. M. FAGGIN & C. A. PEDERSEN. 1994. Infusion of an oxytocin antagonist into the medial preoptic area prior to progesterone inhibits sexual receptivity and increases rejection in female rats. Horm. Behav. **28:** 288-302.
19. CALDWELL, J. D., G. F. JIRIKOWSKI, E. R. GREER & C. A. PEDERSEN. 1989. Medial preoptic area oxytocin and female sexual receptivity. Behav. Neurosci. **103:** 655-662.
20. WITT, D. M. & T. R. INSEL. 1991. Site-specific injections of a selective oxytocin receptor antagonist affects female sexual behavior. Soc. Neurosci. New Orleans, LA.
21. SCHULZE, H. & B. GORZALKA. 1991. Oxytocin effects lordosis frequency and lordosis duration following infusion into the medial-preoptic area and ventormedial hypothalamus of female rats. Neuropeptides **18:** 99-106.
22. MAHALATI, K., K. OKANOYA, D. M. WITT & C. S. CARTER. 1991. Oxytocin inhibits male sexual behavior in prairie voles. Pharmacol. Biochem. Behav. **39:** 219-222.
23. STONEHAM, M. D., B. J. EVERITT, S. HANSEN, S. L. LIGHTMAN & K. TODD. 1985. Oxytocin and sexual behavior in the male rat and rabbit. J. Endocrinol **107:** 97-106.
24. WITT, D. M., J. T. WINSLOW & T. R. INSEL. 1992. Enhanced social interactions in rats following chronic, centrally infused oxytocin. Pharmacol. Biochem. Behav. **43:** 855-861.
25. ELANDS, J., C. BARBERIS, S. JARD, E. TRIBOLLET, J. DREIFUSS, K. BANKOWSKI, M. MANNING & W. SAWYER. 1987. ^{125}I-labelled $d(CH_2)_5[Tyr(Me)^2,Thr^4,Tyr\text{-}NH_2^9]$ OVT: A selective oxytocin receptor ligand. Eur. J. Pharmacol. **147:** 197-207.
26. ELANDS, J., A. BEETSMA, C. BARBERIS & E. R. DE KLOET. 1988. Topography of the oxytocin receptor system in rat brain: An autoradiographical study with a selective radioiodinated oxytocin antagonist. J. Clin. Neuroanat. **1:** 293-302.
27. WITT, D. M., C. S. CARTER & T. R. INSEL. 1991. Oxytocin receptor binding in female prairie voles: Effects of endogenous and exogenous estradiol stimulation. J. Neuroendocrinol. **3:** 155-161.
28. FREUND-MERCIER, M. J., M. E. STOECKEL, J. M. PALACIOS, A. PAZOS, J. M. REICHART, A. PORTE & P. RICHARD. 1987. Pharmacological characteristics and anatomical distribution of [^{3}H]oxytocin-binding sites in the Wistar rat brain studied by autoradiography. Neuroscience **20:** 599-614.
29. TRIBOLLET, E., C. BARBERIS, S. JARD, M. DUBOIS-DAUPHIN & J. J. DREIFUSS. 1988. Localization and pharmacological characterization of high affinity binding sites for vasopressin and oxytocin in the rat brain by light microscopic autoradiography. Brain Res. **442:** 105-118.
30. WITT, D. M., T. R. INSEL & C. S. CARTER. 1991. Estrogen modulation of oxytocin: Effects on sociosexual interactions and CNS receptor binding in prairie voles. *In* Oxytocin in Maternal, Sexual and Social Behavior. C. A. Pedersen, J. D. Caldwell, G. F. Jirikowski & T. R. Insel, Eds.: Ann. N.Y. Acad. Sci. **652:** 445-447.
31. CARTER, C. S., A. C. DEVRIES & L. L. GETZ. 1995. Physiological substrates of mammalian monogamy: The prairie vole model. Neurosci. Biobehav. Rev. **19:** 303-314.
32. INSEL, T. S. & L. E. SHAPIRO. 1992. Oxytocin receptor distribution reflects social organization in monogamous and polygamous voles. Proc. Natl. Acad. Sci. USA **89:** 5981-5985.
33. DE KLOET, E. R., D. A. M. VOORHIUS & J. ELANDS. 1985. Estradiol induces oxytocin receptor binding sites in rat hypothalamic ventromedial nucleus. Eur. J. Pharmacol. **118:** 185-188.
34. DE KLOET, E. R., D. A. M. VOORHIUS, Y. BOSCHMA & J. ELANDS. 1986. Estradiol modulates density of putative "oxytocin receptors" in discrete rat brain regions. Neuroendocrinology **44:** 415-421.

35. INSEL, T. R. 1986. Postpartum increases in brain oxytocin binding. Neuroendocrinology **44:** 515-518.
36. COIRINI, H., A. JOHNSON & B. MCEWEN. 1989. Estradiol modulation of oxytocin binding in the ventromedial hypothalamic nucleus of male and female rats. Neuroendocrinology **50:** 193-198.
37. COIRINI, H., A. E. JOHNSON, M. SCHUMACHER & B. S. MCEWEN. 1992. Sex differences in the regulation of oxytocin receptors by ovarian steroids in the ventromedial hypothalamus of the rat. Neuroendocrinology **55:** 269-275.
38. JOHNSON, A. E., H. COIRINI, G. F. BALL & B. S. MCEWEN. 1989. Anatomical localization of the effects of 17 β-estradiol on oxytocin receptor binding in the ventromedial hypothalamic nucleus. Endocrinology **124:** 207-211.
39. JOHNSON, A. E., H. COIRINI, B. S. MCEWEN & T. R. INSEL. 1989. Testosterone modulates oxytocin binding in the hypothalamus of castrated male rats. Neuroendocrinology **50:** 199-203.
40. JOHNSON, A. E., G. F. BALL, H. COIRINI, C. R. HARBAUGH, B. S. MCEWEN & T. R. INSEL. 1989. Time course of the estradiol-dependent induction of oxytocin receptor binding in the ventromedial hypothalamic nucleus of the rat. Endocrinology **125:** 1414-1419.
41. SCHUMACHER, M., H. COIRINI, M. FRANKFURT & B. S. MCEWEN. 1989. Localized actions of progesterone in hypothalamus involve oxytocin. Proc. Natl. Acad. Sci. USA **86:** 6798-6801.
42. SCHUMACHER, M., H. COIRINI, D. W. PFAFF & B. F. MCEWEN. 1990. Behavioral effects of progesterone associated with rapid modulation of oxytocin receptors. Science **250:** 691-694.
43. TRIBOLLET, E., S. AUDIGIER, M. DUBOIS-DAUPHIN & J. J. DREIFUSS. 1990. Gonadal steroids regulate oxytocin receptors but not vasopressin receptors in the brain of male and female rats. An autoradiographical study. Brain Res. **511:** 129-140.
44. BALE, T. & D. DORSA. 1995. Sex differences in and effects of estrogen on oxytocin receptor messenger ribonucleic acid expression in the ventromedial hypothalamus. Endocrinology **136:** 27-32.
45. BALE, T., D. DORSA & C. JOHNSTON. 1995. Oxytocin receptor mRNA expression in the ventromedial hypothalamus during the estrous cycle. J. Neurosci. **15:** 5058-5064.
46. INSEL, T. R., J. T. WINSLOW & D. M. WITT. 1992. Homologous regulation of brain oxytocin receptors. Endocrinology **130:** 2602-2608.
47. SWANSON, L. & P. SAWCHENKO. 1983. Hypothalamic integration: Organization of the paraventricular and supraoptic nuclei. Ann. Rev. Neurosci. **6:** 269-324.
48. BUIJS, R. M., G. J. DE VRIES, F. W. VAN LEEUWEN & D. F. SWAAB. 1983. Vasopressin and oxytocin: Distribution and putative functions in the brain. *In* The Neurohypophysis: Structure, Function and Control, Progress in Brain Research. B.A. Cross & G. Leng, Eds.: 115-122. Elsevier. Amsterdam.
49. SOFRONIEW, M. V. 1983. Morphology of vasopressin and oxytocin neurones and their central and vascular projections. *In* The Neurohypophysis: Structure, Function and Control, Progress in Brain Research. B. A. Cross & G. Leng, Eds.: 101-114. Elsevier. Amsterdam.
50. BUIJS, R. M. 1978. Intra- and extra-hypothalamic vasopressin and oxytocin pathways in the rat. Cell Tissue Res. **192:** 423-435.
51. AKAISHI, T. & Y. SAKUMA. 1985. Estrogen excites oxytocinergic, but not vasopressinergic cells in the paraventricular nucleus of the female rat hypothalamus. Brain Res. **335:** 302-305.
52. THEODOSIS, D. & D. POULAIN. 1992. Neuronal-glia and synaptic plasticity of the adult oxytocinergic system. *In* Oxytocin in Maternal, Sexual, and Social Behaviors. C. Pedersen, J. Caldwell, G. Jirikowski & T. Insel, Eds. Ann. N.Y. Acad. Sci. **652:** 303-325.

53. Caldwell, J. D., P. J. Brooks, G. F. Jirikowski, A. S. Barakat, P. K. Lund & C. A. Pedersen. 1989. Estrogen alters oxytocin mRNA levels in the preoptic area. J. Neuroendocrinol. **1:** 1-7.
54. Jirikowski, G., J. Caldwell, W. Stumpf & C. Pedersen. 1988. Estradiol influences oxytocin immunoreactive brain systems. Neuroscience **25:** 237-248.
55. Pfaff, D., J. Haldar & S. Chung. 1992. *In situ* hybridization for showing hormone effects on oxytocin mRNA in specific populations of hypothalamic neurons and their possible participation in multiplicative hormonal responses. *In* Oxytocin in Maternal, Sexual, and Social Behaviors. C. Pedersen, J. Caldwell, G. Jirikowski & T. Insel, Eds. Ann. N.Y. Acad. of Sci. **652:** 347-356.
56. Ivell, R. 1986. Biosynthesis of oxytocin in the brain and peripheral organs. *In* Neurobiology of Oxytocin. D. Ganten & D. Pfaff, Eds.: 1-18. Springer-Verlag. Berlin.
57. Carmichael, M. S., R. Humbert, J. Dixen, G. Palmisano, W. Greenleaf & J. M. Davidson. 1987. Plasma oxytocin increases in the human sexual response. J. Clin. Endocrinol. Metab. **64:** 27-31.
58. Kendrick, K. M., E. B. Keverne, C. Chapman & B. A. Baldwin. 1988. Microdialysis measurement of oxytocin, aspartate, γ-aminobutyric acid and glutamate release from olfactory bulb of the sheep during vaginocervical stimulation. Brain Res. **442:** 171-174.
59. Steinman, J. L., J. T. Winslow, G. Sansone, C. Gerdes & T. R. Insel. 1992. Release of oxytocin into spinal cord superfusates in response to vaginocervical stimulation in rats. Soc. Neurosci. **18:** Abstract 194-198.
60. Murphy, M. R., J. R. Seckl, S. Burton, S. A. Checkley & S. L. Lightman. 1987. Changes in oxytocin and vasopressin secretion during sexual activity in men. J. Clin. Endocrinol. Metab. **65:** 738-741.
61. Hughes, A. M., B. J. Everitt, S. L. Lightman & K. Todd. 1987. Oxytocin in the central nervous system and sexual behavior in male rats. Brain Res. **414:** 133-137.
62. Stock, S. & K. Uvnas-Moberg. 1988. Increased plasma levels of oxytocin in response to afferent electrical stimulation of the sciatic ans vagal nerves and in response to touch and pinch in anaesthetized rats. Acta Physiol. Scand. **132:** 29-34.
63. Crowley, W. & W. Armstrong. 1992. Neurochemical regulation of oxytocin secretion in lactation. Endocrinol. Rev. **13:** 33-64.
64. Renaud, L. & C. Bourque. 1991. Neurophysiology and neuropharmacology of hypothalamic magnocellular neurons secreting vasopressin and oxytocin. Prog. Neurobiol. **36:** 131-169.
65. Sheng, M. & M. E. Greenber. 1990. The regulation and function of c-*fos* and other immediate early genes in the nervous system. Neuron **4:** 477-485.
66. Morgan, J. & T. Curran. 1991. Stimulus-transcription coupling in neurons: Role of cellular immediate-early genes. Ann. Rev. Neurosci. **14:** 421-451.
67. Sagar, S. M., F. R. Sharp & T. Curran. 1988. Expression of c-*fos* protein in brain: Metabolic mapping at the cellular level. Science **240:** 1328-1331.
68. Meister, B., M. Villar, S. Ceccatelli & T. Hokfelt. 1990. Localization of chemical messengers in magnocellular neurons of the hypothalamic supraoptic and paraventricular nuclei: An immunohistochemical study using experimental manipulations. Neuroscience **37:** 603-633.
69. Landry, M., A. Trembleau, R. Arai & A. Calas. 1991. Evidence for colocalization of oxytocin mRNA and galanin in magnocellular hypothalamic neurons: A study combining in situ hybridization and immunohistochemistry. Mol. Brain Res. **10:** 91-95.
70. Sawchenko, P., L. Swanson & W. Vale. 1984. Corticotropin-releasing factor:co-expression within distinct subsets of oxytocin-, vasopressin- and neurotensin-immunoreactive neurons in the hypothalamus of the male rat. J. Neurosci. **4:** 1118-1129.
71. Baum, M. & B. Everitt. 1992. Increased expression of c-*fos* in the medial preoptic area after mating in male rats: Role of afferent inputs from the medial amygdala and midbrain central tegmental field. Neuroscience **50:** 627-646.

72. Kollack, S. & S. Newman. 1992. Mating behavior induces selective expression of Fos protein within the chemosensory pathways of the male Syrian hamster brain. Neurosci. Lett. **143:** 223-228.
73. Robertson, G. S., J. G. Pfaus, L. J. Atkinson, H. Matsumura, A. G. Phillips & H. C. Fibiger. 1991. Sexual behavior increases c-*fos* expression in the forebrain of the male rat. Brain Res. **564:** 352-357.
74. Witt, D. M. & T. R. Insel. 1994. Male sexual behavior activates c-fos-like protein in oxytocin neurons in the paraventricular nucleus of the hypothalamus. J. Neuroendocrinol. **6:** 13-18.
75. Wagner, C. K. & L. G. Clemens. 1991. Projections of the paraventricular nucleus of the hypothalamus to the sexually dimorphic lumbosacral region of the spinal cord. Brain Res. **539:** 254-262.
76. Frye, C. & E. Leadbetter. 1994. 5 alpha-reduced progesterone metabolites are essential in hamster VTA for sexual receptivity. Life Sci. **54:** 653-659.
77. Witt, D. M., L. J. Young & D. Crews. 1995. Progesterone modulation of androgen-dependent sexual behavior in male rats. Physiol. Behav. **57:** 307-313.
78. Argiolas, A. 1992. Oxytocin stimulation of penile erection. *In* Oxytocin in Maternal, Sexual, and Social Behavior. C. Pedersen, J. Caldwell, G. Jirikowski & T. Insel, Eds.: Ann. N.Y. Acad. Sci. **652:** 194-203.
79. Witt, D. M. & H. Gainer. 1995. Calcium regulation of hypothalamic Fos gene expression following depolarization. Soc. Neurosci. **21:** 1652.
80. Wray, S. 1992. Organotypic slice explant roller tube cultures. *In* Neuromethods, Vol. 23: Practical Cell Culture Techniques. A. Boulton, G. Baker & W. Walz, Eds.: 201-239. Humana Press. New York, NY.

V
Clinical Perspectives on Social Behavior

22

Integrative Functions of Lactational Hormones in Social Behavior and Stress Management

C. Sue Carter and Margaret Altemus

Historically, and in primitive cultures, women continued to lactate throughout most of their reproductive lives. It is widely accepted that breast feeding offers benefits to the infant. However, the importance of lactation to the behavior and physiology of the mother has only recently been recognized.[1] For example, until this century lactational inhibition of ovulation was a major form of contraception in most human cultures and had important consequences for population control. Modern patterns of lactation[2] and hormonal contraception[3] have reduced the effectiveness of lactational contraception. However, the capacity of breast feeding to inhibit ovarian cyclicity is a clear example of the biological power of the neuroendocrine system responsible for lactation.

Lactation is a defining property of mammals and until modern times was essential to mammalian reproduction. In the research described here we examined the hypothesis that adaptations associated with lactation might facilitate stress management in recently parturient women.

It is from the functions of the mammary glands that the taxonomic classification of Mammalia takes it name. In mammals, physiological and behavioral adaptations associated with lactation are integral components of the female reproductive system. Despite the evolutionary importance of lactation, our understanding of the physiological and behavioral consequences for the mother of this uniquely female process is remarkably incomplete.

Among the neuroendocrine adaptations that accompany both birth and subsequent lactation are hormonal changes that promote selective social interactions, including maternal behaviors and high levels of physical contact. Concurrently, the processes responsible for lactation may reduce maternal reactivity in response to environmental stressors. In the present paper we focus on chronic lactational adaptations that involve

Support from the Department of Defense, National Science Foundation (BNS 7925713, 8506727, and 8719748), and the National Institutes of Health including the Institute of Child Health and Human Development (HD 16679) and the National Institute of Mental Health (MH 45836) has been essential to this research.

the nervous system and the adrenal axis. In addition, we examine the functions of the uniquely mammalian hormone oxytocin, which plays a pivotal role in the integration of the behavioral and physiological processes unique to female physiology. Investigations of the functions of oxytocin have led to a consideration of the actions of its companion neurohypophysial hormone vasopressin. We further speculate that oxytocin and vasopressin and interactions between these hormones might regulate dynamic behavioral states, including the capacity of an individual to respond to both social and physical challenges.

BIOLOGICAL CORRELATES OF LACTATION

Lactation at the level of the breast is primarily under the control of two hormones: prolactin, which is necessary for milk production, and oxytocin, which is responsible for milk ejection.[4] The hormones of pregnancy promote the growth of the mammary glands and duct systems. After birth the breasts initially produce colostrum and do not actually begin to secrete milk until about 2–3 days postpartum. Milk production requires the action of prolactin which stimulates the alveoli of the mammary glands to secrete milk.

Prolactin is a peptide hormone primarily produced by the anterior pituitary gland which is important in maternal milk production. Prolactin synthesis and release are regulated by various hypothalamic inhibitory and releasing factors, including dopamine (sometimes called the prolactin inhibitory factor, PIF). The secretion of prolactin is further facilitated by the stimulus of suckling, which increases the levels of a prolactin-releasing hormone (PRH), also known as vasoactive intestinal peptide. There is evidence implicating prolactin in maternal behavior,[5] and high levels of prolactin are associated with reproductive inhibition.[6] Evidence also indicates that prolactin can reduce activity in the hypothalamic-pituitary-adrenal (HPA) axis.[7,8] However, the behavioral effects of prolactin and the possible actions of prolactin on behavior and the nervous system are generally not well defined.

Oxytocin is a neuropeptide that, among other sites, is synthesized in the paraventricular nucleus and supraoptic nucleus of the hypothalamus. The synthesis of oxytocin and the excitability of oxytocinergic cells are regulated in part by sex steroids including estrogen and progesterone. Oxytocin, from the magnocellular regions of the paraventricular nucleus and supraoptic nucleus, is transported by neurosecretion to the posterior pituitary (neurohypophysis) where it is released in pulses into the circulatory system. Cervical stimulation during parturition and nipple stimulation during nursing are proximate stimuli for the release of oxytocin. In addition, the magnocellular cells that release oxytocin are capable of remarkable morphological plasticity. Like other neurons, oxytocinergic cells are normally separated and thus insulated from each other by glia. However, during parturition and lactation, glial processes retract, allowing the formation of multiple synapses and permitting rapid communication among oxytocinergic cells. Increased connectivity among oxytocin-producing magnocellular neurons facilitates the pulsatile release of this hormone.[9,10] When blood-borne oxytocin reaches the prolactin-primed breast, it causes constriction of the myoepithalial cells of the nipple, and thus it is responsible for the milk letdown or milk ejection reflex. During parturition the major target for oxytocin is the uterus;

the primary action of oxytocin in the uterus also is based on the capacity of this hormone to cause muscle contractions. Oxytocin is named for its ability to facilitate a ''quick birth,'' and it has been recognized since early in the twentieth century that the timing of uterine contractions during birth and subsequent milk ejections during lactation were dependent on the actions of oxytocin.[11] There also is reason to believe that oxytocin is important to maternal behavior[12–16] and to sexual behavior in both males and females,[17,18] and to ejaculatory function in males.[19] In the present paper, we have looked beyond the traditional reproductive functions of oxytocin to speculate on the role of this hormone in the maintenance of behavioral and physiological homeostasis.

STIMULI RELEASING OXYTOCIN

Various types of stimuli associated with social interactions can release oxytocin. As just noted, oxytocin is released during lactation by breast stimulation and can become conditioned to stimuli associated with the infant.[4] Oxytocin is released by genital stimulation and during mating in a variety of species (reviewed in refs. 18,20, and 21). In adult rats, nongenital tactile contact releases oxytocin, even in anesthetized animals.[22] In addition, in both male and female rats, oxytocin is released following emersion in warm water, vibration, electro-acupuncture, and tactile stimulation or massage.[22–24]

Events that are considered ''stressful'' are associated with the release of oxytocin into the peripheral circulation in rats.[25,26] In humans, the effects of stress on the release of oxytocin are less clear. In nonlactating women, oxytocin is released in response to nipple stimulation, but only in the luteal phase of the menstrual cycle. Oxytocin does not increase measurably in humans during exercise[27] or hypertonic saline infusions (Demitrack, personal communication). In one study that did report a stress-induced release of oxytocin, only ''emotionally'' reactive women showed a reliable oxytocin release.[28] In addition, oxytocin treatment in humans tends to inhibit the release of ACTH, whereas in rats oxytocin increases ACTH secretion. Finally, although corticosterone tends to be elevated in lactating rats,[26] it is not elevated in lactating women.[27] The reason for this species differences in peripheral oxytocin responses to stress is not known.

INTERACTIONS BETWEEN SYSTEMS REGULATING LACTATION AND THE ADRENAL AXIS

Lactation is inhibited by stress,[29] and the functions of the adrenal axis in turn are modulated by lactation and the hormonal systems that regulate lactation. However, both oxytocin and vasopressin may be released in response to stress, especially in rats, and both may be considered components of the adrenal stress axis.[26,28]

Neuroendocrine reactivity of the adrenal axis is generally reduced during lactation. It has been known since the early 1970s that lactating female rodents showed reduced adrenal reactivity, often indexed by reduced corticosterone secretion, following exposure to stressors such as ether, surgical trauma, and electric shock.[30–34] In rats, injections of hypertonic saline solution normally are considered stressful and are expected to release glucocorticoids. However, during lactation there is selective inhibition of normal hypothalamic stress responses, including in rats a reduction in gene expression for both corticotropin-releasing hormone (CRH) and enkephalin, an endogenous opiate, and a concomitant reduction in serum levels of corticosterone and oxytocin.[35] During lactation the release of oxytocin in response to exogenous CRH is abolished.[36] In humans, both ACTH[37] and corticosterone levels[38] fall during a bout of breast feeding. Evidence also indicates that peripheral injections of oxytocin can inhibit ACTH and cortisol release in both men and women. In addition, oxytocin injections can inhibit the release of ACTH and/or cortisol, which normally follows treatment with CRH, vasopressin plus CRH, or exercise (reviewed in ref. 37).

Wiesenfeld and associates[39] measured reduced autonomic reactivity in response to infant cries in lactating women. Both skin conductance and heart rate indicated lower levels of sympathetic arousal in lactating versus nonlactating mothers.

The reduced responsivity to stressful experiences associated with lactation may be viewed as an adaptive response which protects a nursing female from overreacting to stressful stimuli and promotes successful lactation. It was found that lactating women interact more positively with their babies, directing more touching and smiling towards their infants than do bottle-feeding mothers.[40] Adler and associates[41] reported more positive moods in nursing versus bottle-feeding mothers.

Altemus and associates[27] examined the effects of physical stress in lactating versus recently delivered, bottle-feeding women. Women in that study were given treadmill exercise to 90% of their VO2 max. The two groups were matched in age and weeks postpartum. The peak blood lactate level, a measure of exercise intensity, was similar in both groups, and lactating and nonlactating subjects had similar basal levels of ACTH and cortisol. ACTH, cortisol, and vasopressin increased following exercise in bottle-feeding women, as would be expected in normal controls. However, the magnitude of the increase in ACTH, cortisol, and vasopressin in response to exercise stress was blunted in the lactating women. Thus, lactating women show marked inhibition of stress hormone secretion in response to exercise, which was not seen in postpartum women who bottle-fed their infants. Taken together these studies suggest for humans and other mammals that lactation and/or oxytocin can reduce physiological reactivity to various stressors.

Lactation also influences the activity of other neural systems that have been implicated in the management of psychological stress. For example, catecholamine responses to stress are reduced in lactating rats.[42] Suckling also increases central production of gamma amino butyric acid (GABA) in rats[43] and sheep.[44] GABA is an inhibitory neurotransmitter, known to play an important role in the regulation of anxiety and behavioral reactivity. Lactating females do not show the expected neuronal activation in cortical neurons following exposure to an excitatory amino acid,[45] suggesting that the functional modifications associated with lactation extend beyond the hypothalamus to include cortical functions.

Because oxytocin and lactation may alter adrenal function and glucocorticoid secretion, immunological consequences might be expected. Recent research on the effects of lactation on immunological parameters is generally uncommon in animals or humans. Among the few studies available is work indicating that lactation is associated with enhanced inflammatory reactions to endotoxin[46] and ozone[47] in rats. Prolactin receptors were described on lymphocytes,[48] and prolactin appears to act as an immune stimulant in several *in vitro* systems and in animal models of inflammatory disease.[49,50] The importance of lactation in the regulation of the immune system deserves additional study.

Clinical research also indicates that biological changes associated with pregnancy and lactation may protect some women from mental disorders. In women with a history of panic disorder, panic symptoms tend to decline in pregnancy and remain low during the lactation period.[51,52] These results suggest that patterns of infant feeding may influence a mother's mental health and thus her ability to deal with the demands of child rearing.

Stress generally has detrimental effects on female reproduction. Despite lactation-associated adaptations to reduce autonomic and adrenal reactivity, as just described, anxiety in the mother can interfere with both birth and lactation.[53–55] For example, Newton and Newton[29,56] found that the amount of milk produced by a nursing woman dropped dramatically (from 168 to 99 g) if she was distracted or stressed by noxious stimulation, such as injection of physiological saline solution. Injection of oxytocin returned milk production to normal levels (153 g). Catecholamine infusion also decreases milk release at the level of the breast, possibly by promoting vasoconstriction.[57]

NEURAL AND BEHAVIORAL EFFECTS OF LACTATION AND OXYTOCIN

In the remainder of this paper we focus on the hypothesis that oxytocin, which is only one of many hormones that are influenced by lactation, has behavioral actions that may be important to our understanding of the processes responsible for management of both social and physical stress.

Lactation and the hormones of lactation, including oxytocin, have various behavioral effects. Temporary impairments of memory and attention were reported in late pregnancy and during early lactation.[58] Research reports indicate that oxytocin administration can be amnesic in humans,[59] whereas vasopressin, which has many antioxytocinergic effects,[60] promotes several kinds of learning[61,62] and may enhance performance in attention-demanding tasks.[63] Oxytocin also may reduce anxiety, as measured in animals by increased exploratory behavior,[64,65] and reduced submissive behavior and freezing. Animals that are treated with high doses of oxytocin exhibit sedation.[65] Oxytocin treatment, administered centrally or peripherally, is followed by long-term lowering of blood pressure in rats.[66] Evidence from rodents demonstrates that oxytocin, probably acting within the CNS, blocks pain.[67–69] The antinociceptive effects of oxytocin are not blocked by naloxone treatment (a specific antagonist for opioid receptors), but are prevented by specific antagonists for oxytocin,[24,67,68] suggesting that the effects are specific to oxytocin and do not require the release of endogenous opiates.

The effects of oxytocin may not be totally independent of the endogenous opiates, however. In rats, oxytocin inhibits the development of tolerance to and other responses to opiates and cocaine. Oxytocin treatment reduces dopamine utilization and decreases the number of apparent binding sites for dopamine. On the basis of these findings, Sarnyai and Kovacs[70] have proposed that oxytocin acts as a neuromodulator of dopaminergic activity, which in turn regulates CNS processes leading to drug addiction. Dopamine release is a component of both the reward system and stress responses. The capacity of oxytocin to modulate dopaminergic activity could be involved in its effect on stress reactivity.

Oxytocinergic and vasopressinergic systems might influence behaviors through effects on other neural pathways and the autonomic system. For example, both hormones have been implicated in the control of the autonomic nervous system, with oxytocin having primarily parasympathetic actions[16] and vasopressin serving as a central and peripheral component of the sympathetic nervous system (reviewed in refs. 63, 71, and 72). The behavioral effects of oxytocin and vasopressin correlate with their autonomic actions, supporting the hypothesis of Uvnäs-Moberg[1,16] that oxytocin and its vagal activities may integrate a variety of metabolic and behavioral systems.

OXYTOCIN, VASOPRESSIN, AND THE EVOLUTION OF STRESS MANAGEMENT

Oxytocin and arginine vasopressin differ from each other in only two of nine amino acids and are generally considered to be mammalian hormones. However, vasopressin-like peptides have been identified in mollusks, and van Kesteren and associates[75] suggest that ''prohormones of the vasopressin/oxytocin superfamily must have been present in the common ancestors of vertebrates and invertebrates.'' Thus, vasopressin-like molecules are ancient, found in both vertebrates and invertebrates, and associated with many ''adaptive'' or homeostatic behaviors.[74]

A large literature, beyond the scope of this chapter, revealed many neurobiological interactions between oxytocin and vasopressin (reviewed in refs. 63, 71, 72, and 73). Most, but not all of this research indicates that vasopressin and oxytocin have antagonistic or opposite functions.

In vertebrates, the release of vasopressin is associated with fluid and temperature regulation, regulation of the cardiovascular and autonomic nervous systems. Vasopressin is a central component of the adrenal stress axis, capable of synergizing with CRH to release ACTH.[76] Vasopressin also directly regulates territorial and defensive behaviors in animals.[77] Central vasopressin levels, as measured in cerebrospinal fluid, are elevated in patients with obsessive-compulsive disorder.[78] In humans the cognitive content of obsessions often includes themes of a defensive or territorial nature. Recent findings, as just described, indicating that lactation is associated with a reduction in anxiety, obsessiveness, and stress reactivity offer preliminary support for the hypothesis that lactation and/or oxytocin can counteract the defensive behavioral patterns associated with stress and the central release of vasopressin. The physiological changes associated with lactation provide a remarkable example of an adaptive state that may favor the interests of the infant over its mother, which is a unique characteristic of mammalian reproduction.

On the basis of these and other observations we speculated that vasopressin might have broad functions associated with defending an organism against both physiological stressors, such as dehydration, hemorrhage, or autonomic challenges, and psychological threats, including aggression from an intruder or other forms of stressful stimulation. The presence of high levels of oxytocin, such as the pulses that accompany parturition, lactation, and sexual behavior, could functionally antagonize the actions of vasopressin. Alternatively, vasopressin, which is released during intense stress, might override the actions of oxytocin, supporting behaviors that would, under the most severe circumstances, promote the survival of the individual.

SUMMARY

For mammalian reproduction to succeed, self-defense and asociality must be subjugated to positive social behaviors, at least during birth, lactation, and sexual behavior. Perhaps the important task of regulating the interaction between social and agonistic behaviors is managed, in part, by interactions between two related neurochemical systems that incorporate oxytocin and vasopressin in their functions.

The neuropeptides oxytocin and vasopressin participate in important reproductive functions, such as parturition and lactation, and homeostatic responses, including modulation of the adrenal axis. Recent evidence also implicates these hormones in social aspects of reproductive behaviors. For example, oxytocin is important for a variety of positive social behaviors, including the regulation of maternal-infant interactions. In adult animals, oxytocin may facilitate both social contact and selective social interactions associated with social attachment and pair bonding,[73] and it participates in the regulation of parasympathetic functions. Vasopressin, in contrast, is associated with behaviors that might be broadly classified as "defensive" including enhanced arousal, attention, or vigilance, increased aggressive behavior, and a general increase in sympathetic functions. On the basis of the literature on the functions of these hormones and our own recent findings, we propose that dynamic interactions between oxytocin and vasopressin are components of a larger system which integrates the neuroendocrine and autonomic changes associated with mammalian social behaviors and the concurrent regulation of the stress axis. In addition, studies of lactating females provide a valuable model for understanding the more general neuroendocrinology of the stress axis.

Peptide hormones, including oxytocin and vasopressin, do not readily cross the blood-brain barrier and must be administered centrally (i.c.v.) to reach the brain. Nasal sprays have been used to promote milk let down and have been used in some behavioral studies,[59,61] but the extent to which such compounds reach the brain is not known. Therefore, virtually nothing is known regarding the effects in humans of centrally administered oxytocin. The study of human lactation, in conjunction with animal research, provides an opportunity to begin to develop viable hypotheses regarding the behavioral effects of oxytocin.

REFERENCES

1. Uvnäs-Moberg, K. 1989. The gastrointestinal tract in growth and reproduction. Sci. Am. **261:** 78-83.
2. Carter, C. S. 1988. Patterns of infant feeding, the mother-infant interaction and stress management. *In* Stress and Coping Across Development. T. M. Field, P. M. McCabe & N. Schneiderman., Eds.: 27-46. L. Erlbaum Assoc. Hillsdale, NJ.
3. Short, R. A. 1984. Breast feeding. Sci. Am. **250:** 35-41.

4. WAKERLEY, J. B., G. CLARKE & A. J. S. SUMMERLEE. 1994. Milk ejection and its control. *In* The Physiology of Reproduction. E. Knobil & J. Neill, Eds.: 2283-2321. Raven Press. New York, NY.
5. BRIDGES, R. S. 1990. Endocrine regulation of parental behavior in rodents. *In* Mammalian Parenting: Biochemical, Neurobiological and Behavioral Determinants. N. A. Krasnegor & R. S. Bridges., Eds.: 93-117. Oxford University Press. New York, N.Y..
6. MCNEILLY, A. S. 1994. *In* The Physiology of Reproduction. E. Knobil & J. Neill, Eds.: 1179-1212. Raven Press. New York, NY.
7. SCHLEIN, P. A., M. X. ZARROW & V. H. DENENBERG. 1974. The role of prolactin in the depressed or "buffered" adrenocorticosteroid response of the rat. J. Endocrinol. **62:** 93-99.
8. ENDORCZI, E. & C. S. NYAKAS. 1972. Pituitary adrenal function during lactation and after LTH (prolactin) administration in the rat. Acta Physiol. Acad. Sci. Hung. **41:** 49-54.
9. THEODOSIS, D. T., L. BONFANTI, S. OLIVE, G. ROUGON & D. A. POULAIN. 1994. Adhesion molecules and structural plasticity of the adult hypothalamo-neurohypophysial system. Psychoneuroendocrinology **19:** 455-462.
10. HATTON, G. I., B. K. MODNEY & A. K. SALM. 1992. Increases in dendritic bundling and dye coupling of supraoptic neurons after the induction of maternal behavior. Ann. N.Y. Acad. Sci. **652:** 142-155.
11. HELLER, H. 1974. History of neurohypophysial research. *In* Handbook of Physiology. Section 7: Endocrinology, Vol. IV. Part 1. R. O. Greep & E. B. Astwood, Eds.: 103-177. American Society of Physiology, Washington, DC.
12. WIDSTROM, A.-M., V. WAHLBERG, A.-S. MATTHIESEN, P. ENEROTH, K. UVNÄS-MOBERG, S. WERNER & J. WINBERG. 1990. Short-term effects of early suckling and touch of the nipple on maternal behaviour. Early Hum. Dev. **21:** 153-163.
13. PEDERSEN, C. A., J. D. CALDWELL, G. PETERSON, C. H. WALKER & G. A. MASON. 1992. Oxytocin activation of maternal behavior in the rat. Ann. N.Y. Acad. Sci. **652:** 58-69.
14. KENDRICK, K. M. & E. B. KEVERNE. 1992. Control of synthesis and release of oxytocin in the sheep brain. Ann. N.Y. Acad. Sci. **652:** 102-121.
15. KEVERNE, E. B. & K. M. KENDRICK. 1992. Oxytocin facilitation of maternal behavior in sheep. Ann. N.Y. Acad. Sci. **652:** 83-101.
16. UVNÄS-MOBERG, K. 1994. Role of efferent and afferent vagal nerve activity during reproduction: Integrating function of oxytocin on metabolism and behaviour. Psychoneuroendocrinology **19:** 687-695.
17. CALDWELL, J. D. 1992. Central oxytocin and female sexual behavior. Ann. N.Y. Acad. Sci. **652:** 166-179.
18. CARTER, C. S. 1992. Oxytocin and sexual behavior. Neurosci. Biobehav. Rev. **16:** 131-144.
19. ARGIOLAS, A. & G. L. GESSA. 1991. Central functions of oxytocin. Neurosci. Biobehav. Rev. **15:** 217-223.
20. CARMICHAEL, M. S., R. HUMBERT, J. DIXEN, G. PALMISANO, W. GREENLEAF & J. M. DAVIDSON. 1987. Plasma oxytocin increases in the human sexual response. J. Endocrinol. Metab. **64:** 27-31.
21. MURPHY, M. R., J. R. SECKL, S. BURTON, S. A. CHECKLEY & S. L. LIGHTMAN. 1987. Changes in oxytocin and vasopressin secretion during sexual activity in men. J. Clin. Endocrinol. Metab. **65:** 738-741.
22. STOCK, S. & K. UVNÄS-MOBERG. 1988. Increased plasma levels of oxytocin in response to afferent electrical stimulation of the sciatic and vagal nerves and in response to touch and pinch in anaesthetized rats. Acta Physiol. Scand. **132:** 29-34.
23. UVNÄS-MOBERG, K., G. BRUZELIUS, P. ALSTER & T. LUNDEBERG. 1993. The antinociceptive effect of non-noxious sensory stimulation is partly mediated through oxytocinergic mechanisms. Acta Physiol. Scand. **149:** 199-204.
24. AGREN, G., T. LUNDEBERG, K. UVNÄS-MOBERG & A. SATO. 1996. The oxytocin antagonist 1-deamino-2-D-Tyr-(Oet)-4-Thr-8-Orn oxytocin reverses the increase in the withdrawal

response latency to thermal nociceptive stimuli following oxytocin administration or massage in rats. Brain Res. In press.

25. Samson, W. K. & R. J. Mogg. 1990. Oxytocin as part of stress responses. *In* Behavioral Aspects of Neuroendocrinology, D. Ganten & D. Pfaff. Eds.: 33-60. Springer-Verlag. Berlin.
26. Lightman, S. L. 1992. Alterations in hypothalamic-pituitary responsiveness during lactation. Ann. N.Y. Acad. Sci. **652:** 340-346.
27. Altemus, M., P. A. Deuster, E. Galliven, C. S. Carter & P. W. Gold. 1995. Suppression of hypothalamic-pituitary-adrenal axis response to stress in lactating women. J. Clin. Endocrinol. Metab. **80:** 2954-2959.
28. Sanders, G., J. Freilicher & S. L. Lightman. 1990. Psychological stress of exposure to uncontrollable noise increases plasma oxytocin in high emotionality women. Psychoneuroendocrinology **15:** 47-58.
29. Newton, M. & N. Newton. 1948. The let-down reflex in human lactation. J. Pediatr. **33:** 698-704.
30. Thoman, E. B., R. L. Conner & S. Levine. 1970. Lactation suppresses adrenal corticosteroid activity and aggressiveness in rats. J. Comp. Physiol. Psychol. **70:** 364-369.
31. Stern, J. M. & S. Levine. 1974. Psychobiological aspects of lactation in rats. *In* Progress in Brain Research, Vol. 41. Integrative Hypothalamic Activity. D. G. Swaab & J. P. Schade, Eds.: 433-444. Elsevier. Amersterdam.
32. Stern, J. M., L. Goldman & S. Levine. 1973. Pituitary adrenal responsiveness during lactation in rats. Neuroendocrinology **12:** 179-191.
33. Stern, J. M. & J. L. Voogt. 1974. Comparison of plasma corticosterone and prolactin levels in cycling and lactating rats. Neuroendocrinology **13:** 173-181.
34. Maestripieri, D. & F. R. D'Amato. 1991. Anxiety and maternal aggression in house mice (*Mus musculus*): A look at interindividual variability. J. Comp. Psychol. **105:** 295-301.
35. Lightman, S. L. & W. S. Young, III. 1989. Lactation inhibits stress-mediated secretion of corticosterone and oxytocin and hypothalamic accumulation of corticotropin-releasing factor and enkephalin messenger ribonucleic acids. Endocrinology **124:** 2358-2364.
36. Patel, H., H. S. Chowdrey & S. L. Lightman. 1991. Lactation abolishes corticotropin-releasing factor-induced oxytocin secretion in the conscious rat. Endocrinology **128:** 725-727.
37. Chiodera, P., C. Salvarani, A. Bacchi-Modena, R. Spallanzani, C. Cigarini, A. Alboni, E. Gardini & V. Coiro. 1991. Relationship between plasma profiles oxytocin and adrenocorticotropic hormone during suckling or breast stimulation in women. Horm. Res. **35:** 119-123.
38. Amico, J., J. M. Johnston & A. H. Vagnucci. 1994. Suckling induced attenuation of plasma cortisol concentrations in postpartum lactating women. Endocrinol. Res. **20:** 79-87.
39. Wiesenfeld, A. R., C. Z. Malatesta, P. B. Whitman, C. Grannose & R. Vile. 1985. Psychophysiological response of breast- and bottle-feeding mothers to their infants' signals. Psychophysiology **22:** 79-86.
40. Dunn, J. B. & M. P. Richards. 1977. Observations on the developing relationship between mother and baby in the neonatal period. *In* Studies in Mother-Infant Interaction. H. R. Scaefeer, Ed.: 427-455. Academic Press. New York, NY.
41. Adler, E. M., A. Cook, D. Davidson, C. West & J. Bancroft. 1986. Hormones, mood and sexuality in lactating women. Br. J. Psychiatry **148:** 74-79.
42. Higuchi, T., H. Negoro & J. Arita. 1989. Reduced responses of prolactin and catecholamine to stress in the lactating rat. J. Endocrinol. **122:** 495-498.
43. Qureshi, G. A., S. Hansen & P. Sodersten. 1987. Offspring control of cerebrospinal fluid GABA concentrations in lactating rats. Neurosci. Lett. **75:** 85-88.
44. Kendrick, K. M., E. B. Keverne, M. R. Hinton & J. A. Goode. 1992. Oxytocin amino acid and monoamine release in the region of the medial preoptic area and bed nucleus

of the stria terminalis of the sheep during parturition and suckling. Brain Res. **569:** 199-209.

45. ABBUD, R., G. E. HOFFMAN & M. S. SMITH. 1993. Cortical refractoriness to N-methyl-D,L-aspartic acid (NMA) stimulation in the lactating rat: recovery after pup removal and blockade of progesterone receptors. Brain Res. **604:** 16-23.
46. GORDON, T., P. A. WEIDEMAN & A. F. GUNNISON. 1993. Increased pulmonary response to inhaled endotoxin in lactating rats. Am. Rev. Resp. Dis. **147:** 1100-1104.
47. GUNNISON, A. F., P. A. WEIDEMAN & M. SOBO. 1992. Enhanced inflammatory response to acute ozone exposure to rats during pregnancy and lactation. Fundam. Appl. Toxicol. **19:** 607-612.
48. BELLUSSI, G., G. MUCCIOLI, C. GHE & C. R. DI. 1987. Prolactin binding sites in human erythrocytes and lymphocytes. Life. Sci. **41:** 951.
49. BERNTON, E., H. BRYANT, J. HOLADAY & J. DAVE. 1992. Prolactin and prolactin secretagogues reverse immunosuppression in mice treated with cysteamine, glucocorticoids, or cyclosporin-A. Brain Behav. Immun. **6:** 394-408.
50. WALKER, S. E. 1993. Prolactin: An immune-stimulating peptide that regulates other immune-modulating hormones. Lupus **2:** 67-69.
51. KLEIN, D. F., A. M. SKROBALA & R. S. GARFINKEL. 1995. Preliminary look at the effects of pregnancy on the course of panic disorder. Anxiety **1:** 227-232.
52. COWLEY, D. S. & P. P. ROY-BYRNE. 1989. Panic disorder during pregnancy. J. Psychosom. Obstet. Gynaecol. **10:** 193-210.
53. GROSVENOR, C. E. & F. MENA. 1967. Effect of auditory, olfactory and optic stimuli upon milk ejection and suckling-induced release of prolactin in lactating rats. Endocrinology **80:** 840-846.
54. NEWTON, N. 1973. Interrelationships between sexual responsiveness, birth, and breast feeding. *In* Contemporary Sexual Behavior: Critical Issues in the 1970s. J. Zubin & J. Money, Eds.: 77-98. Johns Hopkins University Press. Baltimore.
55. NEWTON, N. 1978. The role of the oxytocin reflexes in three interpersonal reproductive acts: Coitus, birth and breastfeeding. *In* Clinical Psychoneuroendocrinology in Reproduction. L. Carenza, P. Pancheri & L. Zichella, Eds.: 411-418. Academic Press. New York.
56. NEWTON, N. 1982. The quantitative effect of oxytocin (pitocin) on human milk yield. Ann. N.Y. Acad. Sci. **652:** 481-483.
57. CROSS, B. A. 1953. Sympathetico-adrenal inhibition of the neuro-hypophysial milk-ejection mechanisms. J. Endocrinol. **9:** 7-18.
58. SILBER, M., O. ALMKVIST, B. LARSSON & K. UVNÄS-MOBERG. 1990. Temporary peripartal impairment in memory and attention and its possible relation to oxytocin concentration. Life Sci. **47:** 57-65.
59. KENNETT, D. J., M. C. DEVLIN & B. M. FERRIER. 1982. Influence of oxytocin on human memory processes: Validation by a control study. Life Sci. **31:** 273-274.
60. BARBERIS, C., S. AUDIGIER, T. DURROUX, J. ELANDS, A. SCHMIDT & S. JARD. 1992. Pharmacology of oxytocin and vasopressin receptors in the central and peripheral nervous system. Ann. N.Y. Acad. Sci. **652:** 39-45.
61. BRUINS, J., R. HUMAN & J. M. VAN REE. 1992. Effect of a single dose of desglycinamide-[Arg8]vasopressin or oxytocin on cognitive processes in young healthy subjects. Peptides **13:** 461-468.
62. DANTZER, R., R. M. BLUTHE, G. F. KOOP & M. LE MOAL. 1987. Modulation of social memory in male rats by neurohypophyseal peptides. Psychopharmacology **91:** 363-368.
63. DE WIED, D., Ed. 1990. Neuropeptides Basics and Perspectives. Amsterdam. Elsevier.
64. ARLETTI, R. & A. BERTOLINI. 1987. Oxytocin acts as an antidepressant in two animal models of depression. Life Sci. **41:** 1725-1730.
65. UVNÄS-MOBERG, K., S. AHLENIUS, V. HILLEGAART & P. ALSTER. 1994. High doses of oxytocin cause sedation and low doses cause an anxiolytic-like effect in male rats. Pharmacol. Biochem. Behav. **49:** 101-106.

66. PETERSSON, M., P. ALSTER, A. LUNDEBERG & K. UVNÄS-MOBERG. 1996. Oxytocin causes a long-term decrease of blood pressure in female and male rats. Physiol. Behav. **60:** 1311-1315.
67. CALDWELL, J. D., G. A. MASON, D. A. STANLEY, G. JERDACK, V. J. HRUBY, P. HILL, A. J. PRANGE, JR. & C. A. PEDERSEN. 1987. Effects of nonapeptide antagonists on oxytocin- and arginine-vasopressin-induced analgesia in mice. Reg. Peptides **18:** 233-241.
68. UVNÄS-MOBERG, K., G. BRUZELIUS, P. ALSTER, I. BILEVICIUTE & T. LUNDEBERG. 1992. Oxytocin increases and a specific oxytocin antagonist decreases pain threshold in male rats. Acta Physiol. Scand. **144:** 487-488.
69. LUNDEBERG, T., K. UVNÄS-MOBERG, G. AGREN & G. BRUZELIUS. 1994. Anti-nociceptive effects of oxytocin in rats and mice. Neurosci. Lett. **170:** 153-157.
70. SARNYAI, Z. & G. L. KOVACS. 1994. Role of oxytocin in the neuroadaptation to drugs of abuse. Psychoneuroendocrinology **19:** 85-117.
71. PEDERSEN, C. A., J. D. CALDWELL, G. F. JIRIKOWSKI & T. R. INSEL, Eds. 1992. Oxytocin in Maternal, Sexual and Social Behaviors. Ann. N.Y. Acad. Sci., Vol. 652. New York, NY.
72. NORTH, W. G., A. M. MOSES & L. SHARE, Eds. 1993. The Neurohypophysis: A Window on Brain Function. Ann. N.Y. Acad. Sci., Vol. 689. New York, NY.
73. CARTER, C. S., A. C. DEVRIES & L. L. GETZ. 1995. Physiological substrates of monogamy: The prairie vole model. Neurosci. Biobehav. Rev. **19:** 303-314.
74. MOORE, F. L. 1987. Behavioral actions of neurohypophysial peptides. *In* Psychobiology of Reproductive Behavior: An Evolutionary Perspective. D. Crews, Ed.: 62-87. Prentice Hall. Englewood Cliffs, NJ.
75. VAN KESTEREN, R. E., A. B. SMIT, R. W. DIRKDS, N. D. DEWITH, W. P. M. GERAERTS & J. JOOSSE. 1992. Evolution of the vasopressin/oxytocin superfamily: Characterization of a cDNA encoding a vasopressin-related precursor, preproconopressin, from the mollusc *Lymnaea stagnalis*. Proc. Natl. Acad. Sci. USA **89:** 4593-4597.
76. WHITNALL, M. H. 1993. Regulation of the hypothalamic corticotropin-releasing hormone neurosecretory system. Prog. Neurobiol. **40:** 573-629.
77. FERRIS, C. 1992. Role of vasopressin in aggressive and dominant/subordinate behavior. Ann. N.Y. Acad. Sci. **652:** 212-226.
78. ALTEMUS, M., T. PIGOTT, K. T. KALOGERAS, M. DEMITRACK, B. DUBBERT, D. L. MURPHY & P. W. GOLD. 1992. Abnormal regulation of corticotrophin-releasing hormone and vasopressin in patients with obsessive-compulsive disorder. Arch. Gen. Psychiatry **49:** 9-20.

23

Psychobiology of Early Social Attachment in Rhesus Monkeys: Clinical Applications

Gary W. Kraemer

The aims of this paper are, first, to review recent theory and research on the psychobiology of attachment with special emphasis on the mother-infant relationship in primates, and second, to discuss how changing perspectives on the causes and effects of affiliation might affect our understanding of developmental psychopathology. To efficiently address the proposed topics, it is necessary to briefly provide a theoretical and historical context.

ETHOLOGICAL CONTROL SYSTEMS THEORY OF ATTACHMENT

Since the late 1960s, the preeminent theory of attachment has been that propounded by Bowlby in collaboration with Ainsworth.[1] Before their contributions, sustenance of the infant was thought to be the primary reason for infant-caregiver interactions. Attachment was viewed as a mechanism that kept caregiver and infant together for this purpose. In contrast, the Bowlby-Ainsworth ethological control systems theory (ECST) of attachment suggested that secure infant-caregiver attachment is necessary for optimal psychosocial development of the infant; and, vice versa, some pathological behavior exhibited by adolescents and adults may be causally related to disruption of early attachment.[2] This conclusion was controversial when first proposed, but these days is taken as being practically common sense by many health care professionals and academicians. Indeed, the basic ideas on which ECST is based are so well accepted that it makes the most sense to explain new or different views in terms of how they differ from ECST.

The ethological control systems theory is based on the premise that there is a genetically encoded imprinting-like motivation for the infant to attach to an object that is also a secure base and a caregiver.[2] A *secure base* has at least three characteristics: (1) it is reliable; (2) it shields the infant from environmental threats; and (3) it is sustaining and provides the infant with resources (e.g., nutrition). *Attachment behavior* involves (at least) visual tracking, maintaining proximity, and seeking contact with the secure

Address for correspondence: Gary W. Kraemer, Harlow Primate Laboratory, University of Wisconsin, 22 N. Charter St., Madison, WI 53715 (tel: 608 263-5076; fax: 608 263-4356; e-mail: gkraemer@mail.soemadison.wisc.edu).

base. This behavior is regulated by "goal-corrected" homeostatic mechanisms in the infant, consisting of internal representations of the external world (i.e., cognitive working models of the caregiver and environment). Having a secure base maximizes the chances of survival and permits the infant to develop veridical internal representations of the external world (*working models*), explore the environment, and develop optimally.[2]

Disruption of usual attachment to a caregiver means that the child does not have a secure base and is prone to incorporation of conflicting models of attachment objects and the environment. It does not explore, acquire knowledge, and develop as it would otherwise. Bowlby[2] cited this as a cause of previously unrecognized childhood depression and anxiety disorders, later vulnerability to adverse responses to usual stressors, and inadequate caregiving when the child becomes a parent. By the latter effect, subsequent offspring are not adequately cared for, so disrupted attachment produces a form of developmental psychopathology that can propagate across generations.[2]

The ethological control systems theory has not altered the way that clinicians view or approach the treatment of problems of childhood psychosocial development in the way Bowlby[2] had wished that it would, however. Bowlby[2] maintained that the reason was that clinicians do not understand the implications of the theory for treatment. Another factor may be that ECST does not encompass major psychobiological problems and phenomena that are of current concern to clinicians, and research on the presumed neurobiological substrates of attachment behavior has produced results that, if not incompatible, are at least not accounted for by ECST. This has led to formulation of the psychobiological attachment theory (PAT).[1,3] PAT expands on ECST with the aim of providing an understanding of attachment useful to both scientists and clinicians, but, in so doing, challenges or demands modifications of three basic assumptions underlying ECST.

MODIFICATIONS OF CORE ASSUMPTIONS OF ATTACHMENT THEORY

As with psychoanalytic theories that preceded it, ECST proposes that there are internal mechanisms in the infant that cause or regulate behavior but are not observable either technically or perhaps theoretically. Among these are the constructs of "drives" and cognitive "working models." The assumptions that require modification in transition from attachment theories based on psychological constructs to psychobiology are in the following areas:

1. *The nature of the "motivation" for infants to develop attachments to caregivers:* Ultimately ECST employs the construct of an innate "drive" to survive and attach as an explanation of the cause of infant behavior. Drives denote unknown causes of the initiation and regulation of behavior. At this point, however, internal causes of behavior are more profitably conceived of as reflecting the actions of neural mechanisms with measurable characteristics and levels of function.

2. *The effect that attachment (or disruption of attachment) has on the constitutional nature of the infant:* If we assume that the only or the most significant long-term effects of attachment are on cognitive working models of the social environment,

TABLE 1. Social Characteristics of Primate Laboratory Rearing Conditions Used in Studies of Attachment in Rhesus Monkeys

Rearing Descriptor	Social Characteristics
Total isolation	No sensory contact with other monkeys, no attachment object
Partial isolation	Monkeys can see, hear, smell, but not touch other monkeys; no attachment object
Surrogate rearing	Monkeys are in partial isolation, but have a cloth-covered inanimate surrogate mother as an attachment object
Peer rearing	Monkeys are reared with like-aged peers; they are not socially isolated, but do not have contact or experience with an adult mother
Mother rearing	Monkeys are reared by their biological mother

then any behavioral effects that might be attributable to altered body physiology are outside of the theory. Indeed, undeniable biological variation that may be observed and cited as a factor in behavior may be assigned to the wrong causal domain, that is, attributable to genetic causes, even though the cause of such variation is actually social-environmental in origin.

3. *The probable mechanism by which the positive effects of secure attachment and negative effects of attachment disruption are transmitted across generations (transgenerational effects)*: If we assume that transgenerational effects are composites of only two domains of causality, altered cognition (working models), and/or temperament (another construct), then the idea of a third or ''interface'' domain with equal stature may be overlooked.[4] Prior attachment theory is silent on what the persisting physiological effects attachment might be. Yet, environmentally produced alteration of primary physiological responsiveness to stressors counts as an interface domain between cognitive regulation of behavior and more basic regulation of response proclivities which may be genetic in origin. Alteration of basic physiologic responses could be one way in which maternal responsiveness to offspring is persistently affected.

A Matter of Perspective

Most reports reviewed herein concern the effects of rearing rhesus monkey infants without real rhesus monkey mothers and then comparing the characteristics of these infants with those that were reared by monkey mothers. Monkeys that were not reared with their mothers were generally reared in conditions that provided a range of nonmaternal social stimulation and interaction (TABLE 1). The more usual view of this research is that rearing in any other circumstances than by a monkey mother in a natural environment counts as environmental, social, or maternal deprivation.[5] From this viewpoint the behavioral and biological differences observed in infants reared in unusual circumstances are referred to as the ''effects of privation'' of one kind or another. Another way to view this research is that the behaviors and characteristics of the socially isolated monkey reveal how the primate nervous system and body develop when there is no social stimulation, no attachment, and no monkey caregivers. (It is important to note that all living rhesus monkeys had some form of a caregiver, otherwise they would not be alive. In the laboratory, socially isolated monkeys have human caregivers; cf. ref. 5).

Rearing monkeys in progressively richer rhesus social environments (i.e., partial isolation, surrogate-rearing, peer-rearing, and finally mother-rearing) allows us to measure the effects of infant attachment and affiliation to members of their own species. That is, with each increment in rearing condition we see the effects of the addition of components of social stimuli that the infant would usually experience, without providing the full complement of usual peri- and postnatal stimulation until the attachment object is a real mother.[4]

This perspective is important because rhesus infants exhibit attachment behaviors towards inanimate objects (diapers and terry cloth covered wooden blocks) and like-aged rhesus infants (peers).[6] When we observe the infant developing under these circumstances, we can measure the effects of having a living or inanimate attachment object per se. The only attachment objects that provide mothering, though, are rhesus monkey mothers. Hence, when we compare surrogate and peer-reared monkeys to mother-reared monkeys, we are comparing the effects of exhibiting attachment behavior towards an unresponsive object, to the effects of being attached to a living being, to the effects of being attached to a living being and being mothered. As a prelude, it turns out that being mothered, and not just being attached to a "secure base," is the most important thing for the psychobiological development of the infant.[4,7] As outlined before, there are three major assumptions underlying attachment theory that will be reconsidered from this perspective.

THE MOTIVATION TO EXHIBIT ATTACHMENT BEHAVIOR

One cornerstone of ECST is that infants are motivated by a drive to survive and are able to recognize and seek a secure base. By implication, infants must be able to identify a secure base and to make contact with that base a goal. Harlow *et al.*'s[6] studies with wire and cloth-covered surrogate mothers indicate, however, that rhesus infants will reliably direct attachment behavior towards inanimate objects. Among these they choose objects with soft and furry surface characteristics rather than those capable of sustaining the infant by feeding it. Rhesus infants are always born to a real mother that is furry and she usually feeds the infant; they are rarely given a choice. What the comparison of the usual ecological reality with Harlow's studies indicates, nonetheless, is that the isolated infant can be presented with an object with certain stimulus characteristics, and it will exhibit its species-typical attachment behavior even though the object is in no way, shape, or form a secure base. Indeed, the monkey preferring a terry cloth surrogate as an attachment object when a wire surrogate or a human feeds it is actually making a counter-survival choice. Rhesus infants also attach to abusive or neglectful rhesus mothers and thereafter exhibit exaggerated attachment behavior towards these insecure bases even when they have other choices.[8] In sum, the rhesus neonate's nervous system and exhibited behavior are not tuned to a more global construct of security that adult humans understand.

Instead, it seems that the neonate's nervous system is preset to exhibit attachment behaviors towards a select and probably species-specific set of stimuli, many of which have no direct survival value but are usually expressed by an object that usually has enormous survival value. This was Bowlby's thought as well. These stimuli and their effects on the nervous system can be viewed as causal factors in the infant's exhibition of attachment behavior, without further endowing the infant with motivations to survive or a concept of security, however. This is where current research in psychobiology departs from ECST constructs.

EFFECT OF ATTACHMENT (OR ITS DISRUPTION) ON THE INFANT

ECST explains the dramatic behavioral response to separation of an infant from its caregiver by proposing that the separation response is related to the role of the mother-infant relationship and "attachment" in survival.[9,10] One implication of this view is that the strength of attachment should be related to the survival value of the attachment object; another is that the nature and magnitude of the response to separation should be proportional to the strength of the attachment.

The behavioral response to mother-infant separation in human and nonhuman primates has often been characterized as occurring in two sequential phases, "protest" and "despair." Protest is manifested by increased activity, agitation, and vocalization. Despair is characterized by inactivity, withdrawal, an increase in self-directed behaviors such as self-mouthing (finger sucking) and self-clasping, adoption of a fetal-like self-enclosed body posture, and often failure to eat.[6,11] Protest and despair are often viewed as variations of a response to loss that differ in severity and time of onset. Exhibition of despair is viewed as a severe and depression-like response to separation and presumably reflects a greater perceived loss.[11]

Psychobiological Causes of the Response to Separation

Despite the appeal of these views, studies in rhesus monkeys indicate that more severe responses to separation (despair) usually occur among infants reared by inadequate or abusive mothers, that is, attachment objects that have reduced survival value by comparison with highly competent mothers. One example is that mother-reared infants are most disturbed by separation and likely to exhibit persistent changes in responses to stressors when environmental circumstances prior to separation degrade the reliability and adequacy of the mother.[12–14] Another example is that rhesus infants reared with inanimate surrogate mothers that do not have any capacity to feed, nurture, or protect the infant generally have more severe responses to separation than do monkeys separated from real mothers.[15]

The psychobiological explanation for the behavioral response to separation per se is that it reveals what happens when the regulatory influences of the attachment object are removed. Hence, real mothers initially provide an external regulatory mechanism for many of the physiological mechanisms that the infant possesses but does not regulate itself.[3] At some point in development the infant becomes self-regulating through the development of internal regulatory mechanisms entrained to the stimuli that the mother provides. This regulation persists in the mother's absence, so mother-reared monkeys usually exhibit few adverse effects of separation. If the infant is attached to an object that does not provide the usual regulating stimuli, such as an inanimate surrogate mother, it may not develop the usual self-regulatory processes. So, severe responses to separation may be better explained by a lack of adequate behavioral and physiological regulatory mechanisms rather than an internal cognitive state, that is, perception of loss.[4,15]

EFFECTS OF MOTHERING ON INFANT CONSTITUTION

Collectively, the psychobiological studies just cited suggest that the monkey mother is usually a potent regulator of the infant's behavior through exhibition of stimuli that the infant is set to respond to in a particular way. It would be a mistake to think of this as a "reflex" in the way we typically think of spinal cord mechanisms. Instead, the idea is that the infant's behavior usually becomes entrained to the mother's and vice versa, in a transactional relationship occurring over time.

One effect of this is that global aspects of the infant's physiology also entrain to the social interactions and environment associated with the mother. Prior attachment theories assume, if only by the default of not addressing the topic, that the regulation of the infant's physiology is a product of genetic endowment. The idea would be that brain homeostatic mechanisms such as those that regulate such primary characteristics as body temperature, metabolic rate and body composition, sleep-cycles, and hormonal responses to stressors, for example, form, develop, and mature according to a preset genetic plan. The environmental factors that would concern us would be those that might interfere with the unfolding of this plan. Exposure to malnutrition, disease, trauma, and toxins would be examples. It might be assumed, then, that as long as infants are genetically sound and are not exposed to biological insults, their physiological constitution should develop normally. Given this assumption it is also true that physiological changes are not likely to be examined if the only insult that the infant has been exposed to is psychosocial deprivation, but has been well cared for in other respects.

It is well established, however, that monkeys reared in social isolation or partial social isolation differ physiologically, behaviorally, and cognitively from socially reared monkeys. A brief list of reported differences[4,16,17] includes altered temperature regulation, immune system function, body weight regulation, and eating patterns (polydipsia and hyperphagia); exhibition of self-injurious behavior, motor stereotypies, hyper- or hypoemotionality, and aggressiveness; failure to be able to use facial expression as a discriminative stimulus in learning tasks, failure to inhibit well learned responses, and failure to be able to detect oddity; and disrupted sexual and maternal behavior. In sum, social privation affects almost every aspect of what it means to be a social monkey, and if the privation extends over the first 6-9 months of postnatal life, most effects persist into adulthood.[1,6]

This is where the reversal of perspective advocated before becomes critical. There are a variety of reasons why monkeys reared in total social isolation might differ physiologically from socially reared monkeys. Among these are that: (1) there are fewer and less complex stimuli coming into the nervous system, so complete social deprivation qualifies as sensory deprivation as well; and (2) the range of motor behavior possible or required is sharply delimited. Under these circumstances general physiological changes might be attributed to gross and persisting differences in sensory stimulation and activity levels rather than to psychosocial deprivation alone. What is necessary, then, is to progressively add more of ''what is missing'' in the isolation environment until the developing infant has what can be assured to be a rich social sensory environment, attachment objects, and is able to or required to engage in all of the motor behavior it is capable of, and yet it is deprived of one critical aspect of usual development–maternal care.

Peer Rearing

Peer-reared monkeys are separated from their biological mothers shortly after birth and reared in a primate nursery for 30 days. During this time and thereafter they are housed with two to three like-aged cagemates. Peer-reared monkeys are not deprived of social stimulation and interaction per se, and they develop strong attachments to their cagemates. Being attached to peers, they are engaging in social behavior with animate warm furry members of their own species. What is missing, then, is the regulatory characteristics of an adult female rhesus monkey.

If the social behavioral development of peer-reared monkeys is compared to that of mother-reared monkeys, six major differences are commonly cited.[6,7,18–25] First, as infants and juveniles, peer-reared monkeys engage in an extraordinary amount of clinging to one another and in self-directed finger and toe sucking (self-directed behavior). This is especially evident if the peer group is exposed to an external ''threat'' such as a human observer. Mother-reared juvenile monkeys, in contrast, cling or huddle together primarily during rest or sleep periods, often threaten in return if threatened, and rarely are found with a finger or toe in their mouths. Experienced observers generally characterize peer-reared monkeys as being considerably more timid, fearful, and emotionally labile than mother-reared monkeys. Second, intragroup interactions appear to be chaotic, with individuals being either inordinately separated from group activity or intensely engaged, with rapid fluctuations between the two. Experienced human observers characterize groups of peer-reared monkeys as being in a chronically higher ''tension'' or ''stress'' state than groups of mother-reared monkeys. Third, peer-reared juvenile monkeys are more likely to have a severe response to separation from there cagemates than are mother-reared monkeys living in peer groups as juveniles. Fourth, the performance of peer-reared monkeys on basic cognitive tasks differs from that of mother-reared monkeys. For example, peer-reared monkeys achieve a higher percentage correct performance on delayed nonmatching to sample tasks, and this may play out in relative inflexibility in changing problem-solving strategies when the nature of the task changes. Fifth, although aggression frequency in groups of peer-reared monkeys is generally lower than that in groups of mother-reared monkeys, when aggressive bouts do occur among peer-reared monkeys, they are likely to be more prolonged and vigorous and more likely to produce wounding and severe injury than they are among mother-reared monkeys. Finally, as adults, peer-reared rhesus females are considerably more likely to reject or neglect their infants.

Psychobiological Effects of Peer Rearing

A number of psychobiological studies in rhesus monkeys have focused on the development of the brain biogenic amine neurotransmitter systems and the hypothalamic-pituitary-adrenal (HPA) axis. Biogenic amine systems in this context refers collectively to the brain norepinephrine (NE), dopamine (DA), and serotonin (5HT) systems. These neurotransmitter and neuroendocrine systems are thought to play a role in brain mechanisms regulating reward (NE and DA), information gating and impulse control (5HT), and response to and adaptation to stress (HPA axis).[1] It has also been suggested that malfunction of the NE, DA, and 5HT systems may be causal factors in some human psychiatric disorders. Thus, it has been suggested that affective disorders may be caused by aberrations in NE and/or 5HT system function and schizophrenia by aberrations in DA system function, and that impulsive violence and suicide may be related to aberrations in 5HT system function in particular (see refs. 1 and 4 and associated commentaries for review). It has also been suggested that aberrations in HPA axis function play a role in depression (see ref. 26).

Considerable interest has been shown in viewing the behavioral effects of separation or social deprivation in rhesus monkeys as analogs or ''models'' of some human psychiatric disorders. For example, a considerable body of research centers on the idea that the despair response to separation may be an analog of some forms of human depression.[22,27] The reason for mentioning this here is to explain why these systems, and not others, are the primary dependent measures found in many studies.[28] What is at issue here, however, is whether these systems are affected by social rearing conditions, attachment, and mothering.

When the latter question is addressed, it is clear that peer-reared monkeys differ from mother-reared monkeys in levels of activity in all of these dependent measures. In nonhuman primates the dependent measures of activity level in these systems are usually derived from measures of the neurotransmitter, hormone, or their metabolites in cerebrospinal fluid (CSF) or blood.[28] The major metabolites of NE, DA, and 5HT (3-methoxy-4-hydroxy phenylglycol [MHPG], homovanillic acid [HVA], and 5-hydroxyindoleacetic acid [5HIAA], respectively) are often measured in lieu of the neurotransmitter for technical reasons, one of which is that the levels of neurotransmitter in CSF are extremely low. A partial summary of results of studies from different laboratories specifically comparing peer- and mother-reared monkeys is presented in TABLE 2.

Overall, the results are not entirely consistent. Primarily, differences in one measure or another are not found in one study or another. Normally, this would worry the scientists involved, but careful scrutiny of the studies supports the following considerations and interpretation.

1. Age is a critical factor. Clarke *et al.*[26] found that peer-reared monkeys had higher levels of CSF NE than did mother-reared monkeys from 1-6 months of age, whereas Kraemer and Clarke[23] report lower CSF NE levels than those in mother-reared monkeys from 9 months of age and up. This indicates a cross-over in the direction of effect at about 7-8 months of age, corresponding to weaning and separation of the mother-reared monkeys from their mother. Beyond this, under baseline conditions, adolescent and young adult (24-48 months of age) peer-reared monkeys

TABLE 2. Biogenic Amine and Hypothalamic-Pituitary-Adrenal Axis Measures in Peer-Reared Monkeys by Comparison to Mother-Reared Monkeys over Stages of Development

Age Range (mo.)	Difference
"Baseline" Conditions	
1-6	No difference in cortisol,[29] no difference in 5HIAA or HVA,[29] higher MHPG[a];[29] higher CSF NE (months 5-6), higher MHPG[30]
8-12	Lower CSF NE, lower HVA, no difference in MHPG, trend to higher 5HIAA ($p < 0.08$), lower cortisol and ACTH[23]
18	No difference in cortisol,[29] higher MHPG[a29]
24 or greater	Lower CSF NE[22]
"Social Separation Stress" Conditions	
1-6	Higher cortisol,[29] lower 5HIAA[b],[29] higher MHPG[29]
8-12	Lower CSF NE[b] and HVA, no difference in MHPG or 5HIAA[30]
18	Higher cortisol,[29] higher 5HIAA[19] (trend),[29] higher MHPG[29]
24 or greater	No difference in 5HIAA,[19] higher MHPG,[19] higher cortisol and ACTH (Clarke, report in preparation)

[a] Higley *et al.*[29] report a main effect of rearing and a main effect of separation on MHPG. The rearing by separation interaction is not reported, so "higher" MHPG is carried in cells of this table as a report by this group.

[b] Difference is due to change in mother-reared group.

at the Harlow Primate Laboratory exhibit lower levels of NE than do mother-reared monkeys and no differences in MHPG.[22]

2. Differences in experimental protocols and laboratory housing facilities and procedures are likely to be a factor. Higley *et al.*[19,29] reliably report higher levels of MHPG in peer-reared monkeys in their experimental protocols, whereas Clarke *et al.*[30] find this effect only in the first 6 months postpartum. Studies measuring MHPG in young adult peer-reared monkeys exposed to repeated separations as juveniles are more consistent with reports by Higley *et al.*, however (Clarke, report in preparation).

3. Social stressors and age of exposure appear to be critical factors. Clarke[26] and Kraemer and Clarke[23] do not report increased cortisol in 6-18-month-old peer-reared monkeys, as do Higley *et al.*[29] However, significant differences exist in the amount of social disruption the monkeys are exposed to across studies and the ages at which stressors are imposed. As with studies measuring MHPG, Clarke (report in preparation) found increased cortisol and ACTH levels in young adult peer-reared monkeys exposed to repeated separations as juveniles, which is consistent with reports by Higley *et al.*[29]

A unifying theme present across studies is that peer-reared monkeys are often found to be biologically different from mother-reared monkeys, but the magnitude and even the direction of difference in dependent measures may vary over development and in relation to prior or ongoing environmental circumstances. One explanation for this, at least in terms of interpreting results obtained by measuring NE and HPA axis activity under a variety of different circumstances, is that depending on the system, receptor and synthetic mechanisms may be inordinately up- or downregulated at various junctures in development in peer-reared monkeys.

For example, juvenile peer-reared monkeys housed in stable social groups generally maintain lower baseline levels of CSF NE and the DA metabolite HVA than do group-housed juvenile mother-reared monkeys.[23] When challenged, however, the behavioral response of peer-reared monkeys to social stressors or drugs that activate NE and DA neurotransmitter systems is exaggerated and inordinate by comparison to mother-reared monkeys. It has been suggested that this hyperresponsiveness may be attributable to postsynaptic receptor upregulation secondary to lower levels of activity that may be maintained over a significant time period.[23] Juvenile peer-reared monkeys housed in stable social groups also maintain lower baseline levels of adrenocorticotropic hormone (ACTH) and cortisol than do mother-reared monkeys, but they have a *blunted* HPA axis response (increase in ACTH and/or cortisol) to psychosocial stressors such as separation from cagemates.[26] Thus, the exaggerated behavioral response to stressors in peer-reared monkeys, perhaps mediated in part by hypersensitive brain NE and/or DA systems, is not paralleled by comparably enhanced or even normal neuroendocrine responses.

Hence, when mother- and peer-reared monkeys are challenged, either a hyper- or a hyporesponse by the peer-reared monkeys is often observed depending on what is being measured. The differences observed after or during challenge may vary in magnitude or even direction from the baseline condition depending on age and experience. Overall, altered responsiveness is present even when there are no measurable differences in baseline values, and this is the feature of peer-reared monkeys that characterizes them across ages and environments. Thus, having peculiarly high or low measures of one neurotransmitter or hormone is not a core biological effect of maternal privation (peer-rearing) that might be related to any "core" aspect of the behavioral disturbances cited before. This conclusion may not be satisfying for those seeking to relate persisting changes in activity levels in one "key" neurochemical or neuroendocrine system to specific aspects of behavior. Biological psychiatrists and neuroscientists often attempt to reduce clinical reasoning about psychiatric disorders or scientific reasoning about complex behaviors to having too much, just the right amount, or too little of one key neurotransmitter or hormone. The effects of maternal attachment, or its disruption, are multivariate and dynamic, however, and not amenable to such reasoning.

PSYCHOBIOLOGICAL ORGANIZATION AND DISORGANIZATION

The major theme espoused in previous sections pertains to concepts of "regulation" and "organization" of neurobiological systems that are presumably caused by interactions with a mother. In turn, the literature cited before suggests that the usual organization of responses to stressors among brain neurochemical and neuroendocrine mechanisms fails to materialize in peer-reared monkeys. Organization implies that indices of activity in individual systems should be within normal limits and that measures of activity among systems that are mechanistically linked should be correlated. Overall, demonstrable covariance in dependent measures of system activity seems critical, because individual measures might be within normal limits as far as one can tell, while usual covariance is nonexistent. Similarly, individual measures of activity might appear to be aberrant, but the usual covariance might still be present. Ideally, both the level of activity in multiple systems and the covariance or correlation among their activity levels over time would be measured. With both sets of information we should be able to ascertain if levels of activity and interrelationships among several brain neurochemical systems account for the behavior of interest.

Multivariate Measures of Organization in Biogenic Amine Systems

The development and actions of the brain 5HT, NE, and DA systems appear usually to be interrelated. Part of the evidence for this is that the levels of these biogenic amines and/or their metabolites in CSF are usually correlated.[29,31,32] Mother-reared offspring tracked from birth to preadolescence exhibit significant and substantial intercorrelations among NE, 5HIAA, and HVA beginning within 2 months after birth and thereafter.[32] Thus, levels of activity in brain biogenic amine systems covary, usually. Also, measures of biogenic amine system activity, primarily measures of NE and/or DA system activity, covary with exhibition of social behavior, social development, and behavioral responses to stressors such as separation from companions.[15,19,32]

It is also important to note that multivariate measures of biogenic amine system activity do not always intercorrelate significantly. For example, many of the interrelationships just cited as developing soon after birth do not materialize in socially isolated rhesus infants.[32] This finding suggests, first, that the correlations among measures that are observed in socially reared monkeys are not attributable to necessarily interlocked neurochemical or transport mechanisms, and second, that important aspects of neurobiological organization are attributable to infant-mother attachment and do not occur if the infant monkey has no mother.[15]

Multivariate Biological Measures in Peer- and Mother-Reared Monkeys

In a prior report Kraemer and Clarke[23] presented behavioral and biological data obtained between 8 and 10 months of age from 48 infant rhesus monkeys (*Macaca mulatta*) who were either mother-or peer-reared for the first 7 months postpartum and then housed in stable peer groups thereafter. One objective of the study was to determine if measures of biogenic amine system activity and measures of ongoing social behavior were related to one another depending on rearing condition. Two CSF samples were taken 3 weeks apart and assayed for levels of NE, HVA, and 5HIAA. Adrenocorticotropic hormone and cortisol were determined in blood samples collected at the same time as the CSF.

The mean duration of behaviors exhibited in the social groups was recorded in 24 five-minute observation sessions conducted over 6 weeks. The intent in analysis of behavior was to focus on general aspects of social behavior and not detailed analysis of individual behaviors. Therefore, behavioral data were collapsed into four categories collectively comprising approximately 90% of the behavior exhibited in social groups (behaviors not included were eating, drinking, self-care behaviors,

TABLE 3. Behavioral and Neurochemical Intercorrelations in Mother-Reared Monkeys (n = 24)[a,b]

	NE	HVA	5HIAA	Inactive	Activity	Social
NE						
HVA	0.38					
5HIAA	0.55*	0.63*				
Inactive	−0.58**	−0.20	−0.27			
Activity	−0.16	0.05	−0.04	−0.04		
Social	−0.57*	−0.24	−0.46*	0.59**	0.23	
Aggression	−0.43**	−0.10	−0.58**	0.33	0.28	0.57**

[a] Reprinted, with permission, from ref. 23.

[b] Correlations (Pearson Product) among behavior duration (activity, social, inactivity measured over 6 weeks, mean out of possible 300 seconds/session), total duration of aggression (seconds), and cerebrospinal fluid concentrations of norepinephrine (NE, pg/ml), homovanillic acid (HVA, ng/ml), and 5-hydroxyindoleacetic acid (5HIAA, ng/ml) in mother-reared juvenile rhesus monkeys. *Significantly different from zero, p <0.05; **significantly different from zero and peer-reared monkeys; p <0.05.

e.g., self-grooming, and "disturbance behaviors," e.g., self-directed behavior and stereotypies). Behavioral categories were: *Activity:* Including locomotion and environmental exploration (manual manipulation of objects); *Social:* Collectively including prosocial behaviors such as grooming, body or manual touching of others, and maintaining proximity (<10 cm) to others; *Inactivity:* Not active and not social; basically, sitting quietly with no others scorable behavior evident; *Aggression:* Biting, fur pulling, and scratching.

In terms of differences in baseline neurochemical and neuroendocrine measures, peer-reared monkeys had lower levels of CSF NE and HVA, lower levels of ACTH and cortisol, and higher levels of activity (and lower durations of inactivity) ($p <$ 0.05 for each measure). The mean level of 5HIAA was higher in peer-reared monkeys, but this difference did not reach conventional significance ($p < 0.08$). TABLES 3 and 4 (reprinted from ref. 23) show the intercorrelations among the behavioral and neurochemical measures for mother- and peer-reared monkeys, respectively.

In TABLE 3, 9 of the 21 intercorrelations among the variables were significantly different from zero in mother-reared monkeys. Of these 9 correlations, 5 were significantly different from correlations among the same measures observed in peer-reared monkeys. The data indicate that inactivity, prosocial behavior, and aggression were negatively correlated with CSF NE levels, and prosocial behavior and aggression were negatively correlated with CSF 5HIAA levels as well. Among neurochemical measures, positive correlations were observed between NE and 5HIAA, and between HVA and 5HIAA. The HVA-5HIAA correlation is commonly observed in mammalian CSF and is thought to reflect some basic linkage between the dopamine and serotonin systems or the mechanisms of transport of these compounds into CSF.[31] Among the behaviors, prosocial behavior was positively correlated with both inactivity and frequency of aggression in mother-reared monkeys. The overall picture is that to the

TABLE 4. Behavioral and Neurochemical Intercorrelations in Peer-Reared Monkeys (n = 23)[a,b]

	NE	HVA	5HIAA	Inactive	Activity	Social
NE						
HVA	0.26					
5HIAA	0.24	0.71*				
Inactive	0.16	−0.25	−0.37			
Activity	0.02	0.17	0.39	−0.54*		
Social	−0.26	−0.14	−0.19	0.17	0.02	
Aggression	0.04	−0.03	−0.14	−0.15	0.07	−0.08

[a] Reprinted, with permission, from ref. 24.

[b] Correlations (Pearson Product) among behavior duration (activity, social, inactivity measured over 6 weeks, mean out of possible 300 seconds/session), total duration of aggression (seconds), and cerebrospinal fluid concentrations of norepinephrine (NE, pg/ml), homovanillic acid (HVA, ng/ml), and 5-hydroxyindoleacetic acid (5HIAA, ng/ml) in peer-reared juvenile rhesus monkeys. *Significantly different from zero, $p < 0.05$; **significantly different from zero and mother-reared monkeys, $p < 0.05$.

degree to which a mother-reared monkey evenly divides its behavior into domains of sitting quietly (inactive) or engaging in social behavior or aggressive bouts (maximizing the measures of each), this is inversely correlated with measures of activity levels in the NE and serotonin systems. The latter two measures are, in turn, correlated with one another.

By contrast, only 2 of 21 correlations were significantly different from zero in peer-reared monkeys. The only significant neurochemical relationship was HVA-5HIAA correlation, and as noted before, this appears to be a feature of functioning mammalian nervous systems per se. The only behaviors that were intercorrelated in peer-reared monkeys were activity and inactivity, and it should be noted that these seemingly "inverse" measures were not negatively correlated in mother-reared monkeys. Overall, the picture one gets is that the manner in which peer-reared monkeys divide their time is not related to measures of neurochemical activity as it is in mother-reared monkeys. Similarly, that a peer-reared monkey engages in more or less prosocial behavior does not translate into also spending more or less time sitting quietly or engaging in aggression, as is the case with mother-reared monkeys.

Perhaps the best way to summarize, then, is that the lack of intercorrelations among behaviors and among behaviors and neurochemical measures in peer-reared monkeys reflects the characterization of these monkeys presented before. Their social behavior strikes the human observer as being chaotic and not as patterned and regulated as that of mother-reared monkeys. If measures of biogenic amine system activity reflect actions of underlying behavior regulatory systems (which is why these measures were collected in the first place), then the conclusion is that activity in these systems does not correspond with behavior in peer-reared monkeys as it does in mother-reared monkeys.

An overwhelming amount of data suggest that brain biogenic amine systems usually play core and central roles in regulating behavior in a variety of mammalian species. What the literature and data cited suggest, then, is that in nonhuman primates, the usual behavioral regulatory characteristics of these systems are not entirely determined by genetic endowment or "hard-wired" into mechanisms that mediate ongoing sensorimotor processing and behavior. Instead, it seems that development of functional competence of these systems, in rhesus monkeys at least, depends on early interactions with a maternal caregiver.

Transgenerational Disorganization?

The competence of a rhesus monkey to adequately rear her own offspring is largely determined by her own rearing experience.[6] Monkeys reared by their mothers are usually competent. As noted before, peer-reared monkeys often neglect or abuse their infants.[33] One explanation for this outcome, consistent with ECST, is that female primates develop a working model of the mother-infant relationship during early development. Stated in other terms, they learn how to mother by being mothered and, perhaps or almost certainly as juveniles and adolescents, by watching older females mother their infants. It seems unlikely, however, that laboratory-housed rhesus infants learn mothering skills from their mothers and then retain and apply this knowledge years later. Also, mother-reared laboratory-housed females usually perform adequately as mothers even if they have never seen another female engaging in maternal behavior with her infant.

A hypothesis consistent with the perspective presented herein is that adequate mothering and mother-infant attachment promote species-typical psychobiological development in offspring and thereby the capacity to respond to and cope with social environmental challenges. Later, this early psychobiological development determines the degree to which new mothers can respond to their own neonates maternally and how rapidly they acquire and exhibit mothering skills. This, in turn, determines how their offspring will fair and so on.

Studies in a variety of mammals, including monkeys, indicate that behavioral responsiveness to young is related to hormonal state.[34] Therefore, the overall suggestion is that the effects of early rearing experience on neurobiological and neuroendocrine development may produce persistent alterations in hormonal state and responsiveness to neonates. Such variation may in large measure account for corresponding transgenerational variation in infant care or neglect in rhesus monkeys. Although this global hypothesis remains to be tested, similar considerations might be applied to understanding transgenerational effects of early privation in humans. Hence, working models of how to care for offspring are important, but there must also be a characteristic parental responsiveness to infants and children.[34] This must coexist with a behavioral and physiological capacity to meet the challenges posed by offspring.[34] This adaptive capacity of the adult may in turn be mediated through neurochemical and neuroendocrine systems that were dependent on earlier maternal care to attain their functional stature.

CONCLUSIONS

When the basic assumptions underlying attachment theory are revised in light of recent data, our understanding of how early attachment and affiliation contribute to psychosocial development changes as well, as does our understanding of the probable relationship between disrupted attachment and disorders of childhood psychosocial development. A theory that provides a clear explanation of what can go wrong with attachment and what happens next is important in understanding: (1) how prevention and early intervention in childhood disorders might best be effected; (2) how treatment in ongoing disorders of childhood development might best be accomplished; (3) how transgenerational effects of disrupted childhood development can be prevented when the child becomes a parent; and (4) how the three preceding factors contribute to our overall understanding of probable causes of psychopathology and its persistence across life span and perhaps generations.

Understanding the mechanisms of attachment and affiliation and the effects of failure of these mechanisms appears to be particularly important when the otherwise competent infant is neglected or abused or when the neurobiologically compromised infant fails to establish an affillative relationship with a caregiver. There are three implications of psychobiological attachment theory that are not easily derived from theories based on psychological constructs.

First, if the competent infant does not attach to a caregiver that provides adequate regulation as part of a transactional relationship, then some of the effects of this will surface in what is traditionally considered to be the individual's basic cognitive processing ability and physiological constitution. That is, the way in which the individual orients to and responds physiologically to social stressors may be altered. The kind of behavioral differences that seem to be most important would be those usually assigned to the domain of "temperament," that is, to approach or withdraw, to be inhibited or uninhibited, shy or reckless, extraverted or neurotic.[4] This is not to say that the dimensions of temperament are entirely environmentally determined, but only that it is both theoretically and clinically important to consider that cognitive processing and physiologic responsiveness may be altered in children who are orphaned, neglected or abused, or who are institutionalized for one reason or another.

Second, and related to the first point, one implication of psychobiological attachment theory is that "failure to attach" when the child is presented with the opportunity is more likely due to failure to perceive and process stimuli in the usual way than to aberrations in "motivation." Considering childhood responses to stressors (such as prolonged separation from the caregiver), the psychobiological perspective is that the unattached child may not be regulating well physiologically and may be unable to perceive or tune to social regulators that may be available.[4]

Third and finally, the neurobiological effects of social environmental factors repeatedly shown to adversely affect social development in rhesus monkeys are not restricted to one neurobiological system. Furthermore, once changes in multiple systems are observed, usually significant interrelationships among measures of the activity of different systems are absent as well. Once usual interrelationships among neurobiological systems degrade, the usual relationship of activity in any particular system to behavior also degrades.[23] It is unlikely that "pharmacological fixes" focusing on one or two aspects of neurochemical function or physiology are going to restore what is basically an organizational problem. By reverse logic, if attachment mechanisms usually afford what is necessary to organize basic sensorimotor and physiologic mechanisms, then therapy for the unattached or neglected child should focus on providing the child with an external regulatory system that is both environmental and interpersonal. The trick here is to acknowledge that the child may not be open to or able to process the usual social stimuli. Finding out what therapeutic approaches can be used to entrain the "disorganized" nervous system thus becomes the focus of new research and development of clinical paradigms based on PAT.

SUMMARY

"Attachment" has been viewed as the process by which the infant bonds to a caregiver and develops and maintains affiliative social relationships. Whereas past theories suggested that the neurobiological mechanisms that enable the infant to engage in regulated social interactions develop autonomously, the more current view is that the organization of cognitive and emotional systems that regulate social behavior depends on early caregiver-infant attachment. It is well known that disruption of caregiver-infant attachment produces abnormal behavior and increases or decreases the activity of different brain neurochemical systems in rhesus monkeys. Furthermore, it has been suggested that these effects might serve as a model for the etiology of some forms of human psychopathology. Current research indicates that caregiver privation alters the development of usual interrelationships among the activity of several neurochemical and neuroendocrine systems and alters basic cognitive processes. In line with the idea that the caregiver usually exerts a potent organizing effect on the infant's psychobiology, the long-standing effects of caregiver privation on behavior and emotionality are probably attributable to changes in multiple regulatory systems and cognitive-emotional integration rather than restricted effects on the activity of any specific set of neurochemical systems.

REFERENCES

1. Kraemer, G. W. 1992. A psychobiological theory of attachment. Behav. Brain Sci. **15:** 493-511.
2. Bowlby, J. 1988. A Secure Base. Basic Books. New York.
3. Hofer, M. A. 1987. Early social relationships: A psychobiologist's view. Child Dev. **58:** 633-647.
4. Kraemer, G. W. 1992. Psychobiological Attachment Theory (PAT) and psychopathology. Behav. Brain Sci. **15:** 525-534.
5. Kagan, J. 1992. The meanings of attachment. Behav. Brain Sci. **15:** 517-518.
6. Harlow, H. F., M. K. Harlow & S. J. Suomi. 1971. From thought to therapy: Lessons from a primate laboratory. Am. Sci. **59:** 538-549.
7. Kraemer, G. W. 1995. The significance of social attachment in primate infants: The caregiver-infant relationship and volition. *In* Motherhood in Human and Nonhuman Primates: Biological and Social Determinants. C. R. Pryce, R. D. Martin & D. Skuse, Eds.: 152-161. Karger. Basel.
8. Sackett, G. P. 1970. Unlearned responses, differential rearing experiences, and the development of social attachments in rhesus monkeys. *In* Primate Behavior: Developments in Field and Laboratory Research, Vol. 1.: 111-140. Academic Press. New York.
9. Ainsworth, M. D. S., M. C. Biehar, E. Waters & S. Wall. 1978. Patterns of Attachment: A Psychological Study of the Strange Situation. Erlbaum. Hillsdale, N.J.
10. Bowlby, J. 1973. Attachment and Loss: Separation, Anxiety, and Anger. Basic Books. New York.
11. Bowlby, J. 1969. Attachment and Loss: Attachment. Basic Books. New York.

12. HINDE, R. A. 1977. Mother-infant separation and the nature of inter-individual relationships: Experiments with rhesus monkeys. Proc. Roy. Soc. Lond. **196:** 29-50.
13. McGINNIS, L. M. 1978. Maternal separation versus removal from group companions in rhesus monkeys. Child Psychol. Psychiatry **8:** 15-27.
14. ROSENBLUM, L. A. & G. S. PAULLY. 1984. The effects of varying environmental demands on maternal and infant behavior. Child Dev. **55:** 305-314.
15. KRAEMER, G. W., M. H. EBERT, D. E. SCHMIDT & W. T. McKINNEY. 1991. Strangers in a strange land: A psychobiological study of mother-infant separation in rhesus monkeys. Child Dev. **62:** 548-566.
16. LUBACH, G. R., E. M. W. KITTRELL & C. L. COE. 1992. Maternal influences on body temperature in the primate infant. Physiol. Behav. **51:** 987-994.
17. LUBACH, G. R., C. L. COE & W. ERSHLER. 1995. Effects of early rearing environment on immune responses of infant rhesus monkeys. Brain Behav. Immun. **9:** 31-46.
18. HARLOW, H. F. 1969. The age-mate or peer affectional system. *In* Advances in the Study of behavior. E. B. Foss, Ed. **2:** 333-383. Academic Press. New York.
19. HIGLEY, J. D., S. J. SUOMI & M. LINNOILA. 1991. CSF monoamine metabolite concentrations vary according to age, rearing, and sex, and are influenced by the stressor of social separation in rhesus monkeys. Psychopharmacology **103:** 551-556.
20. HIGLEY, J. D., M. LINNOILA & S. J. SUOMI. 1994. Ethological contributions: Experiential and genetic contributions to the expression and inhibition of aggression in primates. *In* Handbook of aggressive and destructive behavior in psychiatric patients. M. Hersen, R. T. Ammerman L. Sission, Eds.: 17-32. Plenum Press. New York.
21. KRAEMER, G. W. & W. T. McKINNEY. 1979. Interactions of pharmacological agents which alter biogenic amine metabolism and depression: An analysis of contributing factors within a primate model of depression. J. Affect. Dis. **1:** 33-54.
22. KRAEMER, G. W. 1988. Speculations on the developmental neurobiology of protest and despair. *In* Inquiry into Schizophrenia and Depression: Animal Models of Psychiatric Disorders. P. Simon, P. Soubrie & D. Widlocher, Eds. **11:** 101-147. Karger. Basel.
23. KRAEMER, G. W. & A. S. CLARKE. 1996. Social attachment, brain function, and aggression. Ann. N.Y. Acad. Sci. In press.
24. SUOMI, S. J., H. F. HARLOW & C. J. DOMEK. 1970. Effect of repetitive infant-infant separation of young monkeys. J. Abnorm. Psychol. **76:** 161-172.
25. SUOMI, S. J. 1983. Models of depression in primates. Psychol. Med. **13:** 465-469.
26. CLARKE, A. S. 1993. Social rearing effects on HPA axis activity over early development and in response to stress in young rhesus monkeys. Dev. Psychobiol. **26:** 433-447.
27. KRAEMER, G. W. 1985. The primate social environment, brain neurochemical changes and psychopathology. Trends Neurosci. **8:** 339-340.
28. KRAEMER, G. W. & W. T. McKINNEY. 1988. Animal models in psychiatry: Contributions of research on synaptic mechanisms. *In* Receptors and Ligands in Psychiatry and Neurology. A. K. Sen & T. Lee, Eds.: 459-483. Cambridge University Press. Cambridge.
29. HIGLEY, J. D., S. J. SUOMI & M. LINNOILA. 1992. A longitudinal study of CSF monoamine metabolite and plasma cortisol concentrations in young rhesus monkeys: Effects of early experience, age, sex, and stress on continuity of individual differences. Biol. Psychiatry **32:** 127-145.
30. CLARKE, A. S., D. HEDEKER, M. H. EBERT, D. E. SCHMIDT, W. T. McKINNEY & G. W. KRAEMER. 1996. Rearing experience and biogenic amine activity in infant rhesus monkeys. Biol. Psychiatry. Biol. Psychiatry **40:** 338-352.
31. AGREN, H., I. N. MEFFORD, M. V. RUDORFER, M. LINNOILA & W. POTTER. 1986. Interacting neurotransmitter systems. A non-experimental approach to the 5HIAA-HVA correlation in human CSF. J Psychiatry Res. **20:** 175-193.
32. KRAEMER, G. W., M. H. EBERT, D. E. SCHMIDT & W. T. McKINNEY. 1989. A longitudinal study of the effects of different rearing environments on cerebrospinal fluid norepineph-

rine and biogenic amine metabolites in rhesus monkeys. Neuropsychopharmacology **2:** 175-189.

33. Suomi, S. J. & C. Ripp. 1983. A history of motherless monkey mothering at the University of Wisconsin primate laboratory. *In* Child Abuse: The Non-human Primate Data. M. Reite & N. Caine, Eds.: 49-78. Alan R. Liss. New York.

34. Fleming, A. S., C. Corter & M. Steiner. 1996. Sensory and hormonal control of maternal behavior in rat and human mothers. *In* Motherhood in Human and Nonhuman Primates: Biosocial Determinants.: 106-114. Karger. New York.

24

Psychological and Neuroendocrinological Sequelae of Early Social Deprivation in Institutionalized Children in Romania

Mary Carlson and Felton Earls

ETHICAL FRAMEWORK FOR RESEARCH ON SEVERELY DISADVANTAGED CHILDREN

The situation of infants and children living in state-operated residential institutions in Romania provides a setting in which the consequences of severe social deprivation can be examined. These children experience a form of custodial care in which their medical and nutritional needs are met, but their social and psychological needs are not. The tens of thousands of infants and children from birth to age 3 living in the institutions known as *Leagane* (meaning cradles) are but the leading edge of the hundreds of thousands of children spending much or all of their lives in institutional care. This high prevalence of institutional care for children peaked in the two decades prior to 1990, during the political era of Nicolae Ceausescu. His social and economic policies forced families to bear more children than they wanted or could afford, resulting in around 2% of the population being cared for by the state until they reached the age of 18. Over the 5 years since the fall of Ceausescu's regime, the economic and social instability (resulting from an uncertain transition to a market economy and democratic political rule) has not produced the expected reduction in the rate of admission of infants and children to these institutions.[1]

Romania is not unique among industrialized countries in employing institutional remedies for children affected by complex societal problems. We believe it is scientifically and ethically imperative to analyze the developmental deficits of such children within the context of the social and material resources available to them and their families, that is, not to decouple the social cause from the developmental consequences. We hold that the empirical validity of developmental studies of socially and economically disadvantaged children is threatened when any child is examined in isolation from their immediate social context and those societal factors that have an impact on their families and communities. Study of the deficits or capacities of the decontextualized child can lead to invalid attributions of intrinsic causation within the child (e.g., genes for temperament, IQ) rather than to those sequences of regulatory events that have given rise to the child's phenotypic features. It is this perspective, one that combines ethical and social imperatives with scientific investigation, that provides the rationale for this study.

Studying children in a situation of extreme deprivation provokes such a strong response that pursuing an ethical voice to govern one's work would seem crucial. We intend to go beyond the guidelines required by human studies procedures in the United States and become advocates for these children at the same time that we assess the consequences of their living conditions.[2] In approaching the Romanian situation, the ethical framework that we used to guide this work is the UN Convention on the Rights of the Child (CRC). This was based on its broad coverage of both the needs and capacities of children and youth and the near universal acceptance of its principles.[3] The CRC introduces a level of ethical analysis that legitimately takes children's issues beyond the family into the international political arena, with the awareness that "it is children who pay the heaviest price for our short-sighted economic policies, our political blunders, and our wars."[4]

Children's rights can be characterized in three broad categories: (1) survival (right to basic needs such as shelter, nutrition, and access to medical services); (2) care/protection (right to education, play, culture, leisure, religion, and protection from exploitation, and (3) participation (right to voice, to association, and to information). As a legal document, the intent is that these rights would be specified in national legislation, but as principles for developmental research, clinical medicine, and public health, these rights can be thought of as a framework to guide research, treatment, and services for children without the need for legal sanctions. Of all the categories of rights, participation rights are the most controversial and to us the most important, as they view the child as a citizen. The democratization of children does not separate the child and his/her family, but specifies the rights of families "to provide direction in a manner consistent with the evolving capacities of the child." For young children, caretaker/community participation is critical, as are the developing capacities of the child to initiate and have an opinion in the growth of biological and psychological competence.

EPIGENETIC FACTORS IN BRAIN DEVELOPMENT, DAMAGE, AND SENSORY DEPRIVATION

The demonstration of a direct relation between the tactile modality and social deprivation was established in the laboratory of Harry Harlow where it was shown that tactile contact was a stronger determinant of attachment to a surrogate mother than feeding and that tactile (but not visual or auditory) deprivation was a critical determinant of the autistic-like behavioral syndrome that resulted from early social deprivation.[5] These studies were continued by Mason[6] and many others, including one of the authors.[7]

For the last two decades an important goal of neurophysiological studies of somatic sensory cortex has been to establish cerebral localization of tactile discrimination capacity in primates and to gain an understanding of the role of the tactile system in the development and maintenance of tactile capacity and social behavior.[8] Components of this research program have included studies of the neural and behavioral effects of localized surgical lesions of somatic sensory area of the cerebral neocortex in fetal, infant and juvenile, and adult primates,[9] along with studies of prenatal and early postnatal tactile deprivation (produced by reversible peripheral nerve crush). Unlike research in the visual system in which early deprivation results in enduring modifications of cortical circuitry, these studies of fetal and neonatal macaques with primary somatic sensory cortex (SI) lesions demonstrated a remarkable level of tactile sparing/recovery, and SI topography is not permanently altered after months of perinatal sensory deprivation (studies in progress). Based on anatomic studies in other modalities and other studies of early thalamocortical projections to SI and secondary somatic sensory cortex (SII), this lack of persisting deficits after SI or SII lesions may be due to the stabilization of early exuberant and normally transient pathways.[10] Similarly, months of tactile deprivation in fetal and neonatal macaques have resulted in no permanent cortical changes or lasting sensory deficits. The results of this body of work, much of which has been conducted in the laboratory of the first author, suggest that early tactile deprivation does not work at the level of cortical processing of sensory input. It is in response to the more recently developing work on stress hormone regulation by the hypothalamic-pituitary-adrenal (HPA) system that we aim to better understand how neurodevelopmental events might explain the profound and enduring behavioral consequences of early tactile deprivation in human and nonhuman primates.

NEUROENDOCRINOLOGY OF STRESS, COGNITIVE DEVELOPMENT, AND GROWTH

The proposed studies were conceived from the finding in the HPA system that early tactile deprivation reduced the number of the stress hormone or glucocorticoid (GC) receptor binding sites in the hippocampus and frontal cortex, but not in the hypothalamus, pituitary, septum, or amygdala.[11] A working model of molecular events involved in the upregulation of GC receptors by touch begins with an increase in plasma thyroid levels, leading to an increase in serotonin (5-HT) turnover, followed by increases in cAMP and activation of cycle nucleotide-dependent protein kinases. A transcription factor (AP2) is activated in this cascade in hippocampal neurons within minutes of handling/touch, and the promoter region of the human GC receptor gene has numerous binding sites for AP2, all making a strong case for the role of touch in GC receptor gene regulation.[12] Downregulation of GC receptors in nonhandled rodents results in a compromised negative feedback loop along the HPA axis and chronically elevated levels of circulating GC due to poor reactivity control.[13] Tactile experience beyond the preweaning period in touch-deprived rodents does not compensate for early deprivation, indicating a critical period for this effect.[14] Further studies in these rodents demonstrate that the same hippocampal neurons (CA3 and CA1 pyramidal cells) that characteristically contain GC receptors degenerate prematurely as a consequence of persistently elevated stress hormone levels,[15-17] resulting in forms of memory loss associated with hippocampal damage.[18] The molecular and cellular mechanisms by which these high GC concentrations threaten hippocampal neurons are not ones of direct toxicity but rather of indirect endangerment to make the neurons more vulnerable to any coincident insult (i.e., hypoxia-ischemia, epileptic seizures, hypoglycemia, toxicity, and trauma). Glucocorticoids inhibit glucose utilization in hippocampal neurons, inducing an energetic vulnerability that in combination with activation of an excitatory animo acid/calcium cascade stimulated by the coincidental insult can lead to cell death.[19]

ASSESSMENT OF STRESS HORMONE AND PHYSICAL AND PSYCHOLOGICAL DEVELOPMENT IN 2–3-YEAR-OLD CHILDREN IN *LEAGANE*

In the wake of Ceausescu's assassination in December 1989, images of the severe deprivation experienced by generations of institutionalized infants and children in Romania were shocking. The revelation that infants could be so grossly neglected seemed unfathomable, given the knowledge accumulated over the last century on the detrimental consequences of institutional rearing on both physical growth and psychological development. The muteness, blank facial expressions, social withdrawal, and bizarre stereotypic movements of these infants bore a strong resemblance to the behavior of socially deprived macaques and chimpanzees. Most of the children living since birth in these *Leagane* had experienced severe tactile/social deprivation due to the high child:caretaker ratios and custodial rearing practices. In looking for a population of children in whom to examine stress and HPA system regulation, we discovered an early enrichment program in Iasi, Romania, organized by an American psychologist, Joseph Sparling.[20] In this program, two groups of 2-9-month-old infants were randomly assigned to either a social/educational enrichment condition with a child:caretaker ration of 4 : 1 or left in the standard depriving condition with a child:caretaker ratio of 20 : 1. Our familiarity with recent research in neuroendocrinology showing the effects of touch (or handling) on brain and cognitive development led us to think that examination of HPA system regulation in these infants was an appropriate condition in which to evaluate the rehabilitative potential of this intervention. The results of laboratory studies in rodents point to the importance of tactile/social stimulation during the preweaning period on the development of HPA regulation.[21]

In the 9-month period necessary to obtain funding for this study, this intervention program lost its support. Thus, after a 13-month period of enrichment, children in the intervention group were once again living in the depriving conditions. The children in the intervention group had shown significantly accelerated physical growth and mental/motor development compared to the control group during the enrichment period, but they were no longer superior to the control children in either growth or performance 5–6 months after the program ended (as measured on the Denver Development Screening Test). Measures of weight and height, head, triceps and chest circumference, and mental and motor performance (using the Bayley Scales of Infant Development) revealed that the intervention group had lost the advantage obtained from the previous enrichment experience. At this same time, we measured cortisol (using a noninvasive method of obtaining samples of saliva[22]) to determine its level, diurnal variation, and its reactivity to a stressful event. Salivary samples were taken prior to meals on two consecutive days: at 8 AM, noon and 7 PM on Day 1 and again at 8 AM and noon, and at three closely spaced intervals in the afternoon (5 PM, 6:30 PM, and 7 PM) on Day 2. The afternoon period corresponded to intervals

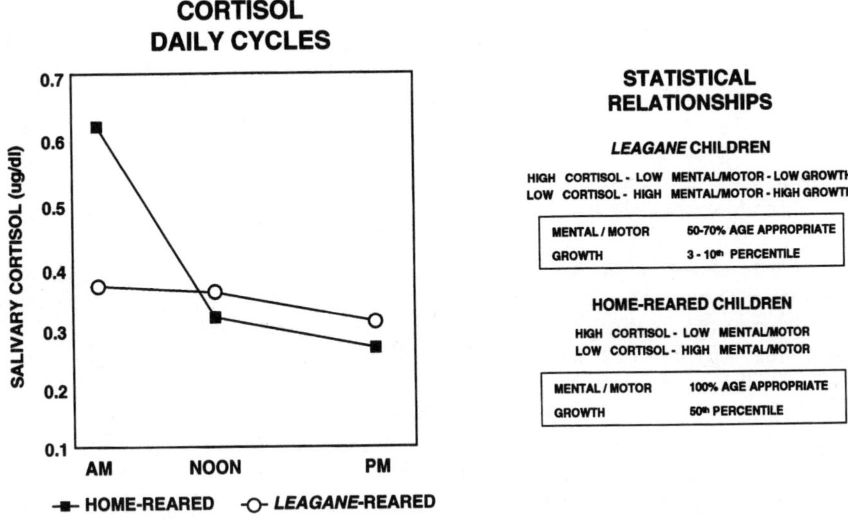

FIGURE 1. Home-reared and *Leagane* children 2 years of age.

before and 15 and 45 minutes after a physical examination, which was introduced as a mild stressor. The AM cortisol levels in the institutionalized *Leagane* children were significantly lower than those in home-reared Romanian children of the same age (FIG. 1) and remained elevated at noon and PM compared to those of the children at home. When the two *Leagane* groups are examined separately (FIG. 2), the control

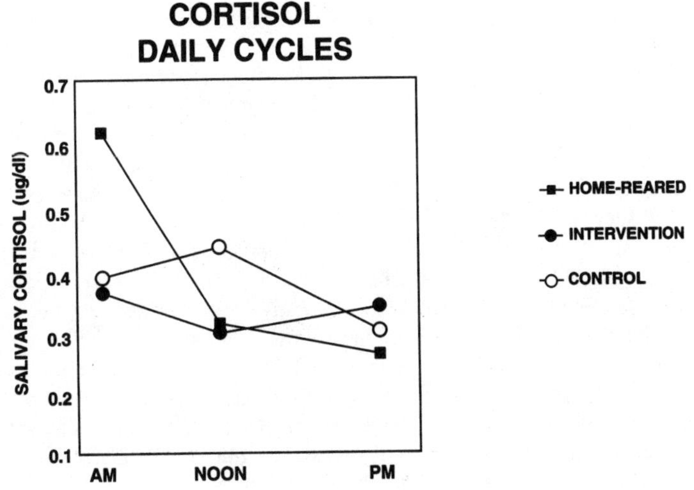

FIGURE 2. Home-reared, intervention, and control *Leagane* children 2 years of age.

group levels can be seen to rise significantly at noon (compared to the intervention group levels). Significant correlations were obtained between levels of cortisol for certain times of day and performance on Denver Tests and Bayley Scales, as well as with physical measures for the *Leagane* children. As a group, the *Leagane* children were strikingly below the Bayley norms and growth norms for their age. Correlations between cortisol and the mental and motor scales of the Bayley (but not with physical growth) were also found for the home-reared children. These children were similar to US children in their psychological performance and physical growth. We have obtained additional measurements from the *Leagane* children as they have moved to pre-school institutions, along with measures of family-reared 2- and 3-year-old children at home and in day-care settings, which we expect to give us insight into the separate contributions of early experience and current context in the regulation of diurnal variation in cortisol secretion and its relationship to mental and motor performance.

Although the rodent studies described above indicate the presence of a critical period for touch to regulate the negative feedback system for glucocorticoids, this intervention program (average age of enrollment at 6 months) may have begun relatively late to confer a significant advantage on development of the HPA system. Studies of the development of stress regulation in normal infants describe a single diurnal pattern emerging at about 12 weeks of age[24] and modulation of stress reactivity occurring at about 4-6 months of age.[25]

STRESS HORMONE AND PSYCHIATRIC AND MEMORY DISORDERS

This study in psychosocially deprived and stressed young children not only carries implications for deficient learning and memory, but also may convey a lifelong vulnerability to certain psychiatric disorders. The results of this research will be compared to clinical studies of psychiatric conditions in adults that reveal similar factors of HPA dysregulation, hippocampal degeneration, and declarative memory loss. A particularly dramatic and paradoxical relationship exists in posttraumatic stress disorder. Patients with this disorder typically have low cortisol levels compared to those of normal individuals or those with other psychiatric diagnoses. One explanation for this phenomenon is that higher levels of the HPA axis (hypothalamus and pituitary) become hypersensitive to circulating levels of cortisol, leading to enhanced negative feedback, thereby inhibiting CRH and ACTH synthesis and/or release responsible for GC secretion in the adrenal gland.[25] The most profound similarity with the work in rodents is the finding of significant hippocampal shrinkage on magnetic resonance imaging (MRI) in patients with posttraumatic stress disorder.[26] The presence of shrinkage is strongly associated with declarative memory deficits, but not other cognitive tasks that are typically spared in patients with temporal lobe amnesia. Both MRI changes in hippocampal volume and verbal memory loss have been associated with the degree of cortisol elevation in Cushing's disease in adults.[27] Elevated endogenous levels of cortisol associated with memory impairment are seen in depressed adults and adolescents,[28] and elevated levels of exogenous glucocorticoids administered for control of asthma have been shown to produce memory deficits and other cognitive changes in children.[29,30]

FUTURE DIRECTIONS

These studies promise to advance the understanding of social factors in the development of HPA regulation in the first few years of life and the impact of this regulation on cognitive, emotional and social development. Although the tragic circumstances of the tens of thousands of infants subjected to profound social deprivation in Romania presents an extreme example, the more normative situation of daily or weekly care facilities in that country suggests wider implications of these findings. We find it remarkable that the categories of rights (survival, care/protection, and participation) that identify both needs and capacities of children, when threatened, are among the most potent activators of the stress hormone system. In the complex and dynamic ecological system in which the child develops, rights can be realized (or violated) by the caretaker and child's access to resources and by their combined capacities to avoid or prevent threats to well-being. Chronic violation of these rights potentially has an impact on life-long HPA regulation and thereby can impair many important biological and psychological functions.

Caution is required in any simple interpretation of these results, as the HPA system is responsive to a wide range of social and nonsocial influences. At least two strong motivations exist to continue the studies so far initiated in the *Leagane* children. The first is to examine in greater detail the situational specificity of the high levels we have so far discovered and to look for changes in HPA activity that might be attributable to changes in caretaking arrangements as children move into different family and educational environments. The other reason is to provide assistance in the massive effort to steer that society in the direction of either drastically improving or altogether eliminating these institutions.

Improving these institutions, as many administrators are striving to accomplish, must be predicated on the assumption that the political and economic climate that characterizes this transitional society will continue to strain the resources of families to care for their children with the ugly consequence that the number of abandoned children will not significantly decrease. Eliminating the *Leagane,* certainly the more desirable alternative, is predicated on a societal determination to find other solutions to care for abandoned infants (e.g., adoption, foster care, and group homes) and to drastically improve the support for families, so that surrendering one's child to the state becomes neither desirable nor necessary.

If our initial findings hold, suggesting that ordinary day care can be particularly stressful for preschool children, then improving the quality of these environments should also be vigorously pursued. The implications for the cognitive and social development of future generations of adults in this society are potentially serious when one considers that most Romanian children spend significant amounts of time in some form of institutional setting. At the same time that we pursue our scientific study of HPA regulation in Romania, we are interested in the applications of this study to other populations of children. One group is represented by Romanian children who have been adopted by caring and relatively affluent families outside of Romania. The results of at least one published account measuring the social adjustment of such a group indicate lasting social deficits (mainly in the form of indiscriminate friendliness) in children who were adopted after spending 9 months or more in a Romanian institution.[31] Another group in whom we are interested are infants and preschool children attending day care of varying quality in the United States. To date, standards for determining what is quality day care remain crude and very poorly regulated. For the most part, standards for licensure are based on structural criteria such as child/staff ratio, caretaker training, and the types of play and educational materials available. From our perspective, quality should be judged primarily on the basis of social relationships, degree of control and predictability experienced by the child, and the level of consistency in expectations and practices shared by different adults in the child's home and school environments. These are attributes that come close to our concept of rights, such that their absence constitutes a violation of needs (and frustration of capacities) required for satisfactory psychological development. As we observed in the *Leagane* of Romania, adequate physical care can be provided, child/staff ratios can even appear appropriate, yet the subjective level of stress experienced by the child is high, as reflected in diurnal patterns of cortisol secretion.

In light of the evidence from studies of social deprivation in animals and humans of the harmful effects on brain functions of high levels of glucocorticoids in early development, we are reviewing the human literature on the constraints that seem to operate in limiting the degree to which recovery from the effects of profound social deprivation are possible.[32] Although this undoubtedly has implications for the nature of affiliative relations in Romanian society, we are increasingly concerned about the consequences of the growing numbers of children under age 5 who live in poverty in this country (a rate that has increased from 15% to 26% over the last 20 years).[33] When this reality is coupled with the increasing rates of maternal employment, which is the objective of "workfare," and the insufficient supply of satisfactory child care arrangements, the enduring negative effects on child well-being for a large segment of American society should be appreciated. These conditions constitute a warning that child rights are being violated. In not more than one context have we witnessed a call for a return to orphanages in this country.[34] Our work is to complete the construction of a framework that consolidates science and ethics in such a way that prevents our public policy from returning to the use of institutional solutions for children and families for complex social and economic deprivations that have their origins in national and global policies.

REFERENCES

1. The Situation of Child and Family in Romania. 1995. The National Committee for Child Protection, Romanian Government and United Nations Children's Fund (UNICEF).
2. Munir, K & F. Earls. 1992. Ethical principles governing research in child and adolescent psychiatry. J. Am. Acad. Child Adolesc. Psychiatry **31:** 408-414.
3. This Document Was Adopted By The U.N. General Assembly in 1989. As of March 1996, 180 member countries have signed or become State Parties to the CRC while the United States is among the 6 countries that have neither signed nor become State Parties to this document.
4. Hammerberg, T. 1992. Making Reality of the Rights of the Child, Save the Children. Sweden.
5. Harlow, H. F. and M. K. Harlow. 1973. Social deprivation in monkeys. *In* Readings from the Scientific American: The Nature and Nurture of Behavior.: 108-116. W. H. Freeman Co. San Francisco.
6. Mason, W. A. 1970. Early deprivation in the biological perspective. *In* Education of the Infant and Young Child. V. H. Denenberg, Ed.: 25-50. Academic Press. New York.

7. RANDOLPH, M. C. & W. A. MASON. 1969. Effects of rearing conditions on distress vocalization in chimpanzees. Folia Primatol. **10:** 103-112.
8. CARLSON, M. 1990. Role of somatic sensory cortex in tactile discrimination in primates. *In* Cerebral Cortex. E. G. Jones & A. Peters, Eds. Vol. **8B:** 451-486. Plenum. New York.
9. CARLSON, M. & H. BURTON. 1988. Recovery of tactile function after damage to primary or secondary somatic sensory cortex in infant *Macaca mulatta.* J. Neurosci. **8:** 833-859.
10. CARLSON, M., D. D. M. O'LEARY & H. BURTON. 1987. Potential role of thalamocortical connections in recovery of tactile function following somatic sensory cortex lesions in infant primates. Soc. Neurosci. Abstr. **13:** 25.2.
11. MEANEY, M. J., R. M. SAPOLSKY & B. S. MCEWEN. 1985. The development of the glucocorticoid receptor system in the rat limbic brain: II. An autoradiographic study. Dev. Brain Res. **18:** 159-164.
12. MEANEY, M. J., S. BHATNAGAR, J. DIORO, S. LAROCQUE, D. FRANCIS, D. O'DONNELL, N. SHANKS, S. SHARMA, J. SMYTHE & V. VIAU. 1993. Molecular basis for the development of individual differences in the hypothalamic-pituitary-adrenal stress response. Cell. Mol. Neurobiol. **13:** 321-347.
13. MEANEY, M. J., D. H. AITKEN, S. SHARMA, S. VIAU & A. SARRIEAU. 1989. Postnatal handling increases hippocampal type II, glucocorticoid receptors and enhances adrenocortical negative-feedback efficacy in the rat. Neuroendocrinology **50:** 597-604.
14. MEANEY, M. J. & D. H. AITKEN. 1985. The effects of early postnatal handling on the development of hippocampal glucocorticoid receptors: Temporal parameters. Dev. Brain Res. **22:** 301-304.
15. SAPOLSKY, R. M., H. UNO, C. S. REBERT & C. E. FINCH. 1990. Hippocampal damage associated with prolonged glucocorticoid exposure in primates. J. Neurosci. **10:** 2897-2902.
16. MCEWEN, B. S., J. ANGULO, H. CAMERON, H. M. CHAO, D. DANIELS, M. N. GANNON, E. GOULD, S. MENDELSON, R. SAKAI, R. SPENCER & C. WOOLLEY. 1992. Paradoxical effects of adrenal steroids on the brain: Protection vs degeneration. Biol. Psychiatry **11:** 177-199.
17. WATANABE, Y., E. GOULD & B. S. MCEWEN. 1992. Stress induces atrophy of apical dendrites of hippocampal CA3 pyramidal neurons. Brain Res. **588:** 341-345.
18. BODNOFF, S. R., A. G. HUMPHREYS, J. C. LEHMAN, D. M. DIAMOND, G. M. ROSE & M. J. MEANEY. 1995. Enduring effects of chronic corticosterone treatment on spatial learning, synaptic plasticity, and hippocampal neuropathology in young and mid-aged rats. J. Neurosci. **15:** 61-69.
19. SAPOLSKY, R. M. 1994. The physiological relevance of glucocorticoid endangerment of the hippocampus. *In* Brain Corticosteroid Receptors: Studies on the Mechanism, Function and Neurotoxicity of Corticosteroid Action. E. R deKloet, E. C. Azmitia, & P. W. Landfield, Eds. Ann. N.Y. Acad. Sci. **746:** 294-307.
20. SPARLING, J., B. BASCOM, M. CIONGRADI, C. DRAGOMIR & A. BODEA. 1992. Programul Screening-Interventie. Paper Presented at the Sixth Annual Conference of Children at Risk. University of Colorado and Pan American Health Organization.
21. MEANEY, M. J., D. H. AITKEN, S. R. BONDNOFF, L. J. INY & R. M. SAPOLSKY. 1985. The effects of postnatal handling on the development of the glucocorticoid receptor systems and stress recovery in the rat. Prog. Neuropsychopharmacol. Biol. Psychol. **9:** 731-734.
22. KIRSCHBAUM, C. & D. H. HELLHAMMER. 1994. Salivary cortisol in psychoneuroendocrine research: Recent developments and applications. Psychoneuroendocrinology. **19:** 313-333.
23. PRICE, D. A., G. C. CLOSE & B. A. FIELDING. 1983. Age of appearance of circadian rhythm in salivary cortisol values in infancy. Arch. Dis. Child. **58:** 454-456.
24. GUNNAR, M., L. HERTSGAARD, M. LARSON & J. RIGATUSO. 1991. Cortisol and behavioral responses to repeated stressor in the human newborn. Dev. Psychobiol. **24:** 487-506.

25. Yehuda, R., B. Kahana, K. Binder-Brynes, S. Southwick, S. Zemelman, J. W. Mason & E. L. Giller. 1995. Low urinary cortisol excretion in holocaust survivors with posttraumatic stress disorder. Am. J. Psychiatry **152:** 1815-1818.
26. Bremner, J. D., P. Randall, T. M. Scott, R. A. Bronen, J. P. Seibyl, S. M. Southwick, R. C. Delaney, G. McCarthy, D. S. Charney & R. B. Innis. 1995. MRI-based measurement of hippocampal volume in patients with combat-related posttraumatic stress disorder. Am. J. Psychiatry **152:** 973-981.
27. Starkman, M. N., S. S. Gebarski, S. Berent & D. E. Schteingart. 1992. Hippocampal formation volume, memory dysfunction and cortisol levels in patients with Cushing's syndrome. Biol. Psychiatry **32:** 756-765.
28. Dahl, R., N. Ryan, J. Puig-Antich, N. Nguyen, M. Al-Shabbout, V. Meyer & J. Perel. 1991. 24-hour cortisol measures in adolescents with major depression: A controlled study. Biol. Psychiatry **30:** 25-36.
29. Bender, B. G., J. A. Lerner & E. Kollasch. 1988. Mood and memory changes in asthmatic children receiving corticosteroids. J. Am. Acad. Child Adol. Psychiatry **27:** 720-725.
30. Rubinow, D. R., R. M. Post, R. Savard & P. W. Gold. 1984. Cortisol hypersecretion and cognitive impairment in depression. Arch. Gen. Psychiatry **41:** 279-283.
31. Carter, K. M., E. Ames & S. Morison. 1995. Attachment security and indiscriminately friendly behavior in children adopted from Romanian orphanages. Dev. and Psychopathol. **7:** 283-294.
32. Earls, F. & M. Carlson. 1996. Recovery from profound social deprivation. In preparation.
33. National Center on Poverty in Children. Annual Report. 1995. Columbia University School of Public Health. New York, NY.
34. Frank, D. A., P. E. Klass, F. Earls & L. Eisenberg. 1996. Infants and orphanages? A view from the Pediatrics and Child Psychiatry. Pediatrics. **97:** 569-578.

25

Affiliation and Neuropsychiatric Disorders: The Deficit Syndrome of Schizophrenia

Brian Kirkpatrick

The revolution in psychiatry spearheaded in the 1950s and 1960s by the Department of Psychiatry at Washington University led to great advances in our understanding of many of the mental illnesses that afflict humanity. The simple early insistence on agreement on diagnosis was the key step necessary for the astonishing increase in our understanding of serious depression, schizophrenia, anxiety disorders, developmental disorders, and other problems. Untold numbers of people around the world have benefited from these advances.

Affiliative behaviors are relevant to several neuropsychiatric disorders. Loss of relationships, or critical relationships,[1–5] increase the subsequent risk of recurrence of major depression, a neurobehavioral syndrome with complex biological changes.[6,7] The experience of ''expressed emotion,'' that is, living with a critical, intrusive person, also increases the risk of exacerbation of psychotic symptoms in patients with schizophrenia.[8] There are also disorders in which it is the nature of the person's affiliative behaviors that is abnormal. Childhood autism is defined in the *Diagnostic and Statistical Manual of the American Psychiatric Association,* Fourth Edition, in part by a lack of seeking social relationships, whereas borderline personality disorder is characterized in part by the particular nature of the person's relationships.[9] The deficit syndrome of schizophrenia, reviewed here, is also defined in part by a lack of interest in relationships.

Thus, the neurobiology of social behavior is one of the ''basic sciences'' of psychiatry. However, changes in complex behaviors can often fruitfully be studied by considering somewhat simpler functions, such as temperature regulation, exchange of nutrients, or attention. A similar situation may be emerging in the study of patients with the deficit syndrome of schizophrenia.

This work was supported in part by Public Health Service grants MH45074, MH35996, MH35996 (supplement), and MH40279 and funding from the National Alliance for Research on Schizophrenia and Depression.

Address for correspondence to: Brian Kirkpatrick, MD, Maryland Psychiatric Research Center, P.O. Box 21247, Baltimore, MD 21228 (tel: 410/455-7662; fax: 410/788-3837).

TABLE 1. Summary of Diagnostic Criteria for Schizophrenia[a]

1. Two or more of the following, each present for a significant portion of time during a 1-month period (or less if successfully treated):
   A. Delusions
   B. Hallucinations
   C. Disorganized speech (e.g., frequent derailment or incoherence)
   D. Grossly disorganized or catatonic behavior
   E. Negative symptoms, i.e., affective flattening, alogia, or avolition
2. Social/occupational dysfunction
3. Continuous signs of the disturbance persist at least 6 months
4. Exclusion of schizoaffective and mood disorder
5. Not due to substance use or a general medical condition
6. If a pervasive developmental disorder is present, the additional diagnosis of schizophrenia is made only if prominent delusions or hallucinations are also present for at least 1 month (or less if successfully treated)

[a] Adapted from the Diagnostic and Statistical Manual of Mental Disorders, Fourth Edition, American Psychiatric Association.[9]

AFFILIATIVE ABNORMALITIES OF THE DEFICIT SYNDROME

The Deficit Syndrome

From the perspective of human suffering and costs to society, schizophrenia is one of the most burdensome illnesses of humanity. The total national direct and indirect costs of schizophrenia were estimated at $65 billion for 1991.[10] It is usually a chronic condition, and many people with schizophrenia exhibit difficulties from childhood to late adult life. It is also very severe in its effects, with many patients unable to work for most of their adult lives. In the United States, schizophrenia may account for 2.5% of total annual health care expenditures, 10% of the totally and permanently disabled population, and at least 14% of homeless people in big cities.[11] Its 1-2% lifetime prevalence[12] makes it one of the most common serious diseases.

Modern diagnostic criteria for schizophrenia are based largely on "positive" psychotic symptoms, such as hallucinations, delusions, and disorganized speech and behavior (TABLE 1), and these problems can impact very seriously on the patient's quality of life. However, patients with schizophrenia also have other sources of distress and impairment. They have an increased risk of both major depressive episodes and suicide,[13] and the coexistence of drug abuse and schizophrenia is approximately twice that expected by chance.[14] Patients with schizophrenia commonly have significant cognitive problems, which typically remain despite improvement, with treatment, of positive symptoms.[15,16]

Evidence has long existed that schizophrenia is not a single disease, but a syndrome composed of groups with differing etiologies and pathophysiologies. A foreshadowing of this concept can be found in the writings of Kraepelin,[17] who at the end of the nineteenth century delineated two major groups within the "functional" psychoses, schizophrenia and affective disorder:

TABLE 2. Diagnostic Criteria for Deficit Syndrome of+Schizophrenia[18,19]

1. At least 2 of the following 6 negative symptoms must be present:
   A. Restricted affect
   B. Diminished emotional range
   C. Poverty of speech
   D. Curbing of interests
   E. Diminished sense of purpose
   F. Diminished social drive
2. Some combination of 2 or more of the negative symptoms listed above must have been present for the preceding 12 months and always present during periods of clinical stability (including chronic psychotic states). These symptoms may or may not be detectable during transient episodes of acute psychotic disorganization or decompensation.
3. Negative symptoms above must be primary, that is, not secondary to factors other than the disease process. Such factors include:
   A. Anxiety
   B. Drug effect
   C. Reaction to suspiciousness (or other psychotic symptoms)
   D. Mental retardation
   E. Depression
4. Patient must meet DSM (3, 3R, or 4) criteria for schizophrenia.

> Now if we make a general survey of the psychic clinical picture of (schizophrenia) . . . there are apparently two principal groups of disorders which characterize the malady. On the one hand we observe a weakening of those emotional activities which permanently form the mainsprings of volition. In connection with this, mental activity and instinct for occupation become mute. The result of this part of the morbid process is emotional dullness, failure of mental activities, loss of mastery over volition, of endeavor, and of ability for independent action. The essence of personality is thereby destroyed, the best and most precious part of its being, as Griesinger once expressed it, torn from her. With the annihilation of personal will, the possibility of further development is lost, which is dependent wholly on the activity of volition. . . . It is worthy of note . . . that memory and acquired mental proficiency may occasionally be preserved in a surprising way when there is complete and final destruction of the personality itself.

A marked decrease in affiliative behaviors is found among patients with schizophrenia who exhibit the "destruction of the personality" described by Kraepelin. These patients exhibit a group of clinical features that, within a chronic schizophrenia sample, are robustly intercorrelated.[18] The diagnostic criteria for this group of impairments, called the deficit syndrome,[19] are given in TABLE 2. This categorization can be made with good interrater reliability, and has proven to be very stable[18,20] (Amador *et al.,* unpublished data). The "decreased social drive" of these patients also has good interrater reliability.[18] This feature is elicited on clinical interview of them and is rated on the basis of clinical interview, observation of their behavior, and the testimony of their clinicians and family members.

Efforts have been made to operationalize this area of psychopathology. Currently the most popular is the concept of "negative symptoms." The instrument most widely used to quantify this area of impairment is the Scale for the Assessment of Negative

Symptoms.[21] However, we review only those studies that have used deficit syndrome criteria to delineate this group of patients, as the correlates of this group are substantially different from those of other conceptualizations of this area of psychopathology, including negative symptoms. In the studies to be cited, the differences between deficit and nondeficit patients could not be attributed to differences in demographics, duration of illness, or to a greater global severity of psychosis (by some measures, patients with the deficit syndrome have slightly *less* severe "positive" psychotic symptoms, that is, hallucinations, delusions, and disorganized thought and behavior).[22–24]

Affiliation in the Deficit Syndrome

In a consideration of the affiliative changes in patients with the deficit syndrome, it is important to distinguish among social withdrawal, poor social skills,[16,25,26] and a decrease in social interests. Patients with schizophrenia have difficulties in all of these.

A person with schizophrenia might withdraw from the company of others for many reasons: psychotic suspiciousness, drug abuse, preoccupation with hallucinations, an adaptive response to overwhelming stimulation, serious depression, demoralization because of rejection by other people, an adaptive response to poor social skills, or lack of interest. The social withdrawal of patients with the deficit syndrome is not caused by these factors.[18,19] They are in fact less severely affected by these factors than are other persons with schizophrenia (to be discussed). Patients with these other causes of social withdrawal are said to have secondary negative symptoms in contrast to the primary negative symptoms of patients with the deficit syndrome.[18,19] The significance and validity of this distinction are found in studies showing that the deficit syndrome (with primary negative symptoms) has clinical and neurobiological correlates that differ from those of negative symptoms as conventionally defined, which includes both primary and secondary negative symptoms.

In addition to the abnormalities found on clinical assessment, patients with the deficit syndrome have higher scores than nondeficit patients on the Chapman Social Anhedonia Scale, which is a self-report scale that measures the pleasure experienced in social interactions.[27] On the other Chapman Psychosis Proneness Scales,[28–30] they also report greater Physical Anhedonia[27] (a measure of the pleasure experienced in such activities as taking a bath, watching a sunset, or listening to music), but they do not differ from nondeficit patients on measures of psychotic-like experiences (Perceptual Aberration and Magical Ideation) or Impulsive Nonconformity.[31]

In clinical populations, anhedonia (the absence of or decrease in the experiencing of pleasure) is usually associated with dysphoria, or emotional pain, especially depression and/or anxiety.[32] There are many reasons for a patient with schizophrenia to be dysphoric, such as the effects of stigmatization, distressing psychotic symptoms, and a decreased ability to function. Indeed, the distress caused by schizophrenia is reflected in an increased risk of suicide among persons who have the disease.[13] Patients with the deficit syndrome are more severely impaired than other patients with schizophrenia relative to their ability to function;[23,24,33] despite this difference, they are *less* dysphoric than are others with schizophrenia (Table 1). In a followup study, at an average of 1.5 years after categorization into deficit and nondeficit groups, outpatients with schizophrenia were assessed by raters blind to this categorization, and patients completed a self-report of depressive mood. On followup, deficit patients exhibited less severe depressive mood on both self-report and clinicians' ratings, as well as lower scores on a general a measure of dysphoria.[22,34] In the Chestnut Lodge study, in which patients were assessed an average of 19 years after admission to a tertiary care center, 10 of 130 nondeficit patients had committed suicide compared to 0 of 44 deficit patients.[33] This difference was not statistically significant, but it is highly suggestive and consistent with other evidence.

If deficit patients, despite what one would expect to be the greater stress associated with their poorer level of function, prove to have a decreased risk of suicide compared to that of other persons with schizophrenia, this would be of considerable clinical and theoretical interest. Despite their greater impairment, which would appear to increase their social stresses, patients with the deficit syndrome may be less responsive to these stressors. The decreased awareness of impairment exhibited by deficit patients (X. Amador *et al.*, unpublished data) and/or the information processing difficulties they exhibit (to be discussed) may be the basis for this paradox.

The content of the delusions of deficit patients is also remarkable. Suspiciousness, which consists of beliefs about the actions and intents of other persons, is very common in schizophrenia and is commonly assessed in research settings. Deficit patients are more impaired than nondeficit patients, and because of their blunted affect (decreased expressive gestures and facial expressiveness), more abnormal in appearance and might therefore have greater reason to be concerned with the intentions of other persons towards them. Nonetheless, they are *less* suspicious than other people with schizophrenia. This difference has been found in multiple datasets.[23,35] In one study, a detailed assessment permitted the categorization of delusions other than suspiciousness into those with an exclusively social content versus other delusions. Deficit patients had less severe social delusions, but did not differ from nondeficit patients relative to other delusions.[35] Moreover, deficit patients did not differ from others patients in the severity of hallucinations or the disorganization of thought and behavior often found in schizophrenia. Thus, the decreased social interests used to define deficit patients (TABLE 1) extend to the content of their delusions; however, it is the nature of their day-to-day relationships and their desire for relationships rather than the content of their delusions that are the basis for rating diminished social drive.

A decrease in affiliation is not the only abnormality that these patients exhibit. Their loss of pleasure and decrease in goal-directed activity extend to areas other than affiliation; for instance, they also report increased physical anhedonia.[31] Furthermore, the identification of a group of neuropsychological impairments in these patients (to be discussed) suggests an information-processing basis for these behavioral abnormalities. Nonetheless, these patients exhibit a decrease in affiliative behaviors that is quite striking, and its clinical features are unique.

NEUROBIOLOGY OF THE DEFICIT SYNDROME

To understand the possible neurobiological basis of the affiliative abnormalities of the deficit syndrome, a brief review of the research on this form of schizophrenia is helpful. The deficit syndrome appears to constitute a separate disease, as patients with the deficit syndrome differ from other patients with schizophrenia relative to the dimensions used to distinguish one disorder from another, including signs and symptoms, course of illness, treatment response, risk and etiological factors, and biological correlates and pathophysiological changes.

Signs and Symptoms

As just noted, the deficit syndrome is defined by characteristic signs and symptoms and the differential diagnosis of these features,[18,19] and subtle differences exist between deficit and nondeficit patients in the content of their delusions.[35] However, the two groups do not differ in the severity of hallucinations, formal thought disorder, all delusions, or global psychosis (hallucinations plus delusions plus formal thought disorder.)[22,36]

Patients with the deficit syndrome appear to be less aware of their impairments (have less "insight") than are other patients with schizophrenia; this difference has been found in two independent studies (Amador *et al.*, unpublished data). Secondary social withdrawal and other secondary negative symptoms are not correlated with awareness of impairment.[36] Despite their greater impairment, deficit patients express less dissatisfaction with their lives (Lehman *et al.*, unpublished data).

Course of Illness

"Premorbid" Abnormalities. It has long been noted that prior to the onset of frank psychosis, there are behavioral and neurological abnormalities in many people who as adults meet criteria for the diagnosis of schizophrenia. In two studies, these "premorbid" abnormalities were shown to be strongly associated with the deficit syndrome in adulthood, most clearly in late adolescence. An inability to maintain or a lack of interest in relationships, especially in late adolescence, is most prominent.[24,37] These studies were limited by dependence on the recall of patients and informants. Deficit patients were also less likely to be married before the onset of frank psychosis; this difference was not confounded by age of onset.[33] It was also reported that prior to neuroleptic exposure, patients with the deficit syndrome more frequently exhibited abnormal movements than did nondeficit patients.[38]

Onset. The observation that an insidious or gradually progressing onset is associated with a lack of emotionality and a poor prognosis is an old one. Fenton and McGlashan[33] found an association between insidious onset and subsequent deficit features, although deficit and nondeficit groups did not differ relative to age of first admission.

Middle Course. During early and middle adult life, the deficit syndrome is very stable relative to both deficit/nondeficit categorization (Amador *et al.*, unpublished data) and characteristic clinical features.[22,34] In this same period, deficit patients have poorer social and occupational function, their equal or lesser severity of positive symptoms notwithstanding.[24] However, they appear to have a *lesser* risk of one of the complications of the illness, namely, drug abuse,[24] and may have a decreased risk of suicide as well.[33] Secondary social withdrawal and other negative symptoms are less robust predictors of drug abuse or its absence than is the deficit syndrome.[24]

Late Course. Some studies have shown that late in life, patients with schizophrenia have on average an improvement in both the severity of psychotic symptoms and their level of function.[39–41] The psychopathology of the deficit syndrome seems more persistent than psychotic symptoms, and late in life deficit patients continue to have poorer function than do nondeficit patients.[20,33] The deficit/nondeficit categorization has also proven to be highly stable in the long term and was a better predictor of long-term outcome than negative symptoms broadly defined.[20]

Treatment Response

Given the widespread use of the typical neuroleptic antipsychotic drugs, it is almost tautological to say that the social withdrawal of deficit patients responds more poorly to these drugs than does that of other people with schizophrenia. The negative symptoms of deficit patients cannot be attributed to neuroleptic side effects.[18,19,42] However, in two studies with the newer ''atypical'' antipsychotic clozapine, which has efficacy greater than do the older drugs, the negative symptoms of deficit patients had a poorer response than did those of nondeficit patients[43] (Conley *et al.*, unpublished, but see Meltzer[44]).

Risk and Etiological Factors

Evidence that genetic factors contribute to the etiology of schizophrenia now includes a replicated linkage to an area on chromosome 6 in some families.[45–50] However, there are no studies on the differential genetic contribution to deficit versus nondeficit forms of the disorder.

Immunological abnormalities have been found in schizophrenia,[51,52] and there are suggestions that these are involved in the pathophysiology of the deficit syndrome. Waltrip *et al.*[53,54] reported an association between the deficit syndrome and antibodies to borna disease virus (unpublished data). The *a priori* hypothesis that borna virus might be involved in the pathophysiology of schizophrenia was based on its characteristics: (1) it is neurotrophic, and (2) in animal models it may persist in an asymptomatic carrier state if the animal is exposed early in life. No other viruses were assessed in this study. Extensive evidence indicates that schizophrenia is a developmental disorder that can be traced to the earliest stages of life. However, this study suggested that only about a third of patients with the deficit syndrome would have this pathology, so the importance of this finding is so far unclear.

There are many reports of an association between schizophrenia and winter birth, and this is usually related to the seasonality of infectious diseases and the impact of infections and the immune response on brain development. Patients born in the winter appear to have a less severe form of the disease and may have features associated with nondeficit rather than deficit schizophrenia.[55–57] In four of five Northern Hemisphere datasets, including one epidemiological sample of first-admission patients, the deficit syndrome was associated with an increase in June/July births (Kirkpatrick *et al.*, unpublished data). Negative symptoms broadly defined did not predict season of birth. Moreover, in a nonpatient study group, deficit syndrome-like features were also found to have a greater severity in subjects born in June/July than in those born in the rest of the year, suggesting this effect may also operate in the schizophrenia spectrum. However, this nonpatient study group was not an epidemiological sample (Kirkpatrick *et al.*, unpublished data).

Biological Correlates and Pathophysiological Changes

Neurocognitive Function. Abnormalities in neurocognitive function have been identified in deficit patients. Several studies found abnormalities in attention and visuospatial processing; the measures used include visual reaction time measures,[58] smooth pursuit eyetracking (Ross *et al.*, unpublished data), span of apprehension, and a degraded-stimulus continuous performance task (Buchanan *et al.*, unpublished data). This information has been supplemented by a study using a structured neurological examination, in which abnormal neurological signs in the realm of sensory integration were more common in deficit than in nondeficit patients.[37] The two schizophrenia groups did not differ in the sequencing of complex motor acts, motor coordination, or miscellaneous signs. In a study in which an extensive neuropsychological battery was administered, poorer test scores were found in deficit than in nondeficit patients; this was most marked in tests thought to be related to frontal and parietal function.[59]

Anatomy. We previously proposed that a dysfunction of one of the parallel, segregated cortical-subcortical circuits that have been delineated in mammals[60] underlies positive psychotic symptoms (the anterior cingulate circuit), whereas dysfunction in another of these circuits (the dorsolateral prefrontal circuit, of which the inferior parietal cortex is a component) underlies the negative symptoms of the deficit syndrome.[61] The evidence for this hypothesis comes from the neurocognitive studies just mentioned as well as structural and functional imaging studies[62,63] (Wolkin *et al.*, unpublished data). Dysfunction in the psychosis circuit would be found in both deficit and nondeficit groups and perhaps in other psychotic disorders as well (such as delusional disorder and psychotic affective disorder). Since the time of our review of this evidence, two unpublished positron emission tomography studies also found a decrease in activation in the inferior parietal cortex in deficit compared to nondeficit patients (Tamminga, Lahti, and Holcomb *et al.*, unpublished data). Animal studies implicating the dorsolateral prefrontal circuit in the control of visuospatial processing and visual attention[64] are consistent with the hypothesis that deficit patients, whose function is particularly impaired in these domains, have an abnormality localized to this circuit.

This hypothesis may be accurate, but evidence suggests that it is also somewhat incomplete. In a test of an *a priori* hypothesis, the volume of cerebellar vermis lobules 8 to 10 was measured in controls and in deficit and nondeficit patients (Summerfelt *et al.*, unpublished data). Deficit patients had significantly larger volumes than did nondeficit patients; neither group differed significantly from controls, but the cell sizes were small.

IS THE DEFICIT SYNDROME SIMPLY MORE OF THE SAME?

We proposed that patients with the deficit syndrome have a distinctive disease, with a pathophysiology separate from those of other patients with schizophrenia. An important alternative explanation for the studies we have reviewed is that deficit syndrome patients simply have a more severe variant of schizophrenia. However, certain findings contradict this interpretation. First, in a study of frontal lobe volume,[62] deficit syndrome patients not only had a greater frontal lobe volume than did nondeficit patients, but did not differ significantly from normal controls. As just noted, deficit patients have *poorer* function on neuropsychological tests associated with frontal lobe damage than do nondeficit patients.[69] This combination of greater volume despite poorer function suggests a different pathophysiology. The finding of a more normal ventricular/brain ratio in deficit than nondeficit patients (Wolkin *et al.*, unpublished data) also contradicts the "more of the same" hypothesis.

The two possible risk factors for the deficit syndrome, season of birth and borna virus antibodies, also suggest a different etiology and therefore imply a different pathophysiology; again, the evidence does not fit easily with the concept of "more of the same." The finding that winter birth is associated with all of schizophrenia and the deficit syndrome with summer birth further implies that winter birth is strongly associated with nondeficit schizophrenia. Thus, there is a "double dissociation" of clinical features and risk factors. The studies of summer birth and the deficit syndrome have been too small to test this hypothesis in a robust fashion; however, data on the nondeficit group from one clinic (with its important potential biases) were consistent with this view.

WHY ARE DEFICIT PATIENTS ASOCIAL?

Patients with the deficit syndrome of schizophrenia have a distinctive profile of affiliative abnormalities. These cannot be attributed to the usual causes of social withdrawal in schizophrenia, such as anxiety, suspiciousness, depression, psychotic disorganization, or drug abuse, as they are *less* psychotic (by some measures), *less* dysphoric, and abuse drugs less than do other patients with schizophrenia who seek out relationships and suffer when these relationships are lost.

Are the information processing abnormalities found in deficit patients the basis of these behavioral abnormalities? This possibility is currently the most likely explanation, but it will be difficult to test definitively. At present there is no effective treatment for either the information processing problems or the clinical features of the deficit syndrome. If future drug treatments reverse the neurocognitive impairments, clinical features, or both, the relationship between these aspects of this disorder may be clarified.

ANIMAL MODELS AND THE DEFICIT SYNDROME

In medicine, animal models can be used as either "assays" or homologs. However, homologous models of the deficit syndrome face serious difficulties, because the naturally occurring human deficit syndrome is associated with psychosis, and modeling psychotic symptoms behaviorally in animals is problematic.

However, an important potential ''assay'' relevant to the deficit syndrome exists that could in theory be developed in animal models, namely, a model for screening pharmaceuticals prior to clinical testing. No medication has currently been shown to treat the clinical features of the deficit syndrome. New drugs for the treatment of schizophrenia move from the laboratory to clinical trials because of their effects in specific animal screening models. These models are poor homologs of the psychopathology of schizophrenia or not homologous at all in terms of phenomenology, but they perform extremely well in predicting antipsychotic efficacy. However, they have not succeeded in selecting treatments for deficit syndrome features; in view of the evidence just summarized, that the neural basis of the deficit syndrome is separate from that of positive psychotic symptoms, this failure is not surprising.

We discussed elsewhere possible animal models for predicting efficacy in the deficit syndrome[65,66] and briefly outline our work on one possible model. We are currently investigating the role of the dorsolateral prefrontal circuit in the control of male parental behavior in the prairie vole. The rationale for this circuit is that areas with homology to the primate circuit, which has been implicated in the pathophysiology of the deficit syndrome, can be found in rodents.[67,68] We chose male parental behavior because it is part of a group of behavioral and developmental features that, on a cross-species basis, tend to be found in mammals, or not, as a group.[69,70] Many features of these clusters are found in humans and the prairie vole, and in contrast to the rat, high levels of male parental behavior occur spontaneously in the vole. We found activation, as measured by Fos peptide expression, in the cortical components of this circuit in male voles that were exposed to a pup (Kirkpatrick *et al.,* unpublished data). (Fos is not expressed or is not detectable in our assay in either exposed or unexposed animals in the thalamic or striatal components of this circuit.) Thus, the behavioral line of reasoning and the anatomic reasoning have shown some convergence.

Much work is needed to clarify whether some variant of this model can predict the efficacy of possible drug treatments of the deficit syndrome. However, if this goal is reached, patients and families whose lives were seriously injured by this disorder would benefit greatly.

ACKNOWLEDGMENTS

Thanks to Robert W. Buchanan, MD, Ericka Pearce, and C. Sue Carter, PhD, for comments on an earlier version of this manuscript.

REFERENCES

1. Okasha, A., A. S. El Akabawi, K. S. Snyder, A. K. Wilson *et al.* 1994. Expressed emotion, perceived criticism, and relapse in depression: A replication in an Egyptian community. Am. J. Psychiatry **151:** 1001-1005.
2. Asarnow, J. R., M. J. Goldstein, M. Tompson & D. Guthrie. 1993. One-year outcomes of depressive disorders in child psychiatric inpatients: Evaluation of the prognostic

power of a brief measure of expressed emotion. J. Child Psychol. Psychiatry **34:** 129-137.

3. Hooley, J. M. & J. D. Teasdale. 1989. Predictors of relapse in unipolar depressives: Expressed emotion, marital distress, and perceived criticism. J. Abnorm. Psychol. **98:** 229-235.
4. Marks, M. M., A. Wieck, A. Seymour, S. A. Checkley & R. Kumar. 1992. Women whose mental illnesses recur after childbirth and partners' levels of expressed emotion during late pregnancy. Br. J. Psychiatry **161:** 211-216.
5. Schwartz, C. E., D. J. Dorer, W. R. Beardslee, P. W. Lavori & M. B. Keller. 1990. Maternal expressed emotion and parental affective disorder. Risk for childhood depressive disorder, substance abuse, or conduct disorder. J. Psychiatr. Res. **24:** 231-250.
6. Keller, M. B. 1994. Depression: A long-term illness. Br. J. Psychiatry **26**(Suppl.): 9-15.
7. Schildkraut, J. J., I. J. Kopin, S. M. Schanberg & J. Durell. 1995. Norepinephrine metabolism and psychoactive drugs in the endogenous depressions. Pharmacopsychiatry **1**(Suppl.): 24-37.
8. Bebbington, P. & L. Kuipers. 1994. The predictive utility of expressed emotion in schizophrenia: An aggregate analysis. Psychol. Med. **24:** 707-718.
9. American Psychiatric Association. 1994. Diagnostic and Statistical Manual of Mental Disorders, 4th Ed. DSM-IV. American Psychiatric Association. Washington, DC.
10. Wyatt, R. J., I. Henter, M. C. Leary & E. Taylor. 1995. An economic evaluation of schizophrenia—1991. Soc. Psychiatry Psychiatr. Epidemiol. **30:** 196-205.
11. Rupp, A. & S. J. Keith. 1993. The costs of schizophrenia. Assessing the burden. Psychiatr. Clin. North Am. **16:** 413-423.
12. Regier, D. A., J. H. Boyd, J. D. Burke, Jr., D. S. Rae *et al.* 1988. One-month prevalence of mental disorders in the United States: Based on five Epidemiologic Catchment Area sites. Arch. Gen. Psychiatry **45:** 977-986.
13. Caldwell, C. B. & I. I. Gottesman. 1992. Schizophrenia—a high risk factor for suicide: Clues to risk reduction. Suicide Life Threatening Behav. **44:** 479-493.
14. Regier, D. A., M. E. Farmer, D. S. Rae, B. Z. Locke *et al.* 1990. Comorbidity of mental disorders with alcohol and other drug abuse. Results from the Epidemiologic Catchment Area (ECA) Study. JAMA **264:** 2511-2518.
15. Gold, J. M. & P. D. Harvey. 1993. Cognitive deficits in schizophrenia. Psychiatr. Clin. North Am. **16:** 295-312.
16. Green, M. F. 1996. What are the functional consequences of neurocognitive deficits in schizophrenia? Am. J. Psychiatry **153:** 321-330.
17. Kraepelin, E. 1971. (1919). Dementia Praecox and Paraphrenia. Robert E. Krieger Publishing Co. Inc. New York.
18. Kirkpatrick, B., R. W. Buchanan, P. D. McKenney, L. D. Alphs & W. T. Carpenter, Jr. 1989. The Schedule for the Deficit Syndrome: An instrument for research in schizophrenia. Psychiatry Res. **30:** 119-124.
19. Carpenter, W. T., Jr., D. W. Heinrichs & A. M. Wagman. 1988. Deficit and nondeficit forms of schizophrenia: The concept. Am. J. Psychiatry **145:** 578-583.
20. Fenton, W. S. & T. H. McGlashan. 1992. Testing systems for assessment of negative symptoms in schizophrenia. Arch. Gen. Psychiatry **49:** 179-184.
21. Amador, X. F., M. Flaum, N. C. Andreasen, D. H. Strauss *et al.* 1994. Awareness of illness in schizophrenia and schizoaffective and mood disorders. Arch. Gen. Psychiatry **51:** 826-836.
22. Kirkpatrick, B., R. W. Buchanan, A. Breier & W. T. Carpenter, Jr. 1993. Case identification and stability of the deficit syndrome of schizophrenia. Psychiatry Res. **47:** 47-56.
23. Kirkpatrick, B., R. Ram & E. J. Bromet. 1996. The deficit syndrome in the Suffolk County Mental Health Project. Schizophr. Res. Submitted.

24. KIRKPATRICK, B., X. F. AMADOR, M. FLAUM, S. A. YALE, J. M. GORMAN, W. T. CARPENTER, JR., M. TOHEN & T. MCGLASHAN. 1996. The deficit syndrome in the DSM-IV Field Trial: I. Alcohol and other drug abuse. Schizophr. Res. In press.
25. LYSAKER, P. H., M. D. BELL, W. S. ZITO & S. M. BIOTY. 1995. Social skills at work. Deficits and predictors of improvement in schizophrenia. J. Nerv. Ment. Dis. **183:** 688-692.
26. HALFORD, W. K. & R. L. HAYES. 1995. Social skills in schizophrenia: Assessing the relationship between social skills, psychopathology and community functioning. Soc. Psychiatry Psychiatr. Epidemiol. **30:** 14-19.
27. CHAPMAN, L. J., J. P. CHAPMAN & M. L. RAULIN. 1976. Scales for physical and social anhedonia. J. Abnorm. Psychol. **85:** 374-382.
28. CHAPMAN, L. J. & J. P. CHAPMAN. 1987. The search for symptoms predictive of schizophrenia. Schizophr. Bull. **13:** 497-503.
29. CHAPMAN, L. J., J. P. CHAPMAN & E. N. MILLER. 1982. Reliabilities and intercorrelations of eight measures of proneness to psychosis. J. Consult. Clin. Psychol. **50:** 187-195.
30. CHAPMAN, L. J., W. S. EDEL & J. P. CHAPMAN. 1980. Physical anhedonia, perceptual aberration, and psychosis proneness. Schizophr. Bull. **6:** 639-653.
31. KIRKPATRICK, B. & R. W. BUCHANAN. 1990. Anhedonia and the deficit syndrome of schizophrenia. Psychiatry Res. **31:** 25-30.
32. FAWCETT, J., D. C. CLARKE, W. A. SCHEFTNER & R. D. GIBBONS. 1983. Assessing anhedonia in psychiatric patients. Arch. Gen. Psychiatry **40:** 79-84.
33. FENTON, W. S. & T. H. MCGLASHAN. 1994. Antecedents, symptoms progression, and long-term outcome of the deficit syndrome in schizophrenia. Am. J. Psychiatry **151:** 351-356.
34. KIRKPATRICK, B., R. W. BUCHANAN, A. BREIER & W. T. CARPENTER, JR. 1994. Depressive symptoms and the deficit syndrome of schizophrenia. J. Nerv. Ment. Dis. **182:** 452-455.
35. KIRKPATRICK, B., X. F. AMADOR, S. A. YALE, J. R. BUSTILLO, R. W. BUCHANAN & M. TOHEN. 1996. The deficit syndrome in the DSM-IV Field Trial: II. Depressive episodes and persecutory beliefs. Schizophr. Res. In press.
36. BUCHANAN, R. W., B. KIRKPATRICK, D. W. HEINRICHS & W. T. CARPENTER, JR. 1990. Clinical correlates of the deficit syndrome of schizophrenia. Am. J. Psychiatry **147:** 290-294.
37. FENTON, W. S., R. J. WYATT & T. H. MCGLASHAN. 1994. Risk factors for spontaneous dyskinesia in schizophrenia. Arch. Gen. Psychiatry **51:** 643-650.
38. ANGST, J. 1988. European long-term followup studies of schizophrenia. Schizophr. Bull. **14:** 501-513.
39. MCGLASHAN, T. H. 1988. A selective review of recent North American long-term followup studies of schizophrenia. Schizophr. Bull. **14:** 515-542.
40. RAM, R., E. J. BROMET, W. W. EATON, C. PATO & J. E. SCHWARTZ. 1992. The natural course of schizophrenia: A review of first-admission studies. Schizophr. Bull. **18:** 185-207.
41. BUSTILLO, J. R., B. KIRKPATRICK & R. W. BUCHANAN. 1995. Neuroleptic treatment and negative symptoms in deficit and nondeficit schizophrenia. Biol. Psychiatry **38:** 64-67.
42. BREIER, A., R. W. BUCHANAN, B. KIRKPATRICK, O. R. DAVIS, D. IRISH, A. SUMMERFELT & W. T. CARPENTER, JR. 1994. Effects of clozapine on positive and negative symptoms in outpatients with schizophrenia. Am. J. Psychiatry **151:** 20-26.
43. MELTZER, H. Y. 1995. Clozapine: Is another view valid? **152:** 821-825.
44. ANTONARAKIS, S. E., J. L. BLOUIN, A. E. PULVER, P. WOLYNIEC *et al.* 1995. Schizophrenia susceptibility and chromosome 6p24-22. Nat. Genet. **11:** 235-236.
45. GURLING, H., G. KALSI, A. HUI-SUI CHEN, M. GREEN *et al.* 1995. Schizophrenia susceptibility and chromosome 6p24-22. Nat. Genet. **11:** 234-235.
46. MOWRY, B. J., D. J. NANCARROW, D. P. LENNON, L. A. SANDKUIJL *et al.* 1995. Schizophrenia susceptibility and chromosome 6p24-22. Nat. Genet. **11:** 233-234.

47. Schwab, S. G., M. Albus, J. Hallmayer, S. Honig *et al.* 1995. Evaluation of a susceptibility gene for schizophrenia on chromosome 6p by multipoint affected sibpair linkage analysis. Nat. Genet. **11:** 325-327.
48. Straub, R. W., C. J. MacLean, F. A. O'Neill, J. Burke *et al.* 1995. A potential vulnerability locus for schizophrenia on chromosome 6p24-22: Evidence for genetic heterogeneity. Nat. Genet. **11:** 287-293.
49. Wang, S., C. E. Sun, C. A. Walczak, J. S. Ziegle *et al.* 1995. Evidence for a susceptibility locus for schizophrenia on chromosome 6pter-p22. Nat. Genet. **10:** 41-46.
50. Rapaport, M. H. & J. B. Lohr. 1994. Serum-soluble interleukin-2 receptors in neuroleptic-naive schizophrenic subjects and in medicated schizophrenic subjects with and without tardive dyskinesia. Acta Psychiatr. **90:** 311-315.
51. Rapaport, M. H., C. G. McAllister, Y. S. Kim, J. H. Han *et al.* 1994. Increased serum soluble interleukin-2 receptors in Caucasian and Korean schizophrenic patients. Biol. Psychiatry **35:** 767-771.
52. Waltrip, R. W., 2nd, R. W. Buchanan, A. Summerfelt, A. Breier *et al.* 1995. Boma disease virus and schizophrenia. Psychiatry Res. **56:** 33-44.
53. Carbone, K. M., S. W. Park, S. A. Rubin, R. W. Waltrip, 2nd & G. B. Vogelsang. 1991. Boma disease: Association with a maturation defect in the cellular immune response. J. Virol. **65:** 6154-6164.
54. Bradbury, T. M. & G. A. Miller. 1985. Season of birth in schizophrenia: A review of evidence, methodology, and etiology. Psychol. Bull. **98:** 569-594.
55. Boyd, J. H., A. E. Pulver & W. Stewart. 1986. Season of birth: Schizophrenia and bipolar disorder. Schizophr. Bull. **12:** 173-186.
56. Eaton, W. W. 1991. Update on the epidemiology of schizophrenia. Epidemiol. Rev. **13:** 320-328.
57. Thaker, G., B. Kirkpatrick, R. W. Buchanan, R. Ellsberry *et al.* 1989. Oculomotor abnormalities and their clinical correlates in schizophrenia. Psychopharmacol. Bull. **25:** 491-497.
58. Buchanan, R. W., M. E. Strauss, B. Kirkpatrick, C. Holstein *et al.* 1994. Neuropsychological impairments in deficit vs. nondeficit forms of schizophrenia. Arch. Gen. Psychiatry **51:** 804-811.
59. Alexander, G. E., M. D. Crutcher & M. R. DeLong. 1990. Basal ganglia-thalamocortical circuits: Parallel substrates for motor, oculomotor, prefrontal and limbic functions. Prog. Brain Res. **85:** 119-146.
60. Carpenter, W. T., Jr., R. W. Buchanan, B. Kirkpatrick, C. Tamminga & F. Wood. 1993. Strong inference, theory testing, and the neuroanatomy of schizophrenia. Arch. Gen. Psychiatry **50:** 825-831.
61. Buchanan, R. W., A. Breier, B. Kirkpatrick, A. Elkashef, R. C. Munson, F. Gellad & W. T. Carpenter. 1993. Structural abnormalities in deficit vs. non-deficit schizophrenia. Am. J. Psychiatry **150:** 59-65.
62. Tamminga, C. A., G. K. Thaker, R. W. Buchanan, B. Kirkpatrick, L. D. Alphs, W. T. Carpenter & T. N. Chase. 1992. Limbic system abnormalities identified in schizophrenia using PET/FDG: and neocortical alterations with deficit syndrome. Arch. Gen. Psychiatry **49:** 522-530.
63. King, V. R. & J. V. Corwin. 1993. Comparisons of hemi-inattention produced by unilateral lesions of the posterior parietal cortex or medial agranular prefrontal cortex in rats: Neglect, extinction, and the role of stimulus distance. Behav. Brain Res. **54:** 117-131.
64. Kirkpatrick, B. 1994. Psychiatric disease and the neurobiology of social behavior. Biol. Psychiatry **36:** 501-502.
65. Kirkpatrick, B. & W. T. Carpenter, Jr. 1995. Drug development and the deficit syndrome of schizophrenia. Biol. Psychiatry **38:** 277-278.
66. Reep, R. L., H. C. Chandler, V. King & J. V. Corwin. 1994. Rat posterior parietal cortex: Topography of corticocortical and thalamic connections. Exp. Brain Res. **100:** 67-84.

67. REEP, R. L., G. S. GOODWIN & J. V. CORWIN. 1990. Topographic organization in the corticocortical connections of medial agranular cortex in rats. J. Comp. Neurol. **294:** 262-280.
68. KLEIMAN, D. G. 1977. Monogamy in mammals. Q. Rev. Biol. **52:** 39-69.
69. DEWSBURY, D. A. 1987. The comparative psychology of monogamy. Nebr. Symp. Motiv. Pap. **35:** 1-50.

Contributors

David H. Abbott
Wisconsin Regional Primate Center
University of Wisconsin
Madison, WI

Margaret Altemus
Mental Retardation Research Center
UCLA School of Medicine
Los Angeles, CA

Filippo Aureli
Department of Psychology
Emory University
Atlanta, GA

Marni Bekkedal
Department of Psychology
Rollins College
Winter Park, FL

Mary Carlson
Department of Neurobiology
Harvard Medical School
Boston, MA

C. Sue Carter
Department of Zoology
University of Maryland
College Park, MD

David Crews
Department Zoology
University of Texas
Austin, TX

A. Courtney DeVries
Department of Zoology
University of Maryland
College Park, MD

Geert J. DeVries
Department of Psychology
University of Massachusetts
Amherst, MA

Alan F. Dixson
Sub-Department of Animal Behavior
Cambridge University
Cambridge, UK

Christine M. Drea
Rockwood Sciences Library
Arcata, CA

Felton Earls
Harvard Medical School
Boston, MA

Laurence G. Frank
Department of Psychology
University of California
Berkeley, CA

Lowell L. Getz
Department of Ecology, Ethology, and Evolution
University of Illinois
Urbana, IL

Stephen E. Glickman
Department of Psychology
University of California
Berkeley, CA

Nigella Hillgarth
Department of Zoology
University of Washington
Seattle, WA

Thomas R. Insel
Yerkes Regional Primate Research Center
Emory University
Atlanta, GA

Jerry Jacobs
Department of Zoology
University of Washington
Seattle, WA

Eric B. Keverne
Sub-Department of Animal Behavior
University of Cambridge
Cambridge, UK

Brian Kirkpatrick
Maryland Psychiatric Research Center
Baltimore, MD

Sara Kollack-Walker
Mental Health Research Institute
University of Michigan
Ann Arbor, MI

Gary W. Kraemer
Department of Kinesiology and Harlow Primate Laboratory
University of Wisconsin
Madison, WI

I. Izja Lederhendler
Behavioral and Integrative Neuroscience
NIMH
Rockville, MD

S. Levine
Department of Psychiatry and Behavioral Sciences
Stanford University School of Medicine
Stanford, CA

D. M. Lyons
Department of Psychiatry and Behavioral Sciences
Stanford University School of Medicine
Stanford, CA

Frances L. Martel
Sub-Department of Animal Behavior
University of Cambridge
Cambridge, UK

William A. Mason
Department of Psychology and California Regional Primate Research Center
University of California, Davis
Davis, CA

Sally P. Mendoza
Department of Psychology and California Regional Primate Research Center
University of California, Davis
Davis, CA

Eric Nelson
Department of Psychology
Bowling Green State University
Bowling Green, OH

Claire M. Nevison
Sub-Department of Animal Behavior
University of Cambridge
Cambridge, UK

Sarah Winans Newman
Department of Psychology
Cornell University
Ithaca, NY

Michael Numan
Department of Psychology
Boston College
Chestnut Hill, MA

Jaak Panksepp
Department of Psychology
Bowling Green State University
Bowling Green, OH

David B. Parfitt
Department of Psychological Neuroscience
Michigan State University
East Lansing, MI

Cort A. Pedersen
Department of Psychiatry
University of North Carolina School of Medicine
Chapel Hill, NC

Stephen W. Porges
Institute for Child Study
University of Maryland
College Park, MD

R. Lucille Roberts
Department of Psychology
University of Maryland
College Park, MD

Wendy Saltzman
Wisconsin Regional Primate Research Center
University of Wisconsin
Madison, WI

A.F. Schatzberg
School of Medicine
Stanford University
Stanford, CA

Nancy J. Schultz-Darken
Wisconsin Regional Primate Research Center
University of Wisconsin
Madison, WI

Teige P. Sheehan
Department of Psychology
Boston College
Chestnut Hill, MA

Tessa E. Smith
Department of Psychology
University of Nebraska
Omaha, NE

Charles T. Snowdon
Department of Psychology
University of Wisconsin
Madison, WI

Pamela L. Tannenbaum
Department of Psychology and Yerkes Regional Primate Research Center
Emory University
Atlanta, GA

Susan E. Taymans
Department of Ecology, Ethology, and Evolution
University of Illinois
Urbana, IL

Kerstin Uvnäs-Moberg
Department of Physiology and Pharmacology
Karolinska Institute
Stockholm, Sweden

Constanza Villalba
Program in Neuroscience and Behavior
Department of Psychology
University of Massachusetts
Amherst, MA

Frans B. M. de Waal
Department of Psychology
Emory University
Atlanta, GA

Kim Wallen
Department of Psychology and
Yerkes Regional Primate Research Center
Emory University
Atlanta, GA

Zuoxin Wang
Department of Psychiatry and Behavioral Sciences and Yerkes Regional Primate Research Center
Emory University
Atlanta, GA

Mary L. Weldele
Department of Psychology
University of California
Berkeley, CA

Jessie R. Williams
Department of Zoology
University of Maryland
College Park, MD

John C. Wingfield
Department of Zoology
University of Washington
Seattle, WA

Diane M. Witt
Department of Psychology
Binghamton University
Binghamton, NY

Sonja I. Yoerg
Department of Psychology
University of California
Berkeley, CA

Larry Young
Department of Psychiatry
Emory University School of Medicine
Atlanta, GA

Cynthia J. Zabel
Redwood Sciences Laboratory
Arcata, CA